Treatment and Management of
CANCER IN THE ELDERLY

BASIC AND CLINICAL ONCOLOGY

Series Editor

Bruce D. Cheson

Professor of Medicine and Oncology
Head of Hematology
Georgetown University
Lombardi Comprehensive Cancer Center
Washington, D.C.

ADDITIONAL VOLUMES IN PREPARATION

Treatment and Management of
CANCER IN THE ELDERLY

edited by

Hyman B. Muss
University of Vermont
Burlington, Vermont, U.S.A.

Carrie P. Hunter
North Potomac, Maryland, U.S.A.

Karen A. Johnson
National Cancer Institute
Bethesda, Maryland, U.S.A.

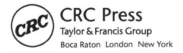

CRC Press
Taylor & Francis Group
Boca Raton London New York

CRC Press is an imprint of the
Taylor & Francis Group, an **informa** business

CRC Press
Taylor & Francis Group
6000 Broken Sound Parkway NW, Suite 300
Boca Raton, FL 33487-2742

First issued in paperback 2019

© 2006 by Taylor & Francis Group, LLC
CRC Press is an imprint of Taylor & Francis Group, an Informa business

No claim to original U.S. Government works

ISBN-13: 978-0-8493-4035-2 (hbk)
ISBN-13: 978-0-367-39096-9 (pbk)

Library of Congress Card Number 2005046656

Library of Congress Cataloging-in-Publication Data

Treatment and management of cancer in the elderly / edited by Hyman Muss, Carrie Hunter, Karen A. Johnson
    p. ; cm.
  Includes bibliographical references and index.
  ISBN-13: 978-0-8493-4035-2 (alk. paper)
  ISBN-10: 0-8493-4035-7 (alk. paper)
  1. Geriatric oncology. I. Muss, Hyman B. II. Hunter, Carrie P., 1947- III. Johnson, Karen A. (Karen Audrey), 1946-
    [DNLM: 1. Aged. 2. Neoplasms--therapy. QZ 266 T7836 2006]

RC281.A34T74 2006
618.97'6994--dc22
                                           2005046656

Visit the Taylor & Francis Web site at
http://www.taylorandfrancis.com

and the CRC Press Web site at
http://www.crcpress.com

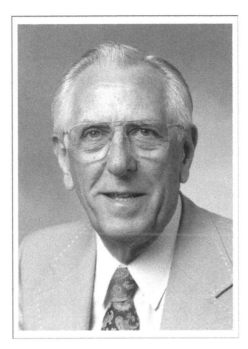

B.J. Kennedy 1921–2003, MD

This text is dedicated to Dr. Byrl James Kennedy, "B.J." to all that knew and loved him. B.J. was one of the fathers of Medical Oncology, a president of the American Society of Clinical Oncology, and among the first to bring awareness of the major issues and challenges in caring for cancer in elders. He would have enjoyed reading this text which helps overcome myths about cancer in older patients and which stresses giving elders information and appropriate options concerning diagnosis, treatment and supportive care. (Photograph courtesy of the American Society of Clinical Oncology).

Preface

Cancer is a disease of aging. Twenty percent of the population in the United States is projected to be aged 65 years and older by year 2030 and the majority of cancers will occur in this age group. Cancer risk increases with age as a result of cumulative genetic, molecular, and biologic changes. In most affluent nations great progress in the prevention and treatment of infectious and childhood disease has led to major increases in longevity, but such gains have come with an increase in the number of people with cancer. The greatest burden of cancer occurs in men and women aged 65 years and older, a population that suffers excess morbidity, reduced quality of life, and economic disparity due to chronic disease. Advancements in the diagnosis and treatment of cancer have resulted in significant reductions in morbidity and improved quality of life, yet these advances have not been adequately shared with the older population. Until recently, cancer in the elderly received little attention. Screening and early detection were offered less frequently to older patients than their younger counterparts. Even now with the greater awareness of the benefits of screening, elders are less likely to receive mammography, colonoscopy and Papanicolaou smears—all procedures associated with decreased mortality—when compared to younger patients. Older patients are also less likely to be offered curative surgery, adjuvant treatment, and treatment for metastases. Some of these decisions in elders are appropriate but in many instances, such undertreatment is representative of long held and mistaken age biases that ultimately lead to poorer outcomes and shortened survival.

We know much more now about the aging process than we did in the past. Shifting demographics, major advances in medical treatment, and improved health and longevity in persons past middle age have led to a gradual transition from a palliative approach to disease management, to an emphasis on curative treatment. Moreover, prevention and risk-reduction for many cancers is now feasible. The awareness of the burden of cancer among elders has led to increased research and support from federal agencies, academic and private institutions, and other public health organizations. In addition to relaxation of eligibility criteria that previously restricted the inclusion of older patients in clinical trials, new trials focusing on the elderly and which include detailed functional and quality of life assessments are now in progress. Data from clinical trials is mandatory for providing optimal care to elders with cancer, and for factoring in the effects of comorbidity and loss of function on cancer treatment. This book brings together a compendium of knowledge on cancer in the elderly that we believe will be useful for health care professionals, researchers, educators, policy makers, and students of public health and preventive medicine.

   Treatment and Management of Cancer in the Elderly addresses major and fundamental issues and problems encountered in delivering cancer care to elderly patients. This compendium builds on our first edition of *Cancer in the Elderly* with an expanded base of knowledge and information on new and current approaches for optimizing cancer care, the results of multi-disciplinary treatments, and strategies for more effective control of cancer in the elderly. The complexity of cancer management is elucidated in chapters that incorporate multi-disciplinary approaches to cancer treatment. The text could be thought of in four parts. Part one includes chapters on epidemiology, the major treatment modalities of surgery, radiation and chemotherapy, and a new chapter on elder law. Part two includes chapters on hematologic malignancy and part three includes chapters on solid tumors. These chapters on site-specific cancers examine the best treatment practices and present results from prevention, adjuvant, neo-adjuvant, and treatment trials. When appropriate, treatment sections on surgery, radiation therapy, chemotherapy, and other modality therapies are included in these chapters. Part four includes chapters on quality of life, geriatric assessment, and comorbidity, and new chapters on exercise, nutrition, management of the frail elderly, end-of-life care, and family support.

   The editors dedicate this work to physicians, nurses, other health professionals, and scientists who will utilize the knowledge gained to improve cancer care management in elderly patients. We also dedicate this work to those elderly cancer patients, their family members, and supporting teams who struggle each day to optimize cancer care with human compassion and dignity.

Hyman B. Muss
Carrie P. Hunter
Karen A. Johnson

Acknowledgment

We express our sincerest thanks to Ms. Linda Norton at the University of Vermont for her help in the preparation of this manuscript.

Contents

Contributors

Ronald D. Adelman Division of Geriatrics and Gerontology, Weill Medical College of Cornell University, New York, New York, U.S.A.

Lodovico Balducci Division of Geriatric Oncology, Department of Interdisciplinary Oncology, University of South Florida and H. Lee Moffitt Cancer Center and Research Institute, Tampa, Florida, U.S.A.

Margot G. Birke Elder Law Solutions, Newburyport, Massachusetts, U.S.A.

Deborah A. Boyle Banner Good Samaritan Medical Center, Phoenix, Arizona, U.S.A.

Robert E. Bristow Department of Gynecology and Obstetrics, The Kelly Gynecologic Oncology Service, The Johns Hopkins Medical Institutions, Baltimore, Maryland, U.S.A.

William J. Brundage Department of Surgery (Otolaryngology), University of Vermont College of Medicine, Burlington, Vermont, U.S.A.

Jeffrey Alan Bubis Dartmouth Hitchcock Medical Center, Lebanon, New Hampshire, U.S.A.

Joseph S. Chan Oregon Health and Science University, Portland, Oregon, U.S.A.

Tara A. Cleary Memorial Sloan Kettering Cancer Center, New York, New York, U.S.A.

Harvey Jay Cohen Duke University Medical Center and Veterans Administration Medical Center, Durham, North Carolina, U.S.A.

Kerry S. Courneya Faculty of Physical Education and Recreation, University of Alberta, Edmonton, Alberta, Canada

Meredith P. Crisp Division of Gynecologic Oncology, Department of Obstetrics and Gynecology, University of Miami School of Medicine, Miami, Florida, U.S.A.

Susan S. Devesa   Descriptive Studies, Biostatistics Branch, Division of Cancer Epidemiology and Genetics, National Cancer Institute, NIH, DHHS, Bethesda, Maryland, U.S.A.

Peter C. Enzinger   Department of Medical Oncology, Dana-Farber Cancer Institute, Department of Medicine, Brigham and Women's Hospital, and Department of Medicine, Harvard Medical School, Boston, Massachusetts, U.S.A.

William B. Ershler   Clinical Research Branch, National Institute on Aging, Harbor Hospital, National Institutes of Health, Baltimore, Maryland, U.S.A.

Martine Extermann   Division of Geriatric Oncology, Department of Interdisciplinary Oncology, University of South Florida and H. Lee Moffitt Cancer Center and Research Institute, Tampa, Florida, U.S.A.

Patricia A. Ganz   UCLA Department of Medicine, Los Angeles, California, U.S.A.

Marc Gautier   Hematology and Oncology, Dartmouth Hitchcock Medical Center, Lebanon, New Hampshire, U.S.A.

Barbara A. Given   College of Nursing, Michigan State University, East Lansing, Michigan, U.S.A.

Charles W. Given   Department of Family Practice, College of Human Medicine, Michigan State University, East Lansing, Michigan, U.S.A.

Steven M. Grunberg   University of Vermont, Vermont Cancer Center, Burlington, Vermont, U.S.A.

Vadim Gushchin   SUNY at Buffalo School of Medicine, Roswell Park Cancer Institute, Buffalo, New York, U.S.A.

Arti Hurria   Memorial Sloan Kettering Cancer Center, New York, New York, U.S.A.

Karen A. Johnson   Breast and Gynecologic Cancer Research Group, Division of Cancer Prevention, National Cancer Institute, Bethesda, Maryland, U.S.A.

John M. Kane III   Department of Breast and Soft Tissue Surgery, SUNY at Buffalo School of Medicine, Roswell Park Cancer Institute, Buffalo, New York, U.S.A.

Kristina H. Karvinen   Faculty of Physical Education and Recreation, University of Alberta, Edmonton, Alberta, Canada

M. Margaret Kemeny   Mount Sinai School of Medicine, Queens Cancer Center, Jamaica, New York, U.S.A.

Gretchen G. Kimmick   Duke University Medical Center, Durham, North Carolina, U.S.A.

Jonathan E. Kolitz Don Monti Division of Oncology/Division of Hematology, North Shore University Hospital, Manhasset, New York, U.S.A.

William G. Kraybill Department of Breast and Soft Tissue Surgery, SUNY at Buffalo School of Medicine, Roswell Park Cancer Institute, Buffalo, New York, U.S.A.

Laura Kruper Department of Surgery, University of Pennsylvania, Philadelphia, Pennsylvania, U.S.A.

Nicholas C. Lambrou Division of Gynecologic Oncology, Department of Obstetrics and Gynecology, University of Miami School of Medicine, Miami, Florida, U.S.A.

Timothy L. Lash Boston University Schools of Medicine and Public Health, Boston, Massachusetts, U.S.A.

Stuart M. Lichtman Memorial Sloan-Kettering Cancer Center, Commack, New York, U.S.A.

Joyce Liu Department of Medical Oncology, Dana Farber Cancer Institute, Boston, Massachusetts, U.S.A.

Dan L. Longo Clinical Research Branch, National Institute on Aging, Harbor Hospital, National Institutes of Health, Baltimore, Maryland, U.S.A.

Ursula Matulonis Department of Medical Oncology, Dana Farber Cancer Institute, Boston, Massachusetts, U.S.A.

Sam Mazj Hematopoietic Stem Cell Transplantation, Stanford University Medical Center, Stanford, California, U.S.A.

Margaret L. McNeely Faculty of Physical Education and Recreation, University of Alberta, Edmonton, Alberta, Canada

Loren K. Mell Department of Radiation and Cellular Oncology, University of Chicago, Chicago, Illinois, U.S.A.

John A. Milner Nutritional Science Research Group, Division of Cancer Prevention, National Cancer Institute, National Institutes of Health, Rockville, Maryland, U.S.A.

David H. Moore Department of Obstetrics and Gynecologic, Indiana University School of Medicine, Indianapolis, Indiana, U.S.A.

Arno J. Mundt Department of Radiation and Cellular Oncology, University of Chicago, Chicago, Illinois, U.S.A.

Arash Naeim UCLA Department of Medicine, Los Angeles, California, U.S.A.

Susan S. Percival Department of Food Science and Human Nutrition, University of Florida, Gainesville, Florida, U.S.A.

George K. Philips   Hematology/Oncology Unit, University of Vermont College of Medicine and Fletcher Allen Health Care, Burlington, Vermont, U.S.A.

David B. Reuben   UCLA Department of Medicine, Los Angeles, California, U.S.A.

Christopher W. Ryan   Oregon Health and Science University, Portland, Oregon, U.S.A.

Homayoon Sanati   UCLA Department of Medicine, Los Angeles, California, U.S.A.

William A. Satariano   School of Public Health, University of California, Berkeley, California, U.S.A.

Lynn M. Schuchter   Division of Hematology and Oncology, Abramson Cancer Center, University of Pennsylvania, Philadelphia, Pennsylvania, U.S.A.

Christopher M. Sellar   Faculty of Physical Education and Recreation, University of Alberta, Edmonton, Alberta, Canada

Pearl H. Seo   Duke University Medical Center and Veterans Affairs Medical Center, Durham, North Carolina, U.S.A.

Nirish S. Shah   Clinical Research Branch, National Institute on Aging, Harbor Hospital, National Institutes of Health, Baltimore, Maryland, U.S.A.

Paula R. Sherwood   School of Nursing, University of Pittsburgh, Pittsburgh, Pennsylvania, U.S.A.

Rebecca A. Silliman   Boston University Schools of Medicine and Public Health, Boston, Massachusetts, U.S.A.

Richard M. Stone   Department of Medicine, Harvard Medical School and Adult Leukemia Program, Department of Adult Oncology, Dana Farber Cancer Institute, Boston, Massachusetts, U.S.A.

Julio Vaquerano   Mount Sinai School of Medicine, Queens Cancer Center, Jamaica, New York, U.S.A.

Nicholas J. Vogelzang   Nevada Cancer Institute, Las Vegas, Nevada, U.S.A.

Sabrina M. Witherby   University of Vermont, Vermont Cancer Center, Burlington, Vermont, U.S.A.

Michael K. K. Wong   Department of Medicine, SUNY at Buffalo School of Medicine, Roswell Park Cancer Institute, Buffalo, New York, U.S.A.

1

Introduction

Lodovico Balducci and Martine Extermann
*Division of Geriatric Oncology, Department of Interdisciplinary Oncology,
University of South Florida and H. Lee Moffitt Cancer Center
and Research Institute, Tampa, Florida, U.S.A.*

The practice of medicine evolves with societal changes. During the last 50 years, healthier lifestyles, medical advances, reduction in birth rate, and absence of a major world conflict have resulted in a progressive aging of the Western and, to a lesser extent, the world population (1). The medical implications of a more prolonged life expectancy include a higher prevalence of chronic diseases and disabilities, the emergence of new diseases and clinical pictures, and a closer interaction of health and social scientists to optimize function and quality of life of older individuals. For example, multiple comorbidities may delay the diagnosis of serious diseases, such as cancer, because early symptoms of cancer may be ascribed to a pre-existing condition, may prevent adequate cancer treatment due to increased risk of therapeutic complications, and may change the goals of treatment from life prolongation to symptom management and function preservation in view of the shortened life expectancy (2). Likewise, the dissolution of the extended family has reduced the pool of family caregivers, so that disabled or ill older individuals depend more and more on the formal support network.

This book addresses the interactions between aging and cancer, cancer being the most common cause of death and disability for older individuals up to age 85 (3). Cancer is a disease of aging, and the aging of the population is the major factor in the increased incidence of cancer during the last five decades. Already, 50% of all malignancies occur in the 12% of the population aged 65 and older. By the year 2030, when the elderly are expected to represent 20% of the entire U.S. population, 70% of all malignancies will occur after age 65 (Fig. 1) (4). It is fair to state that the major burden of cancer is placed on the older population. This finding by itself would justify a book on geriatric oncology. We believe it is important to emphasize four areas where aging of the population may influence the practice of oncology. These include the epidemiology of cancer in the older person, aging and natural history of cancer, evaluation of the older cancer patient, and training in geriatric oncology.

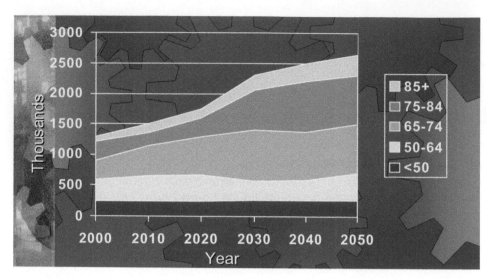

Figure 1   Cancer and aging: cancer burden. *Source*: Modified from Ref. 4.

Epidemiology of cancer and aging. Of special interest are the emerging epidemics of some malignancies in the elderly, changes in the epidemiology of lung and cervical cancer, the stage at presentation of cancer in elderly individuals, and multiple malignancies. Since 1970, the incidence of non-Hodgkin's lymphoma has increased 80% for individuals aged over 60 and that of malignant brain tumors has increased 700% for individuals aged 70 and over (5). A possible explanation of these findings is that the aged represent a natural monitoring system for new environmental carcinogens. That is, older organisms contain a higher number of cells in advanced carcinogenesis than younger organisms and are more susceptible to the action of environmental carcinogens (6). New cancer epidemics due to yet unidentified environmental carcinogens manifest first in older individuals. The increased incidence of brain tumors in the population aged 50 and over, 10 years after it occurred in the elderly, supports this hypothesis (5).

Lung cancer is becoming a disease of the elderly. The median age of lung cancer currently is 71 years (3), up from the age of 60 in 1970. Also, the prevalence of more indolent forms of lung cancer is increasing. The high rate of smoking cessation at middle age is the likely explanation of these findings (7). Deaths from cardiovascular and chronic obstructive lung diseases decline, the appearance of lung cancer is delayed, and its course becomes more indolent with smoking cessation. This evolution may warrant the study of prevention and adjuvant treatment of lung cancer in elderly ex-smokers. Whereas the incidence of cervical cancer decreases after the age of 40, the risk of cancer-related deaths seems to increase with age, which elicits questions concerning the etiology and pathogenesis of cervical cancer in older women and the benefits of screening the elderly for this disease.

Though breast cancer may become more indolent with age, it is more likely to present at an advanced stage in older women (8). Seemingly, older women do not utilize screening mammography adequately. The study of age-related barriers to cancer screening and of strategies to reverse these obstacles may improve the control of breast and other common cancers in this population (9).

In about 10% of cancer patients aged 70 and older, a second and even a third malignancy is observed (10). Except for smoking-related neoplasms, the presence of two different malignancies in the same patient seems to be independent of a common etiology and due to aging alone (10). Yet, the presence of more than one cancer in the same individual involves new decisions related both to prevention and treatment.

Aging and the natural history of cancer. The natural history of several cancers may change with age (3,11). Age is a marker of underlying and only partially defined biological phenomena that may influence cancer behavior. The mechanisms responsible for these changes involve either the neoplastic cell (the seed of cancer) or the tumor host (the soil where the cancer grows). Examples of both mechanisms are recognizable. Acute myelogenous leukemia is more resistant to chemotherapy in older individuals due to a seed mechanism. The prevalence of leukemic cells expressing multidrug resistance and unfavorable cytogenetics increases after the age of 60, and acute leukemia in the elderly is preceded by myelodysplasia in the majority of cases. Breast cancer becomes more indolent with age, due to a combination of seed and soil mechanisms. The prevalence of hormone-receptor-rich, well-differentiated breast cancer increases with age, and at the same time, the reduced production of estrogen (endocrine senescence) may disfavor the growth of breast cancer. Other neoplasms whose prognosis changes with age include non-Hodgkin's lymphoma and ovarian cancer, for which the prognosis worsens, and non-small cell lung cancer, for which it may improve. Mechanisms by which the older tumor host may modulate the growth of cancer include: increased production of inflammatory cytokines, such as interleukin 6 (IL 6) (11), which may stimulate the proliferation of lymphoid malignancies, proliferative senescence of the tumor stroma that releases growth factors and enzymes favoring metastases (12), and immune-senescence that paradoxically may delay the growth of some tumors while favoring the growth of others (13).

Assessment of the older person with cancer. Aging involves a progressive reduction in the functional reserve of multiple organ systems and increased prevalence of comorbidity that may reduce the life expectancy and the tolerance of stress by older individuals (14). In addition, a progressive reduction in personal and social resources, including income, access to transportation, and the number of family members and friends capable of providing home care, may represent barriers to medical interventions. These age-related changes are poorly mirrored in chronologic age and chronologic age is a poor surrogate for the institution of cancer prevention or treatment.

Any intervention aimed to prevent or treat cancer in the elderly should be based on individual life expectancy and tolerance of treatment, and on the availability of adequate resources to face treatment-related emergencies. In addition, reversible situations that may compromise the administration of treatment, including depression, malnutrition, and limited home care support, should be recognized and addressed. The common approach to these questions involves a comprehensive geriatric assessment, including function, other diseases, cognition, nutrition, psychosocial factors, and social support. The geriatric assessment is not fully standardized, however, and the expertise to perform it is limited largely to geriatric centers. In addition, it is time consuming. In the last few years, research on geriatric assessment has focused on screening tests to establish which older individuals need a full assessment, and on laboratory tests that may help predict the risk of death and functional dependence. Of the screening instruments available, that developed by the cardiovascular health study (CHS) deserves special mention because it is simple to execute and has been validated with a large number of subjects and an 11-year follow-up (15).

The CHS concluded that five simple tests allow health care providers to divide the older population into three groups, fit, prefrail, and frail—groups with different risks of mortality, functional dependence, and rates of hospitalization and institutionalization. It appears reasonable to recommend that all individuals aged 65 or 70 years and over undergo the CHS evaluation, and the prefrail and frail group receive a full geriatric assessment. Of the laboratory tests, markers of inflammations, such as IL 6 and C-reactive protein, appear the most promising in predicting risk of death and functional dependence in a home-dwelling population of older individuals (16). Aging has been construed as a progressive chronic inflammation that may undergo sudden exacerbation as a result of disease and trauma.

Training in geriatric oncology. Increasing age is a risk factor for cancer and cancer death, is associated with changes in tumor biology, and generates novel and unique decisional issues related to cancer prevention and treatment, clinical research, including the diversity of older patients, and the recruitment of these patients into clinical trials, and it requires special training in the assessment of older individuals, of the quality of their life during treatment and, perhaps more important, during survival. Aware of these issues, the National Institute of Aging, in combination with the National Cancer Institute, has funded through competitive grants the Institution of Geriatric Oncology Programs and Clinical Research in older individuals with cancer. In the forefront of the educational needs related to aging, the Hartford Foundation has funded a number of fellowships in geriatric oncology in academic cancer centers. The immediate outcome of this effort will be an answer to the most pressing problems, including the enrollment of older individuals in clinical trials of cancer prevention and cancer treatment, a time- and cost-effective assessment of the older patient with cancer, and the definition of biological changes of aging that may influence tumor behavior. It is legitimate to ask also what will be the long-term outcome of this effort, that is, what will be the face of geriatric oncology 10 or 20 years from now. Three models appear to be possible. One involves the institution of a new specialty of geriatric oncology whose practitioners are trained to take care of patients over a certain threshold of age (70 or 75) or, alternatively, of the so-called "prefrail" or "frail" cancer patients. The second model involves a training of all oncologists, beginning in medical school, in the assessment of older individuals. A third model calls for the cooperation of oncologists and aging specialists acting as primary care physicians of older patients. Of course, a combination of the three models is also possible. Irrespective of the most functional health care model, it is encouraging to find that the interactions between aging and cancer are being investigated, and a solution for its problems is being sought. This book may provide an important reference to these efforts.

REFERENCES

1. Yancik RM, Ries L. Cancer in older persons: magnitude of the problem and efforts to advance the aging/cancer research interface. In: Balducci L, Lyman GH, Ershler WB, Extermann M, eds. Comprehensive Geriatric Oncology. London: Taylor and Francis, 2004:38–45.
2. Yancik R, Ganz P, Varricchio CG, Conley B. Perspectives on comorbidity and cancer in older patients: approaches to expand the knowledge base. J Clin Oncol 2001; 19:1147–1151.
3. Jemal A, Murray T, Ward E, et al. Cancer statistics 2005. CA Cancer J Clin 2005; 55:10–30.

4. Edwards BK, Howe HL, Ries LA, et al. Annual report to the nation on the status of cancer, 1973–1999, featuring implications of age and aging on U.S. cancer burden. Cancer 2002; 94:2766–2792.

5. Balducci L, Aapro M. Epidemiology of cancer and aging: clinical and biological implications. In: Balducci L, Extermann M, eds. Biological Basis of Geriatric Oncology. New York: Springer, 2005:1–16.

6. Anisimov W. Biological interactions of aging and carcinogenesis. In: Balducci L, Extermann M, eds. Biological Basis of Geriatric Oncology. New York: Springer, 2005:17–52.

7. Khuder SA, Mutgi AB. Effect of smoking cessation on major histologic types of lung cancer. Chest 2001; 120:1577–1583.

8. Randolph WM, Mahnken JD, Goodwin JS, et al. Using medicare data to estimate the prevalence of breast cancer screening in older women: comparison of different methods to identify screening mammograms. Health Serv Res 2002; 37:1643–1657.

9. Fox SA, Rotzheim RG. Barriers to cancer prevention in the older person. In: Balducci L, Lyman GH, Ershler WB, Extermann M, eds. Comprehensive Geriatric Oncology. London: Taylor and Francis, 2004:376–388.

10. Luciani A, Balducci L. Multiple primary malignancies. Sem Oncol 2004; 31:264–273.

11. Ershler WB. The influence of advanced age on cancer occurrence and growth. In: Balducci L, Extermann M, eds. Biological Bases of Geriatric Oncology. New York: Springer, 2005:75–88.

12. Hornsby PJ. Proliferative senescence and cancer. In: Balducci L, Extermann M, eds. Biological Basis of Geriatric Oncology. New York: Springer, 2005:53–74.

13. Chen JJW, Lin YC, Yao PL, et al. Tumor-associated macrophages: the double-edged sword in cancer progression. J Clin Oncol 2005; 23:953–965.

14. Balducci L, Extermann M. Assessment of the older cancer patient. In: Balducci L, Lyman GH, Ershler WB, Extermann M, eds. Comprehensive Geriatric Oncology. London: Taylor and Francis, 2004:223–235.

15. Fried LP, Tangen CM, Walston J, et al. Frailty in older adults: evidence for a phenotype. J Gerontol Med Sci 2001; 56A:M146–M156.

16. Cohen HJ, Harris F, Pieper CF. Coagulation and activation of inflammatory pathways in the development of functional decline and mortality in the elderly. Am J Med 2003; 114:180–187.

2

The Burden of Cancer in the Elderly

Susan S. Devesa
Descriptive Studies, Biostatistics Branch, Division of Cancer Epidemiology and Genetics, National Cancer Institute, NIH, DHHS, Bethesda, Maryland, U.S.A.

INTRODUCTION

In 2005, it was estimated that a total of 1,372,910 new cases of invasive cancer would be diagnosed in the United States (1); this estimate does not include the more than 1,000,000 cases of basal and squamous cell skin cancer. The majority of these cancers occur at three sites. In men, over 55% of new cases are due to cancers of the prostate (33%), lung and bronchus (13%), and colon and rectum (10%). In women, 55% of new cases are due to cancers of the breast (32%), lung and bronchus (12%), and colon and rectum (11%).

TRENDS IN CANCER

Between 1978 and 2002, the incidence rate in men rose 13% for all cancers combined and 77% for prostate cancer, while declining 20% for lung cancer (2). Among women, the incidence rate increased 15% for all cancers combined, 71% for lung cancer, and 32% for breast cancer. The colorectal cancer incidence rate declined by 17% for both sexes during this period. The risk of developing most cancers increases with advancing age. More than half of all new cancers in 2002 occurred in the population aged 65 years and older. This proportion will increase, due, in large part, to the impact of the baby boom generation, and the burden of cancer will increase as more people live longer.

In the United States, cancer is the second most frequent cause of death, accounting in 2002 for more than 550,000 deaths (23%) and following only deaths due to heart diseases (Table 1) (3). Cancer was the second most frequent cause of death among both males and females overall and at ages 65 to 84. Cancer was the leading cause of death among women aged 20 to 64 and men aged 45 to 64. The most frequent cause of death due to cancer at all ages combined was lung cancer, followed by prostate cancer among males and breast cancer among females, with colorectal cancer the third and pancreatic cancer the fourth among both sexes (Table 2). These patterns are apparent at ages 65 to 84. However, among older males, prostate cancer ranked first, followed by lung, colorectal, and bladder cancers. Among older

Table 1 Reported Deaths for the Five Leading Causes of Death by Age and Sex, United States, 2002

Rank	All ages Male	All ages Female	Ages 0–19 Male	Ages 0–19 Female	Ages 20–44 Male	Ages 20–44 Female	Ages 45–64 Male	Ages 45–64 Female	Ages 65–84 Male	Ages 65–84 Female	Ages 85+ Male	Ages 85+ Female
	All causes: 1,198,982	All causes: 1,244,048	All causes: 32,565	All causes: 21,289	All causes: 100,901	All causes: 50,828	All causes: 259,085	All causes: 166,642	All causes: 580,525	All causes: 550,119	All causes: 225,966	All causes: 455,170
1	Heart diseases: 340,899	Heart diseases: 356,001	Accidents: 8,271	Perinatal conditions: 6,188	Accidents: 28,104	Cancer: 11,448	Cancer: 76,307	Cancer: 66,721	Heart diseases: 175,875	Heart diseases: 150,253	Heart diseases: 80,935	Heart diseases: 169,238
2	Cancer: 288,763	Cancer: 268,501	Perinatal conditions: 8,028	Accidents: 4,171	Heart diseases: 12,180	Accidents: 9,450	Heart diseases: 71,139	Heart diseases: 30,665	Cancer: 167,037	Cancer: 144,782	Cancer: 34,621	Cerebrovascular diseases: 48,096
3	Accidents: 69,183	Cerebrovascular diseases: 100,048	Congenital anomalies: 3,585	Congenital anomalies: 3,233	Suicide: 11,592	Heart diseases: 5,290	Accidents: 16,273	Cerebrovascular diseases: 7,218	Chronic obstructive pulmonary diseases: 39,771	Cerebrovascular diseases: 43,019	Cerebrovascular diseases: 18,316	Cancer: 44,561
4	Cerebrovascular diseases: 62,621	Chronic obstructive pulmonary diseases: 64,101	Homicide: 2,225	Cancer: 989	Cancer: 9,516	Suicide: 2,802	Liver diseases: 9,513	Chronic obstructive pulmonary diseases: 7,177	Cerebrovascular diseases: 33,862	Chronic obstructive pulmonary diseases: 39,258	Chronic obstructive pulmonary diseases: 12,436	Alzheimer's disease: 26,602
5	Chronic obstructive pulmonary diseases: 60,708	Diabetes mellitus: 38,948	Suicide: 1,479	Homicide: 776	Homicide: 9,193	HIV infection: 2,225	Diabetes mellitus: 8,908	Accidents: 6,747	Diabetes mellitus: 18,712	Diabetes mellitus: 21,279	Pneumonia and influenza: 11,199	Pneumonia and influenza: 20,796

Source: From Ref. 3.

Table 2 Reported Deaths for the Five Leading Cancers by Age and Sex, United States, 2002

Rank	All ages	0–19	20–44	45–64	65–84	85+
Males	All cancers: 288,763	All cancers: 1,282	All cancers: 9,516	All cancers: 76,307	All cancers: 167,037	All cancers: 34,621
1	Lung and bronchus: 90,121	Leukemia: 382	Lung and bronchus: 1,488	Lung and bronchus: 25,588	Lung and bronchus: 56,340	Prostate: 8,957
2	Prostate: 30,446	Brain and ONS: 327	Colon and rectum: 964	Colon and rectum: 7,537	Prostate: 19,053	Lung and bronchus: 6,699
3	Colon and rectum: 28,471	Endocrine system: 104	Brain and ONS: 912	Pancreas: 4,538	Colon and rectum: 16,124	Colon and rectum: 3,838
4	Pancreas: 14,876	Bones and joints: 96	Leukemia: 850	Esophagus: 3,506	Pancreas: 8,540	Bladder: 1,791
5	Leukemia: 12,058	Soft tissue: 82	Non-Hodgkin's lymphoma: 679	Liver and IHBD: 3,469	Leukemia: 6,833	Leukemia: 1,597
Females	All cancers: 268,501	All cancers: 989	All cancers: 11,448	All cancers: 66,721	All cancers: 144,782	All cancers: 44,561
1	Lung and bronchus: 67,509	Leukemia: 296	Breast: 3,141	Lung and bronchus: 17,215	Lung and bronchus: 41,960	Colon and rectum: 7,308
2	Breast: 41,514	Brain and ONS: 244	Lung and bronchus: 1,388	Breast: 14,181	Breast: 18,057	Lung and bronchus: 6,943
3	Colon and rectum: 28,132	Endocrine system: 89	Cervix uteri: 890	Colon and rectum: 5,302	Colon and rectum: 14,771	Breast: 6,134
4	Pancreas: 15,387	Bones and joints: 83	Colon and rectum: 748	Ovary: 4,465	Pancreas: 9,202	Pancreas: 2,937
5	Ovary: 14,682	Soft tissue: 71	Leukemia: 625	Pancreas: 3,000	Ovary: 7,860	Non-Hodgkin's lymphoma: 2,164

Note: All cancer categories exclude basal and squamous cell skin cancers and in situ carcinomas except bladder.
Abbreviations: ONS, other nervous system; IHBD, intrahepatic bile duct.
Source: From Ref. 3.

females, colorectal cancer ranked first, followed by lung, breast, and pancreatic cancers. At young ages, leukemia and brain cancer predominated. Among males aged 20 to 64, the predominant cancers were those of the lung and colorectum. Among females, breast cancers exceeded lung cancer at ages 20 to 44, but the reverse occurred at ages 45 to 64. The number of deaths due to cancer rose from about 2300 among those under the age of 20 to more than 300,000 at ages 65 to 84 years, and to 79,000 at ages 85 and older.

In this chapter, we will draw upon descriptive data available from several sources. Much of the incidence and survival data derive from information regarding primary cancers diagnosed among the residents of areas in the United States participating in the Surveillance, Epidemiology, and End Results (SEER) program supported by contracts awarded by the National Cancer Institute, and population estimates based on data from the Census Bureau (4). Mortality data for the United States were based on death certificate information provided by the National Center for Health Statistics. Data provided by the World Health Organization and compiled by the International Agency for Research on Cancer were used to evaluate the international variation in mortality among the elderly (5).

From 1978 to 2002, the total number of cancer cases, excluding superficial skin cancers, diagnosed in the nine SEER areas rose 72%, and the number of deaths in the United States due to cancer rose 41% (Table 3). These increases were due to several factors. The first is the growth in the population size, which increased about 30%. Thus, the crude incidence rate per 100,000 population rose 33%, and the crude mortality rate increased 9%. Rates for most cancers rise with age. Because mortality owing to other causes, notably cardiovascular disease, has declined, people have been living longer, shifting the age distribution toward older ages. A technique called age adjustment accounts for these changes, permitting the comparing of rates as though the population age distributions were the same. Comparison of the age-adjusted rates, a better reflection of the changes in risk, reveals that the incidence rose by a more modest 16%, and the mortality actually declined by 5%.

The projected number of cancer cases is expected to double over the next 50 years, from 1.3 million in 2000 to 2.6 million in 2050, due to population growth

Table 3 Trends in Total Cancers in the United States, 1978 to 2002, All Ages

	1978	2002	% Change
Incidence[a] in 9 SEER areas			
Number of cases	71,921	123,856	72.2
Population	21,035,770	27,219,888	29.4
Crude incidence rate[b]	341.9	455.0	33.1
Age-adjusted incidence rate[b]	407.2	471.4	15.8
Deaths in the United States			
Number of deaths	395,099	557,264	41.0
Population	222,097,449	287,974,001	29.7
Crude mortality rate[b]	177.9	193.5	8.8
Age-adjusted mortality rate[b]	204.4	193.5	−5.3

[a]Excludes basal and squamous cell skin cancers and in situ carcinomas except bladder.
[b]Per 100,000, age-adjusted using the 2000 U.S. population standard.
Source: From Refs. 2 and 3.

and decline in death rates, even with no changes in the current cancer incidence rates (6). The number of incident cancers among the elderly aged 75 and older are projected to almost triple from 389,000 in 2000 to 1,102,000 in 2050, and the number among those aged 85 and older is expected to increase fourfold. The projected increases in the numbers of cancers among the elderly will be of increasing importance to clinicians, researchers, and health care administrators in planning future cancer care and research interventions, as well as health policies and public health campaigns for the elderly.

The incidence of all cancers combined among elderly males aged 65 to 84 years increased 24%, from 2538 per 100,000 person-years during 1978–1982 to 3157 during 1988–1992, before declining 8% to 2899 during 1998–2002 (Fig. 1). Total cancer mortality rose 5% and then decreased 9% during the same time periods. Among elderly females, both incidence and mortality rates were considerably lower, although continuing to rise, over the entire time period. Total cancer incidence rates increased 21%, from 1408 to 1703, and mortality rates rose 13%, from 720 to 813.

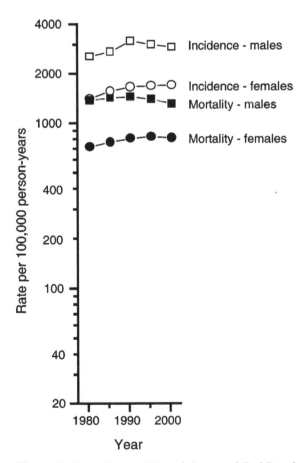

Figure 1 Surveillance, Epidemiology, and End Results (SEER) program incidence in 9 areas and U.S. mortality rates for all cancers combined among the elderly aged 65 to 84 years by sex, 1978–1982 to 1998–2002.

Among elderly males, the rising total cancer incidence rates were driven largely by prostate cancer: rates increased by 78% from the period 1978–1982 to 1988–1992, a period during which many subclinical cases of prostate cancer were diagnosed based on prostate-specific antigen screening along with digital rectal examination (7,8); subsequently, the rates declined 14% by 1998–2002 (Fig. 2A). Lung cancer incidence among elderly males peaked around 1990. This reflects the impact of large declines in prevalence of smoking since 1965, due in large part to successful smoking prevention and cessation public health campaigns (9,10). Colorectal cancer also peaked during the late 1980s; trends varied by subsite, with rates declining for rectal cancer and rising for proximal cancer (11). Rates increased substantially for esophageal and kidney cancers, melanoma, and the lymphomas. The rises in esophageal and kidney cancer incidence are related to smoking and obesity (12–14), whereas increasing melanoma rates are related to ultraviolet radiation and sunburns (15). The rising lymphoma incidence may be related to occupational exposures to pesticides or solvents and to AIDS, particularly among young and middle-aged men; risk also may be associated with diets that are high in animal protein and fat and low in fruits and vegetables (16,17). Rates for stomach cancer have declined, most likely related to reductions in smoking, improved diet, and decreases in the prevalence of *Helicobacter pylori* (12). Decreases in oral cancer rates are also related to declining tobacco use (both cigarette smoking and the use of smokeless tobacco), alcohol consumption, and infection with certain viruses (18). Prostate cancer mortality increases were less dramatic than those for incidence, and the mortality declined notably in recent years. Lung cancer mortality rates also peaked around 1990, and the patterns for the other cancers resembled the incidence trends.

Among elderly females, the most rapid increases in incidence as well as mortality were for lung cancer (Fig. 2B). Lung cancer rates more than doubled from 1978–1982 to 1998–2002, although the rates of increase have diminished in recent years. American women started smoking about 10 years later than American men, and they have not been as successful at quitting (9,19). During the 1980s, the lung cancer mortality rate for women aged 65 to 84 years surpassed both the breast and colorectal cancer mortality rates, and, in the 1990s, lung cancer surpassed colorectal cancer as the second most frequent cancer. Breast cancer incidence rates rose significantly until the 1990s, with a more modest rise in rates since that time; mortality rates have declined 16% since 1990. The rapid increases in the incidence of breast cancer during the 1980s in the United States, and more recently in other countries, were related to mammography screening, although the patterns also reflect disparities in lifestyle and hereditary factors (20,21). As among men, the female rates for melanoma, lymphomas, and kidney cancer also increased substantially, whereas the rates declined notably for stomach and cervix uteri cancers. The declines in the incidence of cervical cancer have been more pronounced for squamous cell carcinomas than adenocarcinomas, at older ages than younger ages, and among blacks than whites (22). The more rapid decreases in mortality than in the incidence rates for corpus uteri cancer are related to improvements in survival, which have varied by race, histologic type, stage, grade, and age group (23). Ovarian cancer incidence trends have differed by histologic type, although improving specificity in pathologic classification probably played a role (24).

The risk of dying from cancer generally increases exponentially with age (Fig. 3). Based on U.S. mortality data for the period 1978–2002, the rates for all cancers combined increased linearly from around the age of 20 to about the age of 60, after which the increases were less rapid. Higher rates among males than females were most evident at the ages of 60 and older. This pattern was repeated for many of the specific forms of cancer, although there were exceptions. For lung cancer, the

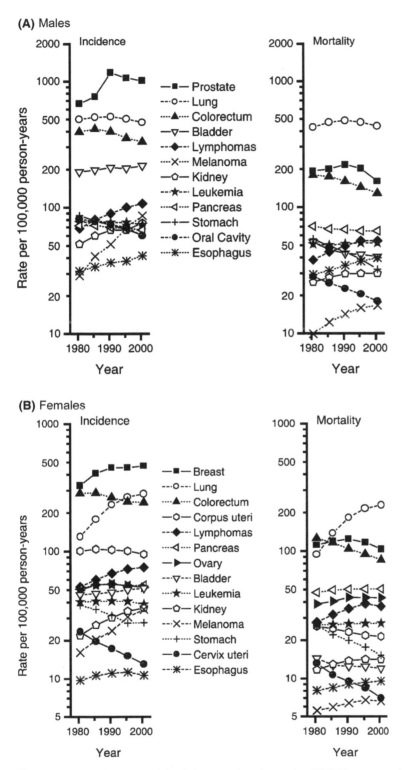

Figure 2 Surveillance, Epidemiology, and End Results (SEER) program incidence in 9 areas and U.S. mortality rates for selected cancers among the elderly aged 65 to 84 years, 1978–1982 to 1998–2002: (**A**) males, (**B**) females. *Note*: Lymphomas include Hodgkin's and non-Hodgkin's lymphoma; oral cavity includes pharynx.

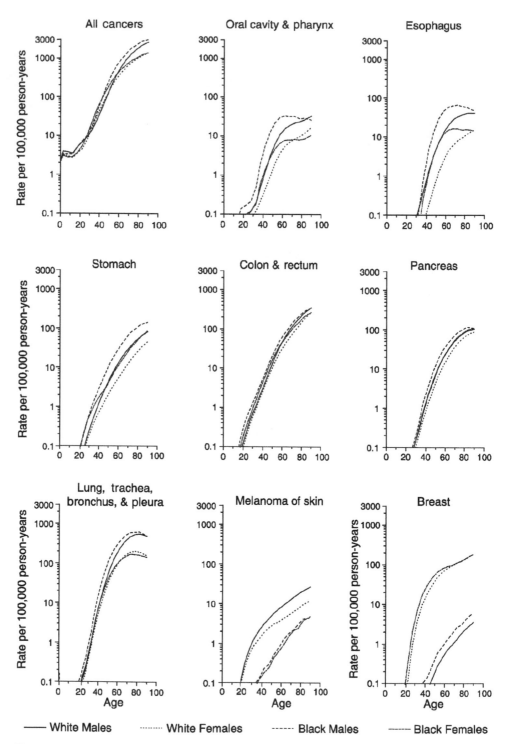

Figure 3 Age-specific mortality rates in the total U.S. population for selected cancers by race and sex, 1978–2002. *Abbreviations*: NOS, not otherwise specified; ONS, other nervous system.

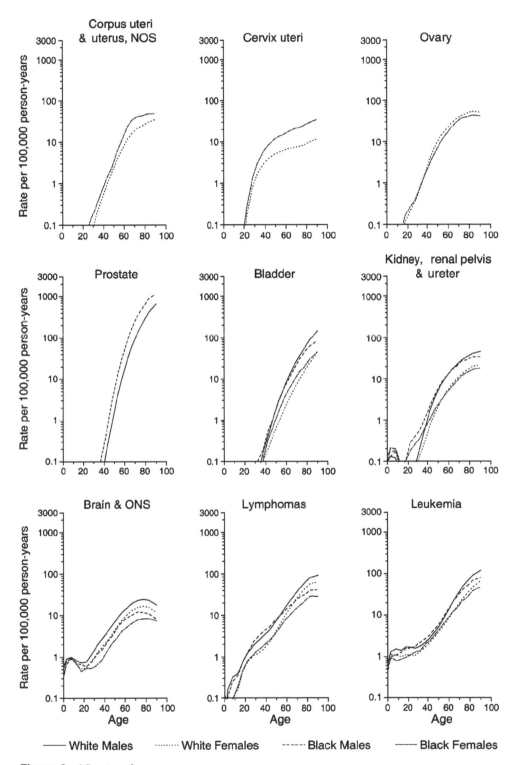

Figure 3 (*Continued*)

male excess was most pronounced at the ages of 40 years and older, with smaller differences at younger ages. Consistently higher rates among blacks than whites were evident for esophageal, stomach, cervix uteri, and prostate cancers, whereas rates among whites were notably higher for melanoma of the skin and corpus uteri cancer. Rates among young people generally were quite low, although bimodal curves were apparent for cancers of the kidney and brain, and for leukemia.

At current rates, the probability at birth of ever developing cancer is 46%, or almost one out of two, for males, and 38%, or more than one out of three, for females (Table 4) (4). At birth, the probability of dying of cancer is more than one out of five. By the age of 60, the probability of eventually developing cancer is also 46% for males, but falls to 33% for females. A male at the age of 60 years has an 18% chance of being diagnosed with prostate cancer, an 8% chance with lung cancer, and a 6% chance

Table 4 Probabilities (%) of Developing (Ever, or After Age 60) or Dying from Cancer by Type of Cancer and Sex, 2000–2002

	Males			Females		
	Developing			Developing		
	Ever	After age 60	Dying	Ever	After age 60	Dying
All cancers	45.67	45.68	23.56	38.09	32.80	19.93
Oral cavity and pharynx	1.38	1.10	0.38	0.68	0.56	0.19
Esophagus	0.76	0.72	0.74	0.25	0.24	0.22
Stomach	1.22	1.21	0.59	0.75	0.71	0.40
Colon and rectum	5.84	5.77	2.36	5.51	5.25	2.23
Liver[a]	0.89	0.76	0.65	0.43	0.39	0.37
Pancreas	1.26	1.24	1.17	1.27	1.24	1.17
Larynx	0.62	0.56	0.23	0.14	0.12	0.06
Lung and bronchus	7.58	7.74	7.25	5.72	5.39	4.92
Melanoma of the skin	1.94	1.56	0.35	1.30	0.76	0.20
Breast	0.12	0.11	0.03	13.22	9.99	2.96
Cervix uteri	–	–	–	0.74	0.34	0.26
Corpus uteri	–	–	–	2.61	2.04	0.51
Ovary	–	–	–	1.48	1.13	1.05
Prostate	17.93	18.48	2.97	–	–	–
Testis	0.36	0.02	0.02	–	–	–
Urinary bladder[b]	3.58	3.72	0.75	1.14	1.10	0.32
Kidney and renal pelvis	1.56	1.37	0.59	0.91	0.76	0.34
Brain and other nervous system	0.65	0.44	0.49	0.50	0.32	0.39
Thyroid	0.35	0.20	0.04	0.97	0.36	0.06
Hodgkin's lymphoma	0.24	0.09	0.05	0.19	0.07	0.04
Non-Hodgkin's lymphoma	2.18	1.88	0.94	1.82	1.57	0.81
Multiple myeloma	0.70	0.68	0.46	0.55	0.51	0.40
Leukemia	1.50	1.34	0.97	1.07	0.89	0.72

Note: Invasive cancer only, unless specified otherwise.
[a]Liver and intrahepatic bile duct.
[b]Urinary bladder (invasive and in situ).
–: Not applicable.
Source: From Ref. 4.

with colorectal cancer during his remaining years. A 60-year-old female has a 10% risk of breast cancer, a 5% risk of colorectal cancer, and a 5% risk of lung cancer during her remaining lifetime. At current rates, 7% of men will die of lung cancer, 3% of prostate cancer, and 2% of colorectal cancer. About 5% of women will die of lung cancer, 3% of breast cancer, and 2% of colorectal cancer.

There is considerable variation in cancer incidence and mortality rates according to racial or ethnic groups (Table 5) (25,26). The racial categories of American Indian or Alaska Native, Asian or Pacific Islander, black, and white are mutually exclusive. The ethnic category Hispanic may include any race; rate are shown for Hispanic and non-Hispanic whites. The highest total cancer incidence rate per 100,000 person-years among males during the period 1992–2002 occurred among blacks, followed by non-Hispanic whites and all whites combined, with lower rates among Hispanic whites and Asian or Pacific Islanders; the rate among American Indians/Alaska Natives was one-half of that among whites. Among females, non-Hispanic whites had the highest total cancer incidence rate, followed by all whites combined, blacks, Hispanic whites, and Asian or Pacific Islanders, with the lowest rate among American Indians/Alaska Natives.

There is also substantial international variation in cancer mortality rates (5,27). Tables 6 and 7 present age-adjusted (world standard) mortality rates during the period 1996–2000, for males and females respectively, for all cancers combined and several cancers among the elderly, defined as those aged 65 to 84 years. Among males, the rates for all cancers combined were highest in Scotland (>1500), followed by the Netherlands, Denmark, the Russian Federation, and the Republic of Korea (all >1400). Total cancer rates were lowest in Sweden, Portugal, and the

Table 5 Cancer Incidence by Racial/Ethnic Group and Sex, 13 SEER Areas 1992–2002

	Males			Females		
	Count	Rate[a]	RR	Count	Rate[a]	RR
All ages						
White	750,056	572.7	1.00	709,057	425.7	1.00
Black	91,547	715.6	1.25	74,496	401.6	0.94
American Indian/Alaska Native	4,008	285.5	0.50	4,349	229.8	0.54
Asian or Pacific Islander	60,499	394.4	0.69	60,175	301.2	0.71
Hispanic white[b]	62,753	442.6	0.77	63,527	319.8	0.75
Non-Hispanic white[b]	580,725	577.9	1.01	550,670	437.7	1.03
Ages 65 and older						
White	463,956	3014.9	1.00	397,720	1760.0	1.00
Black	47,023	3565.0	1.18	34,436	1648.5	0.94
American Indian/Alaska Native	1,917	1515.1	0.50	1,615	942.1	0.54
Asian or Pacific Islander	38,061	2189.0	0.73	26,962	1179.5	0.67
Hispanic white[b]	31,487	2431.1	0.81	24,900	1305.9	0.74
Non-Hispanic white[b]	365,409	3001.8	1.00	318,192	1792.0	1.02

[a]Per 100,000 person-years, age-adjusted using the 2000 U.S. population standard.
[b]Data for Hispanic and non-Hispanic exclude Detroit, Hawaii, Alaska Native Registry, and rural Georgia.
Abbreviation: RR, rate ratio relative to the rate among whites.
Source: From Refs. 25 and 26.

Table 6 International Variation in Mortality Rates[a] for Selected Cancers Among the Elderly (Aged 65 to 84 Years) in Selected Countries, 1996–2000: Males

	All cancers combined	Mouth or pharynx	Esophagus	Stomach	Intestines	Pancreas	Lung	Prostate	Bladder
United States	1187.1	18.2	36.4	30.3	118.3	58.0	420.9	134.2	33.2
Canada	1240.5	22.9	36.2	45.8	131.6	56.4	413.7	143.1	37.1
Denmark	1422.9	25.7	46.3	43.4	189.4	61.7	411.1	200.6	86.0
France	1330.2	47.2	52.4	53.0	143.2	56.9	323.2	142.2	56.8
Germany	1284.0	24.9	28.7	88.2	170.9	64.9	356.5	147.3	52.2
Italy	1359.8	27.6	23.5	102.8	134.5	57.3	430.6	104.2	66.2
Netherlands	1465.2	16.7	49.9	76.1	155.1	57.6	514.6	169.4	57.1
Portugal	1152.2	27.5	31.4	151.1	158.3	45.9	219.4	173.0	47.1
Russian Federation	1420.5	43.2	47.6	235.9	158.5[b]	N/A	444.7	82.3	N/A
Spain	1259.3	29.3	29.8	89.0	144.8	44.6	358.0	124.2	75.6
Sweden	1034.6	13.7	23.9	51.3	121.2	63.6	192.2	219.7	37.8
United Kingdom: England & Wales	1292.4	15.4	66.6	75.6	144.1	51.5	379.8	154.9	55.1
United Kingdom: Scotland	1512.9	23.0	86.6	78.5	177.7	55.2	513.4	151.8	58.6
Australia	1206.5	24.8	39.0	46.6	155.9	51.6	314.9	162.4	34.9
Japan	1253.4	21.2	57.2	234.1	134.9	69.8	299.6	49.9	22.1
Republic of Korea	1409.6	17.5	58.5	328.2	85.5	58.8	384.0	26.1	27.3

[a]Per 100,000 person-years, age-adjusted using the world population standard.
[b]Excluding small intestine.
N/A: Not available.
Source: From Ref. 5.

Table 7 International Variation in Mortality Rates[a] for Selected Cancers Among the Elderly (Aged 65 to 84 Years) in Selected Countries, 1996–2000: Females

	All cancers combined	Stomach	Intestines	Pancreas	Lung	Breast	Cervix uteri	Other uterus	Kidney
United States	745.8	13.8	77.5	44.1	215.1	100.3	7.4	19.7	12.4
Canada	735.9	19.4	77.3	43.6	185.5	108.2	7.2	17.5	12.7
Denmark	974.6	20.1	135.5	54.2	216.8	148.7	18.4	24.7	21.9
France	545.6	18.8	74.2	34.2	43.2	98.2	5.6	24.0	12.3
Germany	687.2	42.5	107.1	45.7	68.8	107.0	10.9	20.9	16.9
Italy	601.4	44.1	72.6	40.1	61.0	94.8	3.3	23.2	10.1
Netherlands	711.6	28.8	95.3	45.9	97.7	128.8	8.9	16.8	18.3
Portugal	521.2	67.8	78.5	27.8	29.2	78.2	8.3	25.9	7.0
Russian Federation	599.8	102.8	97.1[b]	N/A	47.1	71.0	23.0	30.4	N/A
Spain	493.9	36.2	74.6	28.8	25.7	74.5	6.3	20.4	7.9
Sweden	657.2	23.1	84.5	53.8	87.7	81.7	9.5	22.3	20.2
United Kingdom: England & Wales	795.8	28.4	86.9	39.7	170.1	118.7	10.6	16.8	12.8
United Kingdom: Scotland	941.7	39.2	99.0	41.0	261.7	116.6	13.1	14.7	15.3
Australia	647.8	18.8	92.9	40.0	110.0	86.6	9.3	12.9	15.0
Japan	500.3	74.6	69.3	40.7	66.7	25.1	8.0	11.6	4.6
Republic of Korea	507.2	116.6	48.2	32.6	82.2	10.7	12.2	17.8	4.3

[a]Per 100,000 person-years, age-adjusted using the world population standard.
[b]Excluding small intestine.
N/A: Not available.
Source: From Ref. 5.

United States (all <1200). Other countries had rates that were intermediate. These patterns were influenced by variations in the relative frequency of the various forms of cancer. Lung cancer was by far the most common cause of cancer death in every country shown except Sweden; rates ranged from greater than 500 in the Netherlands and Scotland to less than 300 in Japan, Portugal, and Sweden. Intestinal cancer mortality rates were highest in Denmark, followed by Scotland and Germany, with the lowest rates again in the Republic of Korea and the United States. Prostate cancer rates exceeded 100 in all countries except Japan and the Republic of Korea, where the rates were less than 50; rates were highest in Sweden, Denmark, Portugal, and the Netherlands. The patterns for stomach cancer were quite different, with the rate exceeding 300 in the Republic of Korea, 200 in the Russian Federation and Japan, 150 in Portugal, and 100 in Italy, in contrast to a rate of less than 50 in the United States, Denmark, Canada, and Australia. Oral cancers were most frequent in France, pancreatic cancer in Japan and Germany, and bladder cancer in Denmark, Spain, and Italy.

Among elderly females, the rates for all cancers combined were highest in Denmark and Scotland (>900), and lowest in France, Portugal, Spain, the Republic of Korea, Japan, and the Russian Federation (all <600) (Table 7). Lung cancer was the most frequent form of cancer death in the United States, Canada, Denmark, Sweden, the United Kingdom, and Australia; rates ranged from less than 30 in Spain and Portugal to more than 200 in Scotland, Denmark, and the United States. Breast cancer was the most common cancer death in the Netherlands and Germany, with rates exceeding 100, in contrast to a rate of only 25 in Japan and 11 in the Republic of Korea. Intestinal cancer was the first-ranked cancer in Germany, Spain, and Portugal; internationally, rates ranged from 48 in Korea to 136 in Denmark. The leading cancer in Korea, the Russian Federation, and Japan was cancer of the stomach, with rates of 117, 103, and 75, respectively, at least five times that in the United States. Cervix uteri cancer mortality rates were highest in the Russian Federation, Denmark, and Scotland (>13), and lowest in Italy and France (<6). Other uterine cancer rates ranged from less than 15 in Japan, Australia, and Scotland to 30 in the Russian Federation. Kidney cancer rates ranged from less than 10 in the Republic of Korea, Japan, Portugal, and Spain to more than 20 in Denmark and Sweden.

Among patients diagnosed with cancer (all forms combined) in the United States, the five-year relative survival rate, which is adjusted for expected general population mortality, ranged from 53% among black females to 66% among whites (Table 8). These rates were driven by the differing relative frequency of the major forms of cancer and varying survival rates. Survival rates were relatively high among patients diagnosed with cancers of the testis, thyroid, prostate, breast, or corpus uteri, or with melanoma. Patients diagnosed with liver, pancreas, esophagus, or lung cancer fared particularly poorly. Compared with patients of all ages, those diagnosed at the age of 65 years or older in a few instances fared better, such as those diagnosed with breast cancer, but more frequently they did less well. Differences were substantial for those diagnosed with cervix uteri, corpus uteri, ovary, or especially brain cancer, Hodgkin's lymphoma, or leukemia. Survival rates were higher among whites than blacks for most cancers. Black males diagnosed with oral, esophageal, or pancreatic cancer experienced survival rates notably lower than that experienced by the other three racial or gender groups; however, blacks with brain or other nervous system cancers or multiple myeloma had better survival experiences than whites.

The stage of disease at diagnosis varied considerably among the various solid tumors (Table 9). More than 70% of the cancers were still localized to the organ of

Table 8 Five-Year Relative Survival Rates (%) by Race, Sex, and Cancer: All Ages, Ages 65+, SEER Program, 1995–2001

| | All ages | | | | Age 65+ | | | |
| | Whites | | Blacks | | Whites | | Blacks | |
	Males	Females	Males	Females	Males	Females	Males	Females
All cancers	66.5	66.3	58.4	53.2	65.0	55.8	61.2	41.9
Oral cavity and pharynx	61.1	63.1	34.3	52.0	54.8	52.0	27.4	40.6
Esophagus	16.1	16.4	8.6	11.6	13.6	14.3	2.6	6.4
Stomach	19.9	23.9	21.5	24.2	18.6	21.8	19.1	20.6
Colon and rectum	65.6	64.4	55.9	54.3	65.1	63.4	50.9	51.1
Liver[a]	7.4	10.6	5.5	4.6	3.7	6.5	6.4	N/A
Pancreas	4.7	4.2	2.9	5.6	2.9	2.8	0.9	3.9
Larynx	69.5	61.9	53.3	45.2	69.0	54.0	47.1	31.7
Lung and bronchus	13.7	17.7	11.6	15.6	12.0	15.1	10.4	12.8
Melanoma of the skin	90.3	93.5	75.7	78.2	91.5	87.5	55.1	N/A
Breast (female)	–	89.5	–	75.9	–	89.9	–	77.2
Cervix uteri	–	74.6	–	66.1	–	51.9	–	60.2
Corpus uteri	–	86.2	–	61.8	–	80.8	–	50.8
Ovary	–	44.4	–	37.7	–	28.4	–	21.4
Prostate	99.9	–	96.7	–	99.8	–	95.8	–
Testis	96.3	–	87.8	–	76.1	–	N/A	–
Urinary bladder[b]	84.3	78.6	69.7	53.9	81.8	75.5	62.5	51.8
Kidney and renal pelvis	64.7	64.5	61.8	65.9	60.4	55.6	59.9	51.1
Brain and other nervous system	32.1	33.5	37.7	37.5	4.9	6.5	5.3	8.0
Thyroid	94.4	97.7	89.2	95.4	83.6	86.9	N/A	76.6
Hodgkin's lymphoma	84.6	87.7	77.8	83.3	55.9	49.4	N/A	N/A
Non-Hodgkin's lymphoma	59.5	63.3	47.6	59.1	51.9	53.7	41.6	46.7
Multiple myeloma	35.8	28.1	36.3	30.5	27.4	22.3	35.0	23.6
Leukemia	49.6	48.4	39.2	36.9	35.7	36.8	30.2	22.8

Note: Invasive cancer only, unless specified otherwise.
[a]Liver and intrahepatic bile duct.
[b]Urinary bladder (invasive and in situ).
N/A: Not available, –: Not applicable.
Source: From Ref. 4.

origin for those arising in the corpus uteri, prostate, testis, or bladder, and for melanomas of the skin. In contrast, almost 70% of patients diagnosed with ovarian cancer, half of those diagnosed with pancreatic cancer, and 40% of those with lung cancer had distant spread of the disease at the time of diagnosis. The stage of disease strongly influenced subsequent survival. Among females diagnosed with cervix uteri cancer, the five-year relative survival rate exceeded 90% if the cancer was still localized, but it was 17% if there was distant spread; the comparable rates for females with breast cancer were 98% versus 26%, and for males with prostate cancer, 100% versus 34%.

Table 9   Stage Distribution and Five-Year Relative Survival Rates (%) by Stage of Cancer (All Races, Ages, Both Sexes) for Localized, Regional, Distant Disease, SEER Program, 1995–2001

	Stage distribution (%)			Five-year relative survival (%)		
	Local	Regional	Distant	Local	Regional	Distant
Oral cavity and pharynx	34	51	10	82.1	51.3	27.6
Esophagus	26	30	28	31.4	13.8	2.7
Stomach	24	32	32	58.0	21.9	3.1
Colon and rectum	39	38	19	90.4	67.9	9.7
Liver[a]	31	26	22	19.0	6.6	3.4
Pancreas	8	26	52	16.4	7.0	1.8
Larynx	48	45	4	83.8	49.9	18.5
Lung and bronchus	16	37	39	49.5	16.2	2.1
Melanoma of the skin	83	11	3	98.3	63.8	16.0
Breast (female)	63	29	6	97.9	81.3	26.1
Cervix uteri	55	32	8	92.4	54.7	16.5
Corpus uteri	72	16	8	96.1	66.3	25.2
Ovary	19	7	68	93.6	68.1	29.1
Prostate[b]	91	91	5	100.0	100.0	33.5
Testis	71	18	10	99.4	96.3	71.7
Urinary bladder[c]	75	19	3	94.2	48.4	6.2
Kidney and renal pelvis	53	20	22	90.6	60.3	9.7
Thyroid	58	35	5	99.5	96.4	60.0

Note: Invasive cancer only, unless otherwise specified.
[a]Liver and intrahepatic bile duct.
[b]Local and regional combined.
[c]Urinary bladder (invasive and in situ).
Source: From Ref. 4.

HEALTH BEHAVIORS AND RISK FACTORS

Changes in screening practices and lifestyle behaviors impact cancer incidence and mortality. For example, the use of screening procedures to detect early lesions is very important. The large declines in incidence and mortality rates for cancer of the cervix uteri were largely due to increasingly widespread use of the Papanicolaou (Pap) smear and pelvic examinations to detect premalignant treatable lesions (28). The proportion of white non-Hispanic women aged 45 to 64 years who had a Pap smear in the last three years rose from 71% in 1987 to 86% in 2000 (Table 10) (29). The percentages also rose among black non-Hispanic and Hispanic women, whose percentages were lower at each point in time. The screening rates were lower among women aged 65 years and older than among younger women, higher among the nonpoor than the poor, and positively associated with education. The rates increased over time in all the groups. In 2000, screening rates were also lower among women who had no contact with a primary care provider in the past year or who were unmarried (30).

In recent years, mammography screening has become more prevalent (Table 11) (29). The proportion of non-Hispanic white women aged 50 to 64 years who had a mammogram within the past two years more than doubled from 34% in 1987 to 81% by 2000. Rates among non-Hispanic black and Hispanic women were

Table 10 Trends in the Use of Pap Smears by Age Group, Racial/Ethnic Group, and Socioeconomic Group: Percent of Women 45 Years of Age and Older Having a Pap Smear in the Last Three Years

	1987	1994	2000
Ages 45–64 years			
Racial/ethnic group			
White, non-Hispanic	71.2	77.6	85.9
Black, non-Hispanic	76.2	81.9	85.7
Hispanic or Latino	57.7	70.2	77.7
Ages 65 years and older			
Racial/ethnic group			
White, non-Hispanic	51.8	58.4	64.3
Black, non-Hispanic	44.8	60.9	67.3
Hispanic or Latino	41.7	44.1	66.9
Poverty status			
Poor	33.2	44.3	53.9
Near poor or nonpoor	55.8	60.8	66.2
Education			
No high school diploma or GED	44.0	48.0	56.7
High school diploma or GED	55.4	61.4	67.0
Some college or more	59.4	66.9	69.8

Abbreviation: GED, general educational development high school equivalency diploma.
Source: From Ref. 29.

somewhat lower but also rose substantially, from 26% and 23% to 78% and 66%, respectively. Utilization rates among women aged 65 years and older generally were lower than for women aged 50 to 64 years, but mammography participation increased rapidly in all groups and exceeded 65% in each of the racial or ethnic groups in 2000. Poverty status as well as education level influenced the mammography utilization rate.

Cigarette smoking is the predominant cause of lung cancer (31,32). It also increases the risk for cancers of the larynx, oral cavity, pharynx, esophagus, kidney, urinary bladder, pancreas, and cervix uteri. The prevalence of cigarette smoking in 1965 exceeded 50% among adult males and 30% among females (Table 12) (29). Since then, the prevalence of smoking has declined to one-quarter among males and one-fifth or less among females. At each point in time, the prevalence was higher among black than white males, with small racial differences among females. Among persons aged 65 years and older, the smoking prevalence was lower than among the corresponding whole age range, 18 years and older. The prevalence declined over time among males, whereas the rates rose among females till they peaked during the mid-1980s. During 2002, the prevalence of cigarette smoking among black males was more than twice that among the other three racial/gender groups aged 65 years and older.

Although specific dietary factors are less well established as influencing cancer risk, high fruit and vegetable consumption appears to be protective for many cancers (33). Energy balance and physical activity are important, as obesity has been associated with several cancers, including those of the colorectum, corpus uteri, and (in postmenopausal women) breast. Since at least the early 1970s, the proportion of the

Table 11 Trends in Mammography Utilization by Age Group, Racial/Ethnic Group, and Socioeconomic Group: Percent of Women 50 Years of Age and Older Having a Mammogram in the Last Two Years

	1987	1990	1994	2000
Ages 50–64 years				
Racial/ethnic group				
White, non-Hispanic	33.6	58.1	67.5	80.5
Black, non-Hispanic	26.4	48.4	63.6	77.7
Hispanic or Latino	23.0	47.5	60.1	66.4
Ages 65 years and older				
Racial/ethnic group				
White, non-Hispanic	24.0	43.8	54.9	68.3
Black, non-Hispanic	14.1	39.7	61.0	65.5
Hispanic or Latino	N/A	41.1	48.0	68.2
Poverty status				
Poor	13.1	30.8	43.9	54.8
Near poor or nonpoor	25.5	46.2	57.7	69.9
Education				
No high school diploma or GED	16.5	33.0	45.6	57.5
High school diploma or GED	25.9	47.5	59.1	72.0
Some college or more	32.3	56.7	64.3	74.1

N/A: Not available.
Abbreviation: GED, general educational development high school equivalency diploma.
Source: From Ref. 29.

population that is overweight and the proportion that is obese have increased dramatically (Table 13) (29). The proportion overweight or obese is higher among black women than the other racial/gender groups; in recent years, 78% of black non-Hispanic women were overweight and 50% were obese. The proportions have been higher among Mexicans than white non-Hispanics. The percent that is

Table 12 Trends in Cigarette Smoking Prevalence (%) in the United States by Sex and Race: Ages 18 Years and Older, 65 Years and Older

	1965	1974	1985	1995	2002
Ages 18 years and older[a]					
White males	50.4	41.7	31.3	26.2	25.0
Black males	58.8	53.6	40.2	29.4	26.7
White females	33.9	32.0	27.9	23.4	21.1
Black females	31.8	35.6	30.9	23.5	18.3
Ages 65 years and older					
White males	27.7	24.3	18.9	14.1	9.3
Black males	36.4	29.7	27.7	28.5	19.4
White females	9.8	12.3	13.3	11.7	8.5
Black females	7.1	8.9	14.5	13.3	9.4

[a]Age-adjusted using the year 2000 U.S. population standard.
Source: From Ref. 29.

Table 13 Trends in Percent of the Population Aged 20 Years and Older Who Are Overweight or Obese, According to Sex, Race, and Age, United States

	Overweight[a]			Obese[a]		
	1976–1980	1988–1994	1999–2002	1976–1980	1988–1994	1999–2002
Ages 20–74 years[b]						
Males						
White, non-Hispanic	53.8	61.6	69.5	12.4	20.7	28.7
Black, non-Hispanic	51.3	58.2	62.0	16.5	21.3	27.9
Mexican	61.6	69.4	74.1	15.7	24.4	29.0
Females[c]						
White, non-Hispanic	38.7	47.2	57.0	15.4	23.3	31.3
Black, non-Hispanic	62.6	68.5	77.5	31.0	39.1	49.6
Mexican	61.7	69.6	71.4	26.6	36.1	38.9
Sex/age group						
Males						
20–34 years	41.2	47.5	57.4	8.9	14.1	21.7
35–44 years	57.2	65.5	70.5	13.5	21.5	28.5
45–54 years	60.2	66.1	75.7	16.7	23.2	30.6
55–64 years	60.2	70.5	75.4	14.1	27.2	35.5
65–74 years	54.2	68.5	76.2	13.2	24.1	31.9
75 years and older	N/A	56.5	67.4	N/A	13.2	18.0
Females[c]						
20–34 years	27.9	37.0	52.8	11.0	18.5	28.4
35–44 years	40.7	49.6	60.6	17.8	25.5	32.1
45–54 years	48.7	60.3	65.1	19.6	32.4	36.9
55–64 years	53.7	66.3	72.2	22.9	33.7	42.1
65–74 years	59.5	60.3	70.9	21.5	26.9	39.3
75 years and older	N/A	52.3	59.9	N/A	19.2	23.6

[a] Overweight: body mass index ≥ 25; Obese: body mass index ≥ 30.
[b] Age-adjusted using the 2000 U.S. population standard.
[c] Excludes pregnant women.
N/A: not available.
Source: From Ref. 29.

overweight tends to increase with age before peaking around the age of 65. In addition, heredity, past reproductive experiences in women, and the cumulative effects of environmental exposures to carcinogenic agents and chemicals in genetically susceptible individuals contribute to the risk of developing cancer.

FUTURE CHANGES IN TRENDS

The burden of cancer in the elderly will progressively increase in the early part of the 21st century due to the large number of cancers that will be diagnosed as the "baby boom" generation becomes the elderly population in the United States. One in five persons in the United States will be aged 65 years or older by the year 2030, two-thirds more than the 2000 level (34). A large segment will be from minority racial and ethnic subgroups. With increased longevity, a greater proportion of these cancers will occur in men.

Reducing the burden of cancer is a challenge. Cumulative effects over time of risk factors, genetic susceptibility, environmental exposures to carcinogens, and less healthy behaviors or practices increase the risk of cancer. However, several factors are likely to have a major effect on reducing the rates of cancer, including the reduction of smoking and increased consumption of fruits and vegetables. Behavioral change interventions to modify lifestyle habits, such as smoking and diet, and improved preventive health practices can impact cancer rates (35). Cancer is a disease of genetic alterations. Technological advancements in genetics research will make possible the identification of individuals at risk of developing cancer and will influence future trends in cancer incidence and mortality. Advancements in chemoprevention herald a new era in the primary prevention of cancer (36).

The paradigm of cancer in the elderly population is changing and will continue to shift over the next few decades. Recent data show that overall cancer mortality rates are decreasing, a most encouraging sign (37). Cancer death rates, overall, which had increased 0.5% per year during the period 1975–1990, have declined by an average of 1.1% per year since 1993. During the 1990s, mortality rates decreased in both the sexes for colon and rectum, urinary bladder, stomach, and brain cancers. The rates among males also declined for lung, prostate, and oral cancers, while rates among females decreased for breast and cervix uteri cancers, as well as for non-Hodgkin's lymphoma. Continued monitoring of the trends in cancer incidence and mortality will be needed to determine changes in the burden of cancer due to differences in cohorts, risk factors, environmental exposures, and lifestyle habits, as well as the effects of genetic screening and early detection in the aging population.

ACKNOWLEDGMENTS

We thank Mr. John Lahey of IMS, Inc., Rockville, MD for computer support and figure development, and Dr. B.J. Stone for editorial assistance.

REFERENCES

1. Jemal A, Murray T, Ward E, et al. Cancer statistics, 2005. CA Cancer J Clin 2005; 55(1):10–30.
2. Surveillance, Epidemiology, and End Results (SEER) Program. SEER∗Stat Database: Incidence – SEER 9 Regs Public-Use, Nov 2004 Sub (1973–2002), National Cancer Institute, DCCPS, Surveillance Research Program, Cancer Statistics Branch, released April 2005, based on the November 2004 submission. Last accessed on May 21, 2005 (www.seer.cancer.gov).
3. Surveillance, Epidemiology, and End Results (SEER) Program. SEER∗Stat Database: Mortality – All COD, Public-Use With State, Total U.S. (1969–2002), National Cancer Institute, DCCPS, Surveillance Research Program, Cancer Statistics Branch, released April 2005 (www.seer.cancer.gov). Underlying data provided by NCHS (www.cdc.gov/nchs).
4. Ries LAG, Eisner MP, Kosary CL, et al. SEER Cancer Statistics Review, 1975–2002. Bethesda, MD: National Cancer Institute, 2005 (seer.cancer.gov/csr/1975_2002/).
5. Ferlay J, Bray F, Pisani P, Parkin DM. GLOBOCAN, 2002: Cancer incidence, Mortality and Prevalence Worldwide. IARC Cancer Base No. 5 Version 2.0. Lyon, France: IARC Press, 2004 (www-dep.iarc.fr).
6. Edwards BK, Howe HL, Ries LA, et al. Annual report to the nation on the status of cancer, 1973–1999 featuring implications of age and aging on U.S. cancer burden. Cancer 2002; 94(10):2766–2792.

7. Hsing AW, Devesa SS. Trends and patterns of prostate cancer: what do they suggest? Epidemiol Rev 2001; 23(1):3–13.
8. Potosky AL, Feuer EJ, Levin DL. Impact of screening on incidence and mortality of prostate cancer in the United States. Epidemiol Rev 2001; 23(1):181–186.
9. Devesa SS, Bray F, Vizcaino AP, Parkin DM. International lung cancer trends by histologic type: male:female differences diminishing and adenocarcinoma rates rising. Int J Cancer 2005; 117:294–299.
10. Devesa SS, Grauman DJ, Blot WJ, Fraumeni JF Jr. Cancer surveillance series: changing geographic patterns of lung cancer mortality in the United States, 1950 through 1994. J Natl Cancer Inst 1999; 91(12):1040–1050.
11. Troisi RJ, Freedman AN, Devesa SS. Incidence of colorectal carcinoma in the U.S.: an update of trends by gender, race, age, subsite, and stage, 1975–1994. Cancer 1999; 85(8): 1670–1676.
12. Brown LM, Devesa SS. Epidemiologic trends in esophageal and gastric cancer in the United States. Surg Oncol Clin N Am 2002; 11(2):235–256.
13. Chow WH, Devesa SS, Warren JL, Fraumeni JF Jr. Rising incidence of renal cell cancer in the United States. JAMA 1999; 281(17):1628–1631.
14. Mathew A, Devesa SS, Fraumeni JF Jr, Chow WH. Global increases in kidney cancer incidence, 1973–1992. Eur J Cancer Prev 2002; 11(2):171–178.
15. Jemal A, Devesa SS, Hartge P, Tucker MA. Recent trends in cutaneous melanoma incidence among whites in the United States. J Natl Cancer Inst 2001; 93(9):678–683.
16. Eltom MA, Jemal A, Mbulaiteye SM, Devesa SS, Biggar RJ. Trends in Kaposi's sarcoma and non-Hodgkin's lymphoma incidence in the United States from 1973 through 1998. J Natl Cancer Inst 2002; 94(16):1204–1210.
17. Groves FD, Linet MS, Travis LB, Devesa SS. Cancer surveillance series: non-Hodgkin's lymphoma incidence by histologic subtype in the United States from 1978 through 1995. J Natl Cancer Inst 2000; 92(15):1240–1251.
18. Canto MT, Devesa SS. Oral cavity and pharynx cancer incidence rates in the United States, 1975–1998. Oral Oncol 2002; 38(6):610–617.
19. Jemal A, Travis WD, Tarone RE, Travis L, Devesa SS. Lung cancer rates convergence in young men and women in the United States: analysis by birth cohort and histologic type. Int J Cancer 2003; 105(1):101–107.
20. Althuis MD, Dozier JM, Anderson WF, Devesa SS, Brinton LA. Global trends in breast cancer incidence and mortality 1973–1997. Int J Epidemiol 2005; 34(2):405–412.
21. Lacey JV Jr, Devesa SS, Brinton LA. Recent trends in breast cancer incidence and mortality. Environ Mol Mutagen 2002; 39(2–3):82–88.
22. Wang SS, Sherman ME, Hildesheim A, Lacey JV Jr, Devesa S. Cervical adenocarcinoma and squamous cell carcinoma incidence trends among white women and black women in the United States for 1976–2000. Cancer 2004; 100(5):1035–1044.
23. Sherman ME, Devesa SS. Analysis of racial differences in incidence, survival, and mortality for malignant tumors of the uterine corpus. Cancer 2003; 98(1):176–186.
24. Mink PJ, Sherman ME, Devesa SS. Incidence patterns of invasive and borderline ovarian tumors among white women and black women in the United States. Results from the SEER Program, 1978–1998. Cancer 2002; 95(11):2380–2389.
25. Surveillance, Epidemiology, and End Results (SEER) Program. SEER*Stat Database: Incidence–SEER 13 Regs excluding AK Public-Use, Nov 2004 Sub for Hispanics (1992–2002), National Cancer Institute, DCCPS, Surveillance, Research Program, Cancer Statistics Branch, released April 2005, based on the November 2004 submission (www.seer.cancer.gov).
26. Surveillance, Epidemiology, and End Results (SEER) Program. SEER*Stat Database: Incidence-SEER 13 Regs Public-Use, Nov 2004 Sub for Expanded Races (1992–2002), National Cancer Institute, DCCPS, Surveillance Research Program, Cancer Statistics Branch, released April 2005, based on the November 2004 submission (www.seer.cancer.gov).

27. Parkin DM, Bray FI, Devesa SS. Cancer burden in the year 2000. The global picture. Eur J Cancer 2001; 37(suppl 8):S4–S66.
28. National Institutes of Health Consensus Development Conference statement on cervical cancer. April 1–3, 1996. Gynecol Oncol 1997; 66(3):351–361.
29. National Center for Health Statistics. Health, United States, 2004, with Chartbook on Trends in the Health of Americans. Hyattsville, MD: National Center for Health Statistics, 2004 (www.cdc.gov/nchs/hus.htm).
30. Hewitt M, Devesa SS, Breen N. Cervical cancer screening among U.S. women: analyses of the 2000 National Health Interview Survey. Prev Med 2004; 39(2):270–278.
31. Thun MJ, Henley SJ, Calle EE. Tobacco use and cancer: an epidemiologic perspective for geneticists. Oncogene 2002; 21(48):7307–7325.
32. Sasco AJ, Secretan MB, Straif K. Tobacco smoking and cancer: a brief review of recent epidemiological evidence. Lung Cancer 2004; 45(suppl 2):S3–S9.
33. McCullough ML, Giovannucci EL. Diet and cancer prevention. Oncogene 2004; 23(38):6349–6364.
34. U.S. Census Bureau. U.S. Interim Projections by Age, Sex, Race, and Hispanic Origin. Internet release date March 18, 2004 (www.census.gov/ipc/www/usinterimproj/).
35. Eyre H, Kahn R, Robertson RM. Preventing cancer, cardiovascular disease, and diabetes: a common agenda for the American Cancer Society, the American Diabetes Association, and the American Heart Association. CA Cancer J Clin 2004; 54(4):190–207.
36. Tsao AS, Kim ES, Hong WK. Chemoprevention of cancer. CA Cancer J Clin 2004; 54(3):150–180.
37. Jemal A, Clegg LX, Ward E, et al. Annual report to the nation on the status of cancer, 1975–2001, with a special feature regarding survival. Cancer 2004; 101(1):3–27.

3

Surgery in the Elderly Oncology Patient

M. Margaret Kemeny and Julio Vaquerano
Mount Sinai School of Medicine, Queens Cancer Center, Jamaica, New York, U.S.A.

INTRODUCTION

It is projected that by the year 2030, the number of cancers will reach 1.5 million in the elderly (1). Surgery remains the best treatment modality to cure solid tumors, regardless of age. Surgery is instrumental for diagnosis, resection with curative intent, or palliation. The incidence of many solid cancers continues to rise with age. Because the population of the United States is not only growing but also aging, the number of elderly patients with cancers requiring surgical intervention can be expected to rise. In fact, the elderly (65 and older) comprise 14% of the U.S. population and account for 63% of the cancer cases in the United States (2).

Life expectancy is often underestimated for the elderly. According to the National Vital Statistics (3), the life expectancy of a girl born in 2002 is 79.9 years and of a boy, 74.5 years. Furthermore, the life expectancy of a healthy 65-year-old person is an additional 20 years and an 85-year-old, has an additional 6.1 years (4). Inadequate initial therapy for someone diagnosed with cancer at an older age can result in recurrence or metastases and death from cancer; outcomes that may have been preventable or avoidable with correct treatment at the outset.

Surgery is the mainstay of treatment of the tumors most common in the elderly: colorectal, breast, gastric, and pancreatic cancers. Other tumors that also require surgical intervention for optimal therapy are melanoma and hepatobiliary tumors. With adequate preoperative evaluation, surgical treatment for the elderly should not be different from that for the younger groups, and therefore, the standard of care should not be based on age alone. Scientific data from randomized studies is not readily available for the older population because of the exclusion of the elderly from most clinical trials in the past. Studies that are available are retrospective and often display considerable bias in the patients chosen for certain treatments, especially surgical procedures.

Many biases influence the selection of therapy in the elderly. Concerns stem from what is perceived as limited life expectancy, the presence of comorbid disease, decreased functional status, alterations in mental status, limitations in economic resources, and assumed inability to tolerate treatment. The influence of these biases may affect survival from cancer in the elderly.

In one study evaluating survival up to 10 years after the diagnosis in patients over 65 years of age with cancers of the colon, rectum, breast, and prostate, variable factors that influenced survival were health status (comorbidity, functional status, level of activity), socioeconomic status (income and education level), cognitive status, and availability of social support (5). The factor of not receiving definitive therapy for the cancer (with the exception of prostate) was associated with a threefold greater death rate. Inadequate treatment remained a significant factor even after controlling for stage at diagnosis, socioeconomic factors, comorbidity, and physical functioning. These factors should be taken into account to optimize therapy outcome, but they should not necessarily be used to withhold appropriate treatment.

Surgical procedures in particular have been viewed as carrying prohibitive risk in many elderly patients in the past. As the population ages, there is an increased interest in the feasibility and outcome of surgical intervention in the elderly. In fact, the number of articles related to "neoplasm+surgery+elderly" in Pubmed has increased since the 1980s (Fig. 1) (6,7). Numerous studies have shown that surgical procedures can be performed safely in the elderly (8–18). The balance between operative risk and expected cure or palliation is important when treating any patient with cancer, but especially the elderly with cancer. The impact of treatment on the quality of life is also of prime importance. Many cancer operations are complex and extensive with significant risks of morbidity and mortality. In this chapter, we review the current knowledge on risk assessment, breast cancer, gastrointestinal cancers, melanoma, and laparoscopic surgery as they pertain to the elderly population.

RISK ASSESSMENT

Preoperative risk assessment in the elderly continues to evolve with new methods currently under study (6). Studies of operative risk in the elderly are often retrospective and fail to include adequate matched younger controls for comparison. The assessment of risk involves the interaction between the underlying physiological

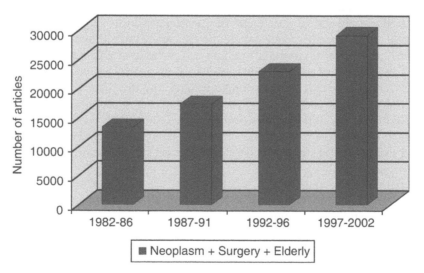

Figure 1 Increase in the number of articles in Pubmed related to "neoplasm+surgery+ elderly." *Source*: From Ref. 7.

status, including normal physiological changes of aging, in addition to physiological changes attributable to comorbidity, and the disease process, the surgical procedure itself, and the anesthesia. Age should not be used as the sole criterion to assess risk or to make therapeutic decisions. Normal physiological changes occur with aging in every major organ system and affect the response to surgical procedures (19). Changes in the physiology of aging are discussed in detail elsewhere in this text.

Operative risk can be assessed in a number of ways. One of the most common scales, used even today, to grade operative risk from anesthesia is the American Society of Anesthesiologists (ASA) General Classification of Physical Status (20). This scale assesses the medical condition of the patient prior to anesthesia and surgery. The physical status of the patient is defined according to five groups.

More accurate measures of specific organ system risk have also been developed. Cardiac events remain a primary cause of perioperative morbidity and mortality. A commonly reported statistic is that patients who have had a myocardial infarction (MI) within three months of surgery have a 30% risk of recurrent MI or cardiac death (21). The risk decreases to 15% after three to six months and to a constant 5% thereafter. Attempts have been made to define cardiac risk more precisely. Nine factors were found to predict independently cardiac complications by multivariate analysis in patients undergoing noncardiac surgery (22). A discriminant-function coefficient was assigned to each factor and a point value derived (Table 1). Four risk categories were defined, based on each patient's point total. The categories correlated well with the risk for cardiac death (Table 2). An age of over 70 does contribute to an increased risk of cardiac complications.

These risk categories were not designed to be exclusionary, but to increase the awareness for potential complications and ensure full preoperative evaluation and attempts to provide interventions to decrease the risk from surgery.

A new method to evaluate the functional life of the oncogeriatric patient and individually predict the risk of cancer surgery is PACE (preoperative assessment of cancer in the elderly). PACE incorporates various tools (Table 3) to predict the outcome of cancer surgery in the elderly. In a pilot study, it has been shown to be feasible, inexpensive, and rarely refused by patients (6). Furthermore, two components that

Table 1 Goldman Criteria for Predicting Postoperative Cardiac Complications

Criteria	Point value
1. S3 gallop or jugular vein distention on preoperative examination	11
2. MI in the preceding six months	10
3. Rhythm other than sinus or premature atrial contractions on preoperative electrocardiogram	7
4. >5 premature ventricular contractions/min documented at any time before operation	7
5. Age > 70 years	5
6. Emergency operation	4
7. Important valvular aortic stenosis	3
8. Intraperitoneal, intrathoracic, or aortic operation	3
9. Poor general medical condition[a]	3

[a]Poa < 60 or pCO_2 > 50 mmHg; K < 3.0 or Cr > 3.0 mg/dL; abnormal SCOT; or patient bedridden from noncardiac causes.
Abbreviations: MI, myocardial infarction; SCOT, signs of chronic liver disease.

Table 2 Goldman Risk Categories for Predicting Postoperative Cardiac Complications

Class	Point total	No or only minor complication (%)	Life-threatening complication (%)	Cardiac death (%)
I	0–5	99	0.7	0.2
II	6–12	93	5	2
III	13–25	86	11	2
IV	≥26	22	22	56

have been significantly associated with increased 30-day morbidity are low performance status (PS) and low performance of activities of daily living (6).

Invasive monitoring to evaluate and optimize hemodynamic function has been advocated in elderly patients prior to major surgery. In one study, 34 of 148 patients (23%) over the age of 65 were found to have an unacceptable risk due to severe cardiopulmonary defects on invasive hemodynamic evaluation, which did not improve with treatment (23). All of the eight patients (of the 34 high-risk patients) who went on to have the originally planned surgery died. However, invasive monitoring is not without risks. A Pulmonary Artery Consensus Conference concluded that routine perioperative pulmonary artery catheter monitoring is not appropriate based on age alone, and further research is needed to define the proper role in geriatric patients (24).

Measures of physiological risk have also been used to predict operative risk in an attempt to take into account multisystem influences aside from just cardiac factors. The Acute Physiology and Chronic Health Evaluation (APACHE) II score originally developed and used for assessing risk in patients in the intensive care unit has been applied for assessing risk in the preoperative setting. Age is included as one of the 12 variables used in the APACHE II score. High preoperative APACHE II scores have been associated with an increase in the morbidity and mortality for patients undergoing major hepatic surgery, pancreatic surgery, and gastric resections (25,26).

Others have attempted to more specifically evaluate the risk of major surgery in the elderly. In one review by Reiss of over 1000 major abdominal operations performed on patients over the age of 70, nearly half were performed for malignant conditions (17). The overall mortality rate was 14%, and five variables were found to

Table 3 Validated Instruments Used with PACE

Mini Mental State Examination
Satariano's Modified Index of Comorbidities
Activities of Daily Living
Instrumental Activities of Daily Living
Geriatric Depression Scale
Brief Fatigue Inventory
Eastern Cooperative Oncology Group Performance Status
American Society of Anesthesiologists Physical Status
POSSUM
Portsmouth POSSUM Modification (see Appendix)

Abbreviations: PACE, preoperative assessment of cancer in the elderly; POSSUM, Physiological and Operative Severity Score for Enumeration of Mortality and Morbidity.

be predictive of increased mortality: (i) patient's age, (ii) modified ASA class, (iii) elective versus emergency surgery, (iv) operation for benign, malignant, operable, or malignant inoperable disease, and (v) major diagnostic group (Table 4). If a patient had two or more features associated with a poor prognosis, the mortality rate was over 50%.

Another series of 795 patients over the age of 90 were evaluated for outcomes of surgery at the Mayo Clinic (27). The 30-day operative mortality was 8.4%. ASA class and emergency surgery correlated well with postoperative morbidity and mortality within 48 hours. Gastrointestinal surgery was associated with an increase in the case fatality within 48 hours. Preoperative renal and biliary dysfunction was associated with increased early postoperative morbidity. However, the overall five-year survival rate was comparable to the rate expected for matched peers.

To minimize the surgical risks in the elderly, careful preoperative assessment of the physiological status and the state of coexisting diseases can be used to guide therapeutic interventions. Optimization of abnormal results prior to, during, or in the postoperative recovery period, would decrease morbidity. Anticipating problems may help recognize certain events before they become irreversible. Morbidity and mortality risks are known to be increased when operating on patients with advanced disease states; moreover, emergency surgery is clearly associated with an increased risk of morbidity and mortality (16,17,27). It has often been reported that there is a delay in diagnosis in elderly patients with malignancies leading to more advanced cancers and emergency presentations. The standard guidelines for the early diagnosis of cancer and treatment should be followed in the elderly. Implementation of these guidelines should decrease late presentation and operative complications.

Table 4 Variables Associated with Increased Risk for Major Abdominal Operations

Risk factor	Mortality rate (%)
ASA I	7.4
III	32.7
Age	
70–74	8.4
75–79	18.9
$\geq$80	23.3
Type of surgery	
Elective	9.7
Emergency	19.7
Condition	
Benign	9.1
Operable malignancy	13.4
Inoperable malignancy	31.4
Diagnosis	
Biliary	2.1
Appendicitis	2.9
Peptic	9.7
Malignant colorectal	12.3
Benign obstruction	22.9
Malignant stomach/esophageal	23.1
Malignant pancreatic	28.1

Abbreviation: ASA, American Society of Anesthesiologists.

BREAST CANCER

The incidence of breast cancer rises with age. Nearly one-third of breast cancers occur in women over the age of 70 (28). One half the deaths are in women over 65 years of age (29). Yet, many studies have demonstrated that breast self-examination, clinical examination by health care providers, and screening mammography are underutilized in the elderly (30–32). Breast cancer biology and screening are discussed elsewhere in this volume.

One of the greatest areas of controversy is whether breast cancer in the elderly should be managed any differently from that in younger women. The fear of treatment morbidity and mortality sometimes prompts a minimalistic approach in the elderly, whereas, at other times, mastectomy is offered with little consideration of the possible desire for breast preservation or reconstruction. The role of axillary dissection, radiation therapy, or adjuvant therapy is also not completely clear.

Randomized trials in both the United States and Europe have shown breast-conserving therapy (BCT) to be equivalent to mastectomy in terms of survival from early-stage breast cancer (33–36). The National Institutes of Health consensus conference also found it to be the preferable method of treating early-stage disease (37). More recently, the 20-year follow-up of the randomized study evaluating breast-conservative surgery confirmed earlier findings of no decrease in disease-free or overall survival with breast-conserving surgery (38). However, BCT is still underutilized for all ages and particularly in the elderly.

The majority of cancers in the elderly are still treated with modified radical mastectomy and very rarely is breast reconstruction performed (39,40). When breast conservation is performed, it is often done without axillary dissection or the use of postoperative radiation, as would be the standard for younger women (39,40). In one retrospective series, the survival of elderly women was found to be lower for those treated with less than standard procedures, although it was not clear what selection criteria were used for determining choice of procedure (40). A lower survival was not demonstrated in a randomized series when lumpectomy alone was performed, although differences in local control rates were clear (41).

There are many factors that influence the use of BCT, including geographical location, race, and hospital characteristics. In one analysis of Medicare patients, geographical variations were marked in the use of BCT (42). In another review of over 18,000 Caucasian women in three age groups—younger than 65, 65 to 74, and older than 74 years—the lowest rate of breast-conserving surgery was in the 65- to 74-year age group (43). In areas of the country where BCT was common in the younger age group, it was less common in the older age group, whereas in areas where it was not commonly used in the younger group, it was more commonly used in the older group. It was postulated that disfiguring surgery was avoided in the younger group, whereas morbidity and mortality were avoided in the older group. But the morbidity and mortality for breast surgery in the elderly are very low (39). The elderly have also been found to have a lower rate of BCT in the treatment of ductal carcinoma in situ (34).

Axillary dissections are primarily done for staging and, secondarily, for local control. The value of preventing distant disease is more controversial, and the procedure does carry risks. But axillary dissections are often omitted in elderly patients with clinically negative axillas (44). Even when node dissections are performed, the number of nodes removed in the elderly is less (45). The morbidity associated with axillary nodal dissection may have played a role in offering this staging technique in the elderly. With the advent of sentinel lymph node (SLN) biopsy, this fear of morbidity should be eliminated. SLN biopsy has been shown to be a safe procedure, with accuracies of 97% in randomized studies (46,47). Furthermore, the safety and feasibility have also been evaluated in the elderly (7). In a series of 241 patients 70 years or older, the SLN was identified in all, with no major complications (7). In this series the SLN was positive for metastasis in 37% of the patients. Using the SLN technique obviates further axillary dissection in SLN-negative patients and therefore decreases the bias of adequate staging in the elderly.

The risk of local recurrence in the axilla is another consideration. In the National Surgical Adjuvant Breast and Bowel Project B-04 trial, 18% of women with clinically negative axillae went on to develop delayed axillary recurrence (48). Delaying the dissection potentially subjects the elderly to an increase in the risk for surgical complications when they are even older and possibly in a more debilitated state. Two randomized trials looked specifically at node dissection in the elderly. In a series of 321 patients with clinically negative axillae and aged over 70 years treated with surgery and tamoxifen without node dissection, the axillary recurrence rate was only 4.3% (49). In a smaller series with node negative axillae, the regional nodal control rate was 82.5% at 103 months after treating the axilla with radiation only (50). The results of the prospective randomized trial (IBCSG-10–93) conducted in Europe will address the role of axillary dissection on disease-free survival, axillary recurrence, and morbidity in the elderly.

Radiation therapy to the breast after breast-conserving surgery for invasive cancer is considered the standard of care. Yet radiation is omitted in many elderly patients after breast-conserving surgery. In one series, even in areas where BCT was used frequently, only 41% of women over the age of 75 had radiation, in contrast to 90% of women younger than 65 years and 86% of women between the ages of 65 and 74 (43). In another report, when surgical therapy was more aggressive and included axillary dissection in the elderly, the use of radiation was also more frequent (39). Concerns have been expressed about whether the elderly will tolerate radiation and whether they will have difficulty completing therapy because of physical restraints in getting to radiation facilities, and whether long-term outcomes are the same as in younger patients. However, studies have provided evidence to refute these concerns (51,52).

Disturbingly, local recurrence rates for breast cancer have been reported to be as high as 35% in the elderly when radiation is not given (53). However, several recent trials have suggested that the risk for local recurrence may, in fact, not be as high in the elderly as in younger patients (54,55). One hypothesis is that tamoxifen, frequently used in this age group, may be protective against local recurrence of breast cancer. A randomized study from the Cancer and Leukemia Group B compared women over the age of 70 with early breast cancer who received lumpectomy plus tamoxifen or lumpectomy followed by tamoxifen plus radiation therapy. All 647 randomized patients were over 70 years with estrogen receptor (ER)-positive tumors less than 2 cm. The group given radiation had a significantly longer time to local or regional recurrence (breast plus axilla) ($P < 0.001$). The time to distant metastases did not differ between the two treatment groups. The five-year disease-free survivals and overall survivals were not significantly different. The conclusions were that radiation therapy improved local control but did not impact on overall survival (56).

For the elderly with breast cancer who have other coexisting medical problems which preclude any form of surgical therapy, and who have a limited life expectancy, it is not unreasonable to treat such patients with tamoxifen alone. Two prospective randomized trials compared tamoxifen alone to surgery alone and found good initial response rates for tamoxifen, although local control rates were worse with tamoxifen than with surgery (53,57).

In an attempt to better define why older women receive less than definitive therapy for breast cancer, one study looked at the extent to which patients' age, marital status, health status, tumor characteristics, and aspects of physician–patient interaction influenced the treatment received (58). The following factors, along with the percentage of patients citing them, were reported as being very important in their choice for therapy: minimizing possibility of recurrence, 100%; physician's recommendation, 96%; quality of life after treatment, 77%; their family's opinion, 52%; what they would have to pay over and above insurance, 28%; and problems they would experience after surgery, 22% (59). The following were found not to be important in the choice: effect of treatment on sexuality, 83%; difficulty getting to and from treatments, 65%; and effects of treatment on appearance, 63%. Patient age, marital status, and the number of times the breast cancer specialist discussed treatment options were independently and significantly associated with the receipt of definitive primary tumor therapy. Older women who were not married and women with whom treatment options were discussed less frequently were less likely to receive definitive primary tumor therapy. The conclusion of the investigators (58) was that older women might be better served if they are offered choices from among definitive therapies, because there is some clinical uncertainty about what is the most appropriate therapy.

Breast cancer treatment in the elderly should not be different from that in younger groups. Breast-conserving surgery has been shown to be safe and effective in treating breast cancer. Sentinel node biopsy may eliminate the need of axillary node dissection in a number of elderly patients. Pharmacotherapy is improving in reducing side effects (aromatase inhibitors) and still decreasing the rates of breast cancer in patients at risk. All these modalities decrease morbidity and are applicable to the elderly.

COLORECTAL CANCER

Colorectal cancer ranks third in the incidence of all cancers in both men and women. Over 104,950 cases of colon cancer and 40,340 cases of rectal cancer are predicted for 2005 (60). According to the National Cancer Data Base in 2001, 58.4% of colon cancer and 44.6% of rectal cancer occurred in individuals over the age of 70 (61).

Symptoms at presentation are reported to be similar in elderly compared to younger patients (62). Although some workers report the location of colon cancers to be similar in elderly and younger patients (63), others report a higher incidence of right-sided lesions and a lower incidence of rectal lesions in elderly patients (62,64,65). In one of these series, more of the elderly presented with anemia, whereas, in the other, the incidence of anemia was the same as in younger patients despite the higher incidence of right-sided lesions (62,64).

The elderly may present with a more advanced stage of colorectal disease, especially those over 80 years of age, and with less differentiated tumors, although it is difficult to document a time delay in diagnosis based on the duration of symptoms (62). Resectability rates are reported to be lower in patients over 80 years of age (62).

Surgical resection of the colon or rectum remains the mainstay of curative therapy for colorectal cancer. It is required in many cases, even in the presence of disseminated disease, to avoid or treat the inevitable complications of obstruction and bleeding. A number of retrospective series have been studied concerning the influence of advanced age on the risk of surgical resection of colorectal cancer.

The risk of perioperative complications is generally reported to be higher in the elderly than in younger patients. Cardiopulmonary complications were increased in one series from 1.8% in patients under the age of 65% to 10.8% in patients 65 to 75 years old, and 8.2% in patients over the age of 75 (12). Anastomotic leak rates were also increased from 4.2% in patients less than 65 years of age to 8.2% in those over 75 years of age (12). Mortality rates are also reported to be higher; however, most series show that age is not an independent factor in predicting mortality (12,66). The cause of death in older patients is systemic complications (mainly cardiopulmonary) in nearly two-thirds of patients, whereas, in the majority of younger patients, postoperative death is caused by anastomotic leakage and other local complications (12). Actual mortality rates for colorectal surgery in the elderly range from 4% to 21% for elective cases to up to 54% for emergency cases (Table 5). Emergency operations are clearly associated with an increased mortality rate.

Mortality rates are high for palliative operations, such as creation of a colostomy (11,67). This procedure is often done as an emergency procedure in an end-stage patient; both factors (colostomy and an emergency procedure) are known to contribute to an increased mortality risk (11,67). Although some workers report the stage at presentation and incidence of performing palliative surgery is the same in the elderly as in younger patients, others report that a greater proportion of the elderly require emergency surgery or present as an emergency (63,64,68). Furthermore, patients presenting as emergencies also tend to have more advanced-stage disease (68). With the increase in mortality associated with emergency operation and advanced-disease stage, it seems advisable to intervene earlier on an elective basis to avoid such problems as bleeding, perforation, and obstruction, and also to avoid colostomy.

The question of whether surgery is indicated in the setting of advanced disease in the elderly is often raised. One small retrospective study found no difference in morbidity or mortality between 43 elderly patients undergoing surgery for advanced

Table 5 Morbidity and Mortality Rates for Elderly Patients Undergoing Colorectal Surgery

Reference	Year	Age	No. of patients	Diagnosis	Total operative mortality (%)	Elective operative mortality (%)	Emergency operative mortality (%)
(66)	1980	>70	141	70% cancer	8.5		
(11)	1985	>70	163	63% cancer	10.4	10.4	23.3
(68)	1986	>70	242	All cancer			38
			197			18	
(63)	1988	>70	171	All cancer	6		
			140			4	
			31				16
(14)	1989	>80	115	All cancer	20		
			93			18	
			22				27
(12)	1991	>75	98	All cancer	8.2	8.2	
		65–75	139		5.8	5.8	
(70)	1991	>80	163	All cancer	15.3	7.4	53.5
(71)	1992	>70	53	All cancer	7.5		
(64)	1994	>70	219	All cancer	6	4	15
(67)	1996	>80	103	All cancer		4.7	41
(72)	2004	>80	180	All cancer	8.9	6.6	15

disease (obstruction, perforation, hemorrhage, or metastases) compared to 39 patients with localized disease (69). Although surgery can be safely performed, one must also consider other factors, such as impact on the quality of life.

Laparoscopic colon resections are now being safely performed for benign and malignant colon diseases. The advantages described from preliminary experience indicate laparoscopic colon resection may lead to a decrease in postoperative pain and ileus (73). A recent multi-institutional prospective randomized trial comparing lapararoscopic-assisted colectomy versus open colectomy for resectable colon cancer has been reported (74). In this trial, 872 patients were randomized, with 428 patients in the open colectomy forming the basis for the final analysis and 435 patients in the laparoscopy group. The patient characteristics were comparable with the mean age of 70 years in the laparoscopy cohort. The majority of the patients had early colon cancer (68% in the open and 71% in the laparoscopic cohort). Significant differences were noted in the size of incision, duration of analgesics required, and shorter length of stay, favoring the laparoscopic colectomy group. However, the duration of surgery was significantly longer for the laparoscopic group, with a median time of 150 minutes, as compared to 95 minutes in the open colectomy group. After a median follow-up of 4.4 years, there was no significant difference in recurrence rates or survival (74). Other studies have showed that minimally invasive colectomy can be performed successfully in the elderly. In one prospective study, 81 laparoscopic colectomies were completed successfully out of 103 patients aged 65 years and older (75). The mean hospital stay was 5.3 days and a complication rate of 25% was reported. Two of the 81 patients died within 30 days of surgery. In another small series of elderly patients with disseminated or metastatic disease and ASA classes III and IV, laparoscopic colon resection was performed with minor morbidities and no mortality (76). Thirty-five recurrences were reported over a two-year period in one review of the literature (77).

Another potential option for palliative treatment and control of obstruction or hemorrhage in patients with advanced rectal cancer is the use of local intraluminal therapies, such as electrofulguration, laser therapy, or cryotherapy (75). Laser therapy is effective for palliation in 85% to 95% of patients, and procedure-related morbidity and mortality rates are low (75).

The patient's quality of life, although more difficult to measure, is an important outcome for any planned treatment. Creating a stoma must be viewed with caution, because it may be difficult for some elderly patients to manage, not only physically but also psychologically. One series examined what patients over 80 years of age did after leaving the hospital following surgery for gastrointestinal tumor (14): 31% went home, 51% convalesced in a specialized home or medical recovery center, 10% went to a nursing home or specialized institution, and 4% required nursing assistance at home or went to a family home. Overall, 83% returned to their homes without any change in their social environment.

Survival after curative resection for colon carcinoma has been reported to be lower for patients over the age of 70 (78). However, in one series, multivariate analysis demonstrated that the three-year survival was influenced by disease stage and type of operation performed (resection vs. palliation), but not age (older than 80 years vs. younger than 80 years) (79). Hospital stay was longer for those over 80 years, and the cost higher (22% increased cost). Another series indicated, using multivariate analysis, that although the physical status and operative mortality were worse in the elderly undergoing surgery for colorectal cancer, for those elderly patients who were fit for surgery, who underwent curative resection, and who survived over 30 days, the five-year survival was as good as that for younger patients (65).

Colorectal Liver Metastases

Liver resection remains the optimal treatment for localized colorectal liver metastasis. Liver resection can lead to a 21% to 48% five-year survival in selected patients (80–85). The safety of performing liver resections has greatly improved in recent years, owing to improvements in techniques of resection and intraoperative and postoperative care. Liver resections are now being performed with mortality rates of less than 5% (80–83,86).

Liver resections can also be performed safely in elderly patients. A number of series have looked at morbidity and mortality rates for older individuals. One reported on 90 patients ranging from 65 to 82 years of age who underwent liver resection (87). The overall mortality rate was 11%, but it was unacceptably high in patients undergoing right trisegmentectomies (30.7%). However, in a series of 61 patients older than 70 years, the morbidity and mortality rates were 41% and 0%, respectively, for first time resections. The mortality increased for repeat liver resections to 7% (88). In this study, 41% of the first time liver resections and 50% of the repeat liver resections were major resections involving three or more segments.

Another report in 1995 reviewed liver resections for colorectal metastases in 128 patients over 70 years of age (8). For patients over 70 years of age, the perioperative mortality rate was lower than in the earlier report at 4%, which was the same as for patients younger than 70 years. Morbidity rates were 42% and 40%, respectively, for patients younger than 70 years and those older than 70 years. Most of the complications in the elderly were cardiopulmonary. In multivariate analysis, three factors were found to be important in predicting complications. These were male sex (2.6×), resection of at least one lobe of the liver (2.4×), and an operating time of greater than 240 minutes (2.3×). Median hospital stay for patients aged 70 years and older was only one day longer than for patients less than 70 years of age. Morbidity, mortality, and intensive care unit admission rates were not statistically different from younger patients.

Long-term survival following liver resection for colorectal metastases is not clearly influenced by age. No statistically significant difference in survival was found between patients older or younger than 60 years in one report (89). In another report, the median survival time was 40 months and the overall five-year survival rate was 35% for patients 70 years and older, and 44 months and 39% for patients younger than 70 years, which was not significantly different (8). In another report, no significant difference was seen in the five-year survival of patients under 70 years of age and those over 70 years at 39% and 36%, respectively ($P = 0.9$) (10). In a large registry series, age greater than 70 years was of borderline significance ($P < 0.05$) in predicting survival, but even these patients had a five-year survival of 18%, compared to an expected 0% for patients not undergoing resection (80).

Although it is not clear what selection criteria are used to choose elderly patients for the major operation of hepatic resection, it is possible to perform the procedure in the elderly with the anticipation that they will survive the surgery and have the same chance of survival from the cancer as do younger individuals.

HEPATOCELLULAR CANCER

Liver and intrahepatic bile duct cancer accounted for 17,550 cases in the United States of America in 2005 (60). Although less common in the American population than in the Asian population, hepatic resection provides the only hope for curing

Table 6 Hepatic Resection for Hepatocellular Cancer in the Elderly

Reference	No. of patients	Age	Hepatic failure[a]	Operative mortality[a]	Five-year survival (%)
(90)	39	> 70	4 (10)	5	51.6
(15)	32	> 70	2 (6.3)	4 (12.5)	17.6
(91)	27	≥65		11 (40.7)	
(92)	37	> 65	1 (2.7)	2 (5)	18.1
(93)	103	> 70		5 (4.9)	51

[a]Numbers in parentheses are percentages.

patients of hepatocellular cancer. The extensive experience with resection of colorectal liver metastases demonstrates that liver resections can be performed safely in the elderly. However, many of the patients with hepatocellular cancer have underlying cirrhosis as an etiological factor, unlike those with metastatic colorectal cancer, making surgical resection more challenging and dangerous. The functional reserve problem encountered with liver resection in the elderly for colorectal metastases, where the liver is otherwise normal, is compounded by the presence of cirrhosis. Several small series have examined the outcome of hepatic resection for hepatocelluar cancer in the elderly (Table 6).

The morbidity and mortality associated with resection for hepatocellular carcinoma in the elderly were comparable to that for younger patients (90,92–94), with the exception of one series (91). In one study of 103 patients 70 years or older with hepatocellular carcinoma, the resectability rate was 84% in the elderly, compared to 88% in the younger group (93). The morbidity and mortality were comparable between the elderly and younger patients: 28.2% versus 23.3%, and 9.7% versus 6.0%, respectively. The presence and severity of cirrhosis as judged by Child's criteria (see Appendix) does seem to influence the rate of operative mortality, and it is advised that patients with advanced cirrhosis be regarded carefully prior to consideration for major hepatic resection (15,93,94). The overall five-year survival has also been reported to be comparable with the younger group, ranging from 24.3% to 51.6% (93).

PANCREATIC CANCER

The incidence of pancreatic cancer rises with age and over two-thirds of patients are over the age of 65 at diagnosis (95–97). The overall survival of all patients with pancreatic cancer is dismal, with five-year survivals of 4% to 5% (96,98). This is attributed in part to the unfortunate fact that the majority of patients with pancreatic cancer are diagnosed late in the course of the disease when surgical resection is no longer feasible. Due to the late presentation, only 9% to 15% are amenable to surgical resection (96,97). This percentage of resectable patients is even lower for those over the age of 70. Although surgical resection is the only potential method of cure, the results remain disappointing. For patients who are able to undergo resection, the mean survival is still only 10.6 to 24.6 months (99). The Whipple operation, or pancreaticoduodenectomy, is the operation of choice for the most common lesions, which are located in the head of the pancreas, as well as for periampullary, duodenal, and distal common bile duct neoplasms. In the past, it was associated with an extremely high complication rate and with a mortality rate as high as 26%. When weighed against the relatively small survival impact seen with successful surgery, many viewed the procedure as an unreasonable option for treatment (100,101). The role of this operation in elderly patients was fraught with even more concern. However, in more recent years, the morbidity and mortality rates associated with the Whipple operation have decreased significantly at specialty centers (102–104). Mortality rates of between 0% and 5% are more commonly reported (102,103,105). In selected elderly patients, mortality rates for surgery are acceptable and even comparable to the younger group (8,106–108).

One review of 138 patients aged over 70 years who underwent pancreatic resection for malignancy reported an operative mortality rate of 6% and morbidity rate of over 40% (8). Univariate analysis revealed that a history of cardiopulmonary disease, an abnormal preoperative electrocardiogram, and an abnormal chest radiograph were predictors of complications. In multivariate analysis, the only factor found to be a significant predictor of complications was a blood loss of more than 2 L. No significant differences were found in length of hospital stay, rate of intensive care unit admission, and morbidity or mortality rates between patients younger than 70 years and those older than 70 years. Median survival was 18 months, and a five-year survival rate of 21% was observed.

In a Veteran's Administration (VA) series of 77 patients between the ages of 70 and 79 with pancreatic cancer, the mortality rate was 14%, and for six patients over the age of 80, no mortalities were observed (108). Several other smaller series of pancreatic resections have also reported mortality rates in patients over 70 years to be 5% to 10%, with morbidity rates of 14% to 48% (109–111). In another small series of selected patients without cardiac, respiratory, or hepatic failure, no difference in morbidity was seen in patients over 70 years undergoing pancreaticoduodenectomy from those less than 70 years (13).

One series from Johns Hopkins reported on 190 consecutive pancreaticoduodenectomies without a single mortality (112). The majority of cases were performed for malignancies. Previously, the Hopkins group had reported on 37 patients in a series who were over the age of 70 (102). No significant differences were found between the length of stay and rate of complications in patients over 70 years compared to younger patients. However, the patients were admittedly carefully selected prior to the operation, as evidenced by no differences in the preoperative medical risk factors between patients under and over the age of 70.

The major causes of morbidity after pancreatic resection are related to complications associated with pancreatic fistula, anastomotic breakdown, and sepsis (13,104,105,112). Other studies have indicated that the routine use of octreotide may help reduce the risk of postoperative morbidity related to pancreatic fistula, pancreatitis, abscess, and sepsis (113,114).

However, survival rates for resection remain limited (103,105). Five-year survival rates are not different in the elderly. One series reported a five-year survival rate for pancreatic cancer of 17% in patients over the age of 70 and 19% in patients less than 70 years of age (107). Periampullary tumor survival rates were better at 38% and 45%, respectively. Another series reported a five-year survival rate for pancreatic cancer of 19% in patients over the age of 80 and 27% in patients less than 80 years of age (P value not significant) (115). Despite limited long-term survival, resection remains superior to bypass or laparotomy alone. In a review of over 3000 patients from the 1970s, a mean survival of 12.7 months for resection, 5.7 months for bypass, and 2.6 months for laparotomy alone were reported (99). In the same review of over 2000 patients from the 1980s, mean survival increased significantly in resected patients to 17 months, whereas bypass (6.6 months) and laparotomy alone (3.1 months) were no different than in the earlier series.

Because the survival rate for resectable disease is still poor, adjuvant chemoradiation therapy has been given. An improvement in survival has been demonstrated in small series (116–118). More recently, preoperative chemoradiation therapy has been used in an attempt to increase resectability rates and survival in patients with pancreatic cancer (119). Preliminary results reveal preoperative therapy is safe and well tolerated (119). No specific information on how the elderly tolerate such treatment is available.

Yet, the majority of patients with pancreatic cancer are unable to undergo resection. Surgery is needed in nearly 50% of patients for palliation of the two common complications that occur in the natural course of the disease, biliary and gastric obstruction (99). Pain often also requires palliation. The mean survival of patients after bypass is considerably lower than after resection at 4.0 to 11.3 months (99). The elderly may not tolerate bypass procedures as well as younger patients do. A VA study did indicate a higher 30-day morbidity and mortality rate and a lower median survival rate after bypass procedures, which was statistically significant for patients over 70 years (104). However, VA patients may have unique characteristics that put them at higher risk. Each patient must be judged on an individual basis, taking into consideration the overall status of the patient and expected benefit.

The operative mortality rate for biliary bypass ranges from 4% to 33% (mean 19%) and survival from 1.5 to 12 months (mean 5.4 months) (120). However, biliary obstruction can be as effectively managed with stents placed endoscopically, percutaneously, or transhepatically, as shown in several randomized series (121–124). Mortality, rates are lower for stent placement than for surgical bypass, and hospital stays are shorter. Although early complication rates are lower, long-term complication rates, such as recurrent jaundice and cholangitis, are more common than with surgical bypass.

Gastric outlet obstruction, although far less common as a presenting symptom, still requires operative bypass for relief. Survival after bypass is often limited and therefore the overall value is questionable (125).

In patients explored for pancreatic resection, 25% to 75% were found to have unresectable disease (102,115,126). In these patients, a decision must be made about whether to perform prophylactic bypass procedures. In the presence of biliary obstruction, an operative biliary bypass may not be needed if a stent is already in place. Some would argue that biliary bypass via choledochoduodenostomy or jejunostomy can often be accomplished with minimal morbidity and avoids future requirements for stent changes and potential infections and episodes of sepsis associated with the presence of stents.

There continues to be controversy regarding the routine performance of prophylactic gastrojejunostomy at the time of exploration. The argument for doing the procedure is that 13% to 17% of patients will go on to develop gastric outlet obstruction in the future (99,120). It is estimated that another 10% to 20% of patients die with duodenal obstruction without undergoing bypass, which might have been prevented if bypass had been done initially. Doing the bypass adds no morbidity to the procedure (99,120). But for a second operation to bypass the patient, a mortality rate of 22% and a mean survival of only three months have been reported (99). In a recent randomized study from the Netherlands comparing single with double bypass, investigators found that the absolute risk reduction for reoperation in the double bypass group was 18%. Gastric outlet obstruction developed in 5.5% of doubled bypass (consisting of gastrojejunostomy and hepatojejunostomy) patients and in 41.4% of singled bypass (consisting of hepatojejunostomy) patients. Furthermore, there was no difference in morbidity, delayed gastric emptying, postoperative length of stay, median survival, and quality of life. In this series, the authors concluded that prophylactic gastrojejunostomy and hepaticojejunostomy is preferable to a single hepaticojejunostomy (126).

In another prospective randomized trial in patients with unresectable periampullary carcinoma, prophylactic gastrojejunostomy was compared to no bypass. In this series, 19% of the nonbypassed patients developed gastric outlet obstruction, while none of the bypassed (gastrojejunostomy) patients developed gastric outlet obstruction (115). No significant difference was noted in terms of morbidity, postoperative length of stay, or survival. Palliative operations for patients with unresectable pancreatic cancer carried a mortality rate of 3.3%, although the morbidity rate was 37% (102). Out of 118 patients in that series, 41 were over 70 years. These were selected patients who were felt to be able to tolerate a Whipple resection, and who were generally in a better overall condition than those patients who were known to have unresectable or advanced disease and who subsequently develop indications for palliative bypass. The decision for a bypass procedure requires careful clinical judgment. If duodenal impingement is obvious at surgery, a bypass should be done. It must be kept in mind that if gastrojejunostomy is done later when the patient is more debilitated, the risk of complications and mortality increases.

The fact that the majority of patients never go on to develop gastric outlet problems, and that some patients will develop clinical gastric outlet obstruction or delayed gastric emptying despite having had a bypass, argues against the performance of routine gastrojejunostomy (99). Recently, the introduction of laparoscopic techniques has provided a new method of performing the bypass with potentially lower morbidity and mortality in debilitated patients.

GASTRIC CANCER

Gastric cancer death rates have been declining over the past 70 years in the United States (from > 40/100,000 in the 1930s to < 10/100,000 in 2000) (60). Nearly 50% of males and 60% of females diagnosed with gastric cancer in the United States are over the age of 70 (40). Surgery is the only curative modality currently available for gastric cancer and, in noncurative situations also, surgery is needed to palliate patients with gastric bleeding and obstruction.

The Japanese and Chinese have looked at the characteristics of gastric cancer in the elderly. Symptoms at presentation and location of disease in the stomach are similar in younger and older patients (127,128). One series reports no difference in histological type, whereas another reports a higher incidence of intestinal-type histology in the elderly (127–129). The macroscopic pattern, according to the Borrmann criteria, appears to be more localized in the elderly, but the occurrence of synchronous multiple primaries is greater and ranges from 7.7% to 13.2% (127,128,130). The incidence of vascular and lymphatic invasion has been reported to be higher in the elderly, whereas there is no difference in the incidence of lymph node metastases and stage at diagnosis (127,128).

Curative surgery for gastric cancer requires either subtotal or total gastrectomy: surgery that is associated with significant operative morbidity and mortality. The exact extent of surgery remains a controversial subject with regard to not only the extent of gastric resection but also the extent of lymphadenectomy required.

Removal of perigastric nodes is termed a Dl resection, whereas removal of more extensive regional lymph nodes outside the perigastric region is termed a D2 resection. It is not clear whether more extensive resections impact on recurrence or survival. It is clear, however, that complication rates are higher after total gastrectomies and after D2 regional node dissections (131,132). In a large prospective randomized trial from the Netherlands, the rate of surgical complications was doubled after D2 resections (131). The rates of nonsurgical complications (with the exception of that of pulmonary complications, which was also doubled in the D2 group) such as cardiac, urinary tract, and thromboembolic were similar.

The morbidity and mortality rates after gastric resections in the elderly appear to be increased compared to those in younger patients (Table 7). Although preoperative risk factors are increased in the elderly with gastric cancer, particularly with factors of a cardiac and pulmonary nature, the majority of complications and deaths are caused by infections, anastomotic leaks, and pulmonary problems as in younger patients (9,131–133). One small series reported no difference in major surgical complications between older and younger patients, but there was a statistically significant increase in overall septic complications and respiratory infections in older patients (133). The occurrence of multiorgan impairment and malnutrition was statistically related to the incidence of postoperative complications, but it was the degree of organ impairment rather than age that was predictive of postoperative complications.

An important factor in deciding about surgical treatment in the elderly is the impact on the quality of life. One series from Japan assessed the quality of life after gastrectomy for gastric cancer in patients aged over 70 years compared to those younger than 70 years (136). No significant difference was found in the amount of food intake or weight change after surgery in the elderly compared to that in younger patients. However, a significant decrease in PS was found. Although PS declined after surgery in both groups, it improved as time passed after the operation in the younger patients. In the older patients, the initial decline in PS after surgery remained relatively constant and did not improve with time. PS was 0 in 79% of elderly patients preoperatively. Postoperatively, only 56% of patients had a PS of 0 at the time of the questionnaire (0 = patient can go out and do full-scale work; 1 = patient's ability is reduced but can look after himself or herself; 2 = patient is in bed more than 50% of daytime and requires others' help in home life; 3 = patient

Table 7 Gastric Resections in the Elderly

Reference (year)	Country	Age	No. of patients	Morbidity (%)	Mortality (%)
(129) (2000)	Taiwan	≥65	433	21.7	5.1
(134) (1997)[a]	USA-MSKCC[b]	> 70	310	47.1	7.1
(135) (1996)	Japan	70–79	341	22	5.3
		≥80[c]	43	23	5
(131) (1995)	Netherlands	> 70	231		
		D1	128	30	7
		D2	103	45	18
(132) (1988)	Norway	≥80	106	34	15

[a]85% > D1 resection.
[b]Memorial Sloan Kettering Cancer Center.
[c]Only limited surgical procedures were performed in this age group.

Table 8 Gastric Cancer Survival After Curative Resection

Reference	No. of patients	Age	Five-year survival (%) cumulative	Age corrected	10-year survival (%)
(135)	480	50–59	66.3[a]	68.9[b]	59[c]
	578	60–69	58.3	63.2	46
	341	70–79	48.6	62.1	27.4
	432	≥80	28	53	4
(127)	232	< 70	49.4[c]		33.6
		> 70	48.6		23.2
(9)	57	< 70	14.5		
	24	≥70	19.4		
(129)	433	≥65	60		

[a]Cumulative survival rates significantly different between age groups.
[b]Age-corrected survival not significantly different between age groups.
[c]Survival not significantly different between age groups.

patient is totally bedridden and always requires others' help). However, most patients were still able to look after themselves. The "health rate" and employment rate were lower after surgery for the elderly, but over half of those who did not return to work felt it was not necessary for them to return rather than it being not possible for physical reasons. The overall conclusion was that the elderly should not be excluded from surgery based on quality of life concerns. In another smaller series of patients over the age of 70 undergoing total gastrectomy, 70% of patients returned to "normal life" after one year, although regaining of body weight was slower than in younger patients (137).

The five-year survival for curatively resected patients with gastric cancer is similar for younger and older patients (Table 8).

MELANOMA

The overall incidence of melanoma in the United States is increasing. In 2005, there were 59,580 new cases of cutaneous melanoma and an estimated 7770 deaths (60). The cumulative lifetime risk of developing melanoma in the United States in 1980 was 1/250 and in 2002 it was 1/68 (138). The percentage of cases occurring in the older population also appears to be increasing. In 1985, 21.2% of cases occurred in patients over 70 years of age (139), and in 1990 this number increased to 27.2% of cases.

The characteristics of melanoma appear to be slightly different in the elderly. Although the extremities are the most common location for melanomas in females, head and neck melanomas become more frequent with advancing age (140,141). In men, truncal melanomas are most common, but again head and neck melanomas become more frequent and surpass truncal melanomas after the age of 70 (140,141). Older patients have also been reported to have thicker melanomas with deeper levels of invasion and an increase in the incidence of ulceration (60,142,143). It is not clear whether this may reflect a delay in the diagnosis or presentation of these lesions in the elderly population.

There is no evidence to suggest that the treatment for the elderly should be any different than that for younger individuals. The treatment is surgical excision. The surgical options include the width of the margins of resection around the primary lesion and the need for regional lymph node dissection.

Randomized trials have shown that the margins of resection are determined by the thickness of the primary melanoma. For lesions less than 1 mm thick, a 1 cm margin is adequate (144,145). For lesions 1 to 4 mm thick, a margin of 2 cm is advised based on the results of the Intergroup Melanoma Surgery Trial (139,146). Age was not used as a criterion for exclusion in this study.

Although age has not been used as a criterion for determining the margins of resection, one large retrospective series did report age to be a significant independent factor in the risk for local recurrence (147). Patients over 60 years of age were found to have a local recurrence rate of 7.8%, patients between the ages of 30 and 59 had a local recurrence rate of 2.5%, and patients less than 30 years of age had a local recurrence rate of 1.2% at a median follow-up of eight years. Other independently significant risk factors for recurrence included tumor thickness, ulceration, and sex. Although an analysis was not performed for potential factors affecting this high recurrence rate, it might be explained by the higher incidence of head and neck melanomas in the elderly with its attendant higher rate of local recurrence. This also raises a concern about adequacy of margins in elderly patients with melanoma. In the prospective randomized trial evaluating margins, no difference was found in the rate of local recurrence for age over 50 versus age less than 50 (146). However, a higher rate of local recurrence was demonstrated for head and neck lesions.

The dissection of regional lymph nodes for melanoma treatment is routine for patients with clinically positive nodes; however, the value of elective node dissection (ELND) for patients with clinically negative lymph nodes has long been debated because regional node dissections have significant long-term complications. The Intergroup Melanoma Surgical Trial for patients with lesions 1 to 4 mm thick showed no significant difference in the 10-year survival for ELND versus nodal observation (77% vs. 73%; $P = 0.12$) (148) 175. The use of SLN biopsy techniques, introduced by Morton in 1992 (149), has made the discussion of ELND moot. Patients now routinely get SLN biopsies for any lesion greater than 1 mm in thickness.

SLN biopsies can be done using one of two techniques or using both. The original technique used a blue dye injected intradermally at the site of the primary melanoma. The regional node basin was explored surgically for the identification of "blue node(s)" and it was removed. These were termed the SLNs. If these nodes were positive for tumor, a full node dissection would be performed. If negative, then no dissection was done. Initial experience with this technique showed the blue dye method was able to identify the SLN in 82% of patients (149). The false-negative rate of the technique in identifying the presence of metastatic disease was 1% (149). Because of technical difficulties with the blue dye, radiolymphoscintigraphy using technetium-labeled sulfur colloid has been utilized to locate the sentinel node (150). Utilizing both techniques, the sentinel node can be harvested 98% of the time (151). Now the dye and the radiolabeling are used conjointly. The sentinel node not only decreases morbidity, but also accurately determines the state of the regional basin. Furthermore, the interim results (after a median of 54 months follow-up) of the Multicenter Selective Lymphadenectomy Trial (MSLT-I) in stage I melanoma showed a 78% five-year disease-free survival with SLN biopsy versus a 73% in the observation group ($P = 0.01$) (152). The MSLT-1 results also showed that the status of the sentinel node is the most important prognostic factor in this cohort of patients. Adjuvant therapy is discussed elsewhere in this text.

LAPAROSCOPY

Laparoscopy is increasingly being used for resection of malignant disease. In the gastrointestinal tract, colon resections for cancer have been shown to be safe and feasible. The benefits of laparoscopy over conventional surgical techniques shown for nononcological surgical procedures include the limited incisions with an attendant decrease in postoperative pain and a decreased hospital stay and recuperation period. Data from the laparoscopic colon resections in the elderly indicate that rates of conversion and complications are not significantly higher than in younger patients (153–155).

While adapting new techniques to the surgical armamentarium, oncological principles must be maintained. The principles of oncologic surgery must be adhered to so as not to compromise the chance for cure. Bowel handling, tumor manipulation, anastomosis formation, attention to margins, and lymph node clearance must be performed with the same delicacy as open procedures.

Concerns exist regarding trocar site recurrences after laparoscopic resection of cancer. Thirty-five port site recurrences after laparoscopic colectomy were reported in one literature review (77). In the same review, 23 recurrences were reported after thoracoscopic resection of pulmonary malignancies and another 31 cases of port site recurrence were reported after other laparoscopic procedures, including procedures for ovarian cancer and unsuspected gallbladder cancer. However, trocar recurrence in recent reports ranges from 0% to 1.3%, which compares with open rates of 0.6% to 0.68% (156).

For some cancers in which there is a high rate of unresectability, such as hepatobiliary, pancreatic, and gastric cancers, diagnostic laparoscopy may avoid unnecessary laparotomy (157,158). Laparoscopic splenectomy has also been used in hematological malignancies (159).

Randomized studies of colon cancer have shown the applicability and feasibility of laparoscopy in colon cancer. Recurrences and overall survival have been reported to be similar (74). Laparoscopy remains a viable option for elderly patients at high risk of developing postoperative complications.

CONCLUSIONS

Surgical intervention in the elderly should no longer be a question. Appropriate evaluation of the existing morbidities and optimization are essential to successful surgical outcomes. Multiple studies have shown the safety and benefit of performing oncologic surgeries in the elderly. As our population ages, more elderly patients will present with cancer, which will require surgical intervention. The data support that the elderly do as well in terms of morbidity and mortality as their younger counterparts. As more institutions evaluate their experience with the elderly, surgical intervention will become the norm, not an alternative.

APPENDIX

Child's Criteria

| | Child's group | | |
	A (minimal)	B (moderate)	C (advanced)
Serum bilirubin (mg%)	< 2.0	2.0–3.0	> 3.0
Serum albumin (g%)	> 3.5	3.0–3.5	< 3.5
Ascites	Absent	Easily controlled	Poorly controlled
Neurologic disorder	None	Minimal	Advanced coma
Nutrition	Excellent	Good	Poor, wasting

Source: From Ref. 147.

Portsmouth POSSUM

This method is utilized to normalize patient data to make direct comparisons of patient outcomes.

POSSUM parameters

Physiological parameters
Age
Cardiac history
Respiratory history
Blood pressure
Pulse rate
Glasgow Coma Score
Hemoglobin level
White cell count
Urea concentration
Sodium level
Potassium level
Electrocardiogram

Operative parameters
Operative severity
Multiple procedures
Total blood loss
Peritoneal soiling
Presence of malignancy

The predictor equation for mortality is: $\ln(R/(1-R)) = -9.065 + (0.1692 \times \text{physiological score}) + (0.1550 \times \text{operative severity score})$. R is the predicted risk of mortality. *Source*: From Ref. 160.

REFERENCES

1. Polednak AP. Projected numbers of cancers diagnosed in the US elderly population, 1990 through 2030. Am J Public Health 1994; 84(8):1313–1316.
2. Kimmick GG, Peterson BL, Kornblith AB, et al. Improving accrual of older persons to cancer treatment trials: a randomized trial comparing an educational intervention with standard information: CALGB 360001. J Clin Oncol 2005; 23(10):2201–2207.
3. Arias E. United States life tables, 2001. Natl Vital Stat Rep 2004; 52(14):1–38.
4. Extermann ML, Balducci, Lyman GH. What threshold for adjuvant therapy in older breast cancer patients? J Clin Oncol 2000; 18(8):1709–1717.
5. Goodwin JS, Samet JM, Hunt WC. Determinants of survival in older cancer patients. J Natl Cancer Inst 1996; 88(15):1031–1038.

6. Audisio RA, Ramesh H, Longo WE, Zbar AP, Pope D. Preoperative assessment of surgical risk in oncogeriatric patients. Oncologist 2005; 10(4):262–268.

7. Audisio RA, Bozzetti F, Gennari R, et al. The surgical management of elderly cancer patients: recommendations of the SIOG surgical task force. Eur J Cancer 2004; 40(7):926–938.

8. Fong Y, Blumgart LH, Fortner JG, Brennan MF. Pancreatic or liver resection for malignancy is safe and effective for the elderly. Ann Surg 1995; 222(4):426–434; discussion 434–437.

9. Bittner R, Schirrow H, Butters M. Total gastrectomy. A 15-year experience with particular reference to the patient over 70 years of age. Arch Surg 1985; 120(10): 1120–1125.

10. Fong Y, Cohen AM, Fortner JG, et al. Liver resection for colorectal metastases. J Clin Oncol 1997; 15(3): 938–946.

11. Greenburg AG, Saik RP, Pridham D. Influence of age on mortality of colon surgery. Am J Surg 1985; 150(1):65–70.

12. Hesterberg R, et al. Risk of elective surgery of colorectal carcinoma in the elderly. Dig Surg 1991; 8:22–27.

13. Kojima Y, Yasukawa H, Katayama K, Note M, Shimada H, Nakagawara G. Postoperative complications and survival after pancreatoduodenectomy in patients aged over 70 years. Surg Today 1992; 22(5):401–404.

14. Morel P, Egeli RA, Wachtl S, Rohner A. Results of operative treatment of gastrointestinal tract tumors in patients over 80 years of age. Arch Surg 1989, 124(6):662–664.

15. Nagasue N, Chang YC, Takemoto Y, Taniura H, Kohno H, Nakamura T. Liver resection in the aged (seventy years or older) with hepatocellular carcinoma. Surgery 1993; 113(2):148–154.

16. Palmberg S, Hirsjarvi E. Mortality in geriatric surgery. With special reference to the type of surgery, anaesthesia, complicating diseases, and prophylaxis of thrombosis. Gerontology 1979; 25(2):103–112.

17. Reiss R, Deutsch AA, Nudelman I. Abdominal surgery in elderly patients: statistical analysis of clinical factors prognostic of mortality in 1,000 cases. Mt Sinai J Med 1987; 54(2):135–140.

18. Lawrence VA, Hazuda HP, Cornell JE, et al. Functional independence after major abdominal surgery in the elderly. J Am Coll Surg 2004; 199(5):762–772.

19. Evers BM, Townsend CM Jr, Thompson JC. Organ physiology of aging. Surg Clin North Am 1994; 74(1):23–39.

20. Dripps RD, Lamont A, Eckenhoff JE. The role of anesthesia in surgical mortality. JAMA 1961; 178:261–266.

21. Goldman L. Cardiac risks and complications of noncardiac surgery. Ann Intern Med 1983; 98(4):504–513.

22. Goldman L, Caldera DL, Nussbaum SR, et al. Multifactorial index of cardiac risk in noncardiac surgical procedures. N Engl J Med 1977; 297(16):845–850.

23. Del Guercio LR, Cohn JD. Monitoring operative risk in the elderly. JAMA 1980; 243(13):1350–1355.

24. Pulmonary Artery Catheter Consensus conference: consensus statement. Crit Care Med 1997; 25(6):910–925.

25. Gagner M. Value of preoperative physiologic assessment in outcome of patients undergoing major surgical procedures. Surg Clin North Am 1991; 71(6):1141–1150.

26. Gagner M, Franco D, Vons C, Smadja C, Rossi RL, Braasch JW. Analysis of morbidity and mortality rates in right hepatectomy with the preoperative APACHE II score. Surgery 1991; 110(3):487–492.

27. Hosking MP, Warner MA, Lobdell CM, Offord KP, Melton LJ III. Outcomes of surgery in patients 90 years of age and older. JAMA 1989; 261(13):1909–1915.

28. Osteen RT, Karnell LH. The National Cancer Data Base report on breast cancer. Cancer 1994; 73(7):1994–2000.

29. Yancik R, Ries LA. Cancer in older persons. Magnitude of the problem—how do we apply what we know? Cancer 1994; 74(7 suppl):1995–2003.

30. Weinberger M, Saunders AF, Samsa GP, et al. Breast cancer screening in older women: practices and barriers reported by primary care physicians. J Am Geriatr Soc 1991; 39(1):22–29.

31. Vincent AL, Bradham D, Hoercherl S, McTague D. Survey of clinical breast examinations and use of screening mammography in Florida. South Med J 1995; 88(7): 731–736.

32. Leathar DS, Roberts MM. Older women's attitudes towards breast disease, self examination, and screening facilities: implications for communication. Br Med J (Clin Res Ed) 1985; 290(6469):668–670.

33. Winchester DP, Menck HR, Osteen RT, Kraybill W. Treatment trends for ductal carcinoma in situ of the breast. Ann Surg Oncol 1995; 2(3):207–213.

34. Ernster VL, Barclay J, Kerlikowske K, Grady D, Henderson C. Incidence of and treatment for ductal carcinoma in situ of the breast. JAMA 1996; 275(12):913–918.

35. Singletary SE, Shallenberger R, Guinee VF. Breast cancer in the elderly. Ann Surg 1993; 218(5):667–671.

36. Pujol P, Hilsenbeck SG, Chamness GC, Elledge RM. Rising levels of estrogen receptor in breast cancer over 2 decades. Cancer 1994; 74(5):1601–1606.

37. NIH consensus conference. Treatment of early-stage breast cancer. JAMA 1991; 265(3):391–395.

38. Fisher B, Anderson S, Bryant J, et al. Twenty-year follow-up of a randomized trial comparing total mastectomy, lumpectomy, and lumpectomy plus irradiation for the treatment of invasive breast cancer. N Engl J Med 2002; 347(16):1233–1241.

39. Busch E, Kemeny M, Fremgen A, Osteen RT, Winchester DP, Clive RE. Patterns of breast cancer care in the elderly. Cancer 1996; 78(1):101–111.

40. Wanebo HJ, Cole B, Chung M, et al. Is surgical management compromised in elderly patients with breast cancer? Ann Surg 1997; 225(5):579–586; discussion 586–589.

41. Fisher B, et al. Reanalysis and results after 12 years of follow-up in a randomized clinical trial comparing total mastectomy with lumpectomy with or without irradiation in the treatment of breast cancer. N Engl J Med 1995; 333(22):1456–1461.

42. Nattinger AB, et al. Geographic variation in the use of breast-conserving treatment for breast cancer. N Engl J Med 1992; 326(17):1102–1107.

43. Farrow DC, Hunt WC, Samet JM. Geographic variation in the treatment of localized breast cancer. N Engl J Med 1992; 326(17):1097–1101.

44. Davis SJ, et al. Characteristics of breast cancer in women over 80 years of age. Am J Surg 1985; 150(6):655–658.

45. Chu J, et al. The effect of age on the care of women with breast cancer in community hospitals. J Gerontol 1987; 42(2):185–190.

46. Gennari R, et al. Sentinel node biopsy in elderly breast cancer patients. Surg Oncol 2004; 13(4):193–196.

47. Krag D, et al. The sentinel node in breast cancer—a multicenter validation study. N Engl J Med 1998; 339(14):941–946.

48. Fisher B, et al. Ten-year results of a randomized clinical trial comparing radical mastectomy and total mastectomy with or without radiation. N Engl J Med 1985; 312(11):674–681.

49. Martelli G, et al. Long-term follow-up of elderly patients with operable breast cancer treated with surgery without axillary dissection plus adjuvant tamoxifen. Br J Cancer 1995; 72(5):1251–1255.

50. Wazer DE, et al. Breast conservation in elderly women for clinically negative axillary lymph nodes without axillary dissection. Cancer 1994; 74(3):878–883.

51. Swanson RS, Sawicka J, Wood WC. Treatment of carcinoma of the breast in the older geriatric patient. Surg Gynecol Obstet 1991; 173(6):465–469.

52. Peschel RE, et al. The effect of advanced age on the efficacy of radiation therapy for early breast cancer, local prostate cancer and grade III-IV gliomas. Int J Radiat Oncol Biol Phys 1993; 26(3):539–544.
53. Robertson JF, et al. Mastectomy or tamoxifen as initial therapy for operable breast cancer in elderly patients: 5-year follow-up. Eur J Cancer 1992; 28A(4–5):908–910.
54. Veronesi U, et al. Radiotherapy after breast-preserving surgery in women with localized cancer of the breast. N Engl J Med 1993; 328(22):1587–1591.
55. Liljegren G, et al. Sector resection with or without postoperative radiotherapy for stage I breast cancer: five-year results of a randomized trial. Uppsala-Orebro Breast Cancer Study Group. J Natl Cancer Inst 1994; 86(9):717–722.
56. Hughes KS, et al. Lumpectomy plus tamoxifen with or without irradiation in women 70 years of age or older with early breast cancer. N Engl J Med 2004; 351(10):971–977.
57. Bates T, et al. Breast cancer in elderly women: a Cancer Research Campaign trial comparing treatment with tamoxifen and optimal surgery with tamoxifen alone. The Elderly Breast Cancer Working Party. Br J Surg 1991; 78(5):591–594.
58. Silliman RA, et al. The impact of age, marital status, and physician-patient interactions on the care of older women with breast carcinoma. Cancer 1997; 80(7):1326–1334.
59. Landis SH, et al. Cancer statistics, 1999. CA Cancer J Clin 1999; 49(1): 8–31:1.
60. Jemal A, et al. Cancer statistics, 2005. CA Cancer J Clin 2005; 55(1):10–30.
61. Patterns of Diagnosis and treatment for selected cancers Diagnosed 1997–2001. NCDB 2001.
62. Kemppainen M, et al. Characteristics of colorectal cancer in elderly patients. Gerontology 1993; 39(4):222–227.
63. Irvin TT. Prognosis of colorectal cancer in the elderly. Br J Surg 1988; 75(5):419–421.
64. Mulcahy HE, et al. Prognosis of elderly patients with large bowel cancer. Br J Surg 1994; 81(5):736–738.
65. Kingston RD, et al. The outcome of surgery for colorectal cancer in the elderly: a 12-year review from the Trafford Database. Eur J Surg Oncol 1995; 21(5):514–516.
66. Boyd JB, Bradford B Jr, Watne AL. Operative risk factors of colon resection in the elderly. Ann Surg 1980; 192(6):743–746.
67. Spivak H, et al. Colorectal surgery in octogenarians. J Am Coll Surg 1996; 183(1):46–50.
68. Waldron RP, et al. Emergency presentation and mortality from colorectal cancer in the elderly. Br J Surg 1986; 73(3):214–216.
69. Fitzgerald SD, et al. Advanced colorectal neoplasia in the high-risk elderly patient: is surgical resection justified? Dis Colon Rectum 1993; 36(2):161–166.
70. Amaud JP, et al. Colorectal cancer in patients over 80 years of age. Dis Colon Rectum 1991; 34(10):896–898.
71. Vivi AA, et al. Surgical treatment of colon and rectum adenocarcinoma in elderly patients. J Surg Oncol 1992; 51(3):203–206.
72. Clark AJ, et al. Assessment of outcomes after colorectal cancer resection in the elderly as a rationale for screening and early detection. Br J Surg 2004; 91(10):1345–1351.
73. Huscher C, et al. Laparoscopic colorectal resection. A multicenter Italian study. Surg Endosc 1996; 10(9):875–879.
74. A comparison of laparoscopically assisted and open colectomy for colon cancer. N Engl J Med 2004; 350(20):2050–2059.
75. Dohmoto M, Hunerbein M, Schlag PM. Palliative endoscopic therapy of rectal carcinoma. Eur J Cancer 1996; 32A(1):25–29.
76. Vara-Thorbeck C, et al. Indications and advantages of laparoscopy-assisted colon resection for carcinoma in elderly patients. Surg Laparosc Endosc 1994; 4(2):110–118.
77. Johnstone PA, et al. Port site recurrences after laparoscopic and thoracoscopic procedures in malignancy. J Clin Oncol 1996; 14(6):1950–1956.
78. Gardner B, et al. The influence of age upon the survival of adult patients with carcinoma of the colon. Surg Gynecol Obstet 1981; 153(3):366–368.

79. Hobler KE. Colon surgery for cancer in the very elderly. Cost and 3-year survival. Ann Surg 1986; 203(2):129–131.
80. Hughes KS, et al. Resection of the liver for colorectal carcinoma metastases: a multi-institutional study of indications for resection. Surgery 1988; 103:278–288.
81. Nordlinger B, et al. Surgical resection of colorectal carcinoma metastases to the liver. A prognostic scoring system to improve case selection, based on 1568 patients. Association Francaise de Chirurgie. Cancer 1996; 77(7):1254–1262.
82. Rosen CB, et al. Perioperative blood transfusion and determinants of survival after liver resection for metastatic colorectal carcinoma. Ann Surg 1992; 216(4):493–504; discussion 504–505.
83. Sugihara K, et al. Pattern of recurrence after hepatic resection for colorectal metastases. Br J Surg 1993; 80(8):1032–1035.
84. Scheele J, et al. Indicators of prognosis after hepatic resection for colorectal secondaries. Surgery 1991; 110(1):13–29.
85. van Ooijen B, et al. Hepatic resections for colorectal metastases in The Netherlands. A multi-institutional 10-year study. Cancer 1992; 70(1):28–34.
86. Dimick JB, et al. National trends in the use and outcomes of hepatic resection. J Am Coll Surg 2004; 199(1):31–38.
87. Fortner JG, Lincer RM. Hepatic resection in the elderly. Ann Surg 1990; 211(2): 141–145.
88. Zacharias T, et al. First and repeat resection of colorectal liver metastases in elderly patients. Ann Surg 2004; 240(5):858–865.
89. Scheele J, et al. Resection of colorectal liver metastases. World J Surg 1995; 19(1): 59–71.
90. Takenaka K, et al. Liver resection for hepatocellular carcinoma in the elderly. Arch Surg 1994; 129(8):846–850.
91. Yanaga K, et al. Hepatic resection for hepatocellular carcinoma in elderly patients. Am J Surg 1988; 155(2):238–241.
92. Ezaki T, Yukaya H, Ogawa Y. Evaluation of hepatic resection for hepatocellular carcinoma in the elderly. Br J Surg 1987; 74(6):471–473.
93. Hanazaki K, et al. Hepatic resection for hepatocellular carcinoma in the elderly. J Am Coll Surg 2001; 192(1):38–46.
94. Dohmen K, et al. Optimal treatment strategy for elderly patients with hepatocellular carcinoma. J Gastroenterol Hepatol 2004; 19(8):859–865.
95. al-Sharaf K, Andren-Sandberg A, Ihse I. Subtotal pancreatectomy for cancer can be safe in the elderly. Eur J Surg 1999; 165(3):230–235.
96. Niederhuber JE, Brennan MF, Menck HR. The National Cancer Data Base report on pancreatic cancer. Cancer 1995; 76(9):1671–1677.
97. Shore S, et al. Cancer in the elderly: pancreatic cancer. Surg Oncol 2004; 13(4):201–210.
98. Parker SL, et al. Cancer statistics, 1997. CA Cancer J Clin 1997; 47(1):5–27.
99. Watanapa P, Williamson RC. Surgical palliation for pancreatic cancer: developments during the past two decades. Br J Surg 1992; 79(1):8–20.
100. Connolly MM, et al. Survival in 1001 patients with carcinoma of the pancreas. Ann Surg 1987; 206(3):366–373.
101. Edis AJ, Kiernan PD, Taylor WF. Attempted curative resection of ductal carcinoma of the pancreas: review of Mayo Clinic experience, 1951–1975. Mayo Clin Proc 1980; 55(9):531–536.
102. Cameron JL, et al. One hundred and forty-five consecutive pancreaticoduodenectomies without mortality. Ann Surg 1993; 217(5):430–435; discussion 435–438.
103. Michelassi F, et al. Experience with 647 consecutive tumors of the duodenum, ampulla, head of the pancreas, and distal common bile duct. Ann Surg 1989; 210(4):544–554; discussion 554–556.
104. Wade TP, et al. Complications and outcomes in the treatment of pancreatic adenocarcinoma in the United States veteran. J Am Coll Surg 1994; 179(1):38–48.

105. Trede M, Schwall G, Saeger HD. Survival after pancreatoduodenectomy. 118 consecutive resections without an operative mortality. Ann Surg 1990; 211(4):447–458.

106. Lightner AM, et al. Pancreatic resection in the elderly. J Am Coll Surg 2004; 198(5):697–706.

107. Hannoun L, et al. A report of forty-four instances of pancreaticoduodenal resection in patients more than seventy years of age. Surg Gynecol Obstet 1993; 177(6):556–560.

108. Wade TP, et al. The Whipple resection for cancer in U.S. Department of Veterans Affairs Hospitals. Ann Surg 1995; 221(3):241–248.

109. Delcore R, Thomas JH, Hermreck AS. Pancreaticoduodenectomy for malignant pancreatic and periampullary neoplasms in elderly patients. Am J Surg 1991; 162(6): 532–535; discussion 535–536.

110. Kairaluoma MI, Kiviniemi H, Stahlberg M. Pancreatic resection for carcinoma of the pancreas and the periampullary region in patients over 70 years of age. Br J Surg 1987; 74(2):116–118.

111. Spencer MP, Sarr MG, Nagorney DM. Radical pancreatectomy for pancreatic cancer in the elderly. Is it safe and justified? Ann Surg 1990; 212(2):140–143.

112. Yeo CJ, et al. Six hundred fifty consecutive pancreaticoduodenectomies in the 1990s: pathology, complications, and outcomes. Ann Surg 1997; 226(3):248–257; discussion 257–260.

113. Buchler M, et al. Role of octreotide in the prevention of postoperative complications following pancreatic resection. Am J Surg 1992; 163(1):125–130; discussion 130–131.

114. Bassi C, et al. Prophylaxis of complications after pancreatic surgery: results of a multicenter trial in Italy. Italian Study Group. Digestion 1994; 55(suppl 1):41–47.

115. Lillemoe KD, et al. Is prophylactic gastrojejunostomy indicated for unresectable periampullary cancer? A prospective randomized trial. Ann Surg 1999; 230(3):322–328; discussion 328–330.

116. Further evidence of effective adjuvant combined radiation and chemotherapy following curative resection of pancreatic cancer. Gastrointestinal Tumor Study Group. Cancer 1987; 59(12):2006–2010.

117. Kalser MH, Ellenberg SS. Pancreatic cancer. Adjuvant combined radiation and chemotherapy following curative resection. Arch Surg 1985; 120(8):899–903.

118. Whittington R, et al. Adjuvant therapy of resected adenocarcinoma of the pancreas. Int J Radiat Oncol Biol Phys 1991; 21(5):1137–1143.

119. Hoffman JP, et al. A pilot study of preoperative chemoradiation for patients with localized adenocarcinoma of the pancreas. Am J Surg 1995; 169(1):71–77; discussion 77–78.

120. Sarr MG, Cameron JL. Surgical management of unresectable carcinoma of the pancreas. Surgery 1982; 91(2):123–133.

121. Dowsett JF, et al. Endoscopic biliary therapy using the combined percutaneous and endoscopic technique. Gastroenterology 1989; 96(4):1180–1186.

122. Bornman PC, et al. Prospective controlled trial of transhepatic biliary endoprosthesis versus bypass surgery for incurable carcinoma of head of pancreas. Lancet 1986; 1(8472):69–71.

123. Andersen JR, et al. Randomised trial of endoscopic endoprosthesis versus operative bypass in malignant obstructive jaundice. Gut 1989; 30(8):1132–1135.

124. Shepherd HA, et al. Endoscopic biliary endoprosthesis in the palliation of malignant obstruction of the distal common bile duct: a randomized trial. Br J Surg 1988; 75(12):1166–1168.

125. Weaver DW, et al. Gastrojejunostomy: is it helpful for patients with pancreatic cancer? Surgery 1987; 102(4):608–613.

126. Van Heek NT, et al. The need for a prophylactic gastrojejunostomy for unresectable periampullary cancer: a prospective randomized multicenter trial with special focus on assessment of quality of life. Ann Surg 2003; 238(6):894–902; discussion 902–905.

127. Bandoh T, Isoyama T, Toyoshima H. Total gastrectomy for gastric cancer in the elderly. Surgery 1991; 109(2):136–142.

128. Kitamura K, et al. Clinicopathological characteristics of gastric cancer in the elderly. Br J Cancer 1996; 73(6):798–802.
129. Wu CW, et al. Surgical mortality, survival, and quality of life after resection for gastric cancer in the elderly. World J Surg 2000; 24(4):465–472.
130. Maehara Y, et al. Age-related characteristics of gastric carcinoma in young and elderly patients. Cancer 1996; 77(9):1774–1780.
131. Bonenkamp JJ, et al. Randomised comparison of morbidity after D1 and D2 dissection for gastric cancer in 996 Dutch patients. Lancet 1995; 345(8952):745–748.
132. Viste A, et al. Postoperative complications and mortality after surgery for gastric cancer. Ann Surg 1988; 207(1):7–13.
133. Pacelli F, et al. Risk factors in relation to postoperative complications and mortality after total gastrectomy in aged patients. Am Surg 1991; 57(6):341–345.
134. Schwarz RE, Karpeh MS, Brennan MF. Factors predicting hospitalization after operative treatment for gastric carcinoma in patients older than 70 years. J Am Coll Surg 1997; 184(1):9–15.
135. Tsujitani S, et al. Limited operation for gastric cancer in the elderly. Br J Surg 1996; 83(6):836–839.
136. Habu H, et al. Quality of postoperative life in gastric cancer patients seventy years of age and over. Int Surg 1988; 73(2):82–86.
137. Koga S, et al. Total gastrectomy in the aged with special reference to postoperative convalescence and return to normal life. Dig Surg 1985; 2:31–35.
138. Lens MB, Dawes M. Global perspectives of contemporary epidemiological trends of cutaneous malignant melanoma. Br J Dermatol 2004; 150(2):179–185.
139. Balch CM, et al. Efficacy of 2-cm surgical margins for intermediate-thickness melanomas (1 to 4 mm). Results of a multi-institutional randomized surgical trial. Ann Surg 1993; 218(3):262–267; discussion 267–269.
140. Thorn M, et al. The association between anatomic site and survival in malignant melanoma. An analysis of 12,353 cases from the Swedish Cancer Registry. Eur J Cancer Clin Oncol 1989; 25(3):483–491.
141. Kemeny MM, et al. Superior survival of young women with malignant melanoma. Am J Surg 1998; 175(6):437–444; discussion 444–445.
142. Masback A, et al. Cutaneous malignant melanoma in southern Sweden 1965, 1975, and 1985. Prognostic factors and histologic correlations. Cancer 1997; 79(2):275–283.
143. Austin PF, et al. Age as a prognostic factor in the malignant melanoma population. Ann Surg Oncol 1994; 1(6):487–494.
144. Veronesi U, et al. Thin stage I primary cutaneous malignant melanoma. Comparison of excision with margins of 1 or 3 cm. N Engl J Med 1988; 318(18):1159–1162.
145. Veronesi U, Cascinelli N. Narrow excision (1-cm margin). A safe procedure for thin cutaneous melanoma. Arch Surg 1991; 126(4):438–441.
146. Balch CM, et al. Efficacy of an elective regional lymph node dissection of 1 to 4 mm thick melanomas for patients 60 years of age and younger. Ann Surg 1996; 224(3):255–263; discussion 263–266.
147. Urist MM, et al. The influence of surgical margins and prognostic factors predicting the risk of local recurrence in 3445 patients with primary cutaneous melanoma. Cancer 1985; 55(6):1398–1402.
148. Balch CM, et al. Long-term results of a multi-institutional randomized trial comparing prognostic factors and surgical results for intermediate thickness melanomas (1.0 to 4.0 mm). Intergroup Melanoma Surgical Trial. Ann Surg Oncol 2000; 7(2):87–97.
149. Morton DL, et al. Technical details of intraoperative lymphatic mapping for early stage melanoma. Arch Surg 1992; 127(4):392–399.
150. Krag DN, et al. Minimal-access surgery for staging of malignant melanoma. Arch Surg 1995; 130(6):654–658; discussion 659–660.
151. Leong SP. The role of sentinel lymph nodes in malignant melanoma. Surg Clin North Am 2000; 80(6):1741–1757.

152. Morton DL, et al. Interim results of the Multicenter Selective Lymphadenectomy Trial (MSLT-I) in clinical stage I melanoma in ASCO. 2005.
153. Law WL, Chu KW, Tung PH. Laparoscopic colorectal resection: a safe option for elderly patients. J Am Coll Surg 2002; 195(6):768–773.
154. Delgado S, et al. Could age be an indication for laparoscopic colectomy in colorectal cancer? Surg Endosc 2000; 14(1):22–26.
155. Veldkamp R, et al. Laparoscopic resection of colonic cancer. Scand J Surg 2003; 92(1):97–103.
156. Lacy AM, et al. Laparoscopy-assisted colectomy versus open colectomy for treatment of non-metastatic colon cancer: a randomised trial. Lancet 2002; 359(9325):2224–2229.
157. Callery MP, et al. Staging laparoscopy with laparoscopic ultrasonography: optimizing resectability in hepatobiliary and pancreatic malignancy. J Am Coll Surg 1997; 185(1):33–39.
158. Burke EC, et al. Laparoscopy in the management of gastric adenocarcinoma. Ann Surg 1997; 225(3):262–267.
159. Flowers JL, et al. Laparoscopic splenectomy in patients with hematologic diseases. Ann Surg 1996; 224(1):19–28.
160. Prytherch DR, et al. POSSUM and Portsmouth POSSUM for predicting mortality. Br J Surg 1998; 85:1217–1220.

4

Radiation Therapy in the Older Cancer Patient

Loren K. Mell and Arno J. Mundt
*Department of Radiation and Cellular Oncology, University of Chicago,
Chicago, Illinois, U.S.A.*

INTRODUCTION

Radiation therapy (RT) has long occupied an important role in the treatment of cancer. In fact, the first cancer patient was treated with radiation in early 1896, shortly following Roentgen's discovery of X rays. Techniques for RT planning and delivery have evolved considerably over the past century. Today, ionizing radiation is used in the treatment of a wide variety of benign and malignant diseases arising in virtually every organ system in the body.

According to the U.S. National Cancer Institute (1), approximately one-half of all patients diagnosed with cancer undergo RT at some point during the course of their disease. Given the increasing incidence of most malignancies with age (2), it is not surprising that the majority of cancer patients currently undergoing RT are older. Thus, what is true of RT in the treatment of cancer patients generally also applies to its use in the elderly. However, many challenging issues regarding the care of the older cancer patient require special consideration, including prognosis, treatment selection, RT-related toxicities, management of comorbidities, and complicated social factors.

As the U.S. population ages and life expectancy increases, the average age of patients receiving RT is likely to increase as well, and issues particular to elderly cancer patients will take on even greater importance. Correspondingly, there is a growing need to better our understanding of these issues and some have called for greater emphasis on radiation oncology research specific to the elderly (3). The following chapter discusses these issues and highlights aspects of radiation oncology specifically related to aging and to caring for the heterogeneous and unique population of older cancer patients. Particular emphasis is placed on new and emerging RT technologies designed to shorten treatment and reduce normal tissue toxicity, which have special relevance to the older cancer patient.

RADIATION ONCOLOGY PRINCIPLES

Radiation oncology is a field devoted to the use of ionizing radiation in the treatment of benign and malignant disease. Most clinical applications of RT involve the delivery of high-energy photons (X rays), which exert their therapeutic effects by generating reactive oxygen species, which in turn induce DNA damage and cellular death in diseased tissue. Electron beam irradiation is also frequently used to treat superficial tumors. Some centers specialize in RT with heavy particles, such as protons and neutrons, which have specific clinical applications. However, the mechanism of DNA damage and biologic effects differ greatly between photons and heavy particles. Interested readers are referred elsewhere for a more detailed discussion of these topics (4).

Two main approaches are currently used in clinical radiation oncology: teletherapy and brachytherapy. Teletherapy, or external beam RT, is the more common method. Modern teletherapy is most often delivered with high-energy photons and electrons generated by a linear accelerator (Fig. 1). In the past, photon irradiation was frequently administered with gamma rays from a large source of radioactive cobalt-60 (^{60}Co). Brachytherapy involves the use of radioactive isotopes placed within a patient. As these isotopes decay, high-energy X rays (known as gamma rays) or electrons (beta particles) are emitted which deposit dose directly into the tumor and surrounding tissues.

Conventional teletherapy is typically delivered with a limited number of beams (e.g., 2–4) directed upon the treatment site. For example, conventional pelvic irradiation is delivered with four beams (two opposed lateral and two opposed anterior–posterior beams). Angled or oblique beams are frequently used as well; for example, tangential beams are used in breast cancer patients to minimize dose to the underlying lung. During treatment, patients are immobilized on the treatment table and the machine head (gantry) rotates around the patient. Treatment beams are typically shaped by using collimators or customized "blocks" placed in the beam's path to further reduce the dose delivered to surrounding normal tissues. Total treatment time

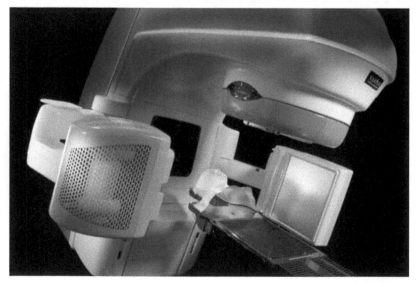

Figure 1 Varian clinac (Varian Medical Systems, Palo Alto, California, U.S.A.). *Source*: Courtesy of L. Scott Johnson, Varian Medical Systems.

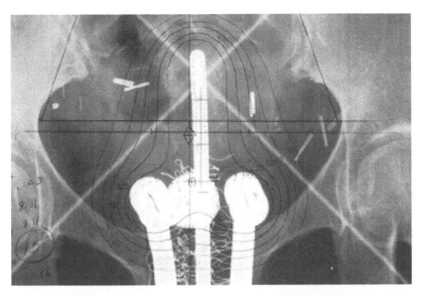

Figure 2 Anterior–posterior X ray of a Fletcher-Suit-Delclos applicator in a patient with cervical cancer. The central tandem is placed within the uterus and the two ovoids (colpostats) are placed within the vaginal fornices next to the cervix. Radioactive sources placed within the tandem and ovoids deliver high doses to the cervix and the uterus.

typically ranges from four to seven weeks, with most patients receiving therapy Monday through Friday of each week. In some situations, a single fraction (e.g., radiosurgery) or limited number of fractions (e.g., hypofractionated RT) may be delivered.

Commonly used isotopes for brachytherapy include cesium-137 (^{137}Cs), iridium-198 (^{198}Ir), and iodine-125 (^{125}I). Sources are placed within an existing cavity in close proximity to a tumor (intracavitary brachytherapy) or directly within the tumor itself (interstitial brachytherapy). Numerous specialized applicators have been developed to aid the proper placement of radioactive sources. One well-known device is the Fletcher-Suit-Delclos applicator, used in women with cervical cancer (Fig. 2). This metal applicator is positioned in the operating room with the patient under anesthesia; sources are subsequently inserted in a shielded room ("after-loaded") once treatment planning is complete, minimizing exposure of the staff. Sources are then left in place for one to four days and removed along with the applicator. Alternatively, short-lived isotopes may be inserted permanently within the patient, such as in prostate "seed" implants.

Multiple special external beam and brachytherapy approaches that improve the quality and delivery of RT have been introduced over the years. A detailed discussion of several such approaches relevant to the treatment of the older cancer patient is presented later in this chapter (see section on "Special Radiation Technologies and Procedures in the Elderly").

GENERAL ISSUES IN GERIATRIC RADIOTHERAPY

Many elderly cancer patients do not receive RT even when it is indicated (5,6), despite the potential benefits of both palliative and curative treatment (7,8). One reason for this is that elderly cancer patients are less likely to receive standard or curative therapy in general (5,6,9–11). In some cases, this is clearly appropriate, such as a patient with a poor performance status and a short life expectancy. Elderly patients frequently have deficiencies in organ function that preclude the use of curative RT (such as a large lung mass in a patient with severe chronic pulmonary disease). A relative emphasis on quality rather than quantity of life also tends to weigh against the aggressiveness of therapeutic recommendations in this population. It may be falsely assumed, however, that tumors in the elderly are biologically less aggressive; while true in some sites such as breast and possibly lung (12), this is not true in most other sites (13).

Logistical barriers to accessing care may also prevent elderly cancer patients from receiving treatment (14). Limited access to and dependency upon others for transportation, impaired functional status and/or cognitive function, and deficiencies in social support all constitute barriers to providing RT in elderly cancer patients (14,15). However, at least one study suggests that elderly cancer patients may actually have fewer and less severe psychosocial problems, and make fewer demands on time and resources than do younger patients (16).

Physician or patient biases and misconceptions may also prevent access to treatment (17). For example, Newcomb and Carbone surveyed 507 women with newly diagnosed breast carcinoma; controlling for stage, women older than 65 were less likely to have received breast conservation therapy, have adjuvant therapy offered, agree to adjuvant therapy when offered, or undergo consultation with a medical and/or radiation oncologist (18). Concerns about the potential side effects of therapy significantly influenced treatment recommendations and selection for elderly patients.

It may be assumed that elderly patients are less likely to tolerate RT, particularly aggressive regimens. However, many retrospective series demonstrate that, at least for appropriately selected patients, this is not the case (19–26). For example, Huguenin et al. reported on 210 patients with cancer arising from a variety of sites, with a median age of 79.3 (21). Patients tolerated aggressive treatment regimens including concurrent chemoradiation, hyperfractionated and accelerated RT, high radiation doses, and large treatment volumes, with rates of toxicity comparable with those seen in younger patients. The principal concern raised in this study was the need for attention to supportive care to address complications such as dehydration. Similarly, an analysis by Zachariah et al. reported that of 191 patients older than 80 undergoing RT, primarily with head and neck, breast, thoracic, or pelvic malignancies, 94% completed treatment as planned without severe acute complications (23).

Some technical considerations complicate the delivery of RT in elderly patients. Older patients with cognitive deficits may have difficulty cooperating with daily setup or may have difficulty remaining still during treatment, which compromises the efficacy of RT. Practical complexities may also arise, for example, in patients with prostheses or implantable cardiac devices, where radiation beam arrangements may have to be altered and more sensitive dosimetric devices employed. There does not appear to be bias, however, with respect to how RT treatment is planned or delivered based on age (27). Older patients should expect the same access to state-of-the-art therapies as younger cancer patients.

IN VITRO AND ANIMAL DATA

The relationship between radiation toxicity and age has been explored in a number of laboratory systems and animal models, with most studies focusing on the response of normal tissue as a function of age. Data analyzing the properties of "tumors" as they relate to host age are more limited. One study has suggested that tumors grown in older mice have a higher proportion of hypoxic cells (thus conferring greater resistance to radiation) (28). Studies of in vitro sensitivity of malignant glioma cells to nitrosureas show higher resistance in patients older than 50 (29); to our knowledge, however, experiments have not shown decreased "radiosensitivity" of glioma cells as a function of age (30).

With the exception of data on total body irradiation (TBI), most studies do not show a difference in RT-related toxicity on the basis of age alone (Fig. 3) (31).

Radiosensitivity of fibroblasts does not appear to be a function of age (31,32); similarly, lymphocytes of breast cancer patients do not exhibit changes in radiosensitivity with respect to host age (33). Hopewell and Young observed no difference in the severity of skin reactions based on age in pigs exposed to a range of radiation doses (34). Data in mice also do not reveal significant age-dependent changes in skin radiosensitivity (35). Landuyt and van der Schueren reported that lip mucosal desquamation and the capacity of mucosal cells to repair radiation damage were independent of age in irradiated mice (36).

Rosen et al. observed no differences in cell survival and repair of sublethal damage as a function of age in cultures of rat aortic smooth muscle cells (37). Sargent and Burns reached the opposite conclusion, however, noting that DNA repair in rat epidermal cells following radiation diminishes with age (38). Diminished capacity for DNA repair appears to be associated with cellular aging (39). Telomere shortening may play a fundamental role in cellular aging and senescence, and tumorigenesis is associated with telomerase activity (40).

At least two studies have shown a "decrease" in radiosensitivity of tissues as a function of age. Moulder and Fish observed that renal radiosensitivity was lower in adult rats compared to young rats, while Hamlet and Hopewell showed that advanced age was associated with less skin sensitivity and a shorter duration of skin healing in rats (41,42).

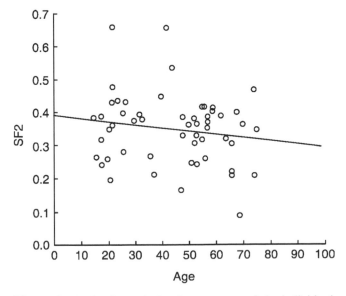

Figure 3 Lack of correlation between age of the individuals and in vitro fibroblast radiosensitivity ($P=0.31$; $r=-0.17$). SF2 = proportion of surviving cells (surviving fraction) after irradiation with a single dose of 2 Gy. *Source*: From Ref. 31.

Results of studies of gastrointestinal (GI) toxicity secondary to radiation have been mixed. Hamilton and Franks saw no difference in the radiosensitivity of GI mucosal cells in 4- versus 24-month-old mice; however, regenerating crypt colonies in older mice were smaller, suggesting a lower rate of repopulation (43). Olofsen-van Acht et al. studied rectal complications in rats exposed to high-dose single fractions of radiation [22 and 39 Gray (Gy)] and found that the incidence of ulceration and vascular occlusion was higher in older rats (44). However, a recent study from the same laboratory using fractionated radiation exposures (such as are administered in clinical RT) concluded that radiation-induced rectal complications in rats were independent of age (45).

Crosfill et al. found a rapid decrease in the TBI dose, resulting in 50% mortality (LD_{50}) in mice after age 40 weeks (46). Similarly, Hursh and Casarett noted a higher mortality in 16- versus 6-month-old rats exposed to identical TBI doses (47); others have reported similar findings for TBI. Lamproglou et al. showed that progressive and irreversible memory loss occurred in elderly rats more often than in young rats when whole brain irradiation was administered in ten 3 Gy fractions over 12 days; however, learning dysfunction did not seem to be age-dependent (48). It could be concluded from the available in vitro and animal data that normal tissue radiation-induced toxicity differs little with age, yet this relationship is likely to be more relevant when large treatment volumes or large fraction sizes are involved.

CLINICAL RADIATION ONCOLOGY IN THE ELDERLY

Central Nervous System Tumors

RT is useful in the treatment of a variety of tumors involving the central nervous system (CNS). It can be administered as adjuvant therapy following surgical resection, as definitive (curative) treatment in patients with partially resected or unresectable tumors, or in patients who are poor operative candidates. RT is also often effective for palliation in patients with CNS tumors, particularly in patients with brain metastases. Unlike most tumors arising from other sites, age has been independently associated with poorer outcomes in some CNS tumors, even after controlling for other strongly confounding prognostic factors such as performance status (49–52).

Much of the literature relating age and outcomes following RT in patients with CNS tumors has focused on patients with malignant gliomas. It is clear from large series such as the RT Oncology Group (RTOG) recursive partitioning analysis that age is an independent prognostic indicator of survival (Table 1) (49). The poorer prognosis according to age does not appear to be explained by either the bias in access to care (53) or intrinsic radioresistance of the gliomas arising in elderly patients (30).

Postoperative RT improves survival in malignant glioma patients (54), and retrospective series in older patients (ages >65–70 years) support an advantage to adjuvant RT over surgery or biopsy alone in this group as well (55–58). Some studies suggest, however, that the magnitude of the benefit in elderly glioma patients is modest at best and may not justify a conventional six-week course of RT (56,58). A more abbreviated treatment course (hypofractionated RT) may be appropriate in elderly patients with glioblastoma multiforme (GBM) (59–61). Roa et al. randomized 100 GBM patients aged over 60 years to either 60 Gy in 30 fractions over six weeks (standard) or 40 Gy in 15 fractions over three weeks (hypofractionated). Median and six-month overall survivals were similar in both arms (5.1 vs. 5.6 months and 44.7% vs. 41.7%

Table 1 RPA of Patients with Malignant Glioma Treated on RTOG Trials

RPA class	Definition	Median survival time (mo)	One-year survival rate (%)	Three-year survival rate (%)	Five-year survival rate (%)
III	Age < 50, KPS ≥ 90	17.1	70	20	14
IV	Age < 50, KPS < 90	11.2	46	7	4
	Age ≥ 50, KPS ≥ 70, G/STR, W+				
V + VI	Age ≥ 50, KPS ≥ 70, G/STR, W-	7.5	28	1	0
	Age ≥ 50, KPS ≥ 70, biopsy				
	Age ≥ 50, KPS < 70				

Age is prognostic independent of performance status (KPS), extent of resection [gross vs. subtotal resection (G/STR) vs. biopsy alone], and neurologic function [working (W+) or not working (W−)].
Abbreviations: KPS, Karnofsky performance status; RPA, recursive-partitioning analysis; RTOG, radiation therapy oncology group.
Source: From Ref. 49.

for the six-week and three-week arms, respectively). Post-treatment increases in corticosteroid use were less common in the hypofractionated arm compared to the standard arm (23% vs. 49%, respectively, $P = 0.02$).

In the light of two recent randomized trials showing a survival benefit to the addition of temozolomide, adjuvant irradiation with concurrent use of temozolomide ($75 \, mg/m^2$/day) followed by six cycles of temozolomide ($150–200 \, mg/m^2$ every 28 days) is now considered by many the standard of care for GBM (62,63). The individual benefits of surgery, RT, and the use of temozolomide in the treatment of elderly patients with high-grade malignant glioma appear marginal (56,64–67). However, aggressive combined modality therapy can significantly prolong survival, and many advocate this approach irrespective of chronologic age (68,69).

Some have advocated temozolomide as monotherapy for elderly patients (70,71). In a retrospective analysis of 86 patients aged 70 or older with either GBM or anaplastic astrocytoma, Glantz et al. noted no difference in one-year overall survivals for patients treated with temozolomide monotherapy versus RT alone (11.9% vs. 9.3%, $P = 0.198$) (70). Two European randomized trials evaluating RT versus temozolomide as first-line adjuvant therapy in elderly GBM patients are ongoing. The efficacy of monotherapy with temozolomide over placebo or best supportive care for this group of patients, however, has not yet been established. It may therefore be more appropriate to observe patients who are unable to receive standard therapy or adjuvant short-course RT until temozolomide as monotherapy has been proven effective.

Other common primary CNS tumors in elderly patients include meningiomas, pituitary adenomas, and schwannomas. Retrospective series comprising large numbers of elderly patients with these tumors have demonstrated excellent tumor control with low rates of adverse sequelae following RT (72–76). Primary CNS lymphoma is also frequently treated with RT, with moderate success (51). Some investigators advocate chemotherapy alone in these patients due to concerns over late neurotoxic sequelae following whole brain irradiation (77). Studies of cognitive outcomes in elderly patients undergoing brain radiation support the assertion that cognitive decline following cranial RT is worse in older cancer patients, particularly with high doses and large treatment volumes or fraction sizes (78,79).

Head and Neck Cancer

Given the large volumes of mucosa irradiated in many head and neck cancer patients, concerns are often raised regarding the tolerance of RT in elderly patients. The available data, however, fail to demonstrate a correlation between increasing age and RT-related toxicity in these patients (80,81).

In a comprehensive review of 1307 head and neck cancer patients undergoing RT (156, age 70 or above), Pignon et al. evaluated acute and chronic toxicities in various age groups ranging from 50 to 75 years and above. No differences were seen in either acute mucosal toxicities or weight loss >10% in the different age groups. A higher incidence of functional (grade 3–4) acute toxicity was seen, however, in older patients. Of patients evaluable for late toxicity, increasing age was not correlated with more frequent or severe chronic sequelae (82).

Schofield et al. reviewed toxicity rates in 98 head and neck cancer patients aged 80 or higher undergoing definitive RT. Treatment tolerance was similar to that seen in younger patients, with only three patients (3%) developing severe late sequelae (83). Of note, comparable tumor control and survival rates were seen between older and younger patients—a finding consistent with other reports (80), despite the fact that lower radiation doses are often delivered to elderly head and neck cancer patients (81).

Increasing attention has been focused on the use of more aggressive approaches in head and neck cancer patients, notably accelerated fractionation schedules, which deliver higher radiation doses in shorter overall times. While associated with improved outcomes, higher rates of toxicity are common (84). To assess the feasibility of this approach in the elderly, Allal et al. reviewed the outcomes of 120 patients (32% aged 70 years or higher) treated with an accelerated concomitant boost approach (85). All patients received 50.4 Gy in 1.8 Gy daily fractions to the primary and bilateral neck. Beginning at the end of week 2, a second dose of 1.5 Gy (total, 19.5 Gy) was delivered to the initial involved sites as a second daily fraction. The total dose to involved sites was thus 69.9 Gy over 38 days. While treatment breaks were more common using this approach in older patients (7% vs. 0%, $P = 0.03$), all patients treated, regardless of age, were able to successfully complete therapy as planned. Moreover, no significant differences were seen in terms of acute toxicities based on age, including the need for nasogastric tube or percutaneous gastrostomy feeding (26% elderly, 23% younger patients). Rates of weight loss were comparable in the two groups. Severe late complications were less frequent in older patients (3% vs. 10%); however, this difference did not reach statistical significance ($P = 0.43$). These results suggest that properly selected elderly head and neck cancer patients can tolerate more aggressive fractionation regimens.

More recently, concomitant chemoradiotherapy approaches in head and neck cancer patients have been explored, either definitively or following surgery (86,87). As with altered fractionation regimens, improved outcomes can be achieved using this approach. However, such benefits are seen at the expense of increased toxicity, and the feasibility of such approaches in the elderly is questioned. Moreover, most combined modality regimens evaluated to date have been cisplatin-based, which may not be an ideal approach in elderly patients, particularly those with multiple comorbidities.

Such concerns have led some investigators to evaluate alternative (non-cisplatin-based) chemoradiotherapy approaches in elderly head and neck cancer patients. Kodaira et al. recently reported the results of a phase I trial evaluating weekly administration of docetaxel and concomitant RT in elderly and/or patients with multiple comorbidities precluding cisplatin use (88). The maximum tolerated dose of docetaxel in these patients was $14 \, mg/m^2/week$, with the most common dose-limiting toxicity being stomatitis within the irradiated field. Prospective clinical trials are clearly needed to evaluate the efficacy of this approach, as well as the feasibility of other non-cisplatin-based concomitant regimens, in elderly head and neck cancer patients.

Lung Cancer

Elderly lung cancer patients frequently have poor pulmonary function and comorbidities that make them poor operative candidates. In otherwise good operative candidates, surgical resection is considered standard treatment and has been associated with similar risk of morbidity and mortality in elderly compared to younger patients (89,90). Despite this, definitive local therapy is often underutilized (91,92). Chemotherapy can prolong survival in elderly patients but is probably underutilized as well (93).

Postoperative RT with concurrent chemotherapy (typically carboplatin/taxol or cisplatin/etoposide) is generally recommended in patients with resected locally advanced non-small cell lung cancer (NSCLC). In some cases, neoadjuvant chemotherapy or chemoradiotherapy may be delivered prior to surgery. In patients with inoperable locally advanced disease, definitive RT alone or concurrent or sequential chemoradiotherapy is frequently recommended. Results from a randomized trial comparing RT versus chemoradiotherapy in patients older than 70 with stage III NSCLC, which is currently underway in Japan, will hopefully provide further information on treating elderly patients with combined modality therapy.

The ability of elderly NSCLC patients to tolerate aggressive combined modality treatment regimens has been explored in several analyses. Elderly patients have been shown to tolerate curative RT regimens (94), even aggressive ones such as concurrent chemotherapy and accelerated hyperfractionated radiation (95), with acceptable toxicity and comparable outcomes when compared to younger patients (95–100). For example, Pignon et al. analyzed outcomes in 1208 patients undergoing thoracic irradiation enrolled on six European Organization for Research on Treatment of Cancer randomized trials and found no evidence that advancing age was associated with higher rates or greater severity of acute or late pneumonitis, esophagitis, weakness, or alteration in performance status. Weight loss, however, was significantly worse in older patients (96). Koga et al. also observed no difference in the frequency of radiation pneumonitis, but a nonsignificant trend toward greater severity of pneumonitis in NSCLC patients older than 70 (98).

Others have observed differences in toxicity in NSCLC based on age. Schild et al. evaluated outcomes in 246 locally advanced NSCLC patients undergoing chemoradiotherapy (101). Grade 4 myelosuppression and pneumonitis were significantly more common in patients older than 70 compared to younger patients [myelosuppression: 78% vs. 56% ($P < 0.01$), respectively; pneumonitis: 6% vs. 1% ($P < 0.01$), respectively]. Survival rates, however, were equivalent, supporting the use of aggressive approaches in appropriately selected older patients. Movsas et al., however, studied a large group of elderly patients with inoperable advanced NSCLC and found that quality-adjusted survival was significantly better for patients treated with RT alone compared to chemoradiotherapy, mainly due to high rates of esophagitis with chemoradiotherapy (102).

A possible means of reducing the severity of RT-related toxicity in elderly NSCLC patients undergoing RT with or without concomitant chemotherapy is the use of the cytoprotector amifostine (Ethyol®, Medimmune Inc., Gaithersburg, Maryland, U.S.A.). Amifostine has been found in several randomized trials to reduce the incidence of esophagitis and pneumonitis in irradiated patients with advanced NSCLC (103–105). Of note, a recent RTOG randomized trial evaluating the addition of amifostine in patients undergoing hyperfractionated twice-daily RT found that patients' experience of dysphagia was reduced with amifostine administration, particularly in patients older than 65 (106). However, other measures of esophagitis were not significantly different between the treatment and control groups. Acute side effects, particularly nausea, hypotension, and drug rash, were worse for patients receiving amifostine. The risk of hypotension can be significantly reduced with subcutaneous administration (106). Concerns have been raised regarding the potential of amifostine also to protect tumor, thereby reducing local control; however, available clinical data to date do not support this concern (104,106,107).

Elderly patients with early stage medically inoperable NSCLC are appropriate candidates for definitive RT, and exhibit comparable outcomes compared to younger patients (108,109). Multiple studies show that high rates of local control can be achieved with RT in these patients, particularly with doses above 60 Gy (Table 2; Fig. 4) (110–115). Severe chronic obstructive pulmonary disease, other comorbidities, and distant metastasis represent significant competing mortality risks, however, in these patients, leading to low rates of long-term survival. Studies of high-dose single or oligofractionated radiation using extracranial stereotactic techniques have also been promising and significantly shorten the duration of RT (116–118), which may be advantageous in elderly patients (see section on "Stereotactive Radiosurgery"). Despite the administration of doses as high as 20 Gy per fraction in some studies, toxicity is quite low (117). Analyses in patients who refuse surgery but are otherwise good operative candidates show survival rates comparable with those seen in patients with the same clinical stage undergoing resection (118). Longer follow-up, however, is needed to evaluate long-term survival rates and assess late toxicity.

Similar to studies of NSCLC, conflicting data exist regarding acute toxicity secondary to RT in elderly patients with small cell lung cancer (SCLC). While Schild et al. observed a higher rate of pneumonitis and treatment-related death in patients aged 70 or older compared to younger patients, the absolute incidence of pneumonitis (6.0%) and mortality (5.6%) were relatively low (119). A large study from Quon et al. did not find evidence of difference in outcomes or toxicity as a function of age (120), and Jeremic et al. reported acceptable rates of toxicity in a study of elderly SCLC patients undergoing accelerated hyperfractionated RT with cisplatin and etoposide (121). Five-year survival in these series was less than 20%, pointing to the need for more effective therapy; however, age itself does not appear to be an appropriate independent criterion for treatment selection.

As in younger patients, prophylactic cranial irradiation (PCI) should be offered to patients with limited stage SCLC who achieve a complete response to chemotherapy and RT. Tai et al. analyzed neurotoxicity in 66 patients undergoing PCI (median age: 64 years); only six patients had chronic neurologic symptoms, some of which may have existed prior to therapy (122).

Table 2 Studies of Definitive RT in Medically Inoperable Stage I NSCLC

N	Age (med.)	Dose	%T1	%T2	Grade 3–5 Tox. (%)	5YOS (%)	CSS%	LC%	References
152	74	60–69 Gy	29	41	0	10	20–55 (2yr)	67 (>70 Gy)	(110)
141	70	64 Gy (med.)	54	46	1.5	13	29–30 (5yr)	–	(111)
108	74	60–65 Gy	47	53	0	15	13–40 (3yr)	52	(112)
103	67	60 Gy (med.)	31	59	1	13	50 (5yr)	–	(113)
77	72	60 Gy (med.)	32	68	Rare	14	17–30 (3yr)	56	(114)
53	73	63 Gy (med.)	38	62	8	6	33 (3yr)	75 (>65 Gy)	(115)

N, number of patients; med., median; T1, T2, T stage; Tox., toxicity.
Abbreviations: CSS, cause-specific survival; LC, local control; NSCLC, non-small cell lung cancer; 5YOS: five-year overall survival; RT, radiation therapy.
Source: From Ref. 111.

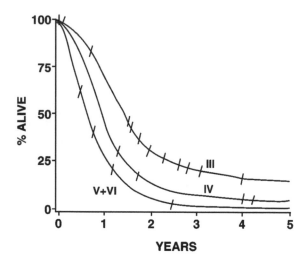

Figure 4 Overall survival by recursive partitioning analysis class for patients with malignant glioma treated on RTOG trials. *Abbreviation*: RTOG, radiation therapy oncology group. *Source*: From Ref. 49.

Breast Cancer

Although the use of RT in elderly breast cancer patients has increased over the past several decades (123), the proportion of elderly women treated with breast-conserving surgery without adjuvant RT has increased as well, because breast-conserving surgery has become increasingly favored over mastectomy (124). Multiple studies have established that older breast cancer patients are less likely than younger patients to receive RT following breast-conserving surgery (27,125–127), especially elderly African-American women (128).

The disuse of RT partly owes to the fact that older women generally are treated less aggressively and are less likely to receive standard or curative treatment for their breast cancer (129–134). While less aggressive treatment is often justified in elderly patients based on clinical and pathologic factors and patient preference (135,136), several studies convincingly show that age is an independent predictor of treatment selection, suggesting that age bias is partly to blame (126,131). Better physician communication regarding treatment options can influence patient awareness and treatment selection, particularly when it comes to adjuvant RT (137,138).

Several randomized trials have shown that adjuvant RT significantly reduces the probability of local recurrence following breast-conserving surgery (139,140), including trials confined to postmenopausal patients (141). Even in node-negative patients with tumors less than 1 cm who receive tamoxifen, however, there is a significant local recurrence risk (approximately 2% per year), which can be reduced to approximately 0.5% per year with adjuvant RT (142). Retrospective series in elderly patients also show high rates of survival, local control, and recurrence-free survival in elderly patients treated with RT (52,143–146). There is no evidence from randomized trials, however, that adjuvant radiation affects overall survival in node-negative breast cancer.

Whether the benefit of RT is applicable to elderly breast cancer patients, however, has been questioned (139). For example, a large randomized trial showed a benefit to adjuvant RT following quadrantectomy for early breast cancer, reducing the 10-year risk of recurrence in the ipsilateral breast from 23.5% to 5.8%; however, the benefit was only seen in women less than 65 years of age (139). Much effort has been devoted to defining a low-risk subgroup of women with early breast cancer in which RT may be appropriately omitted following lumpectomy. A recent randomized trial tested the benefit of adjuvant RT in node-negative patients older than 70, with estrogen receptor-positive tumors less than 2 cm, treated with lumpectomy and tamoxifen. The five-year local recurrence rate in patients treated with lumpectomy and tamoxifen alone was low (4%, 95% confidence interval 2–7%). Adjuvant RT reduced the recurrence to 1% (147). With longer follow-up, however, the recurrence rate in patients not receiving RT will likely rise. In fit elderly patients with a reasonably long life expectancy, many radiation oncologists would still advocate adjuvant RT.

Elderly women with ductal carcinoma in situ (DCIS) may be at lower risk of recurrence compared to younger women, even controlling for margin status, tumor size, and grade (148–150). Patients at low risk for recurrence include those with negative margins >1 cm, low histologic grade, and size <1.5 cm (151). Whether RT should be omitted in this low-risk subgroup is unclear and has not been prospectively evaluated. Several randomized trials show that recurrence rates for DCIS can be quite high, and RT reduces the risk of both non-invasive and invasive carcinoma in the ipsilateral breast by approximately 50% (152–154).

When single-modality adjuvant therapy is being considered (e.g., tamoxifen vs. RT), the relative benefits and downsides of each should be taken into account. The predominant downsides to adjuvant RT in early breast cancer are the inconvenience of a long treatment course, the discomfort of acute skin toxicity, and long-term effects on cosmesis. Lymphedema, pneumonitis, cardiotoxicity, and second malignancies (e.g., angiosarcoma) are rare complications. Tamoxifen, however, has its own set of potential adverse effects such as hot flashes, weight gain, vaginal discharge, thromboembolic events, and endometrial cancer (155). Aromatase inhibitors can cause arthralgia and have adverse effects on bone density—a potential concern in elderly women at risk for fracture (156,157). These risks should be carefully weighed and discussed thoroughly with elderly patients, and the treatment procedure should be tailored to the needs of the individual patient.

Methods of shortening the duration of breast RT can particularly benefit elderly patients, who otherwise might be deterred from undergoing a prolonged treatment course. A current area of exploration and controversy is partial breast irradiation (PBI) (see section on "HDR Brachytherapy") which can significantly shorten treatment, for example, from six weeks of daily treatment to five days of twice-daily treatment. Several PBI approaches are under investigation, involving intracavitary (158) or interstitial brachytherapy (159), three-dimensional (3-D)-conformal or intensity-modulated external beam radiation (160), or intraoperative electron beam therapy (161). Much of the controversy centers around the risk of "elsewhere" failure in the breast, i.e., the recurrence risk in a different quadrant, outside the treated volume, that may be prevented in whole breast irradiation, but not PBI. A related concern is the definition of the adequate treatment volume because it has been noted that most recurrences occur near the site of tumor resection. A randomized trial, National Surgical Adjuvant Breast Project (NSABP) -B39/RTOG 0413, is currently underway comparing PBI with whole breast RT in the adjuvant treatment of early breast cancer or DCIS (see section on "HDR Brachytherapy").

Shortening treatment by altering the fractionation scheme, such as with hypofractionation or treating with an accelerated concomitant boost, has also been used at some centers (162). However, larger fraction sizes tend to worsen cosmesis (163). Modern techniques using 3-D planning can improve dose homogeneity within the breast, reducing the risk for poor cosmetic outcome. It is unclear whether elderly patients are particularly susceptible to the adverse cosmetic effects of RT. While some studies have found worse cosmetic outcomes according to age (164,165), others have not observed this relationship (163,166). Cosmesis in elderly patients is generally at its worst in the first few years following RT, but frequently improves, so that by four years, it is can be difficult to distinguish cosmetic differences compared to nonirradiated controls (147).

In postmenopausal patients with advanced breast cancer (large tumor size, node positivity), adjuvant RT improves overall survival (167). When radiation is given to the axilla and supraclavicular fossa, shoulder stiffness and brachial plexopathy are potential complications. In studies of these complications, elderly patients have been found to be at excess risk for shoulder stiffness, but decreased risk of brachial plexopathy (168,169). The risk of lymphedema rises when RT is given to the axilla, particularly a dissected axilla (170). Some evidence suggests that elderly women are at excess risk of lymphedema (171). Axillary RT alone is associated with a relatively low risk of lymphedema and has comparable control rates to surgery (172); thus, the use of RT instead of surgery to address the axilla may be an appropriate management strategy in select cases.

In recurrent or locoregionally advanced breast cancer, definitive RT is sometimes used (173), often with hyperthermia (174), which may benefit elderly women who are poor surgical candidates. Hyperthermia has also been used to treat patients who require re-irradiation (175). The addition of hyperthermia can improve control of superficial tumors, with response rates approaching 80% to 90% and local control approaching 70% to 80% (174,175).

GI Cancer

Patients with GI tumors commonly undergo RT, delivered either alone or in combination with surgery, chemotherapy, or both. Treatment typically involves the use of large RT fields encompassing considerable volumes of normal tissues, exposing patients to a wide variety of toxicities. To date, multiple investigators have reported on the outcomes and toxicities in elderly GI tumor patients undergoing RT, particularly in patients with esophageal cancer (176–179). Less information is available on RT in elderly patients with other GI tumors, apart from rectal (180) and anal (181) carcinoma.

In a large Japanese Patterns of Care study, Tanisada et al. evaluated the outcomes of 336 esophageal cancer patients undergoing definitive RT (179). Patients were divided into three age groups: young (119 patients, < 65 years), intermediate (94 patients, 65–74 years), and elderly (123 patients, ≥75 years). While radiation doses were comparable with the majority of patients in each age group receiving curative doses (≥60 Gy), chemotherapy was less commonly delivered in elderly (19%) compared to young (50%) and intermediate (40%) age patients ($P = 0.001$). On multivariate analysis, the only factors correlated with survival were performance status, stage, and radiation dose. Age was not found to be a prognostic factor for survival. Moreover, no significant differences were seen in terms of acute and chronic toxicities between the three age groups. The five-year cumulative risk of chronic toxicity in the young, intermediate, and elderly groups was 22%, 21%, and 26%, respectively ($P = 0.69$). Others have reported similar results (176,177).

Given the increasing interest focused on preoperative chemoradiotherapy in esophageal cancer in recent years, Rice et al. at M.D. Anderson Cancer Center evaluated the tolerance of this approach in the elderly (178). Between 1997 and 2002, 200 esophageal cancer patients underwent preoperative therapy (almost exclusively chemoradiotherapy). Patients were divided into two groups based on age at diagnosis: nonirradiated (age <70) and elderly (age ≥70). Treatment was comparable between the two groups, apart from the increased use of triplet chemotherapy in younger patients. Overall, treatment was well tolerated in both age groups, with nearly identical rates of perioperative mortality (4% nonelderly, 2% elderly). The only differences were more frequent postoperative transfusions and arrhythmias in the elderly group. On multivariate analysis, however, age was not correlated with the development of treatment-related complications. Moreover, no significant difference was seen in terms of survival based on age. While not appropriate for all elderly esophageal cancer patients, such results suggest that an aggressive combined modality approach can be considered in properly selected patients.

Despite strong evidence demonstrating improved outcomes in rectal/rectosigmoid cancer patients treated with postoperative RT, multiple investigators have shown that elderly rectal cancer patients are less likely to receive it (182,183). Although presumably withheld due to toxicity concerns, the available data do not support this belief. In a review of 224 patients (ages 20–81 years) undergoing surgery and adjuvant RT at M.D. Anderson Cancer Center, complications were seen in 25.8% of patients, predominantly small bowel obstructions. While correlated with various patient and treatment factors (notably the presence of adhesions), no correlation was seen between increasing age and treatment-related sequelae (180).

Unlike other GI tumors, the preferred treatment of anal carcinoma is concomitant chemoradiotherapy; surgery is reserved solely for the salvage of treatment failures. Concomitant chemoradiotherapy is quite successful in these patients, with local control rates exceeding 80% in most series (184). However, toxicity is common, particularly with regimens containing mitomycin-C and 5-flouorouracil (5-FU). Nevertheless, such approaches appear feasible in properly selected elderly patients. Valenti et al. treated 17 elderly anorectal cancer patients (ages 75–90 years) with mitomycin-C (10 mg/m^2 on day 1), 5-FU (1000 mg/m^2 days 1–4 continuous infusion), and concomitant pelvic-inguinal RT (38–45 Gy) (181). Overall, treatment was well tolerated with three patients (18%) developing grade 3 acute toxicity. Only one patient was unable to complete treatment as planned. At a median follow-up of 26 months, no severe late toxicities were noted. Overall, 16 patients (94%) experienced greater than 50% reduction in the size of the tumor, with six achieving a complete response. Twelve (70%) were able to preserve sphincter function.

Genitourinary Cancers

Numerous investigators have reported excellent long-term outcomes of elderly prostate cancer patients treated with definitive RT, with outcomes comparable with those seen in younger men (52,185–188). In a matched cohort study, Huguenin et al. noted similar five-year cause-specific survival rates in patients aged over 74 years (78%) compared to younger patients (82%). Moreover, the risk of local tumor progression was nearly identical (15% older and 14% younger patients) (186). Johnstone et al. noted no correlation between increasing age and biochemical disease-free survival in a cohort of 1018 stage T1–3 prostate cancer patients treated with definitive RT without androgen blockade (187). In contrast, D'Amico et al. found that advancing age was predictive of death from prostate cancer following definitive RT, but only in men with high-risk features (189).

Considerable attention has also been focused on the impact of increasing age on the risk of RT-related sequelae in prostate cancer patients undergoing definitive RT. Most investigators have noted no correlation between advancing age and either acute or chronic RT sequelae. Jani et al. at the University of Chicago compared genitourinary (GU) and GI toxicity in four different age groups (<60, 60–69, 70–74, and ≥75 years) in 527 prostate cancer patients undergoing definitive RT. No difference was seen in terms of acute and chronic toxicities (190). Huguenin et al. performed a detailed quality-of-life analysis in irradiated prostate cancer patients and found no differences based on age (186). Of note, Liu et al. found that maximal GI and GU symptoms develop earlier in older prostate patients, although the overall frequency and severity of symptoms were similar to that seen in younger patients (191).

A possible "treatment" option proposed for elderly prostate cancer patients is watchful waiting, namely, reserving intervention to the time of disease progression. This is an appealing choice in elderly patients with multiple comorbidities and a limited life expectancy (192). The watchful waiting approach, however, is not appropriate in men with high-risk disease who have a reasonably long life expectancy. Neulander et al. evaluated watchful waiting in 54 elderly localized prostate cancer patients (193). At a median follow-up of 47 months, 28 patients (52%) developed disease progression, biochemical, clinical, or both. Median time to progression was 35 months. Predictors for disease progression included age greater than 75 years, Gleason score, and prostate-specific antigen (PSA). The authors conclude that watchful waiting may not be appropriate for elderly patients with a good performance status and Gleason score ≥6 and/or PSA ≥10 ng/mL. Given the excellent outcome and low toxicity profile of RT in elderly patients, a more prudent approach would be to offer definitive RT.

For invasive bladder cancer, aggressive treatment with combined modality therapies has been shown to be well tolerated in appropriately selected elderly patients (194–196). In patients with multiple comorbidities who are unable to undergo systemic chemotherapy, definitive RT alone should be considered, because it is associated with long-term cures in a modest percentage of patients (197,198). Santacaterina et al. treated 45 elderly patients (ages 70–85 years) with RT alone due to significant comorbidities precluding combined modality therapy (198). No patient developed significant acute morbidity or severe late sequelae. The three- and five-year survival rates of the entire group were 36% and 19.5%, respectively. Others have proposed the use of a split course RT approach in poor performance status bladder cancer patients in an effort to improve treatment tolerance (199,200). In a series of 89 stage T1–4 patients treated with 10 to 12 fractions of split course RT (total dose, 31.5–57.7 Gy), 28 (31%) achieved a complete response (200). Significant late toxicities were noted in seven patients (8%).

Gynecologic Cancer

Controversy exists regarding the impact of age on the outcome of irradiated gynecologic patients. Most of the available data focuses on women with cervical cancer undergoing definitive RT, consisting of both pelvic RT and intracavitary brachytherapy. In some reports, a correlation is seen between age and survival, with older patients experiencing poorer outcomes (201–203). However, in several detailed studies from Japan and the United States focusing on women undergoing comparable treatment, differences in outcome have not been seen (204–208), suggesting that observed outcome disparities based on age may be due, at least in part, to less aggressive treatment in older patients.

Sakurai et al. evaluated outcomes in 380 cervical cancer patients undergoing pelvic RT and intracavitary brachytherapy (207). Patients were divided into three age groups: less than 70 (215 patients), 70 to 79 (124 patients) and greater than 80 years (41 patients). The five-year actuarial cause-specific survivals of the three groups were 68%, 70%, and 65%, respectively. Of note, no significant differences were seen in pelvic recurrence. Mitchell et al. compared outcomes in 60 elderly cervical cancer patients (age greater than 70) with those in 338 patients aged 35 to 69 years (208). Elderly women were noted to have a higher rate of significant comorbidities resulting in more frequent treatment breaks and/or the inability to undergo intracavitary brachytherapy. After controlling for treatment differences, however, outcomes of the older and younger patients were similar.

A commonly held belief is that advancing age is also an adverse prognostic factor in endometrial cancer (209). However, outcome differences based on age may be simply due to the higher prevalence of adverse pathologic features in older women, including deep myometrial invasion, grade 3 tumors, cervical involvement, extrauterine disease, and unfavorable histologies (210). Observed differences may also result from the propensity to perform less complete surgical staging and to deliver less aggressive treatment in older women. In a review of 455 endometrial cancer patients undergoing primary surgery with or without adjuvant RT, Mundt et al. noted a nonsignificant trend to a poorer outcome in older patients (211). The five-year disease-free survivals in women aged less than 60, between 60 and 69, and over 70 years were 74.3%, 70.2%, and 60.3%, respectively ($P = 0.08$). However, after controlling for differences in pathologic features and treatment, increasing age was not associated with a higher risk of recurrence in the multivariate model ($P = 0.21$). In contrast, Alektiar et al. found an association between increasing age and outcome in pathologic stage I and II endometrial cancer patients undergoing adjuvant pelvic RT and/or vaginal brachytherapy (212). On multivariate analysis, age over 70 was associated with a poorer locoregional control, disease-free survival, and cause-specific survival.

Several provocative papers have been published over the years reporting frequent and serious acute and chronic RT-related sequelae in elderly gynecologic cancer patients undergoing pelvic RT. For example, Grant et al. reviewed the toxicity of pelvic irradiation in 31 gynecologic cancer patients aged 75 or higher (213). Of these, 10 (32%) failed to complete treatment secondary to acute symptoms and four (13%) purportedly died from treatment toxicity. However, many patients were treated with unconventional fractionation schemes (including large daily fractions), which certainly contributed to these poor results.

A large number of reports have been published over the years which contradict these results, noting comparable toxicity profiles between younger and older gynecologic patients undergoing RT (205,207,208,210,212,214–216). One exception is Corn et al. who noted a higher incidence of RT-related sequelae in older endometrial cancer patients in a review of 235 patients treated with adjuvant RT (217). Severe sequelae were seen in 11% of women aged over 65 versus 2% of patients aged 65 years or younger—a difference that remained significant in the multivariate analysis controlling for other patient and treatment factors. Of note, in a review of two large patterns of care studies focusing on cervical cancer, Lanciano et al. noted an inverse relationship between increasing age and the risk of severe toxicity, with the highest rates seen in women "below" the age of 40 (218). Taken together, the preponderance of the available data fails to support the belief that RT is more toxic in older gynecologic patients.

Unlike in other malignancies, brachytherapy plays an important role in the treatment of gynecologic tumors, notably cervical and endometrial cancers. Given that intracavitary brachytherapy has been traditionally delivered using low-dose-rate (LDR) approaches, patients typically must undergo general anesthesia and prolonged periods of bed rest, exposing themselves to numerous potential sequelae ranging from uterine perforation to pulmonary embolism. To assess the impact of age on such toxicity, Wollschlaeger et al. studied the type, frequency, and severity of in-hospital problems as a function of increasing age in 170 LDR gynecologic brachytherapy performed in cervical cancer patients (219). No differences were reported in the incidence or severity of infectious, GI, pulmonary, cardiac, or thromboembolic events between patients younger than 65 years versus those older than 65 years. Similarly, Chao et al. evaluated 150 brachytherapy insertions in 96 medically inoperable stage I endometrial cancer patients (40, age >75) and noted significant sequelae in only four (3%), albeit most had multiple and often significant comorbidities (220). In contrast, Lanciano et al. analyzed 95 gynecologic brachytherapy treatments and found that age over 50 years was highly correlated with acute sequelae (221). In fact, age >50 years remained the only significant factor on the multivariate analysis controlling for other confounding factors including comorbidities.

As described later in this chapter, newer brachytherapy techniques, notably high-dose-rate (HDR), which obviate the need for general anesthesia and prolonged bed rest (see Section on "Special Radiation Technologies and Procedures in the Elderly"), may help reduce the risk of significant acute toxicity in elderly gynecologic patients undergoing brachytherapy. Nonetheless, HDR approaches remain associated with potential significant acute sequelae, particularly in patients with severe comorbidities (222).

An unfortunate practice resulting from concerns over potential RT toxicity in elderly gynecologic patients is the withholding of "adjuvant" RT in gynecologic patients found to have high-risk features at the time of hysterectomy. This is particularly commonplace in elderly patients with endometrial cancer. Citron et al. reviewed the outcomes of 79 stage I and II endometrial cancer patients aged 75 or above undergoing definitive surgery with or without adjuvant RT (210). Adverse pathologic features were common, including deep myometrial invasion (47%), grade 3 disease (28%), and unfavorable histologies (15%). In fact, 46 (58%) patients were noted to have one or more adverse pathologic features. Despite strong evidence supporting its use (223,224), only 67% of the high risk patients ultimately received adjuvant RT, predominantly due to concerns over potential toxicity. At a median follow-up of 35 months, the five-year pelvic control rates in patients treated with and without adjuvant RT were 97% and 73.1%, respectively ($P = 0.02$). In the high-risk patients, corresponding pelvic controls were 97% and 47%, respectively ($P = 0.0001$) (Fig. 5). Moreover, adjuvant RT was associated with improved disease-free and overall survivals in these patients. When delivered, RT was well tolerated with only one patient developing a severe toxicity. Given the excellent outcome and low risk of significant toxicity in high-risk elderly endometrial cancer patients, adjuvant RT should be routinely administered in these patients to reduce their risk of relapse.

Lymphoma

Traditionally, RT has occupied a central role in the management of patients with Hodgkin's disease (HD) and non-Hodgkin's lymphoma (NHL). In both, particularly

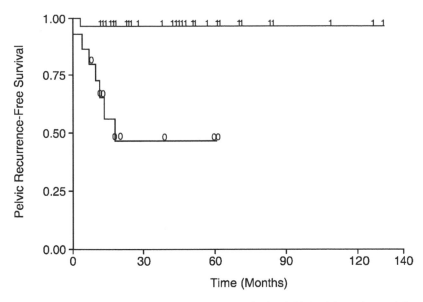

Figure 5 Five-year pelvic relapse-free survival of high-risk endometrial cancer patients treated with adjuvant radiotherapy (1) versus surgery alone (0) ($P < 0.001$ by log rank test). *Source*: From Ref. 213.

in HD, treatment consisted of wide-field irradiation volumes (e.g., total nodal, mantle, and inverted Y fields). Although more commonly diagnosed in younger patients, several investigators have evaluated the outcomes of elderly HD patients undergoing wide-field irradiation techniques, demonstrating the feasibility and success of this approach in properly selected patients (225,226). In a review of 29 stage I and II HD patients aged 60 or above, Zeitman et al. noted that 14 (48%) received optimal staging (laparotomy and/or complete radiographic workup) and optimal treatment (wide-field treatment, total doses of 36–44 Gy) (225). Of these, none relapsed at a median follow-up of 4.75 years. In contrast, 10 of 15 of the suboptimally staged and/or treated patients relapsed. The five-year overall survivals of the optimally and suboptimally managed patients were 61% and 19%, respectively ($P < 0.001$). Corresponding disease-free survivals were 100% and 39%, respectively ($P < 0.01$). Treatment was tolerated even in the radically treated group, with 3 of 14 patients experiencing significant acute toxicity resulting in unplanned treatment breaks and only one developing a significant late toxicity.

Today, the management of both HD and NHL patients has shifted away from the use of wide-field definitive RT to primary chemotherapy approaches (227). When delivered, RT generally consists of localized (limited) treatment volumes, i.e., involved field RT or extended field RT (EFRT), following chemotherapy. Several investigators have reported promising results with acceptable toxicity profiles utilizing such combinations of chemotherapy and limited volume irradiation in elderly patients (228,229).

It should be remembered, however, that localized RT is always a viable treatment option for many elderly lymphoma patients unable to tolerate systemic chemotherapy. In fact, in properly selected elderly NHL patients, limited volume RT alone can be curative (230,231). Wylie et al. reviewed the outcomes of 81 elderly (median age, 78 years) stage I and II NHL patients unable to undergo chemotherapy who were treated with EFRT alone (230). At a median follow-up of 3.9 years, the five-year disease-free and overall survivals of the entire group were 31% and 33%, respectively. However, a favorable subset of patients was identified (age ≤80 years, stage I disease, lactate dehydrogenase levels ≤500), with five-year disease-free and overall survivals of 56% and 62%, respectively.

Skin Cancer

While RT is commonly used in the treatment of skin cancer, no published series has focused exclusively on tolerance and outcome of elderly skin cancer patients undergoing RT. However, series of predominantly elderly patients report excellent tumor control and low rates of toxicity. Lovett et al. reviewed the outcome of 339 primarily elderly (majority in their 70s and 80s) skin cancer patients treated with RT at Washington University (232). Treatment was tolerated well with severe late sequelae seen in only 5.5% of patients. Overall, 92% of patients had excellent or good cosmesis.

A special concern in elderly patients is the problem of neglected skin cancers. Because of their indolent nature, skin cancers may go unnoticed or frankly ignored, while ultimately becoming quite large. Elderly nursing home patients or victims of elder abuse may be especially at risk for neglected cancers, which can be painful and can bleed profusely. Even large tumors can be treated effectively with a short course of RT, typically three weeks' duration, with both curative and palliative effects (Fig. 6).

Metastatic Disease

In elderly cancer patients in whom cure is not possible, palliation of symptoms in an effort to improve patient quality of life is of paramount importance. In patients with painful bone metastases, RT is an effective means of palliation (233), alleviating pain in approximately 70% of patients (234). Short course regimens with high daily fractions are typically used; even a single fraction of 8 Gy can lead to effective and durable palliation of bone metastases. Toxicity is mild and self-limited, regardless of patient age (235). An appealing approach to palliation of diffuse bone metastases in the elderly is treatment with injectable radionuclides strontium-89 or samarium-153. These are one-time treatments with few side effects; myelosuppression is the principal toxicity (236).

RT is also commonly used in the palliative treatment of metastases to other disease sites in elderly cancer patients. Brain metastases are typically treated with short courses of RT, typically 30 Gy in 10 fractions. Few acute sequelae are expected, even in the older patients (235). RT is also commonly used to treat metastatic vertebral lesions resulting in impingement or compression of the spinal cord, an infrequent but devastating event in the elderly cancer patient. Other indications for palliative RT in the elderly include symptomatic liver metastases (237), orbital metastases (238), and carcinomatous meningitis (239). Palliative RT is also beneficial in the treatment of elderly patients with symptomatic locally advanced disease (240,241).

Benign Conditions

Various benign conditions arising in the older patient can also be successfully treated with RT, including macular degeneration (242), pterygium (243), Grave's

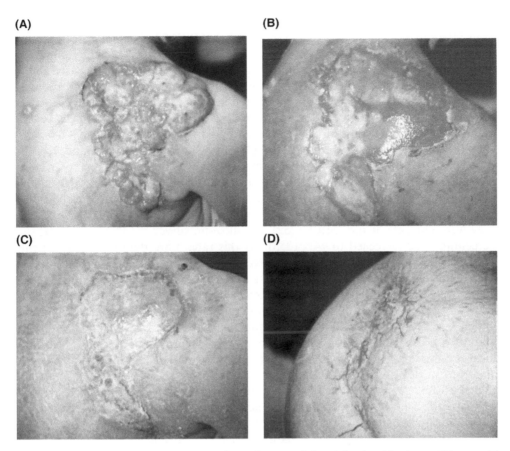

Figure 6 Neglected skin squamous cell carcinoma of the right shoulder in an 85-year-old female nursing home resident: (**A**) prior to RT, and (**B**) immediately following RT. The patient was treated with opposed oblique 6 MV photon fields to 45 Gy in 3 Gy daily fractions. Daily bolus was applied to raise the surface dose: (**C**) six weeks following RT, and (**D**) one year following RT. *Abbreviation*: RT, radiation therapy. *Source*: Courtesy of Azhar Awan, M.D., University of Chicago, Department of Radiation and Cellular Oncology, Chicago, IL.

opthalmoplegia (244), and Peyronie's disease (245). Prophylactic RT is also commonly administered in select arthroplasty patients to prevent the development of heterotopic ossification (246). Until recently, intracoronary irradiation (brachytherapy) was popular in the treatment of patients with in-stent restenosis (247). This approach, however, has given way to the use of drug-eluting stents (248).

SPECIAL RADIATION TECHNOLOGIES AND PROCEDURES IN THE ELDERLY

Intensity-Modulated RT

Despite tremendous technologic advancements in radiation oncology achieved over the last century, the basic approach to the planning and delivery of RT has remained relatively unchanged. After determining the site to be treated, a limited number of treatment beams are selected. Beam parameters are then altered iteratively in order to produce a treatment plan that best irradiates the target tissues while avoiding, whenever possible, normal tissues.

In recent years, however, a novel approach to RT planning and delivery has been introduced, known as intensity-modulated RT (IMRT). Unlike conventional techniques, IMRT conforms the prescription dose to the shape of the target in three dimensions, thereby reducing the volume of normal tissues irradiated. Based on an "inverse" approach, modulated beams are generated using computerized optimization software (249). These beams are delivered at most centers on a linear accelerator equipped with a multileaf collimator, whose "leaves" move in and out of the beam's path under computer control. When cast into a patient, highly conformal dose distributions are achieved. Example IMRT plans are shown in Figures 7 and 8.

Until recently, IMRT was performed at only a limited number of centers around the world. However, with the increasing availability of commercialized planning systems, IMRT is now widely performed in the United States and abroad. In a 2002 practice survey of radiation oncologists in the United States, 32% stated that they were currently using IMRT (252). A follow-up survey in 2004 found that this percentage had increased to 74% (253). At this rate, more than 90% of practicing radiation oncologists may be using this technology by mid-2006.

Multiple investigators have demonstrated the benefits of IMRT in a wide variety of tumor sites. To date, the greatest experience has been in the treatment of head and neck cancer. Lee et al. reported the outcome of 67 nasopharyngeal carcinoma patients treated with IMRT (254). Seventy percent had stage III and IV disease and 50 patients received concomitant chemoradiotherapy. The four-year actuarial local progression-free, locoregional progression-free, and distant metastasis progression-free survivals were 97%, 98%, and 66%, respectively. Grade 3 and 4 chronic toxicities were seen in eight patients. In a subsequent report, these same investigators reported the outcomes of 150 head and neck cancer patients treated with IMRT—most had tumors of the nasopharynx or oropharynx (255). The three-year actuarial local control of the definitive RT patients was 95%; in postoperative patients; the two-year local control rate was 83%. Chao et al. reported treatment outcomes in

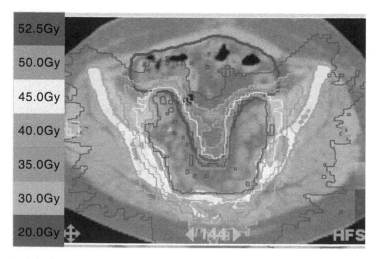

Figure 7 IMRT plan in a cervical cancer patient. The isodose lines are superimposed over an axial computed tomography image in the upper pelvis. The high-dose isodose lines conform to the laterally placed iliac lymph node regions and posteriorly to the presacral region, sparing the centrally placed small bowel. *Abbreviation*: IMRT, intensity-modulated radiation therapy. *Source*: From Ref. 250.

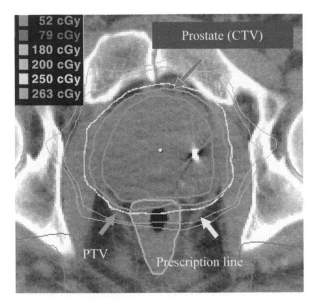

Figure 8 IMRT plan in a prostate cancer patient treated with hypofractionated IMRT. *Abbreviations*: IMRT, intensity-modulated radiation therapy; CTV, clinical treatment volume; PTV, planning treatment volume. *Source*: From Ref. 251.

41 head and neck IMRT patients, focusing on salivary gland function (256). Objective and subjective improvements were seen in both xerostomia and quality of life.

Favorable outcomes have also been seen using IMRT in the treatment of prostate cancer. Zelefsky et al. reviewed 171 localized prostate cancer patients treated with IMRT and compared their outcomes with those seen in conventionally treated patients (257). Significant reductions were seen using IMRT in terms of the volume of bladder and rectum irradiated to high doses. Moreover, grade 2 rectal bleeding was significantly lower in the IMRT group. The two-year actuarial risk of grade 2 rectal bleeding was 2% for IMRT versus 10% for conventional RT ($P < 0.001$). In an update of their experience, these same investigators reported on the outcome of 772 patients (258). Most patients received doses of 81 Gy or above, a dose significantly higher than that conventionally given in the treatment of prostate cancer. Nonetheless, acute grade 2 or higher rectal toxicity was seen in only 4.5% of patients. The three-year actuarial biochemical disease-free survivals were 92%, 86%, and 81%, respectively.

Promising results have also been reported using IMRT in other tumor sites arising in older cancer patients, including breast cancer (259), gynecologic tumors (260), pancreatic cancer (261), brain tumors (262), and soft tissue sarcomas (263).

IMRT has considerable potential in the treatment of the older cancer patient. Sparing of normal tissues may reduce the risk and severity of RT-related toxicities, improving the delivery of treatment and the quality of life of the patient (254–260). Highly conformal IMRT plans may also allow the delivery of higher than conventional doses, improving tumor control (257,258). IMRT may provide a safe and effective means of "reducing" the overall treatment time in select tumor site without increased toxicity (264,265). At the Cleveland Clinic, localized prostate cancer patients were treated with a short-course (hypofractionated) IMRT approach consisting of 70 Gy in 2.5 Gy daily fractions (265). In their most recent analysis, Djemil et al.

reported on 100 T1–3 patients with a median follow-up of 43 months (266). The six-year actuarial relapse-free survival of the entire group was 88%. Treatment was well tolerated, with no patient experiencing grade 3 or higher acute toxicity. The four-year actuarial risk of grade 2 or higher rectal sequelae was 6%.

IMRT may also provide an effective means of "re-treating" patients who have had a recurrence within a previously irradiated field, providing increased options for these patients. Milker-Zabel et al. treated 18 previously irradiated patients with recurrent spinal metastases (267). The median prior RT dose was 38 Gy. The median reirradiation dose was 39.6 Gy. With a median follow-up of 12.3 months, 95% of patients were locally controlled, with 81% experiencing pain relief. No grade 3 acute or late toxicities were noted. Current clinical trials are underway, evaluating IMRT in the treatment of a wide variety of disease sites in patients in the United States, Europe, and Asia.

HDR Brachytherapy

Since its inception, brachytherapy has traditionally been performed using LDR approaches, whereby treatment is delivered over several hours to days. In women with cervical cancer, for example, treatment is delivered in multiple sessions, each lasting two to four days. Given the concerns over radiation exposure, treatment must be delivered as an inpatient therapy with the patient confined to a specially shielded, private room. Visitors are not allowed and interaction with the hospital staff is minimized. In many patients, strict bed rest is required in order to avoid displacement of the brachytherapy applicator (Fig. 9).

In recent years, increasing attention has turned to the use of HDR brachytherapy approaches, whereby treatment is delivered over a few minutes using a high-activity [198]Ir source. Such an approach has several important advantages in the elderly. Foremost, it obviates the need for an inpatient hospitalization as well as prolonged bed rest. This is particularly appealing in older patients at high risk for deep venous thromboses and pulmonary emboli. HDR brachytherapy also avoids isolation of elderly patients from friends and family, a particular concern in patients suffering from cognitive deficits.

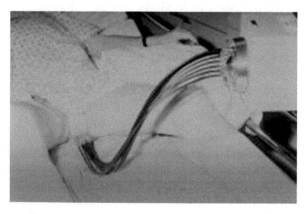

Figure 9 Patient with prostate cancer undergoing HDR brachytherapy. Needles are inserted transperineally under ultrasound guidance and after-loaded with HDR [192]Ir. *Abbreviations*: HDR, high-dose-rate; ^{192}Ir, iridium-192. *Source*: Courtesy of Douglas A. Kelly, Cancer Treatment Centers of America, Tulsa, Oklahoma, U.S.A.

HDR brachytherapy is currently being used in a large number of tumor sites. One of its most popular use is in the treatment of gynecologic malignancies. Multiple investigators have reported excellent tumor control and low complication rates using HDR following surgery (268) and in conjunction with external beam RT in cervical and endometrial cancers (269,270). HDR is also commonly used in the treatment of patients with prostate cancer (271), soft tissue sarcoma (272), and head and neck cancers (273).

Another increasingly common use of HDR brachytherapy is in the treatment of breast cancer. While adjuvant irradiation has traditionally been delivered to the entire breast via external beam RT, PBI approaches such as the Mammosite® brachytherapy device (Cytyc Corporation, Marlborough, Massachusetts, U.S.) are gaining in popularity (Fig. 10). Support for PBI is provided by the fact that patterns of failure studies have demonstrated that the majority of tumor recurrences occur within or near the lumpectomy site (274–276).

Mammosite is an intracavitary brachytherapy approach, whereby treatment is delivered to the lumpectomy site and nearby surrounding tissues following breast-conserving surgery. At the time of lumpectomy (or later, under ultrasound guidance), a balloon catheter is placed within the surgical cavity. Once in place, the balloon is inflated and an HDR source is inserted; delivery of treatment is over a few minutes, typically twice daily over five days.

The appeal of Mammosite in breast cancer patients in general and in the elderly in particular is clear. Unlike the six-week course of whole breast RT, Mammosite is performed over five days. Mammosite also reduces the risk of adverse acute and chronic sequelae, including prolonged fatigue, which is common during and after whole breast RT. While still in its infancy, Mammosite use is growing rapidly, with over 10,000 women treated to date, and with numerous favorable clinical reports (277,278). A large prospective randomized trial (NSABP-39) is currently underway, comparing whole breast irradiation and PBI. The results of this important trial will help determine the optimal RT approach in early-stage breast cancer patients (young and elderly alike).

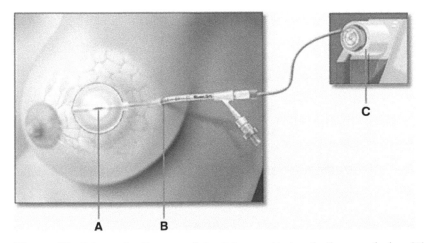

Figure 10 Schematic diagram of the Mammosite brachytherapy device. (**A**) Radioactive source inserted into balloon. (**B**) Mammosite catheter inserted at the time of lumpectomy or shortly thereafter. (**C**) High dose rate brachytherapy afterloading device. *Source*: Courtesy of Proxima Therapeutics, Alpharetta, Georgia, USA.

Stereotactic Radiosurgery

Stereotactic radiosurgery (SRS) is a specialized external beam technique whereby a large, single dose (or limited number of doses) of radiation is delivered to a small volume with high precision. Initially proposed by Leksell in the late 1940s, SRS was only available at a limited number of centers until recent years. In patients with intracranial tumors, SRS is delivered with either a dedicated ^{60}Co unit (Gamma Knife, Elekta Corporation, Stockholm, Sweden) (Fig. 11) or a modified linear accelerator. Multiple beams (or arcs) are used to conform the prescription dose to the target lesion(s); rapid dose falloff results in sparing of surrounding normal tissues. Immobilization is ensured with the aid of surgical pins in the patient's skull or with a relocatable head frame (Fig. 12).

SRS is an appealing approach in older patients because it provides a noninvasive alternative to surgery. Excellent control rates with low toxicity have been reported in a wide variety of brain tumors, including meningiomas, which are commonly diagnosed in the older patient (279). SRS also provides an effective, low-risk means of treating brain metastases in patients with lung, breast, and other malignancies. At a median follow-up of 8.8 months, Schomas et al. reported a local control rate of 88.6% in 80 patients (126 brain metastases) undergoing SRS (280). Other investigators have similarly reported excellent control rates with low rates of toxicity (281,282).

At most centers, SRS is delivered as a "boost" following whole brain RT (WBRT). The benefits of the combined approach were demonstrated in a randomized trial performed by Kondziolka et al. in patients with two to four brain lesions (283). Local control rates at one year following WBRT alone versus WBRT plus SRS were 0% and 92%, respectively, prompting the study to close early. Corresponding median times to local failure were 6 and 36 months, respectively ($P = 0.0005$).

Interest has been raised in the use of SRS alone, particularly in patients with a limited number of metastases, due to concerns over the adverse neurocognitive effects of WBRT. In fact, at some centers, such patients undergo SRS alone and,

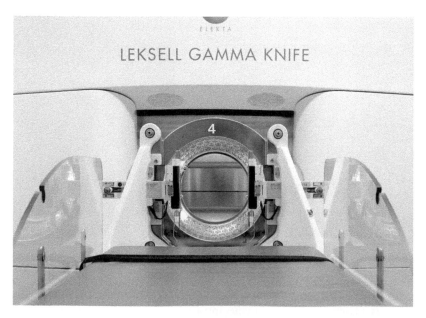

Figure 11   Gamma knife unit. *Source*: Courtesy of Elekta Corporation, Stockholm, Sweden.

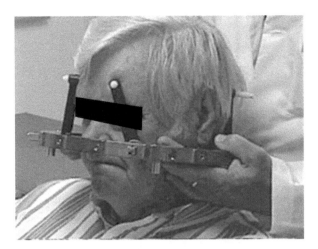

Figure 12 Head-ring used for SRS. During treatment, the ring is secured to the treatment couch to minimize patient movement. *Abbreviation*: SRS, stereotactic radiosurgery. *Source*: Courtesy of John M. Buatti, University of Iowa, Iowa City, Iowa, U.S.A.

if other metastases develop, SRS is repeated (with or without WBRT). The American College of Surgeons Oncology Group is currently conducting a randomized trial comparing SRS alone versus SRS plus WBRT in this setting.

SRS may also have a role in the treatment of select extracranial sites. Its use in the treatment of early stage lung cancer has been explored as an alternative to surgical resection (284,285). Other potential uses of extracranial SRS are in patients with extracranial metastatic disease, reducing the need for prolonged courses of palliative RT or chemotherapy (286).

Prostate Seed Implants

Prostate seed implantation is a form of interstitial brachytherapy that involves the placement of radioactive "seeds" directly into the prostate gland. Radioactive isotopes ^{125}I or palladium-103 (^{103}Pd) with short half-lives are placed permanently, delivering treatment as they decay (Fig. 13).

Although it was first performed in the early 1900s, interest in this approach did not develop until the 1960s (287). Unfortunately, at that time, seeds were implanted under direct vision at the same time as the pelvic lymphadenectomy. Results were disappointing, most likely due to inadequate coverage of the prostate, and thus the approach was largely abandoned. In the 1980s, however, Blasko and coworkers popularized the transperineal approach under real-time ultrasound guidance, ensuring accurate positioning and improved dose coverage. At some centers, seed implants are also used as a "boost" in conjunction with external beam RT (287b).

Prostate seed implantation is an important treatment modality in the elderly prostate cancer patient because for it provides an alternative to both surgery and a prolonged course of external beam RT. Reported control rates have been comparable to both radical prostatectomy and external beam RT in early stage patients, with low rates of toxicity (289,290), apart from transient acute bladder symptoms (291). Excellent long-term outcomes have also been reported in high-risk patients. Merrick et al. recently reviewed the outcomes of 46 high-risk patients (T1c–T2b, Gleason Score 8–9, PSA ≤ 20 ng/mL) treated with external beam irradiation plus

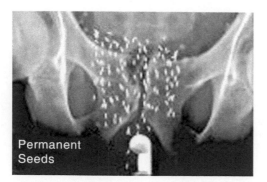

Permanent
Seeds

Figure 13   Anterior–posterior radiograph of the pelvis in a patient treated with LDR permanent prostate brachytherapy, illustrating seeds within the prostate gland. *Abbreviation*: LDR,
low-dose-rate. *Source*: Courtesy of Douglas A. Kelly, Cancer Treatment Centers of America,
Tulsa, Oklahoma, U.S.A.

[103]Pd seed implantation (292). Median patient age was 69.7 years. Thirteen patients
received six months of hormonal therapy. The seven-year actuarial biochemical
relapse-free survival of the entire group was 84.8%, with biochemical relapse defined
as any posttreatment PSA greater than 0.4 ng/mL or three consecutive rises. These
results suggest that such an approach may be appropriate in the properly selected
elderly localized prostate cancer patient. It should be noted that men with baseline
poor urinary function are not ideal candidates and should instead be treated with
external beam RT.

CONCLUSIONS

RT has long played, and continues to play, an important role in the treatment of the
older cancer patient. Although it is commonly believed that the elderly are at high
risk for the development of acute and chronic RT-related sequelae, the majority
of the available laboratory and clinical data do not support this view. In fact, RT
is beneficial and generally well-tolerated in the majority of older cancer patients.
Treatment decisions should instead be based on the general health and performance
status of the individual patient. Age per se should not be used as a reason to withhold definitive, adjuvant, or palliative RT.

It should be noted that elderly cancer patients often encounter particular barriers to receiving RT in many clinical situations when it is indicated. Awareness of
these issues is an important aspect of caring for the older cancer patient. Newer therapeutic technologies may also provide a means of reducing some of these barriers
and of improving the quality of life of the patients treated. Further research is
needed to clearly define the optimal role of RT in this important and growing group
of patients.

REFERENCES

1. http://cis.nci.nih.gov/fact/7_1.htm. Accessed May 26, 2005.
2. United States cancer statistics: 2001 Incidence and Mortality.

3. Yancik R, Yates JW, Cumberlin R. Research recommendations for radiation therapy in older cancer patients. Report from the National Institute on Aging, National Cancer Institute, and American College of Radiology Workshop: radiation therapy and cancer in older persons. Int J Radiat Oncol Biol Phys 1999; 43:3–5.

4. Mundt AJ, Roeske JC, Chung T, Weichselbaum RR. Principles of radiation oncology. In: Holland J, Frei E, Weichselbaum RR, eds. Cancer Medicine. Toronto, Canada: B. C. Decker, 2005:1223–1257.

5. Mor V, Masterson-Allen S, Goldberg RJ, Cummings FJ, Glicksman AS, Fretwell MD. Relationship between age at diagnosis and treatments received by cancer patients. J Am Geriatr Soc 1985; 33:585–589.

6. Samet J, Hunt WC, Key C, Humble CG, Goodwin JS. Choice of cancer therapy varies with age of patient. JAMA 1986; 255:3385–3390.

7. Goodwin JS, Samet JM, Hunt WC. Determinants of survival in older cancer patients. J Natl Cancer Inst 1996; 88:1031–1038.

8. Lash TL, Silliman RA, Guadagnoli E, Mor V. The effect of less than definitive care on breast carcinoma recurrence and mortality. Cancer 2000; 89:1739–1747.

9. Yancik R, Wesley MN, Ries LA, Havlik RJ, Edwards BK, Yates JW. Effect of age and comorbidity in postmenopausal breast cancer patients aged 55 years and older. JAMA 2001; 285:885–892.

10. O'Connell JB, Maggard MA, Ko CY. Cancer-directed surgery for localized disease: decreased use in the elderly. Ann Surg Oncol 2004; 11:962–969.

11. Silliman RA, Guadagnoli E, Weitberg AB, Mor V. Age as a predictor of diagnostic and initial treatment intensity in newly diagnosed breast cancer patients. J Gerontol 1989; 44:M46–M50.

12. Teeter SM, Holmes FF, McFarlane MJ. Lung carcinoma in the elderly population. Influence of histology on the inverse relationship of stage to age. Cancer 1987; 60:1331–1336.

13. Holmes FF. Clinical evidence for change in tumor aggressiveness with age. In: Balducci L, Lyman GH, Ershler WB, eds. Geriatric Oncology. Philadelphia: JB Lipincott Company, 1992:86–91.

14. Goodwin JS, Hunt WC, Samet JM. Determinants of cancer therapy in elderly patients. Cancer 1993; 72:594–601.

15. Goodwin JS, Hunt WC, Samet JM. A population-based study of functional status and social support networks of elderly patients newly diagnosed with cancer. Arch Intern Med 1991; 151:366–370.

16. Mor V, Allen S, Malin M. The psychosocial impact of cancer on older versus younger patients and their families. Cancer 1994; 74(suppl 7):2118–2127.

17. Berkman B, Rohan B, Sampson S. Myths and biases related to cancer in the elderly. Cancer 1994; 74(suppl 7):2004–2008.

18. Newcomb PA, Carbone PP. Cancer treatment and age: patient perspectives. J Natl Cancer Inst 1993; 85:1580–1584.

19. Wasil T, Lichtman SM, Gupta V, Rush S. Radiation therapy in cancer patients 80 years of age and older. Am J Clin Oncol 2000; 23:526–530.

20. Olmi P, Ausili-Cefaro G. Radiotherapy in the elderly: a multicentric prospective study on 2060 patients referred to 37 Italian radiation therapy centers. Rays 1997; 22(suppl 1): 53–56.

21. Huguenin P, Glanzmann C, Lutolf UM. Acute toxicity of curative radiotherapy in elderly patients. Strahlenther Onkol 1996; 172:658–663.

22. Given CW, Given BA, Stommel M. The impact of age, treatment, and symptoms on the physical and mental health of cancer patients. A longitudinal perspective. Cancer 1994; 74(suppl 7):2128–2138.

23. Zachariah B, Balducci L, Venkattaramanabalaji GV, Casey L, Greenberg HM, DelRegato JA. Radiotherapy for cancer patients aged 80 and older: a study of effectiveness and side effects. Int J Radiat Oncol Biol Phys 1997; 39:1125–1129.

24. Nozaki M, Murakami Y, Furuta M, Izawa Y, Iwasaki N. Radiation therapy for cancer in elderly patients over 80 years of age. Radiat Med 1998; 16:491–494.

25. Oguchi M, Ikeda H, Watanabe T, et al. Experiences of 23 patients > or = 90 years of age treated with radiation therapy. Int J Radiat Oncol Biol Phys 1998; 41:407–413.

26. Mitsuhashi N, Hayakawa K, Yamakawa M, et al. Cancer in patients aged 90 years or older: radiation therapy. Radiology 1999; 211:829–833.

27. Steinfeld AD, Diamond JJ, Hanks GE, Coia LR, Kramer S. Patient age as a factor in radiotherapy. Data from the Pattern of Care study. J Am Geriatr Soc 1989; 37(4): 335–338.

28. Rockwell S, Hughes CS, Kennedy KA. Effect of host age on microenvironmental heterogeneity and efficacy of combined modality therapy in solid tumors. Int J Radiat Oncol Biol Phys 1991; 20:259–263.

29. Rosenblum ML, Gerosa M, Dougherty DV, et al. Age-related chemosensitivity of stem cells from human malignant brain tumours. Lancet 1982; 1:885–887.

30. Taghian A, Ramsay J, Allalunis-Turner J, et al. Intrinsic radiation sensitivity may not be the major determinant of the poor clinical outcome of glioblastoma multiforme. Int J Radiat Oncol Biol Phys 1993; 25:243–249.

31. Rudat V, Dietz A, Conradt C, Weber KJ, Flentje M. In vitro radiosensitivity of primary human fibroblasts. Lack of correlation with acute radiation toxicity in patients with head and neck cancer. Radiother Oncol 1997; 43:181–188.

32. Little JB, Nove J, Strong LC, Nichols WW. Survival of human diploid skin fibroblasts from normal individuals after X-irradiation. Int J Radiat Biol 1988; 54:899–910.

33. Baeyens A, Van Den Broecke R, Makar A, Thierens H, De Ridder L, Vral A. Chromo-somal radiosensitivity in breast cancer patients: influence of age of onset of the disease. Oncol Rep 2005; 13:347–353.

34. Hopewell JW, Young CM. The effect of field size on the reaction of pig skin to single doses of X rays. Br J Radiol 1982; 55:356–361.

35. Masuda K, Matsuura K, Withers HR, Hunter N. Age dependency of response of the mouse skin to single and multifractionated gamma irradiation. Radiother Oncol 1986; 7:147–153.

36. Landuyt W, van der Schueren E. Effect of age on the radiation-induced repopulation in mouse lip mucosa. Strahlenther Onkol 1991; 167:41–45.

37. Rosen EM, Goldberg ID, Myrick KV, Levenson SE. Radiation survival of vascular smooth muscle cells as a function of age. Int J Radiat Biol Relat Stud Phys Chem Med 1985; 48:71–79.

38. Sargent EV, Burns FJ. Repair of radiation-induced DNA damage in rat epidermis as a function of age. Radiat Res 1985; 102(2):176–181.

39. Wong KK, Chang S, Weiler SR, et al. Telomere dysfunction impairs DNA repair and enhances sensitivity to ionizing radiation. Nat Genet 2000; 26:85–88.

40. Campisi J. Senescent cells, tumor suppression, and organismal aging: good citizens, bad neighbors. Cell 2005; 120:513–522.

41. Moulder JE, Fish BL. Age dependence of radiation nephropathy in the rat. Radiat Res 1997; 147:349–353.

42. Hamlet R, Hopewell JW. The differential response of the skin in young and old rats to a combination of X-rays and "wet" or "dry" hyperthermia. Int J Radiat Biol Relat Stud Phys Chem Med 1986; 50:853–859.

43. Hamilton E, Franks LM. Cell proliferation and ageing in mouse colon. II. Late effects of repeated x-irradiation in young and old mice. Eur J Cancer 1980; 16:663–669.

44. Olofsen-van Acht MJ, van Hooije CM, van den Aardweg GJ, Levendag PC, van Velthuysen ML. Effect of age on radiation-induced early changes of rat rectum. A histological time sequence. Radiother Oncol 2001; 59:71–79.

45. van den Aardweg GJ, Olofsen-van Acht MJ, van Hooije CM, Levendag PC. Radiation-induced rectal complications are not influenced by age: a dose fractionation study in the rat. Radiat Res 2003; 159:642–650.

46. Crosfill ML, Lindop PJ, Rotblat J. Variation of sensitivity to ionizing radiation with age. Nature 1959; 183:1729–1730.

47. Hursh JB, Casarett GW. The lethal effect of acute x-irradiation on rats as a function of age. Br J Radiol 1956; 29:169–171.

48. Lamproglou I, Baillet F, Boisserie G, Mazeron JJ, Delattre JY. The influence of age on radiation-induced cognitive deficit: experimental studies on brain irradiation of 30 Gy in 10 sessions and 12 hours in the Wistar rat at $1\frac{1}{2}$, 4, and 18 months age. Can J Physiol Pharmacol 2002; 80:679–685.

49. Shaw E, Seiferheld W, Scott C, et al. Reexamining the radiation therapy oncology group (RTOG) recursive partitioning analysis (RPA) for glioblastoma multiforme (GBM) patients [abstr]. Proc Am Soc Thera Rad Oncol (ASTRO), Int J Radiat Oncol Biol Phys 2003; 57(2):S135–S136.

50. Barker FG II, Chang SM, Larson DA, et al. Age and radiation response in glioblastoma multiforme. Neurosurgery 2001; 49:1288–1297.

51. Shibamoto Y, Ogino H, Hasegawa M. Results of radiation monotherapy for primary central nervous system lymphoma in the 1990s. Int J Radiat Oncol Biol Phys 2005; 62:809–813.

52. Peschel RE, Wilson L, Haffty B, Papadopoulos D, Rosenzweig K, Feltes M. The effect of advanced age on the efficacy of radiation therapy for early breast cancer, local prostate cancer and grade III-IV gliomas. Int J Radiat Oncol Biol Phys 1993; 26(3): 539–544.

53. Lutterbach J, Bartelt S, Momm F, Becker G, Frommhold H, Ostertag C. Is older age associated with a worse prognosis due to different patterns of care? A long-term study of 1346 patients with glioblastomas or brain metastases. Cancer 2005; 103: 1234–1244.

54. Walker MD, Green SB, Byar DP, et al. Randomized comparisons of radiotherapy and nitrosoureas for the treatment of malignant glioma after surgery. N Engl J Med 1980; 303:1323–1329.

55. Marijnen CA, van den Berg SM, van Duinen SG, Voormolen JH, Noordijk EM. Radiotherapy is effective in patients with glioblastoma multiforme with a limited prognosis and in patients above 70 years of age: a retrospective single institution analysis. Radiother Oncol 2005; 75(2):210–216.

56. Villa S, Vinolas N, Verger E, et al. Efficacy of radiotherapy for malignant gliomas in elderly patients. Int J Radiat Oncol Biol Phys 1998; 42:977–980.

57. Mohan DS, Suh JH, Phan JL, Kupelian PA, Cohen BH, Barnett GH. Outcome in elderly patients undergoing definitive surgery and radiation therapy for supratentorial glioblastoma multiforme at a tertiary care institution. Int J Radiat Oncol Biol Phys 1998; 42:981–987.

58. Meckling S, Dold O, Forsyth PA, Brasher P, Hagen NA. Malignant supratentorial glioma in the elderly: is radiotherapy useful? Neurology 1996; 47:901–905.

59. Chang EL, Yi W, Allen PK, Levin VA, Sawaya RE, Maor MH. Hypofractionated radiotherapy for elderly or younger low-performance status glioblastoma patients: outcome and prognostic factors. Int J Radiat Oncol Biol Phys 2003; 56:519–528.

60. Phillips C, Guiney M, Smith J, Hughes P, Narayan K, Quong G. A randomized trial comparing 35 Gy in ten fractions with 60 Gy in 30 fractions of cerebral irradiation for glioblastoma multiforme and older patients with anaplastic astrocytoma. Radiother Oncol 2003; 68:23–26.

61. Roa W, Brasher PM, Bauman G, et al. Abbreviated course of radiation therapy in older patients with glioblastoma multiforme: a prospective randomized clinical trial. J Clin Oncol 2004; 22:1583–1588.

62. Stupp R, Mason WP, van den Bent MJ, et al. European Organisation for Research and Treatment of Cancer Brain Tumor and Radiotherapy Groups; National Cancer Institute of Canada Clinical Trials Group. Radiotherapy plus concomitant and adjuvant temozolomide for glioblastoma. N Engl J Med 2005; 352:987–996.

63. Athanassiou H, Synodinou M, Maragoudakis E, et al. Randomized phase II study of temozolomide and radiotherapy compared with radiotherapy alone in newly diagnosed glioblastoma multiforme. J Clin Oncol 2005; 23:2372–2377.

64. Kelly PJ, Hunt C. The limited value of cytoreductive surgery in elderly patients with malignant gliomas. Neurosurgery 1994; 34:62–66.

65. Vuorinen V, Hinkka S, Farkkila M, Jaaskelainen J. Debulking or biopsy of malignant glioma in elderly people—a randomised study. Acta Neurochir (Wien) 2003; 145:5–10.

66. Muacevic A, Kreth FW. Quality-adjusted survival after tumor resection and/or radiation therapy for elderly patients with glioblastoma multiforme. J Neurol 2003; 250: 561–568.

67. Chinot OL, Barrie M, Frauger E, et al. Phase II study of temozolomide without radiotherapy in newly diagnosed glioblastoma multiforme in an elderly population. Cancer 2004; 100:2208–2214.

68. Shaw EG. Nothing ventured, nothing gained: treatment of glioblastoma multiforme in the elderly. J Clin Oncol 2004; 22:1540–1541.

69. Brandes AA, Vastola F, Basso U, et al. A prospective study on glioblastoma in the elderly. Cancer 2003; 97:657–662.

70. Glantz M, Chamberlain M, Liu Q, Litofsky NS, Recht LD. Temozolomide as an alternative to irradiation for elderly patients with newly diagnosed malignant gliomas. Cancer 2003; 97:2262–2266.

71. Chamberlain MC, Recht LD, Glantz M. Regarding "abbreviated course of radiation therapy in older patients with glioblastoma multiforme: a prospective randomized clinical trial." J Clin Oncol 2005; 23:1587–1588.

72. Mirimanoff RO, Dosoretz DE, Linggood RM, Ojemann RG, Martuza RL. Meningioma: analysis of recurrence and progression following neurosurgical resection. J Neurosurg 1985; 62:18–24.

73. Mendenhall WM, Morris CG, Amdur RJ, Foote KD, Friedman WA. Radiotherapy alone or after subtotal resection for benign skull base meningiomas. Cancer 2003; 98:1473–1482.

74. Connell PP, Macdonald RL, Mansur DB, Nicholas MK, Mundt AJ. Tumor size predicts control of benign meningiomas treated with radiotherapy. Neurosurgery 1999; 44:1194–1199.

75. Sheehan JP, Niranjan A, Sheehan JM, et al. Stereotactic radiosurgery for pituitary adenomas: an intermediate review of its safety, efficacy, and role in the neurosurgical treatment armamentarium. J Neurosurg 2005; 102:678–691.

76. Chung WY, Liu KD, Shiau CY, et al. Gamma knife surgery for vestibular schwannoma: 10-year experience of 195 cases. J Neurosurg 2005; 102(suppl):87–96.

77. Freilich RJ, Delattre JY, Monjour A, DeAngelis LM. Chemotherapy without radiation therapy as initial treatment for primary CNS lymphoma in older patients. Neurology 1996; 46:435–439.

78. Maire JP, Coudin B, Guerin J, Caudry M. Neuropsychologic impairment in adults with brain tumors. Am J Clin Oncol 1987; 10:156–162.

79. Laack NN, Brown PD. Cognitive sequelae of brain radiation in adults. Semin Oncol 2004; 31:702–713.

80. Lusinchi A, Bourhis J, Wibault P, Le Ridant AM, Eschwege F. Radiation therapy for head and neck cancers in the elderly. Int J Radiat Oncol Biol Phys 1990; 18:819–823.

81. Chin R, Fisher RJ, Smee RI, Barton MB. Oropharyngeal cancer in the elderly. Int J Radiat Oncol Biol Phys 1995; 32:1007–1016.

82. Pignon T, Horiot JC, van den Bogaert W, Van Glabbeke M, Scalliet P. No age limit for radical radiotherapy in head and neck tumours. Eur J Cancer 1996; 32A(12):2075–2081.

83. Schofield CP, Sykes AJ, Slevin NJ, Rashid NZ. Radiotherapy for head and neck cancer in elderly patients. Radiother Oncol 2003; 69:37–42.

84. Horiot JC, Bontemps P, van den Bogaert W, et al. Accelerated fractionation (AF) compared to conventional fractionation (CF) improves loco-regional control in the

radiotherapy of advanced head and neck cancers: results of the EORTC 22851 randomized trial. Radiother Oncol 1997; 44:111–121.

85. Allal AS, Maire D, Becker M, Dulguerov P. Feasibility and early results of accelerated radiotherapy for head and neck carcinoma in the elderly. Cancer 2000; 88:648–652.

86. Garden AS, Harris J, Vokes EE, et al. Preliminary results of Radiation Therapy Oncology Group 97–03: a randomized phase II trial of concurrent radiation and chemotherapy for advanced squamous cell carcinomas of the head and neck. J Clin Oncol 2004; 22:2856–2864.

87. Cooper JS, Pajak TF, Forastiere AA, et al. Postoperative concurrent radiotherapy and chemotherapy for high-risk squamous-cell carcinoma of the head and neck. N Engl J Med 2004; 350:1937–1944.

88. Kodaira T, Fuwa N, Furutani K, Tachibana H, Yamazaki T. Phase I trial of weekly docetaxel and concurrent radiotherapy for head and neck cancer in elderly patients or patients with complications. Jpn J Clin Oncol 2005; 35:173–176.

89. Harvey JC, Erdman C, Pisch J, Beattie EJ. Surgical treatment of non-small cell lung cancer in patients older than seventy years. J Surg Oncol 1995; 60(4):247–249.

90. Birim O, Zuydendorp HM, Maat AP, Kappetein AP, Eijkemans MJ, Bogers AJ. Lung resection for non-small-cell lung cancer in patients older than 70: mortality, morbidity, and late survival compared with the general population. Ann Thorac Surg 2003; 76(6):1796–1801.

91. Smith TJ, Penberthy L, Desch CE, et al. Differences in initial treatment patterns and outcomes of lung cancer in the elderly. Lung Cancer 1995; 13(3):235–252.

92. Guadagnoli E, Weitberg A, Mor V, Silliman RA, Glicksman AS, Cummings FJ. The influence of patient age on the diagnosis and treatment of lung and colorectal cancer. Arch Intern Med 1990; 150(7):1485–1490.

93. Ramsey SD, Howlader N, Etzioni RD, Donato B. Chemotherapy use, outcomes, and costs for older persons with advanced non-small-cell lung cancer: evidence from surveillance, epidemiology and end results-Medicare. J Clin Oncol 2004; 22(24):4971–4978.

94. Gava A, Bertossi L, Zorat PL, et al. Radiotherapy in the elderly with lung carcinoma: the experience of the Italian "Geriatric Radiation Oncology Group." Rays 1997; 22(suppl 1):61–65.

95. Jeremic B, Shibamoto Y, Milicic B, et al. A phase II study of concurrent accelerated hyperfractionated radiotherapy and carboplatin/oral etoposide for elderly patients with stage III non-small-cell lung cancer. Int J Radiat Oncol Biol Phys 1999; 44(2):343–348.

96. Pignon T, Gregor A, Schaake Koning C, Roussel A, Van Glabbeke M, Scalliet P. Age has no impact on acute and late toxicity of curative thoracic radiotherapy. Radiother Oncol 1998; 46(3):239–248.

97. Kusumoto S, Koga K, Tsukino H, Nagamachi S, Nishikawa K, Watanabe K. Comparison of survival of patients with lung cancer between elderly (greater than or equal to 70) and younger (70 greater than) age groups. Jpn J Clin Oncol 1986; 16(4):319–323.

98. Koga K, Kusumoto S, Watanabe K, Nishikawa K, Harada K, Ebihara. Age factor relevant to the development of radiation pneumonitis in radiotherapy of lung cancer. Int J Radiat Oncol Biol Phys 1988; 14(2):367–371.

99. Pergolizzi S, Santacaterina A, Renzis CD, et al. Older people with non small cell lung cancer in clinical stage IIIA and co-morbid conditions. Is curative irradiation feasible? Final results of a prospective study. Lung Cancer 2002; 37(2):201–206.

100. Hayakawa K, Mitsuhashi N, Katano S, et al. High-dose radiation therapy for elderly patients with inoperable or unresectable non-small cell lung cancer. Lung Cancer 2001; 32(1):81–88.

101. Schild SE, Stella PJ, Geyer SM, et al. The outcome of combined-modality therapy for stage III non-small-cell lung cancer in the elderly. J Clin Oncol 2003; 21(17):3201–3206.

102. Movsas B, Scott C, Sause W, et al. The benefit of treatment intensification is age and histology-dependent in patients with locally advanced non-small cell lung cancer

(NSCLC): a quality-adjusted survival analysis of radiation therapy oncology group (RTOG) chemoradiation studies. Int J Radiat Oncol Biol Phys 1999; 45(5):1143–1149.

103. Antonadou D, Throuvalas N, Petridis A, Bolanos N, Sagriotis A, Synodinou M. Effect of amifostine on toxicities associated with radiochemotherapy in patients with locally advanced non-small-cell lung cancer. Int J Radiat Oncol Biol Phys 2003; 57(2):402–408.

104. Komaki R, Lee JS, Milas L, et al. Effects of amifostine on acute toxicity from concurrent chemotherapy and radiotherapy for inoperable non-small-cell lung cancer: report of a randomized comparative trial. Int J Radiat Oncol Biol Phys 2004; 58:1369–1377.

105. Koukourakis MI, Kyrias G, Kakolyris S, et al. Subcutaneous administration of amifostine during fractionated radiotherapy: a randomized phase II study. J Clin Oncol 2000; 18(11):2226–2233.

106. Movsas B, Scott C, Langer C, et al. Randomized trial of amifostine in locally advanced non-small-cell lung cancer patients receiving chemotherapy and hyperfractionated radiation: radiation therapy oncology group trial 98–01. J Clin Oncol 2005; 23(10): 2145–2154.

107. Malik R, Mell LK, Mundt AJ. Meta-analysis of the effect of amifostine on response rates in advanced non-small cell lung cancer patients treated on randomized trials. American Society for Therapeutic Radiology and Oncology (ASTRO), Denver, Colorado, October 2005.

108. Gauden SJ, Tripcony L. The curative treatment by radiation therapy alone of stage I non-small cell lung cancer in a geriatric population. Lung Cancer 2001; 32(1):71–79.

109. Furuta M, Hayakawa K, Katano S, et al. Radiation therapy for stage I-II non-small cell lung cancer in patients aged 75 years and older. Jpn J Clin Oncol 1996; 26(2):95–98.

110. Dosoretz DE, Katin MJ, Blitzer PH, et al. Radiation therapy in the management of medically inoperable carcinoma of the lung: results and implications for future treatment strategies. Int J Radiat Oncol Biol Phys 1992; 24(1):3–9.

111. Sibley GS, Jamieson TA, Marks LB, Anscher MS, Prosnitz LR. Radiotherapy alone for medically inoperable stage I non-small-cell lung cancer: the Duke experience. Int J Radiat Oncol Biol Phys 1998; 40(1):149–154.

112. Krol AD, Aussems P, Noordijk EM, Hermans J, Leer JW. Local irradiation alone for peripheral stage I lung cancer: could we omit the elective regional nodal irradiation? Int J Radiat Oncol Biol Phys 1996; 34(2):297–302.

113. Graham MV, Purdy JA, Emami B, Matthews JW, Harms WB. Preliminary results of a prospective trial using three dimensional radiotherapy for lung cancer. Int J Radiat Oncol Biol Phys 1995; 33(5):993–1000.

114. Sandler HM, Curran WJ Jr, Turrisi AT. The influence of tumor size and pre-treatment staging on outcome following radiation therapy alone for stage I non-small cell lung cancer. Int J Radiat Oncol Biol Phys 1990; 19(1):9–13.

115. Kaskowitz L, Graham MV, Emami B, Halverson KJ, Rush C. Radiation therapy alone for stage I non-small cell lung cancer. Int J Radiat Oncol Biol Phys 1993; 27(3):517–523.

116. Blomgren H, Lax I, Naslund I, Svanstrom R. Stereotactic high dose fraction radiation therapy of extracranial tumors using an accelerator. Clinical experience of the first thirty-one patients. Acta Oncol 1995; 34(6):861–870.

117. Timmerman R, Papiez L, McGarry R, et al. Extracranial stereotactic radioablation: results of a phase I study in medically inoperable stage I non-small cell lung cancer. Chest 2003; 124(5):1946–1955.

118. Onishi H, Araki T, Shirato H, et al. Stereotactic hypofractionated high-dose irradiation for stage I nonsmall cell lung carcinoma: clinical outcomes in 245 subjects in a Japanese multiinstitutional study. Cancer 2004; 101(7):1623–1631.

119. Schild SE, Stella PJ, Brooks BJ, et al. Results of combined-modality therapy for limited-stage small cell lung carcinoma in the elderly. Cancer 2005; 103(11):2349–2354.

120. Quon H, Shepherd FA, Payne DG, et al. The influence of age on the delivery, tolerance, and efficacy of thoracic irradiation in the combined modality treatment of limited stage small cell lung cancer. Int J Radiat Oncol Biol Phys 1999; 43(1):39–45.

121. Jeremic B, Shibamoto Y, Acimovic L, Milisavljevic S. Carboplatin, etoposide, and accelerated hyperfractionated radiotherapy for elderly patients with limited small cell lung carcinoma: a phase II study. Cancer 1998; 82(5):836–841.

122. Tai TH, Yu E, Dickof P, et al. Prophylactic cranial irradiation revisited: cost-effectiveness and quality of life in small-cell lung cancer. Int J Radiat Oncol Biol Phys 2002; 52(1):68–74.

123. Busch E, Kemeny M, Fremgen A, Osteen RT, Winchester DP, Clive RE. Patterns of breast cancer care in the elderly. Cancer 1996; 78(1):101–111.

124. Du X, Freeman JL, Freeman DH, Syblik DA, Goodwin JS. Temporal and regional variation in the use of breast-conserving surgery and radiotherapy for older women with early-stage breast cancer from 1983 to 1995. J Gerontol A Biol Sci Med Sci 1999; 54(9):M474–M478.

125. Kantorowitz DA, Poulter CA, Sischy B, et al. Treatment of breast cancer among elderly women with segmental mastectomy or segmental mastectomy plus postoperative radiotherapy. Int J Radiat Oncol Biol Phys 1988; 15(2):263–270.

126. Ballard-Barbash R, Potosky AL, Harlan LC, Harlan LC, Nayfield SG, Kessler LG. Factors associated with surgical and radiation therapy for early stage breast cancer in older women. J Natl Cancer Inst 1996; 88(11):716–726.

127. Joslyn SA. Radiation therapy and patient age in the survival from early-stage breast cancer. Int J Radiat Oncol Biol Phys 1999; 44(4):821–826.

128. Mandelblatt JS, Kerner JF, Hadley J, et al. Variations in breast carcinoma treatment in older medicare beneficiaries: is it black or white. Cancer 2002; 95(7):1401–1414.

129. Merchant TE, McCormick D, Yahalom J, Borgen P. The influence of older age on breast cancer treatment decisions and outcome. Int J Radiat Oncol Biol Phys 1996; 34(3):565–570.

130. Goodwin JS, Samet JM. Care received by older women diagnosed with breast cancer. Cancer Control 1994; 1(4):313–319.

131. Newschaffer CJ, Penberthy L, Desch CE, Retchin SM, Whittemore M. The effect of age and comorbidity in the treatment of elderly women with nonmetastatic breast cancer. Arch Intern Med 1996; 156(1):85–90.

132. Hebert-Croteau N, Brisson J, Latreille J, Latreille J, Blanchette C, Deschenes L. Compliance with consensus recommendations for the treatment of early stage breast carcinoma in elderly women. Cancer 1999; 85(5):1104–1113.

133. Truong PT, Wong E, Bernstein V, Berthelet E, Kader HA. Adjuvant radiation therapy after breast-conserving surgery in elderly women with early-stage breast cancer: controversy or consensus? Clin Breast Cancer 2004; 4(6):407–414.

134. Giordano SH, Hortobagyi GN, Kau SW, Kau SW, Theriault RL, Bondy ML. Breast cancer treatment guidelines in older women. J Clin Oncol 2005; 23(4):783–791.

135. Gajdos C, Tartter PI, Bleiweiss IJ, Lopchinsky RA, Bernstein JL. The consequence of undertreating breast cancer in the elderly. J Am Coll Surg 2001; 192(6):698–707.

136. Velanovich V, Gabel M, Walker EM, et al. Causes for the undertreatment of elderly breast cancer patients: tailoring treatments to individual patients. J Am Coll Surg 2002; 194(1):8–13.

137. Liang W, Burnett CB, Rowland JH, et al. Communication between physicians and older women with localized breast cancer, implications for treatment and patient satisfaction. J Clin Oncol 2002; 20(4):1008–1016.

138. Silliman RA, Troyan SL, Guadagnoli E, Kaplan SH, Greenfield S. The impact of age, marital status, and physician-patient interactions on the care of older women with breast carcinoma. Cancer 1997; 80(7):1326–1334.

139. Veronesi U, Marubini E, Mariani L, et al. Radiotherapy after breast-conserving surgery in small breast carcinoma: long-term results of a randomized trial. Ann Oncol 2001; 12(7):997–1003.

140. Fisher B, Anderson S, Bryant J, et al. Twenty-year follow-up of a randomized trial comparing total mastectomy, lumpectomy, and lumpectomy plus irradiation for the treatment of invasive breast cancer. N Engl J Med 2002; 347(16):1233–1241.

141. Fyles AW, McCready DR, Manchul LA, et al. Tamoxifen with or without breast irradiation in women 50 years of age or older with early breast cancer. N Engl J Med 2004; 351(10):963–970.
142. Fisher B, Bryant J, Dignam JJ, et al. Tamoxifen, radiation therapy, or both for prevention of ipsilateral breast tumor recurrence after lumpectomy in women with invasive breast cancers of one centimeter or less. J Clin Oncol 2002; 20(20):4141–4149.
143. Truong PT, Lee J, Kader HA, Speers CH, Olivotto IA. Locoregional recurrence risks in elderly breast cancer patients treated with mastectomy without adjuvant radiotherapy. Eur J Cancer 2005; 41(9):1267–1277.
144. Ugnat AM, Xie L, Morriss J, Semenciw R, Mao Y. Survival of women with breast cancer in Ottawa, Canada: variation with age, stage, histology, grade, and treatment. Br J Cancer 2004; 90(6):1138–1143.
145. Vlastos G, Mirza NQ, Meric F, et al. Breast conservation therapy as a treatment option for the elderly. The M.D. Anderson experience. Cancer 2001; 92(5):1092–1100.
146. Toonkel LM, Fix I, Jacobson LH, Bamberg N. Management of elderly patients with primary breast cancer. Int J Radiat Oncol Biol Phys 1988; 14(4):677–681.
147. Hughes KS, Schnaper LA, Berry D, et al. Lumpectomy plus tamoxifen with or without irradiation in women 70 years of age or older with early breast cancer. N Engl J Med 2004; 351(10):971–977.
148. Gold HT, Dick AW. Variations in treatment for ductal carcinoma in situ in elderly women. Med Care 2004; 42(3):267–275.
149. Vicini FA, Recht A. Age at diagnosis and outcome for women with ductal carcinoma-in-situ of the breast: a critical review of the literature. J Clin Oncol 2002; 20(11):2736–2744.
150. Van Zee KJ, Liberman L, Samli B, et al. Long term follow-up of women with ductal carcinoma in situ treated with breast-conserving surgery: the effect of age. Cancer 1999; 86(9):1757–1767.
151. Silverstein MJ, Buchanan C. Ductal carcinoma in situ: USC/Van Nuys Prognostic Index and the impact of margin status. Breast 2003; 12(6):457–471.
152. Fisher ER, Dingnam J, Tan-Chiu E, et al. Pathologic findings from the National Surgical Adjuvant Breast Project (NSABP) eight year update of protocol B-17: intraductal carcinoma. Cancer 1999; 86:429–438.
153. Julien JP, Bijker N, Fentiman I, et al. Radiotherapy in breast conserving treatment for ductal carcinoma in situ: first results of EORTC randomized phase III trial 853. Lancet 2000; 355:528–533.
154. U.K. Coordinating Committee on Cancer Research (UKCCCR), Ductal Carcinoma in situ (DCIS), working party on behalf of the DCIS trialists in the U.K., Australia, and New Zealand. Radiotherapy and tamoxifen in women with completely excised ductal carcinoma in situ of the breast in the U.K., Australia, and New Zealand: randomized controlled trial. Lancet 2003; 362:95–102.
155. Shapiro CL, Recht A. Side effects of adjuvant treatment of breast cancer. N Engl J Med 2001; 344(26):1997–2008.
156. Howell A, Cuzick J, Baum M, et al. Results of the ATAC (arimidex, tamoxifen, alone or in combination) trial after completion of 5 years' adjuvant treatment for breast cancer. Lancet 2005; 365(9453):60–62.
157. Lonning PE, Geisler J, Krag LE, et al. Effects of exemestane administered for 2 years versus placebo on bone mineral density, bone biomarkers, and plasma lipids in patients with surgically resected early breast cancer. J Clin Oncol 2005; 23(22):5126–5137.
158. Dickler A, Kirk MC, Chu J, Nguyen C. The Mammosite breast brachytherapy applicator: a review of technique and outcomes. Brachytherapy 2005; 4(2):130–136.
159. Polgar C, Strnad V, Major T. Brachytherapy for partial breast irradiation: the European experience. Semin Radiat Oncol 2005; 15(2):116–122.
160. Formenti SC, Truong MT, Goldberg JD, et al. Prone accelerated partial breast irradiation after breast-conserving surgery: preliminary clinical results and dose-volume histogram analysis. Int J Radiat Oncol Biol Phys 2004; 60(2):493–504.

161. Veronesi U, Orecchia R, Luini A, et al. Full-dose intraoperative radiotherapy with electrons during breast-conserving surgery: experience with 590 cases. Ann Surg 2005; 242(1):101–106.

162. Lief EP, DeWyngaert JK, Lymberis SC, et al. Accelerated concomitant boost: emerging technology. In: Mundt AJ, Roeske JC, eds. Intensity Modulated Radiation Therapy: A Clinical Perspective. Toronto, Ontario: BC Decker, 2004.

163. Turesson I, Nyman J, Holmberg E, Oden A. Prognostic factors for acute and late skin reactions in radiotherapy patients. Int J Radiat Oncol Biol Phys 1996; 36(5): 1065–1075.

164. Steeves RA, Phromratanapongse P, Wolberg WH, Tormey DC. Cosmesis and local control after irradiation in women treated conservatively for breast cancer. Arch Surg 1989; 124(12):1369–1373.

165. Pezner RD, Patterson MP, Lipsett JA, et al. Factors affecting cosmetic outcome in breast-conserving cancer treatment—objective quantitative assessment. Breast Cancer Res Treat 1992; 20(2):85–92.

166. Wyckoff J, Greenberg H, Sanderson R, Wallach P, Balducci L. Breast irradiation in the older woman: a toxicity study. J Am Geriatr Soc 1994; 42(2):150–152.

167. Overgaard M, Jensen MB, Overgaard J, et al. Postoperative radiotherapy in high-risk postmenopausal breast-cancer patients given adjuvant tamoxifen: Danish Breast Cancer Cooperative Group DBCG 82c randomised trial. Lancet 1999; 353(9165):1641–1648.

168. Bentzen SM, Overgaard M, Thames HD. Fractionation sensitivity of a functional endpoint: impaired shoulder movement after post-mastectomy radiotherapy. Int J Radiat Oncol Biol Phys 1989; 17(3):531–537.

169. Olsen NK, Pfeiffer P, Johannsen L, Schroder H, Rose C. Radiation-induced brachial plexopathy: neurological follow-up in 161 recurrence-free breast cancer patients. Int J Radiat Oncol Biol Phys 1993; 26(1):43–49.

170. Erickson VS, Pearson ML, Ganz PA, Adams J, Kahn KL. Arm edema in breast cancer patients. J Natl Cancer Inst 2001; 93(2):96–111.

171. Pezner RD, Patterson MP, Hill LR, et al. Arm lymphedema in patients treated conservatively for breast cancer: relationship to patient age and axillary node dissection technique. Int J Radiat Oncol Biol Phys 1986; 12(12):2079–2083.

172. Louis-Sylvestre C, Clough K, Asselain B, et al. Axillary treatment in conservative management of operable breast cancer: dissection or radiotherapy? Results of a randomized study with 15 years of follow-up. J Clin Oncol 2004; 22(1):97–101.

173. Martin LM, le Pechoux C, Calitchi E, et al. Management of breast cancer in the elderly. Eur J Cancer 1994; 30A(5):590–596.

174. Vernon CC, Hand JW, Field SB, et al. Radiotherapy with or without hyperthermia in the treatment of superficial localized breast cancer: results from five randomized controlled trials. International Collaborative Hyperthermia Group. Int J Radiat Oncol Biol Phys 1996; 35(4):731–744.

175. Feyerabend T, Wiedemann GJ, Jager B, Vesely H, Mahlmann B, Richter E. Local hyperthermia, radiation, and chemotherapy in recurrent breast cancer is feasible and effective except for inflammatory disease. Int J Radiat Oncol Biol Phys 2001; 49(5):1317–1325.

176. Hishikawa Y, Kurisu K, Taniguchi M, Kamikonya N, Miura T. High-dose-rate intraluminal brachytherapy for esophageal cancer: 10 years experience in Hyogo College of Medicine. Radiother Oncol 1991; 21:107–114.

177. Yamakawa M, Shiojima K, Takahashi M, et al. Radiation therapy for esophageal cancer in patients over 80 years old. Int J Radiat Oncol Biol Phys 1994; 30:1225–1232.

178. Rice DC, Correa AM, Vaporciyan AA, et al. Preoperative chemoradiotherapy prior to esophagectomy in elderly patients is not associated with increased morbidity. Ann Thor Surg 2005; 79:391–397.

179. Tanisada K, Teshima T, Ikeda H, et al. A preliminary outcome analysis of the Patterns of Care Study in Japan for esophageal cancer patients with special reference to age: non surgery group. Int J Radiat Oncol Biol Phys 2000; 46:1223–1233.

180. Mak AC, Rich TA, Schultheiss TE, Kavanagh B, Ota DM, Romsdahl MM. Late complications of postoperative radiation therapy for cancer of the rectum and rectosigmoid. Int J Radiat Oncol Biol Phys 1994; 28:597–603.
181. Valenti V, Morganti AG, Luzi S, et al. Is chemoradiation feasible in elderly patients? A study of 17 patients with anorectal carcinoma. Cancer 1997; 80:1387–1392.
182. Coburn MC, Pricolo VE, Soderberg CH. Factors affecting prognosis and management of carcinoma of the colon and rectum in patients more than eighty years of age. J Am Coll Surg 1994; 179:65–69.
183. Neugat AI, Fleischauer AT, Sundararajan V. Use of adjuvant chemotherapy and radiation therapy for rectal cancer among the elderly: a population-based study. J Clin Oncol 2002; 20:2643–2650.
184. Eng C, Abbruzzese J, Minsky BD. Chemotherapy and radiation of anal canal cancer: the first approach. Surg Oncol Clin N Am 2004; 13:309–320.
185. Hanks GE, Hanlon A, Owen JB, Schultheiss TE. Patterns of radiation treatment of elderly patients with prostate cancer. Cancer 1994; 74:2174–2177.
186. Huguenin PU, Bitterli M, Lutolf UM, Bernhard J, Glanzmann C. Localized prostate cancer in elderly patients. Outcome after radiation therapy compared to matched younger patients. Strahlenther Onkol 1999; 175:554–558.
187. Johnstone PA, Riffenburgh RH, Moul JW, et al. Effect of age on biochemical disease-free outcome in patients with T1–3 prostate cancer treated with definitive radiotherapy in equal-access health care system: a radiation oncology report of the Department of Defense Center for Prostate Disease Research. Int J Radiat Oncol Biol Phys 2003; 55:964–969.
188. Villa S, Bedini N, Fallai C, Olmi P. External beam radiotherapy in elderly patients with clinically localized prostate adenocarcinoma: age is not a problem. Crit Rev Oncol Hematol 2003; 48:215–225.
189. D'Amico AV, Cote K, Loffredo M, Renshaw AA, Chen MH. Advanced age at diagnosis is an independent predictor of time to death from prostate carcinoma for patients undergoing external beam radiation therapy for clinically localized prostate carcinoma. Cancer 2003; 97:56–62.
190. Jani AB, Parikh SD, Vijayakumar S, Gratzle J. Analysis of influence of age on acute and chronic radiotherapy toxicity in treatment of prostate cancer. Urology 2005; 65:1157–1162.
191. Liu L, Glicksman AS, Coachman N, Kuten A. Low acute gastrointestinal and genitourinary toxicities in whole pelvis irradiation of prostate cancer. Int J Radiat Oncol Biol Phys 1997; 38:65–71.
192. Steinberg GD, Bales GT, Brendler CB. An analysis of watchful waiting for clinically localized prostate cancer. J Urol 1998; 159:1431–1436.
193. Neulander EZ, Duncan RC, Tiguert R, Posey JT, Soloway MS. Deferred treatment of localized prostate cancer in the elderly: the impact of the age and stage at the time of diagnosis on the treatment decision. BJU Int 2000; 85:699–704.
194. Veronesi A, Lo RG, Carbone A, et al. Multimodal treatment of locally advanced transitional cell bladder carcinoma in elderly patients. Eur J Cancer 1994; 30A:918–920.
195. Arias F, Duenas M, Martinez E, et al. Radical chemoradiotherapy for elderly patients with bladder carcinoma invading muscle. Cancer 1997; 80:115–120.
196. Kageyama Y, Okada Y, Arai G, et al. Preoperative concurrent chemoradiotherapy against muscle-invasive bladder cancer: results of partial cystectomy in elderly or high-risk patients. Jpn J Clin Oncol 2000; 30:553–556.
197. Smaaland R, Akslen LA, Tonder B, Mehus A, Lote K, Albrektsen G. Radical radiation treatment of invasive and locally advanced bladder carcinoma in elderly patients. Br J Urol 1991; 67:61–69.
198. Santacaterina A, Settineri N, De Renzis C, et al. Muscle-invasive bladder cancer in elderly-unfit patients with concomitant illness: can curative radiotherapy therapy be delivered? Tumori 2002; 88:390–394.

199. Phillips HA, Howard GC. The treatment of bladder cancer in the elderly. Radiother Oncol 1998; 46:334–335.

200. Vrouvas J, Dodwell D, Ash D, Probst H. Split course radiotherapy for bladder cancer in elderly unfit patients. Clin Oncol (R Coll Radiol) 1995; 7:193–195.

201. Benstead K, Cowie VJ, Blair V, Hunter RD. Stage III carcinoma of the cervix. The importance of increasing age and extent of parametrial infiltration. Radiother Oncol 1986; 5:271–276.

202. Bolli JA, Maners A. Age as a prognostic factor in cancer of the cervix: the UAMS experience. J Ark Med Soc 1992; 89:79–83.

203. Kapp DS, Fischer D, Gutierrez E, Kohorn EI, Schwartz PE. Pretreatment prognostic factors in carcinoma of the uterine cervix: a multivariate analysis of the effect of age, stage, histology and blood counts on survival. Int J Radiat Oncol Biol Phys 1983; 9:445–455.

204. Minagawa Y, Kigawa J, Itamochi H, Terakawa N. The outcome of radiation therapy in elderly patients with advanced cervical cancer. Int J Gynaecol Obstet 1997; 58:305–309.

205. Mitsuhashi N, Takahashi M, Nozaki M, et al. Squamous cell carcinoma of the uterine cervix: radiation therapy for patients aged 70 years and older. Radiology 1995; 194:141–145.

206. Mann WJ, Levy D, Hatch KD, Shingleton HM, Soong SJ. Prognostic significance of age in stage I carcinoma of the cervix. South Med J 1980; 73:1186–1188.

207. Sakurai H, Mitsuhashi N, Takahashi M, et al. Radiation therapy for elderly patients with squamous cell carcinoma of the uterine cervix. Gynecol Oncol 2000; 77:116–120.

208. Mitchell PA, Waggoner S, Rotmensch J, Mundt AJ. Cervical cancer in the elderly treated with radiation therapy. Gynecol Oncol 1998; 71:291–298.

209. Farley JH, Nycum LR, Birrer MJ, Park RC, Taylor RR. Age-specific survival of women with endometrioid adenocarcinoma of the uterus. Gynecol Oncol 2000; 79:86–89.

210. Citron JR, Sutton H, Yamada SD, Mehta N, Mundt AJ. Pathologic stage I-II endometrial carcinoma in the elderly: radiotherapy indications and outcome. Int J Radiat Oncol Biol Phys 2004; 59:1432–1438.

211. Mundt AJ, Waggoner S, Yamada SD, Rotmensch J, Connell PP. Age as a prognostic factor for recurrence in patients with endometrial carcinoma. Gynecol Oncol 2000; 79:79–85.

212. Alektiar KM, Ventratraman E, Abu-Rustum N, Barakat RR. Is endometrial carcinoma intrinsically more aggressive in elderly patients? Cancer 2003; 98:2368–2377.

213. Grant PT, Jeffrey JF, Fraser RC, Tompkins MG, Filbee JF, Wong OS. Pelvic radiation therapy for gynecologic malignancy in geriatric patients. Gynecol Oncol 1989; 33:185–188.

214. Pignon T, Horiot JC, Bolla M, et al. Age is not a limiting factor for radical radiotherapy in pelvic malignancies. Radiother Oncol 1997; 42:107–120.

215. Huguenin P, Baumert B, Lutolf UM, Wight E, Glanzmann C. Curative radiotherapy in elderly patients with endometrial cancer. Patterns of relapse, toxicity, and quality of life. Strahlenther Onkol 1999; 185:309–314.

216. Huguenin PU, Glanzman C, Hammer F, Lutolf UM. Endometrial carcinoma in patients aged 75 years or older: outcome and complications after postoperative radiotherapy or radiotherapy alone. Strahlenther Onkol 1992; 168:567–572.

217. Corn BW, Lanciano RM, Greven KM, et al. Impact of improved irradiation technique, age, and lymph node sampling on the severe complication rate of surgically staged endometrial cancer patients: a multivariate analysis. J Clin Oncol 1994; 12:510–515.

218. Lanciano RM, Martz K, Montana GS, Hanks GE. Influence of age, prior abdominal surgery, fraction size, and dose on complications after radiation therapy for squamous cell cancer of the uterine cervix. A patterns of care study. Cancer 1992; 69:2124–2130.

219. Wollschlaeger K, Connell PP, Waggoner S, Rotmensch J, Mundt AJ. Acute problems during low-dose-rate intracavitary brachytherapy for cervical carcinoma. Gynecol Oncol 2000; 76:67–72.

220. Chao CK, Grigsby PW, Perez CA, Mutch DG, Herzog T, Camel HM. Medically inoperable stage I endometrial carcinoma: a few dilemmas in radiotherapeutic management. Int J Radiat Oncol Biol Phys 1996; 34:27–33.
221. Lanciano RM, Won M, Coia LR, Hanks GE. Pretreatment and treatment factors associated with improved outcome in squamous cell carcinoma of the uterine cervix: a final report of the 1973 and 1978 patterns of care studies. Int J Radiat Oncol Biol Phys 1991; 20:667–673.
222. Petereit DS, Sarkovia JN, Chappell RJ, et al. Perioperative morbidity and mortality of high-dose-rate gynecologic brachytherapy. Int J Radiat Oncol Biol Phys 1998; 42: 1025–1031.
223. Keys HM, Roberts JA, Brunetto VL, et al. A phase III trial of surgery with or without adjunctive external pelvic radiation therapy in intermediate risk endometrial adenocarcinoma: a Gynecologic Oncology Group study. Gynecol Oncol 2004; 92:744–751.
224. Creutzberg CL, van Putten WC, Koper PC, et al. Surgery and postoperative radiotherapy versus surgery alone for patients with stage-I endometrial carcinoma: multicentre randomized trial. PORTEC Study Group. Postoperative radiation therapy in endometrial cancer. Lancet 2000; 355:1404–1411.
225. Zeitman AL, Linggood RM, Brookes AR, Convery K, Piro A. Radiation therapy in the management of early stage Hodgkin's disease presenting in later life. Cancer 1991; 68:1869–1873.
226. Austin-Seymour MM, Hoppe RT, Cox RS, Rosenberg SA, Kaplan HS. Hodgkin's disease in patients over sixty years old. Ann Intern Med 1984; 199:13–18.
227. Feugier P, Van Hoof A, Sebban C, et al. Long-term results of the R-CHOP study in the treatment of elderly patients with diffuse large B-cell lymphoma: a study by the Groupe d'Etude des Lymphomes de l'Adulte. J Clin Oncol 2005; 23:4117–4126.
228. De Sanctis V, Martelli M, Osti MF, et al. Feasibility and results of a multimodality approach in elderly patients with localized intermediate to high-grade non-Hodgkin's lymphomas. Tumori 2004; 90:289–293.
229. Shenkier TN, Voss N, Fairey R, et al. Brief chemotherapy and involved-region irradiation for limited-stage diffuse large-cell lymphoma: an 18 year experience from the British Columbia Cancer Agency. J Clin Oncol 2002; 20:197–204.
230. Wylie JP, Cowan RA, Deakin DP. The role of radiotherapy in the treatment of localised intermediate and high-grade non-Hodgkin's lymphoma in elderly patients. Radiother Oncol 1998; 49:9–14.
231. Saito Y, Yoshikawa D, Yamada T, et al. Non-Hodgkin's lymphoma of stage I and II in elderly patients: a retrospective study in comparison with younger patients. Nippon Igaku Hoshasen Gakkai Zasshi 1995; 55:576–581.
232. Lovett RM, Perez CA, Shapiro SJ, Garcia DM. External irradiation of epithelial skin cancer. Int J Radiat Oncol Biol Phys 1990; 18:235–242.
233. Mandoliti G, Polico C, Capirci C, et al. Radiation therapy of bone metastases in the elderly: a multicentric survey of the Italian "Geriatric Radiation Oncology Group." Rays 1997; 22(suppl 1):57–60.
234. Price PA, Hoskins PJ, Easton D. Low dose single fraction radiotherapy in the treatment of metastatic bone pain: a pilot study. Radiother Oncol 1988; 12:297–301.
235. Crocker I, Prosnitz L. Radiation therapy of the elderly. Clin Geriatr Med 1987; 3: 473–481.
236. Scher HI, Chung LW. Bone metastases: improving the therapeutic index. Semin Oncol 1994; 21:630–656.
237. Leibel SA, Pajak TF, Massullo V, et al. A comparison of misonidazole sensitized radiation therapy to radiation therapy alone for the palliation of hepatic metastases: results of a Radiation Therapy Oncology Group randomized prospective trial. Int J Radiat Oncol Biol Phys 1987; 13:1057–1062.
238. Dobrowsky W. Treatment of choroids metastases. Br J Radiol 1988; 61:140–144.

239. Zachariah B, Zachariah SB, Varghese R, Balducci L. Carcinomatous meningitis: clinical manifestations and management. Int J Clin Pharmacol Ther 1985; 33:7–12.

240. Rees GJ, Devrell CE, Barley VL, Newman HF. Palliative radiotherapy for lung cancer: two versus five fractions. Clin Oncol 1997; 9:90–95.

241. Adelson MD, Wharton JT, Delclos L, Copeland L, Gershenson D. Palliative radiotherapy for ovarian cancer. Int J Radiat Oncol Biol Phys 1987; 13:17–21.

242. Berson AM, Finger PT, Sherr DL, Emery R, Alfieri AA, Bosworth JL. Radiotherapy for age-related macular degeneration: technique and preliminary subjective response. Int J Radiat Oncol Biol Phys 1996; 36:861–866.

243. van den Brenck HA. Results of prophylactic postoperative irradiation in 1300 cases of pterygium. Am J Roentgenol 1968; 103:723–727.

244. Donaldson SS, Bagshaw MS, Kriss JP. Supervoltage orbital radiotherapy for Graves' ophthalmopathy. J Clin Endocrinol Metabol 1973; 37:276–279.

245. Mira JG, Chahbazian CM, del Regato JA. The value of radiotherapy for Peyronie's disease: presentation of 56 new cases studies and review of the literature. Int J Radiat Oncol Biol Phys 1980; 6:161–165.

246. Anthony P, Keys H, McCollister E. Prevention of heterotopic bone formation with early postoperative irradiation in high risk patients undergoing total hip arthroplasty: comparison of 10 Gy vs. 20 Gy schedules. Int J Radiat Oncol Biol Phys 1987; 3:365–369.

247. Saleem MA, Aronow WS, Ravipati G. Intracoronary brachytherapy for treatment of in-stent restenosis. Cardiol Rev 2005; 13:139–141.

248. Belardi JA, Cura F, Albertal M. Use of drug-eluting stents for the treatment of in-stent restenosis in routine clinical practice. Coron Artery Dis 2005; 16:327–330.

249. Xing L, Wu Q, Yang Y, et al. The physics of IMRT. In: Mundt AJ, Roeske JC, eds. Intensity Modulated Radiation Therapy: A Clinical Perspective. Toronto: BC Decker, 2005:20–52.

250. Mell LK, Roeske JC, Mehta N, Mundt AJ. Gynecologic cancer: overview. In: Mundt AJ, Roeske JC, eds. Intensity Modulated Radiation Therapy: A Clinical Perspective. Toronto: BC Decker, 2005.

251. Kupelian P, Willoughby T. Hypofractionated IMRT: case study. In: Mundt AJ, Roeske JC, eds. Intensity Modulated Radiation Therapy: A Clinical Perspective. Toronto: BC Decker, 2005.

252. Mell LK, Roeske JC, Mundt AJ. Survey of intensity modulated radiation therapy use in the United States. Cancer 2003; 98:204–211.

253. Mell LK, Mundt AJ. Survey of IMRT use in the United States, 2004. Cancer 2005; 104:1296–1303.

254. Lee NK, Xia P, Quivey IM, et al. Intensity-modulated radiotherapy in the treatment of nasopharyngeal carcinoma: an update of the UCSF experience. Int J Radiat Oncol Biol Phys 2002; 53:12–22.

255. Lee N, Xia P, Fischbein NJ, Akazawa P, Akazawa C, Quivey JM. Intensity-modulated radiation therapy for head-and-neck cancer: the UCSF experience focusing on target volume delineation. Int J Radiat Oncol Biol Phys 2003; 57:49–60.

256. Chao KS, Deasy JO, Markman J, et al. A prospective study of salivary function sparing in patients with head and neck cancers receiving intensity-modulated or 3-dimensional radiation therapy: initial results. Int J Radiat Oncol Biol Phys 2001; 49:907–916.

257. Zelefsky MJ, Fuks Z, Happersett L, et al. Clinical experience with intensity modulated radiation therapy (IMRT) in prostate cancer. Radiother Oncol 2000; 55:139–140.

258. Zelefsky MJ, Fuks Z, Hunt M, et al. High-dose intensity modulated radiation therapy for prostate cancer: early toxicity and biochemical outcome in 772 patients. Int J Radiat Oncol Biol Phys 2002; 53:1111–1116.

259. Vicini FA, Sharpe M, Kestin L, et al. Optimizing breast cancer treatment efficacy with intensity-modulated radiotherapy. Int J Radiat Oncol Biol Phys 2002; 54:1336–1344.

260. Mundt AJ, Mell LK, Roeske JC. Preliminary analysis of chronic gastrointestinal toxicity in gynecology patients treated with intensity-modulated whole pelvic radiation therapy. Int J Radiat Oncol Biol Phys 2003; 56:1354–1360.

261. Milano MT, Chmura SJ, Garofalo MC. Intensity-modulated radiotherapy in treatment of pancreatic and bile duct malignancies: toxicity and clinical outcome. Int J Radiat Oncol Biol Phys 2004; 59:445–453.

262. Uy NM, Woo SY, The BS. Intensity-modulated radiation therapy (IMRT) for meningioma. Int J Radiat Oncol Biol Phys 2002; 53:1265–1270.

263. Hong L, Alektiar KM, Hunt M. Intensity-modulated radiotherapy for soft tissue sarcoma of the thigh. Int J Radiat Oncol Biol Phys 2004; 59:752–759.

264. DeWyngaert J, Lymberis SC, MacDonald S, et al. Accelerated IMRT with concomitant boost after breast-conserving therapy (BCT): preliminary clinical results and dose volume (DVH) analysis. Int J Radiat Oncol Biol Phys 2004; 60:493–504.

265. Kupelian PA, Reddy CA, Carlson TP, Altsman KA, Willoughby TR. Preliminary observations on biochemical relapse-free survival rates after short-course intensity-modulated radiotherapy (70 Gy at 2.5 Gy per fractions) for localized prostate cancer. Int J Radiat Oncol Biol Phys 2002; 53:904–912.

266. Djemil T, Reddy CA, Willoughby TR, Kupelian PA. Hypofractionated intensity-modulated radiation therapy (70 Gy at 2.5 Gy per fraction) for localized prostate cancer. Int J Radiat Oncol Biol Phys 2003; 57:S275–S276.

267. Milker-Zabel S, Zabel A, Thilmann C, Schlegel W, Wannenmacher M, Debus J. Clinical results of re-treatment of vertebral bone metastases by stereotactic conformal radiotherapy and intensity-modulated radiotherapy. Int J Radiat Oncol Biol Phys 2003; 55:315–324.

268. Alektiar KM, Venkatraman E, Chi DS, Barakat RR. Intravaginal brachytherapy alone for intermediate-risk endometrial cancer. Int J Radiat Oncol Biol Phys 2005; 62:111–117.

269. Nguyen TV, Petereit DG. High-dose-rate brachytherapy for medically inoperable stage I endometrial cancer. Gynecol Oncol 1998; 71:196–203.

270. Toita T, Moromizato H, Ogawa K, et al. Concurrent chemoradiotherapy using high-dose-rate intracavitary brachytherapy for uterine cervical cancer. Gynecol Oncol 2005; 96:665–670.

271. Vicini FA, Vargas C, Edmundson G, Kestin L, Martinez A. The role of high-dose rate brachytherapy in locally advanced prostate cancer. Semin Radiat Oncol 2003; 13: 98–108.

272. Chun M, Kang S, Kim BS, Oh YT. High dose rate interstitial brachytherapy in soft tissue sarcoma: technical aspects and results. Jpn J Clin Oncol 2001; 31:279–283.

273. Kakimoto N, Inoue T, Inoue T, et al. Results of low- and high-dose-rate interstitial brachytherapy for T3 mobile tongue cancer. Radiother Oncol 2003; 68:123–128.

274. Lillegren G, Holmberg L, Adami H, Westman G, Graffman S, Bergh J. Sector resection with or without post-operative radiotherapy for stage I breast cancer: five-year results of a randomized trial. J Natl Cancer Inst 1994; 86:717–722.

275. Crile G, Esselstyn CB. Factors influencing local recurrence of cancer after partial mastectomy. Cleve Clin J Med 1990; 57:143–146.

276. Fisher B, Anderson S. Conservative surgery for the management of invasive and non-invasive carcinoma of the breast. NSABP trials. World J Surg 1994; 18:63–69.

277. Stolier AJ, Fuhrman GM, Scroggins TG, Boyer CI. Post-lumpectomy insertion of the Mammosite brachytherapy device using the scar entry technique: initial experience and technical considerations. Breast J 2005; 11:199–203.

278. Dowlatshahi K, Snider HC, Gittleman MA, Nguyen C, Vigneri PM, Franklin RL. Early experience with balloon brachytherapy for breast cancer. Arch Surg 2004; 139:603–607.

279. Pollock BE. Stereotactic radiosurgery for intracranial meningiomas: indications and results. Neurosurg Focus 2003; 14:4–8.

280. Schomas DA, Roeske JC, Macdonald RL, Sweeney PJ, Mehta N, Mundt AJ. Predictors of tumor control in patients treated with linac-based stereotactic radiosurgery for metastatic disease to the brain. Am J Clin Oncol 2005; 28:180–187.

281. Selek U, Chang EL, Hassenbusch SJ, et al. Stereotactic radiosurgical treatment in 103 patients for 153 cerebral melanoma metastases. Int J Radiat Oncol Biol Phys 2004; 59:1097–1106.

282. Shehata MK, Young B, Reid B, et al. Stereotactic radiosurgery of 468 brain metastases ≤2 cm: implications for SRS dose and whole brain radiation therapy. Int J Radiat Oncol Biol Phys 2004; 59:87–93.

283. Kondziolka D, Patel A, Lunsford LD, et al. Stereotactic radiosurgery plus whole brain radiotherapy versus radiotherapy alone for patients with multiple brain metastases. Int J Radiat Oncol Biol Phys 1999; 45:427–434.

284. Takayama K, Nagata Y, Negoro Y, et al. Treatment planning of stereotactic radiotherapy for solitary lung tumor. Int J Radiat Oncol Biol Phys 2005; 61:1565–1571.

285. Ohashi T, Takeda A, Shigematsu N, et al. Differences in pulmonary function before versus 1 year after hypofractionated stereotactic radiotherapy for small peripheral lung tumors. Int J Radiat Oncol Biol Phys 2005; 62:1003–1008.

286. De Salles AA, Pedroso AG, Medin P, et al. Spinal lesions treated with Novalis shaped beam intensity-modulated radiosurgery and stereotactic radiotherapy. J Neurosurg 2004; 101(suppl 3):435–440.

287a. Holm HH. The history of interstitial brachytherapy of prostatic cancer. Semin Surg Oncol 1997; 13:431–437.

287b. Blasko JC, Gramm PD, Ragde H. Branchy therapy and organ preservation in the management of carcroma of the prostate. Semin Radiat Oncol 1993; 3:240–249.

288. Sathya JR, Davis IR, Julian JA, et al. Randomized trial comparing iridium implant plus external-beam radiation therapy with external-beam radiation therapy alone in node-negative locally advanced cancer of the prostate. J Clin Oncol 2005; 23:1192–1199.

289. Potters L, Morgenstern C, Calugaru E, et al. Twelve-year outcomes following permanent prostate brachytherapy in patients with clinically localized prostate cancer. J Urol 2005; 173:1562–1566.

290. Sharkey J, Cantor A, Solc Z, et al. 103Pd brachytherapy versus radical prostatectomy in patients with clinically localized prostate cancer: a 12-year experience from a single group practice. Brachytherapy 2005; 4:34–44.

291. Merrick GS, Butler WM, Wallner KE, et al. The impact of radiation dose to the urethra on brachytherapy-related dysuria. Brachytherapy 2005; 4:45–50.

292. Merrick GS, Butler WM, Wallner KE, et al. Permanent interstitial brachytherapy for clinically organ-confined high-grade prostate cancer with a pretreatment PSA < 20 ng/mL. Am J Clin Oncol 2004; 27:611–615.

5

Chemotherapeutic Treatment Issues in the Elderly

Marc Gautier
Hematology and Oncology, Dartmouth Hitchcock Medical Center, Lebanon, New Hampshire, U.S.A.

Harvey Jay Cohen
Duke University Medical Center and Veterans Administration Medical Center, Durham, North Carolina, U.S.A.

Jeffrey Alan Bubis
Dartmouth Hitchcock Medical Center, Lebanon, New Hampshire, U.S.A.

INTRODUCTION

Approximately 50% of all malignancies occur in people over 65 years. Chemotherapy has demonstrated beneficial effects in the treatment of cancer, but it has principally been studied in patients under the age of 65. The question remains, how does chemotherapy affect elderly patients, who are frequently afflicted with cancer? In this chapter, we discuss the age-related changes in pharmacokinetics and pharmacodynamics that can alter the outcome of chemotherapy.

Much of what we know about the use of chemotherapeutic drugs in cancer patients is derived from clinical trials. When new chemotherapeutic drugs are initially studied in human beings, they are studied in phase I trials. The goal of these studies is to determine the maximum tolerated dose of the chemotherapeutic agent. Once the appropriate dose of the chemotherapeutic drug is established, phase II studies attempt to determine if there is any activity against specific diseases. Frequently, elderly patients are excluded from these early studies, and thus, in the case of many drugs, there is limited knowledge of the effect of the normal processes of aging on drug metabolism and activity (1).

Phase I and II studies provide a great deal of information about how a given drug interacts with the human system, but these studies usually show a high degree of inter-patient variability. This variability is sometimes due to measurable differences in organ function, but is more frequently due to unknown processes. It is manifested by variable responses and toxicity with the same dose of chemotherapy in different patients.

The standard practice is to dose chemotherapy in a uniform fashion by calculating the dose on the basis of the body surface area of an individual patient. The origin of this practice stems not so much from the point of view of reducing intra-patient variability, but was an attempt to control the dose of drug when moving from animal studies to humans. This chapter seeks to examine some of the sources of the variability among patients receiving chemotherapy. We also suggest how chemother-apeutic doses should be adjusted in the face of known determinants of this variabil-ity. A clear message from the data is that age alone is a poor predictor of the variability among patients. In fact, in older age groups, the intrapatient variability is even higher than that seen in younger age groups.

One other issue needs to be explored in understanding the use of chemotherapy in elderly patients. The narrow therapeutic index of most chemotherapeutic drugs is well known to patients and physicians alike. Frequently, we must confront the question, "Is the benefit worth the toxicity?" To approach that issue, one needs to know the goal of chemotherapy. In modern oncology, there are several accepted roles for the use of chemotherapy. Chemotherapy is frequently used after surgery or radiation in the adjuvant setting. Chemotherapy also can be used alone with curative intent. Frequently, palliation is the only goal for chemotherapy. One important perception among oncologists is that chemotherapy is less effective and more toxic in elderly patients. With the impression of this altered ratio of toxicity to benefit, there is some tendency to avoid doses of chemotherapy that would be more likely to provide a cure, and a subtle shift toward the use of chemotherapy as a palliative, or not at all.

The tendency to shy away from the use of intensive chemotherapy with advanc-ing age has been noted by several investigators (2,3). Although the dose of chem-otherapy can be associated with both toxicity and response rates, modification of the dose of chemotherapy is almost always contingent upon toxicity considerations. Because toxicity can be life threatening, many oncologists avoid doses of chemo-therapy that they believe will be associated with significant toxicity. There are clear examples where aggressive chemotherapy is less well tolerated in older patients than in younger patients [for example, acute myelogenous leukemia (AML) induction therapy] (4). However, multiple studies have demonstrated that older patients can tolerate standard-dose chemotherapy with toxicity similar to that seen in younger patients (5). Moreover, some studies suggest that older patients have less emotional distress associated with receiving chemotherapy (6). Despite these data, many older patients continue to have "adjusted" regimens owing to concerns that age alone will place them at risk for toxicity from chemotherapy.

PHARMACOKINETICS

The term pharmacokinetics describes the principles that apply to the handling (i.e., absorption, distribution, metabolism, and excretion) of drugs in the body. These prin-ciples can be summarized in the following fashion: (a) an optimal outcome is likely if the drug concentration in the serum reaches a target level; (b) there are several defin-able interactions that account for the differences among patients in achieving a target drug level; and (c) thus, a wide range of drug doses may be required to achieve the opti-mal clinical response in different patients. These principles do not expressly consider the factors involved in obtaining the clinical response. Pharmacodynamics is the study of the interactions between these serum levels of drugs and outcomes over time (see section on "Pharmacodynamics"). We will examine each of the four pharmacokinetic factors listed above and assess how aging affects each process.

Absorption

Most cancer chemotherapy is delivered intravenously; however, there are many drugs that are delivered orally, either as single agents or in combinations. Melphalan, cyclophosphamide, methotrexate, and capecitabine are commonly used for a variety of neoplasms that occur in the elderly. Other drugs that have been available intravenously may now be more advantageously used in an oral regimen. Etoposide is an example of a drug that may be more active in a variety of diseases if given in low doses orally over three weeks.

For many reasons, including convenience, it may be preferable to use the oral route of administration in chemotherapy. However, aging affects gastrointestinal physiology in a variety of ways (7). It is clear that gastric acidity decreases with age. The amount of secretions from the intestinal tract also decreases with age. Absorptive surface area, splanchnic blood flow, and bowel motility have less clear alterations with aging. In younger patients, there is a wide variation in the absorption of these oral medicines. In elderly patients, one can expect the same wide variability without any clinically relevant change due to aging (8). Most investigators recommend following the effects of the oral medicine to confirm adequate absorption. Practically, for example, in the use of melphalan for multiple myeloma, one should check the white blood cell count (WBC) two to three weeks after the dose is administered orally to confirm a 50% decrease in the WBC. If the WBC has not fallen this much, then the oral dose needs to be increased to account for the observed lack of absorption. For many drugs, serum levels can be checked to assure adequate absorption (9).

Distribution

Once the chemotherapeutic drug has reached the systemic circulation, either by parental administration or by oral dosing, there are some changes in the distribution of the drug that are predictable with aging. There are well-described changes in body composition that occur with aging (8). There is an increase in the percentage of body weight due to fat and a decrease of muscle and water. The fat content is estimated to increase from 15% of body weight to 30%, whereas intracellular water decreases from 42% to 33%, from the ages of 25 to 75. This will alter distribution volumes for both fat- and water-soluble compounds.

Another factor affecting distribution is related to the binding of certain drugs by plasma proteins. Albumin decreases with age by about 15%. Chronic illness, such as cancer, and poor nutritional status can also significantly lower the level of serum albumin. For drugs that are tightly protein-bound, the amount of free drug available to interact with target receptors will be affected by this change in albumin level. Drugs such as etoposide are clearly affected by this mechanism. Although this is not isolated to elderly patients, it does point out the need to individualize therapy and to consider elderly patients as a subset (10). The frequency of other drug use in the elderly population raises the likelihood of drug–drug interactions via competition for binding sites on albumin. This is more likely to occur in elderly patients than in younger patients because of the frequency of the use of polypharmacy in elderly patients (11).

Despite these clear-cut and predictable changes that occur in the factors controlling distribution in elderly patients, there is little actual data to aid in adjusting the dose of chemotherapy. Nonetheless, these principles should be taken into account by the physician caring for elderly patients.

Metabolism

Once the drug has achieved serum levels and has been distributed into the body compartments, the terminal phase of the drug's presence in the body is primarily related to metabolism and excretion. Activation of the drug is a large component of the metabolism of many drugs. Any alteration in activation or metabolism of a drug will affect the exposure of the patient to the drug.

Hepatic metabolism is a critical element in the pharmacokinetics of many drugs. It is dependent on three critical elements: (a) hepatic blood flow, (b) liver size, and (c) activity of drug-metabolizing enzymes. Each of these elements can be affected by the normal process of aging (12). There is an abundance of data confirming that hepatic blood flow decreases with age. There are also data showing that liver size decreases with age. The amount of decrease in the size of the liver approaches 20% to 40% and may account for the majority of the alterations in the hepatic metabolism of drugs in elderly patients.

Despite the involvement of other enzymes, cytochrome p450—a family of over 60 enzymes—is one of the most prominent enzyme systems in the mechanisms responsible for so-called "hepatic" metabolism. The rate at which these reactions occur varies from patient to patient; this is the result of the inherent variability of these enzymes—there are literally hundreds of genetic variations. Drug–drug interactions involving p450 generally result from either enzyme inhibition or induction and become exponentially more complicated as the number of drugs in the system increase. Chemotherapy drugs known to be substrates of p450 include cyclophosphamide, paclitaxel, decetaxel, ironotecan, vincristine, and the hormonal agent, tamoxifen; ThioTEPA is an inhibitor of p450.

The results of studies examining age-related changes in the drug-metabolizing enzymes within the liver have been controversial (13). Animal models have given mixed results. Some liver enzyme functions appear to decrease with age in some animals but not in others. Specific information regarding chemotherapeutic drug processing by the hepatic enzyme systems in older patients is not available, but one rudimentary study did look at the influence of polypharmacy with p450-metabolized drugs in elderly cancer patients receiving chemotherapy. In this study, a nonstatistically significant trend toward worsening nonhematologic toxicity was noted (14).

Given that there is an agreed change in some hepatic functions associated with advancing age, one would expect that there have been evaluations of specific chemotherapeutic drugs in patients of advanced age. Unfortunately, there is a lack of clinical data regarding age-related changes in the pharmacokinetics of chemotherapeutic drugs. There is interest in these issues, and they are being evaluated in pharmacokinetic phase II studies in elderly patients. To this point, we have only examined age-related changes in liver function. In the setting of known hepatic dysfunction, there is additional information; however, there is much disagreement regarding the measurements of the alterations in hepatic function to best reflect drug metabolism. "Liver function tests," as commonly obtained, do not accurately reflect the ability of the liver to metabolize drugs. Furthermore, other drugs, such as barbiturates, will significantly affect metabolism without altering routine liver function studies. Nonetheless, recommendations regarding dose adjustments of chemotherapy based on liver abnormalities and concomitant medications can be made. Table 1 outlines some of the recommendations that can be made for dose adjustments in the face of known hepatic dysfunction for some common chemotherapeutic drugs.

Table 1 Recommended Dose Adjustments for Selected Agents

Drug	Clearance mechanism	Dose modification
Alkylating agents		
Cyclophosphamide	Renal	Decrease 50% if Cr Cx $< 25\,\mathrm{mL/min/m^2}$
Cisplatin	Renal	Decrease proportional to Cr Cx
Chlorambucil	Metabolic	No recommendations
Antimetabolites		
Methotrexate	Renal	Decrease if Cr Cx $< 60\,\mathrm{mL/min/m^2}$
Fluorouracil	Metabolic	No recommendations
Capecitabine	Renal	Decrease proportional to Cr Cx
Fludarabine	Renal/metabolic	Decrease proportional to Cr Cx
Hydroxyurea	Renal/metabolic	Decrease proportional to Cr Cx
Plant derivatives		
Vincristine	Metabolic	Decrease 50% if bilirubin > 1.5ULN
Etoposide	Renal/metabolic	Decrease proportional to Cr Cx and consider dose adjustment with impaired liver function
Paclitaxel/docetaxel	Metabolic	Consider dose adjustment with impaired liver function
Antitumor antibiotics		
Doxorubicin	Metabolic	Decrease 50% if bilirubin 1.2–3.0 mg/dl Decrease 75% if bilirubin 3.1–5.1 mg/dl Discontinue if 10–20% decline in ejection fraction
Bleomycin	Renal	Decrease 50–75% if Cr Cx $< 25\,\mathrm{mL/min/m^2}$ Discontinue if DLCO falls below 30–35% of pretreatment value

Abbreviations: Cr Cx, creatinine clearance; ULN, upper limits of normal; DLCO, diffusion capacity.

Excretion

The clearest example of age-related decline in organ function relates to the excretion phase of drug handling. There is a clear age-related decrease in renal function as demonstrated by a decrease in the glomerular filtration rate (GFR). The importance of altered renal function on the kinetics of chemotherapeutic drugs is most clear for carboplatin and methotrexate. The key feature, though, is related to altered renal function—and not to age. Thus, a younger patient with a reduced GFR should have a dose adjustment greater than that of an older person with an intact GFR. This continues to confirm the impression that age alone is a poor indicator for adjustment of chemotherapy, and that the alterations in underlying organ function are the critical elements to optimize individual therapy.

Other drugs are thought to be affected by renal excretion as well. Dose adjustment recommendations have been made despite a lack of rigorous clinical data relating these dose adjustments to optimal clinical outcomes. Nonetheless, Table 1 includes frequently recommended dose adjustments in the setting of renal dysfunction.

Some drugs undergo both hepatic metabolism and hepatic excretion via bile. The anthracyclines are most closely associated with biliary excretion. Once again, the relationship of biliary excretion to age is questionable. Animal studies do not associate decreases in biliary excretion with aging. Thus, no specific age adjustments for drugs that have a significant biliary excretion are required. However, in the setting of significant hepatic dysfunction (as demonstrated by an elevated bilirubin), drugs that undergo significant excretion in the bile should be dose adjusted. Table 1 has common recommendations.

PHARMACODYNAMICS

Now that we have evaluated some of the common changes in pharmacokinetics, we will evaluate what is known about the pharmacodynamic changes that occur with aging. Recall that pharmacokinetics describes the behavior of the drug in the body, whereas pharmacodynamics more accurately describes what the drug does to the body. The field of pharmacodynamics is quite complex and there are limited amounts of data specific to elderly patients and chemotherapy.

One reason for the difficulties in studying pharmacodynamics is that frequently only serum levels of drugs are measured, and this may not reflect the level of drug exposure at the target site. Age-related changes in a variety of cellular processes may account for some pharmacodynamic alterations. We know, for example, that the changes in autonomic nervous system function with age render elderly patients more sensitive to the toxicity of beta-blockers. Unfortunately, there is little mechanistic data exploring these issues for cancer chemotherapy.

Several suggestions have been made to account for the pharmacodynamic alterations with aging (13). Changes in P-glycoprotein drug expulsion, abnormal protein synthesis and membrane transport, abnormal DNA repair, and altered drug receptors or target enzymes have all been implicated to account for some pharmacodynamic variability. As noted, however, there are no direct clinical data to prove these claims.

AGE AND TOXICITY OF CHEMOTHERAPY

In this section, we will initially evaluate the clinical data that suggests a difference in end-organ susceptibility to chemotherapy with advancing age. Subsequently, we will evaluate specific agents and classes of chemotherapies (e.g., anthracycline cardiotoxicity). The observed age-related changes in chemotherapeutic sensitivity may have many sources. We will evaluate some of the organ sensitivity that has been noted. The most common age-related chemotherapeutic sensitivity appears to be myelosuppression (15).

Attempting to differentiate the process of aging from comorbid illnesses can be quite difficult. Myelosuppression, which does appear to be more common in the elderly after chemotherapy, has not clearly been associated with age alone. When one examines the bone marrow function of healthy elderly people, there is little discernible decline with age. There have been a variety of studies examining the effects of aging on stem cell number, hematopoietic stroma, and growth factors in normal volunteers. These studies have not clearly shown a decrease in function with advancing age. This implies that any changes may be related to other comorbid illnesses and not to the aging process itself.

Clinically, excessive hematological toxicity has been noted in elderly patients. This may be due to an age-related decrease in stem cell renewal capabilities that manifest when the marrow homeostasis is perturbed—such as results from chemotherapy.

In a series of studies reviewing large numbers of patients and a variety of treatment regimens, an increased incidence of hematologic toxicity was noted in the elderly (16). In a study of over 16,000 patients, excessive hematologic side effects in older patients were associated with certain chemotherapeutic drugs [actinomycin, doxorubicin, methotrexate, methyl-N-(2-chloroethyl)-N'-cyclonitrosourea, vinblastine, and etoposide]. Most of these drugs undergo biliary excretion, and this may account for their excess toxicity. Other studies have demonstrated comparable hematological toxicity for younger and older patients with a variety of chemotherapeutic regimens, such as the combination of cyclophosphamide, methotrexate, and fluorouracil for breast cancer, provided the dose is adjusted for the GFR (17). There are some specific regimens that are frequently associated with excessive hematological toxicity in the elderly.

Induction chemotherapy for acute myeloid leukemia (AML) has been associated with higher early death rates in older patients, principally due to the complications of myelosupression. An Eastern Cooperative Oncology Group study evaluated elderly patients with AML, comparing higher-dose induction chemotherapy to low-dose treatment (18). Although there was no difference in the complete response rate (28%), early deaths were more common in the induction arm (60%) compared to the low-dose arm (25%). The results of this study are typical of studies demonstrating excessive toxicity due to chemotherapy in the hematopoietic organ of elderly patients.

Support for hematologic toxicity is now available. The efficacy of hematopoietic growth factors (e.g., granulocyte colony stimulating factor, granulocyte-macrophage colony stimulating factor, and erythropoietin) is independent of age (19). No longer is dose modification the only option for the management or prevention of hematologic toxicity. Although this has not directly translated into improved outcomes for patients, it has made dose-dense and dose-intense therapy possible. Patients with diseases where dose intensity is associated with higher rates of cure and improved survival, such as AML, multiple myeloma, Hodgkin's and non-Hodgkin's lymphomas, and breast cancer, have benefited from this (20–24). Additionally, dose-density has led to improved outcomes in patients with breast cancer and is a viable therapeutic option in lymphoma (25–27).

Gastrointestinal complaints are frequent in patients taking chemotherapy. Nausea and vomiting are common. Mucositis, usually manifested by a sore mouth, may be more common in the elderly. At least one study suggests that patients older than 65 years treated with 5-fluorouracil (5-FU) had increased rates of mucositis (28). Regardless of the frequency of mucositis, elderly patients are less tolerant to the complications of mucositis, including dehydration, which can accompany lack of oral intake.

Cardiac toxicity is a serious problem, especially in association with anthracycline therapy. Low-output congestive heart failure occurring with high total doses of doxorubicin is the typical clinical scenario. It appears that age may predispose the patient to this toxicity, even at lower total doses of doxorubicin in patients aged over 70 (29). Whether this represents subclinical cardiac disease or reflects the normal physiological aging process resulting in a lack of homeostatic reserve is unclear. Nonetheless, current recommendations advise that elderly patients receive a lower total dose of doxorubicin than younger patients. The mechanism of doxorubicin cardiotoxicity is related to the generation of oxygen-free radicals.

The free-radical scavenger dexrazoxane was approved by the Food and Drug Administration (FDA) for administration to women with breast cancer who had received a cumulative doxorubicin dose of $300 \, mg/m^2$, but would benefit from continued anthracycline therapy. Despite its effectiveness at preventing anthracy-cline-induced cardiac toxicity, it has not gained widespread use. Initially, this was likely due to concerns about lower response rates in patients receiving dexrazoxane compared to those who do not (30). However, further research has not supported this and it is contrary to other data; its use remains supported by a meta-analysis of all available data from randomized trials (31). However unfounded, concerns about its tumor-protective effect do remain. There are no specific studies of dexro-zoxane to prevent cardiac injury in elderly patients.

Few chemotherapy drugs are toxic to the pulmonary system. Bleomycin is the most common drug associated with pulmonary toxicity. At least one study has sug-gested an increased rate of pulmonary toxicity in patients over the age of 70 receiving bleomycin (32). Age-related declines in the elasticity of lung tissue make this toxicity more morbid when it does occur. The pulmonary toxicity associated with bleomycin, like doxorubicin, is associated with high cumulative total doses. No formal recom-mendations are available for dose adjustments in elderly patients.

Although we know there is an age-related decline in renal function, as mani-fested by a decrease in the GFR, there is little evidence to suggest that there is an age-associated increased risk of renal dysfunction from chemotherapy, even with an agent that is heavily associated with renal toxicity, such as cisplatin. Caution should be exercised when prescribing cisplatin to patients with poor renal function, regardless of age.

Neurologic toxicity, principally neuropathy, is a major concern. Although many chemotherapeutic agents are known to be associated with neuropathy (platinum com-pounds, vincas, and taxanes), there is scant evidence relating this risk to advancing age. Some studies have shown a higher rate of peripheral neuropathy in older patients, but clearly, comorbid illnesses, such as diabetes, increase the likelihood of developing peripheral neuropathy, which can sometimes produce profound functional impair-ment. Conclusive data associating age and central nervous system (CNS) toxicity are limited to cerebellar toxicity associated with high doses of cytarabine used in the induction chemotherapy for AML (33). Dose reduction is routine for elderly patients receiving cytarabine in high doses for AML, particularly patients with impaired renal function, as these patients are particularly at risk for CNS dysfunction, including, but not limited to, confusion, generalized encephalopathy, and psychosis (34).

DRUGS

Chemotherapeutic agents are frequently classified into general categories. Although there is no standard system for categorizing chemotherapeutic agents, most are clas-sified according to mechanisms of action. Even though we have limited knowledge about all the mechanisms of action of most chemotherapeutic agents, this is a useful system. Common categories include the alkylating agents (e.g., cyclophosphamide) and antimetabolites (e.g., methotrexate). Some antineoplastic agents are classified according to their derivation. Plant derivatives (e.g., paclitaxel) and antibiotics (e.g., doxorubicin) are also useful chemotherapeutic agents. We will examine the most commonly used agents by category. We will also briefly review characteristic mechanisms of action and general toxicity associated with each class of drug. These issues and others pertaining to the use of chemotherapy in the elderly have been well reviewed in detail by a variety of investigators and the interested reader is referred to these sources for more information (35–40).

Alkylating Agents

Alkylating agents have been classic chemotherapeutic agents since their development as part of chemical warfare during World War I. These chemicals produce highly reactive compounds that form a covalent bond between the two strands of DNA, and other alterations to the DNA structure. Although they seem to be more active against actively dividing cells—possibly because these cells have less time to repair any alkylator damage to the DNA before the next division—alkylating agents are thought to be cell cycle phase nonspecific (will kill both actively dividing and resting cells). This makes these compounds effective against neoplasms with small growth fractions. The most commonly used alkylating agents include cyclophosphamide, chlorabmucil, melphalan, carboplatin, and cisplatin.

Alkylating agents come in a variety of preparations, including intravenous and oral formulations. There is a wide dose range, and both cyclophosphamide and melphalan are used in low oral doses as well as very high-dose therapies, as in bone marrow transplant regimens. Toxicity is dose-related and includes moderate nausea and myelotoxicity. Cyclophosphamide causes a serious cystitis via its metabolite, acrolein; this can be prevented with judicious use of fluids, forced diuresis, and mesna, a chemoprotectant that binds with acrolein, and is eliminated via the urine. Secondary malignancy, especially leukemia, is a well-recognized complication of exposure to these agents and is likely due to the intercalation of these alkylating agents into DNA of normal host cells, causing genetic changes leading to this malignant process.

Although alkylating agents share a common mechanism of action, they have a variety of other characteristics that are quite divergent because of different chemical structures. Thus, pharmacokinetic differences exist among agents with regard to renal clearance (carboplatin) and the requirement for hepatic metabolism to be active (cyclophosphamide). Because of these differences, there is less cross-resistance within the class of alkylating agents than other classes of chemotherapeutic agents.

Antimetabolites

The antimetabolites represent the best-studied class of cancer therapeutic agents. Methotrexate is widely used in clinical situations with activity against a variety of neoplasms (e.g., leukemia, lymphoma, breast cancer, and osteogenic sarcoma) as well as nonmalignant disorders (e.g., psoriasis, rheumatoid arthritis, graft-vs.-host disease, etc.). Methotrexate exerts its wide therapeutic activity via its ability to act as a folate antagonist. Although there are several possible ways to act as a folate antagonist, the major mechanism is via inhibition of the dihydrofolate reductase enzyme in the target cell. This depletes the cell of the available reduced folates and inhibits de novo synthesis of purines and pyrimidines.

High doses of methotrexate can be given safely with an increased therapeutic window by providing a rescue dose of reduced folic acid (leucovorin) several hours after the methotrexate. Toxicity from methotrexate includes myelotoxicity and gastrointestinal mucosal irritation. Chronic low-dose oral methotrexate can cause severe hepatotoxicity.

Other critical intracellular pathways have been successfully targeted. The development of analogues to both purines and pyrimidines, the essential building blocks of DNA, has resulted in active chemotherapeutic agents. The pyrimidine analogue fluorouracil is widely used in colorectal carcinoma. Cytosine arabinoside (araC) is a nucleoside analogue of deoxycytidine and is active against a variety of hematological malignancies. Although the impact of age on azacitadine, a pyrimidine analogue, has not been formally studied, this drug is particularly useful in the treatment of elderly patients with myelodysplastic syndrome and AML. Purine analogues include mercap-topurine, thioguanine, and hydroxyurea. The relatively newly discovered purine ana-logues 2-fluoroadenosine-5-phosphate (fludarabine), 2-chlorodeoxyadenosine, and deoxycoformycin (pentostatin), have further expanded this class of drugs.

Fluorouracil is a commonly used analogue of pyrimidine. There are many potential sites of action of fluorouracil. Fluorouracil requires intracellular activation to exert its antitumor effect. The major target appears to be thymidylate synthase, and the setting of reduced folate availability can further augment antitumor activity. There are other mechanisms that explain fluorouracil's antitumor activity. Unfortu-nately, resistance is common, and each of the mechanisms of action can be evaded by tumor cells. The major toxicity from fluorouracil is dose-related and specifically affects the gastrointestinal mucosa and myeloid elements. Toxicity is related to the schedule of administration of the drug. Diarrhea can be severe and life threatening, especially when a regimen of continuous infusion is used. When leucovorin is used to augment the activity of fluorouracil, gastrointestinal symptoms are increased.

Capecitabine is an orally administered prodrug of 5'-deoxy-5-fluorouridine, which generates 5-FU selectively in tumor cells. It is FDA-approved for treatment of metastatic breast cancer and early stage and metastatic colon cancer. No formal studies have been done examining the pharmacokinetics of capecitabine in the elderly, but patients with hepatic and/or renal dysfunction should receive the drug in a dose-reduced fashion.

Fludarabine, a nucleoside analogue, has become important in the treatment of cancer because of its activity in hematologic malignancies such as chronic lymphocy-tic leukemia (the frequency of which is increased in the elderly population) and the low-grade lymphomas. Fludarabine is active against DNA polymerase-α and acts to stop DNA chain growth. It also decreases concentrations of critical nucleotides. Fludarabine causes significant myelosuppression and, in high doses, causes severe neurotoxicity. The drug is cleared by the kidney, and the dose should be decreased as creatinine clearance decreases (Table 1).

Gemcitabine is an intravenously administered deoxycytidine antimetabolite closely related to araC, but different in its spectrum of activity. Unlike its cousin, whose use is limited to the treatment of hematologic malignancies, gemcitabine is used primar-ily to treat solid tumors (although it may be the most active single agent in previously treated Hodgkin's lymphoma) (41). It has shown activity in cancers of the pancreas, lung (both non-small-cell and small-cell variants), breast, and ovary, amongst others.

Gemcitabine undergoes intracellular conversion and phosphorylation to the nucleotide gemcitabine triphosphate, which competes with deoxycytidine triphos-hate for incorporation into DNA. Elimination is primarily renal, but there are no dosing guidelines for patients with renal or hepatic impairment. Gemcitabine elimination varies according to age and gender, with the half-life of gemcitabine in 79-year-old patients being nearly twice as that of 29-year-old patients (2004). This is important given that the dose-limiting toxicity of gemcitabine is myelosuppress-ion, particularly thrombocytopenia; in an effort to avoid this, some suggest a less frequent schedule of gemcitabine administration.

Plant Derivatives

Many chemotherapeutic agents are natural products that originated from plants. There are three commonly used classes of drugs in this category. The vinca alkaloids (e.g., vincristine), the epipodophyllotoxins (e.g., etoposide), and taxanes (e.g., taxol) will be discussed.

The vincas are active in a wide range of cancers. The mechanism of action involves a disruption of microtubular assembly. Vincristine is one member of this family. The drug binds to tubulin and prevents mitosis, which is dependent on the microtubular assembly process for productive cell division. Vincristine is primarily metabolized in the liver. There is a high degree of protein binding and binding to the cellular elements (platelets) in the blood stream. Toxicity is principally peripheral neuropathy, which is age related and occurs more frequently in older patients. Vinorelbine, a relatively newer vinca alkaloid, is less toxic to the peripheral nerves but has more hematologic toxicity. Its activity profile has made it an attractive drug for use in elderly patients with breast cancer and it has been shown to improve survival of elderly patients with non-small-cell lung cancer (42). The drugs in this family are vesicants and can cause significant local damage if extravasation occurs.

Etoposide represents the family of drugs from the mandrake plant, the epipodophyllotoxins. Like the vincas, etoposide exerts its antineoplastic activity via disruption of the microtubular assembly process, although the site of action is different from that of the vincas. Etoposide also has an additional mechanism of action; by binding to and disrupting topoisomerase II, etoposide induces direct strand breakage in DNA. This is probably the more clinically relevant action as an antineoplastic agent.

Etoposide appears to be cleared by a combination of renal and metabolic processes. Because of significant protein binding, the dose should be adjusted for patients with both renal and hepatic insufficiency. The major dose-limiting toxicity has been myelosupression. Because of the DNA strand breakage, etoposide has been associated with secondary malignancies, including leukemia.

The bark of the yew tree yielded a family of compounds known as the taxanes. This family of drugs includes paclitaxel (semisynthetic, from the bark of the Pacific yew) and docetaxel (semisynthetic, from the bark of the European yew). These drugs, which have very different toxicity profiles, have wide spectrums of activity including cancers of the ovary, breast, lung, head and neck, and pancreas. These drugs also act via microtubule assembly; they promote the assembly and prevent the normal depolymerization. The taxanes are hepatically metabolized and excreted in the bile and thus require dose adjustments in the setting of hepatic insufficiency (43).

A high percentage of hypersensitivity reactions initially limited the wide use of paclitaxel, but with adequate premedications, these can be controlled. A new formulation of paclitaxel (abraxane) that delivers the drug in an albumin-bound injectable suspension instead of using the Cremaphor® solvent, thereby reducing the risk of hypersensitivity, and possibly increasing the antitumor activity is used. Toxicity of the taxanes is dose-dependent and is primarily reflected in bone marrow suppression, particularly neutropenia. Neurologic toxicity can also occur with the taxanes; docetaxel may also cause edema. Although there are few studies that examine toxicity of the taxanes in an elderly population, no data support dose modifications based on age, although docetaxel-induced neutropenia may be more prevalent in patients over the age of 65 (44,45).

Antitumor Antibiotics

Several chemotherapeutic drugs have been derived from antibiotics. The anthracyclines have been extensively studied. These agents are widely active and are used in a variety of tumors. They were originally isolated from the *Streptomyces* species of bacteria. Although doxorubicin and daunorubicin were the first two drugs in this family, there are now many representative anthracyclines. Other antitumor antibiotics include bleomycin and mitomycin C, but we will focus on anthracyclines in this section.

The anthracyclines are active in a wide range of tumors, including breast cancer, lung cancer, and sarcomas, as well as leukemias and lymphomas. The mechanism of action continues to be studied. Topoisomerase II inhibition with resultant DNA strand breakage appears to be an important mechanism. Additionally, the formation of oxygen radicals also enhances cytotoxicity. The anthracyclines appear to be metabolized significantly in the liver with minimal renal clearance. Dose adjustments on the basis of serum bilirubin are necessary.

The major toxicity from the anthracyclines includes myelosuppression and mucositis. The drugs are vesicants and local reactions can be severe. Cardiac toxicity is related to the cumulative dose over time and appears to be directly related to oxygen radical development. Pre-existing cardiac dysfunction increases the risk of cardiac toxicity secondary to the drug. The antitumor antibiotics are also subject to the multidrug resistance (MDR) pump (see section on Drug Resistance and Supportive Care). As such, resistance to these agents is frequently shared with other naturally occurring compounds.

Targeted Therapy

Recently, novel, targeted therapies have been developed to treat malignancies. The first of these was rituximab, a genetically engineered chimeric murine/human monoclonal immunoglobulin (Ig) G that binds specifically to CD20, a B-lymphocyte differentiation antigen on pre-B and mature B-lymphocytes. CD20 regulates early pathways in the activation process for cell cycle initiation and differentiation. Rituximab has proven to be effective in the treatment of patients with a variety of lymphoproliferative disorders and its use is currently being investigated in the treatment of some autoimmune disorders. It is administered intravenously and is well tolerated. Patients should receive prophylaxis against hypersensitivity reactions with acetaminophen and antihistamines. Infusion rates are increased as tolerated, and rituximab does not require dose modifications for impairment of hepatic or renal function.

In a randomized study targeting elderly patients with this drug because of their historically poor survival with standard therapy, treatment-naive patients with diffuse large B-cell non-Hodgkin's lymphoma were randomized to receive either standard cyclophosphamide, adriamycin, vincristine, and prednisone (CHOP) chemotherapy or the same regimen combined with rituximab (R-CHOP), and overall and event-free survival benefits were found in the R-CHOP cohort. Additionally, patients receiving R-CHOP had significantly reduced risks of treatment failure and death. All of this was achieved without greater toxicity than that associated with standard CHOP (46).

Trastuzumab, a recombinant, DNA-derived humanized monoclonal antibody against the human epidermal growth factor 2 (HER2) protein, was approved by the FDA in 1998, for the treatment of metastatic breast carcinoma that overexpresses HER2. In the pivotal trial that led to its approval, the drug was administered to patients in combination with chemotherapy and patients receiving it had a significantly longer time to progression, higher overall response rate, and longer median survival in comparison to those patients receiving chemotherapy alone. The major side effect of trastuzumab is cardiac dysfunction (typically of low grade), particularly when it is administered with an anthracycline. While the contribution of age was not examined in the original study, a retrospective analysis was performed and it was found that patients aged over 60 were almost twice as likely to experience cardiac dysfunction as those patients under the age of 60 (21% vs. 11%) (47). More recently, trastuzumab has shown major benefit in patients with early stage breast cancer.

Caution is advised when considering patients with significant pre-existing cardiac dysfunction. All patients receiving trastuzumab should undergo clinical surveillance for signs of cardiac dysfunction and an appropriate workup should be pursued in those who develop it. Symptoms are typically responsive to standard medical therapy and therapy can often be resumed once stability is achieved.

Gemtuzumab ozogamicin is a recombinant humanized IgG_4 kappa antibody to the CD33 antigen conjugated with the cytotoxic antitumor antibiotic, calicheamicin, and is used in the treatment of myeloid leukemias. It was approved by the FDA in 2000 for the treatment of AML patients 60 years of age and older in first relapse who are not considered candidates for cytotoxic therapy. No differences have been found in the pharmacokinetics of this drug based on gender or age (48). Caution should be taken in its administration though, due to the associated prolonged period of neutropenia following administration.

Gefitinib is an oral, selective epidermal growth factor receptor (EGFR)-tyrosine kinase inhibitor approved for use in patients who have failed both platinum-based and docetaxel-based therapies for non-small-cell lung cancer. It has been studied in elderly patients who have received as few as one prior treatment regimen (chemotherapy or radiotherapy) in an experimental fashion, and has shown modest activity and good tolerability (49). Dermatitis, usually mild, is its most common toxicity. Interstitial lung disease is very rarely seen, but can be fatal. No toxicities were greater in the elderly population than those seen in younger patients in other studies. When treating these patients in a palliative fashion, it is an excellent addition to one's armamentarium.

As our understanding of the molecular basis of cancer expands, more molecular targets are coming into focus. Several additional agents aimed at tumor vasculature [vascular endothelial growth factor (VEGF)/EGFR] and intracellular signaling (tyrosine kinases, the proteosome, etc.) have been developed. Agents that have recently been approved by the FDA include: (i) bevacizumab, a VEGF inhibitor (for metastatic colorectal cancer in combination with a fluorouracil-based regimen); (ii) cetuximab an EGFR inhibitor (for patients with irinotecan-refractory metastatic colorectal cancer); (iii) bortezomib, a proteosome inhibitor (for the treatment of patients with refractory multiple myeloma); (iv) erlotinib an EGFR-tyrosine kinase inhibitor (for treatment of patients with metastatic non-small-cell lung cancer); and (v) imatinib mesylate, a tyrosine kinase inhibitor (for the treatment of metastatic gastrointestinal stromal tumors and chronic myelogenous leukemia). There have been no published studies to prompt concerns regarding toxicities specific to the elderly population. Dosing should not be adjusted based on age.

Hormonal Agents

Hormonal therapy with tamoxifen or an aromatase inhibitor is the most important component of adjuvant therapy for breast cancer and the primary initial modality for patients with hormone-receptor-positive metastatic disease. Hormonal agents are also the primary therapeutic modality for metastatic prostate cancer. There is a paucity of data regarding specific toxicities of these agents in the elderly population; however, their side-effect profiles are well known and clinicians should be aware of these when caring for patients in this population.

Tamoxifen and the aromatase inhibitors are frequently associated with menopausal symptoms like hot flashes and vaginal dryness. Tamoxifen decreases antithrombin III activity by 10% and increases sex-hormone-binding globulin. Because of this, there is an increased risk of thrombosis and stroke, 87% of which occurred in women over the age of 50 years in the National Surgical Adjuvant Breast and Bowel Project-P1 trial (50,51).

Anastrozole, a nonsteroidal, fourth-generation aromatase inhibitor was the first agent in its class to be compared head-to-head with tamoxifen in a randomized fashion. Tamoxifen and anastrozole are associated with musculoskeletal pain, but anastrozole appears to increase the likelihood of musculoskeletal events and bone fractures (52). Additionally, patients taking anastrozole are more likely to have hypercholesterolemia.

Drug Resistance and Supportive Care

Many of the naturally occurring anticancer drugs share a common mechanism of resistance. The MDR pump has the ability to actively pump chemotherapy drugs out of the target cells. Many cancer cells become resistant to the chemotherapeutic drugs through this mechanism. Elderly patients may be particularly prone to this problem. In AML, for example, older patients have greater expression of the MDR gene product than the younger patients. Methods to reverse resistance have focused on poisoning the MDR pump and represent an active area of research.

Chemotherapeutic treatments for cancer patients have long been associated with significant toxicity. Elderly patients have frequently suffered from many of the toxicities as previously noted. It is hoped that advances in supportive care will provide improvements in the toxicity to the therapeutic ratio of the chemotherapeutic drugs.

One of the major advances in supportive care for chemotherapy has been the discovery of recombinant growth factors for hematopoietic cells. Currently, treatments to improve the neutrophil count are approved by the U.S. FDA. There has been extensive commentary on the appropriateness of the use of these growth factors. In acute leukemia, these growth factors can speed the recovery of neutrophil counts for patients going through high doses of chemotherapy but they do not appear to impart improved survival (53). Importantly, the use of myeloid growth factors appears to be safe without clinically significant stimulation of the leukemic process.

Clinically important end points such as a decrease in the number of hospital days, fewer antibiotic days, and cost savings are important and can be improved with the use of these growth factors. Nonetheless, until there are clear survival benefits, there will be continued debate regarding the appropriateness of these expensive factors. The American Society of Clinical Oncology (ASCO) has formulated guidelines for the use of these growth factors (54). The interested reader is referred to that publication. Although there are no specific recommendations based on age alone (outside the situation in acute leukemia), the general recommendations (i.e., prophylaxis is recommended when the risk of febrile neutropenia exceeds 40%) in those guidelines are appropriate for elderly patients with cancer. Others recommend the use of growth factors in elderly patients, in particular, the use of primary prophylaxis in patients receiving CHOP, or CHOP-like regimens (39).

Recombinant human erythropoietin has been useful in the treatment of elderly patients with severe anemia—both treatment related and unrelated—and it can be effective in the setting of transfusion dependency. ASCO and National Comprehensive Cancer Network guidelines are available to advise usage (55,56).

SUMMARY

Pharmaceutical agents are an important part of the armamentarium for cancer therapy. With appropriate administration and monitoring, they can be used effectively for elderly cancer patients in adjuvant, curative, and palliative settings.

REFERENCES

1. Borkowski JM, Duerr M, et al. Relation between age and clearance rate of nine investigational anticancer drugs from phase I pharmacokinetic data. Cancer Chemother Pharmacol 1994; 33:493–496.
2. Mor V, Masterson-Allen S, et al. Relationship between age at diagnosis and treatment received by cancer patients. J Am Geriatr Soc 1985; 33:585–589.
3. Samet J, Hunt WC, et al. Choice of cancer therapy varies with age of patient. JAMA 1986; 255(24):3385–3390.
4. Champlin RE, Gajewski JL, et al. Treatment of acute myelogenous leukemia in the elderly. Semin Oncol 1989; 16:51–56.
5. Leslie WT. Chemotherapy in older cancer patients. Oncology 1992; 6(2):74–80.
6. Nerenz DR, Lov RR, et al. Psychosocial consequences of cancer chemotherapy for elderly patients. Health Serv Res 1986; 6(2):961 976.
7. Vestal RE, Montamat SC, et al. Drugs in special patient groups: the elderly. In: Melmon KL, Hoffmann BB, Nierenberg DW, eds. Basic Principles in Therapeutics. New York: McGraw-Hill, 1992:851–874.
8. Vestal RE. Aging and pharmacology. Cancer 1997; 80(7):1302–1310.
9. Gautier M, Cohen HJ. Multiple myeloma in the elderly. J Am Geriatr Soc 1994; 42:46.
10. Verbeeck RK, Cardinal JA, et al. Effect of age and sex on the plasma binding of acidic and basic drugs. Eur J Clin Pharmacol 1984; 27:91–97.
11. Chrischilles EA, Foley DJ, et al. Use of medications by persons 65 and over: data from the established populations for epidemiologic studies of the elderly. J Gerontol 1992; 47:M137–M144.
12. Woodhouse K, Wynne HA. Age-related changes in hepatic function. Implications for drug therapy. Drugs Aging 1992; 2:243–255.
13. Ratain MJ, Schilsky RL, et al. Pharmacodynamics in cancer therapy. J Clin Oncol 1990; 8(10):1739–1753.
14. Extermann M, Yoder J, et al. Influence of p450-metabolized concomitant medications on toxicity from chemotherapy in older cancer patients. Proc Am Soc Clin Oncol 2003; 22:730.
15. Walsh SJ, Begg CB, et al. Cancer chemotherapy in the elderly. Semin Oncol 1989; 16(1):66–75.
16. Begg CB, Elson PJ, et al. A study of excess hematologic toxicity in elderly patients treated on cancer chemotherapy protocols. In: Yancik R, ed. Cancer in the Elderly: Approaches to Early Detection and Treatment. New York: Springer-Verlag, 1989:149–163.
17. Gelman RS, Taylor SG. Cyclophosphamide, methotrexate, and 5-fluorouracil chemotherapy in women more than 65 years old with advanced breast cancer: the elimination of age trends in toxicity by using doses based on creatinine clearance. J Clin Oncol 1984; 2(12):1404–1413.
18. Kahn SB, Begg CB, et al. Full dose versus attenuated dose daunorubicin, cytosine arabinoside, and 6-thioguanine in the treatment of acute nonlymphocytic leukemia in the elderly. J Clin Oncol 1984; 2(8):865–870.
19. Vose JM. Cytokine use in the older patient. Semin Oncol 1995; 22(1):6–8.
20. Philip T, Guglielmi C, Chauvin F, et al. Autologous bone marrow transplantation versus conventional chemotherapy (DHAP) in relapsed non-Hodgkin lymphoma (NHL): final analysis of the PARMA randomized study (216 patients). Proc Am Soc Clin Oncol 1995; 14:390.

21. Attal M, Harousseau JL, et al. A prospective, randomized trial of autologous bone mar-
     row transplantation and chemotherapy in multiple myeloma. Intergroupe francais du
     myelome. N Engl J Med 1996; 335(2):91–97.
22. Josting A, Reiser M, et al. Treatment of primary progressive Hodgkin's and aggressive
     non-Hodgkin's lymphoma: Is there a chance for cure? J Clin Oncol 2000; 18(2):332–339.
23. Bonneterre J, Roche H, et al. French Adjuvant Study Group 05 trial (FEC 50 vs. FEC
     100): 10-year update of benefit/risk ratio after adjuvant chemotherapy (CT) in node-
     positive (N+), early breast cancer (EBC) patients (pts). Proc Am Soc Clin Oncol 2003;
     22:24.
24. Novitzky N, Thomas V, et al. Increasing dose intensity of anthracycline antibiotics
     improves outcome in patients with acute myelogenous leukemia. Am J Hematol 2004;
     76(4):319–329.
25. Balzarotti M, Spina M, et al. Intensified CHOP regimen in aggressive lymphomas: max-
     imal dose intensity and dose density of doxorubicin and cyclophosphamide. Ann Oncol
     2002; 13(9):1341–1346.
26. Itoh K, Ohtsu T, et al. Randomized phase II study of biweekly CHOP and dose-escalated
     CHOP with prophylactic use of lenograstim (glycosylated G-CSF) in aggressive non-
     Hodgkin's lymphoma: Japan Clinical Oncology Group Study 9505. Ann Oncol 2002;
     13(9):1347–1355.
27. Citron ML, Berry DA, et al. Randomized trial of dose-dense versus conventionally
     scheduled and sequential versus concurrent combination chemotherapy as postoperative
     adjuvant treatment of node-positive primary breast cancer: first report of Intergroup
     Trial C9741/Cancer and Leukemia Group B Trial 9741. J Clin Oncol 2003;
     21(8):1431–1439.
28. Brower M, Asbury R, et al. Adjuvant chemotherapy of colorectal cancer in the elderly.
     Population-based experience. Proc Am Soc Clin Oncol 1993; 12:195.
29. Van Hoff DD, Layard MW, et al. Risk factors for doxorubicin-induced congestive heart
     failure. Ann Intern Med 1979; 91:710–717.
30. Swain SM, Whaley F, et al. Cardioprotection with dexrazoxane for doxorubicin-
     containing therapy in advanced breast cancer. J Clin Oncol 1997; 15(4):1318–1332.
31. Seymour L, Bramwell V. Use of dexrazoxane as a cardioprotectant in patients receiving
     doxorubicin or epirubicin chemotherapy for the treatment of cancer (Practice guideline
     report no. 12-5). Cancer Care Ontario 2004:23.
32. Ginsberg SL, Comis RL. The pulmonary toxicity of antineoplastic agents. Semin Oncol
     1982; 9:34–41.
33. Damon LE, Mass R, et al. The association between high-dose cytarabine neurotoxicity
     and renal insufficiency. J Clin Oncol 1989; 7(10):1563–1568.
34. Baker WJ, Royer GL Jr, et al. Cytarabine and neurologic toxicity. J Clin Oncol 1991;
     9(4):679–693.
35. Balducci L, Extermann M. Cancer chemotherapy in the older patient. Cancer 1997;
     80(7):65–71.
36. Conti JA, Christman K. Cancer chemotherapy in the elderly. J Clin Gastroenterol 1997;
     21(1):65–71.
37. Lichtman SM. Recent developments in the pharmacology of anticancer drugs in the
     elderly. Curr Opin Oncol 1998; 10(6):572–579.
38. Vincenzi B, Santini D, et al. The antineoplastic treatment in the elderly. Clin Terapeutica
     2002; 153(3):207–215.
39. Balducci L. New paradigms for treating elderly patients with cancer: the comprehensive
     geriatric assessment and guidelines for supportive care. J Support Oncol 2003; 1(4 suppl
     2):30–37.
40. Balducci L, Carreca I. Supportive care of the older cancer patient. Crit Rev Oncol
     Hematol 2003; 48(suppl):S65–S70.
41. Santoro A, Bredenfeld H, et al. Gemcitabine in the treatment of refractory Hodgkin's
     disease: results of a multicenter phase II study. J Clin Oncol 2000; 18(13):2615–2619.

42. Effects of vinorelbine on quality of life and survival of elderly patients with advanced non-small-cell lung cancer. The Elderly Lung Cancer Vinorelbine Italian Study Group. J Natl Cancer Inst 1999; 91(1):66–72.

43. Venook AP, Egorin MJ, et al. Phase I and pharmacokinetic trial of paclitaxel in patients with hepatic dysfunction: Cancer and Leukemia Group B 9264. J Clin Oncol 1998; 16:1811–1819.

44. Lichtman SM, Gal D, et al. No increased risk of Taxol toxicity in older patients. J Am Geriatr Soc 1996; 44:472–474.

45. Ten Tije AJ, Verweij J, et al. Prospective evaluation of the pharmacokinetics and toxicity profile of docetaxel in the elderly. J Clin Oncol 2005; 23(6):1070–1077.

46. Coiffier B, Lepage E, et al. CHOP chemotherapy plus rituximab compared with CHOP alone in elderly patients with diffuse large-B-cell lymphoma [see comment]. N Engl J Med 2002; 346(4):235–242.

47. Fyfe G, Mass R, et al. Survival benefit of Herceptin (trastuzumab) and chemotherapy in older (age > 60) patients. Br Ca Res Treat 2001; 269(3):abs 526.

48. Korth-Bradley JM, Dowell JA, et al. Impact of age and gender on the pharmacokinetics of gemtuzumab ozogamicin. Pharmacotherapy 2001; 21(10):1175–1180.

49. Gridelli C, Maione P, et al. Gefitinib in elderly and unfit patients affected by advanced non-small-cell lung cancer. Br J Cancer 2003; 89(10):1827–1829.

50. Dunn BK, Ford LG. Breast cancer prevention: results of the National Surgical Adjuvant Breast and Bowel Project (NSABP) breast cancer prevention trial (NSABP P-1: BCPT). Eur J Cancer 2000; 36(suppl 4):S49–S50.

51. Kinsinger LS, Harris R, et al. Chemoprevention of breast cancer: a summary of the evidence for the U.S. Preventive Services Task Force. Ann Intern Med 2002; 137(1):59–69.

52. Baum M, Budzar AU, et al. Anastrozole alone or in combination with tamoxifen versus tamoxifen alone for adjuvant treatment of postmenopausal women with early breast cancer: first results of the ATAC randomized trial. Lancet 2002; 359(9324):2131–2139.

53. Dombret H, Chastang C, et al. A controlled study of recombinant human granulocyte colony-stimulating factor in elderly patients after treatment for acute myelogenous leukemia. N Engl J Med 1993; 332:1678–1683.

54. Ozer H, Armitage JO, et al. Update of recommendations for the use of hematopoietic colony-stimulating factors: evidence-based, clinical practice guidelines. J Clin Oncol 2000; 18(20):3558–3585.

55. Rizzo JD, Lichtin AE, et al. Use of epoetin in patients with cancer: evidence-based clinical practice guidelines of the American Society of Clinical Oncology and the American Society of Hematology. J Clin Oncol 2002; 20(19):4083–4107.

56. Sabbatini P, Cella D, et al. NCCN cancer and treatment-related anemia guidelines 2004.

6

Legal Issues in Caring for the Elderly

Margot G. Birke
Elder Law Solutions, Newburyport, Massachusetts, U.S.A.

INTRODUCTION

Over the course of the 20th century, the elder population has increased from three to thirty-five million. In 1900, the number of "old old," those 85 years and above, was just over 100,000. In the year 2000, this number had swelled to 4.2 million. In 2003, those 65 years and older accounted for slightly over 12% of the total population of the United States.

In 2011, the "Baby Boomer" generation will turn 65, causing the number of elderly to increase dramatically between 2010 and 2030. The older population is projected to grow to 71.5 million by 2030, or to approximately 20% of the overall population. Even with these statistics, the United States is a younger country than Italy or Japan, and slightly younger than Europe (1).

The U.S. health care system and overall social structure will be significantly impacted by this increase in the elder cohort. A better understanding of the wide spectrum of laws that govern the medical care, living arrangements, and overall ability of elders in our society to live independently, or to be cared for, is necessary for those who in any way service this diverse group of individuals.

This chapter will provide an overview of the field of elder law, advance directives for health care and finances, guardianship, Health Insurance Portability and Accountability Act (HIPAA), and veteran's Aid and Attendance benefits. Medicare, an entitlement program established under Title XVIII of the Social Security Act in 1965 (2), will also be discussed along with Medicaid, a welfare program also developed in 1965 as Title XIX of the Social Security Act (3); Social Security Disability Insurance; Supplemental Security Income; and assisted living and continuing care communities.

ELDER LAW

Elder law is a specialty area of law directing its services to the specific needs of older clients and to clients with disabilities. Elder law attorneys practice in multiple areas including estate planning, Medicare, Medicaid, Social Security benefits, retirement income planning, disability planning, probate and estate administration, guardianship, and decision making through the use of durable powers of attorney, advanced directives, wills, and trusts. Elder law is a holistic and interdisciplinary practice that blends traditional estate planning with maximizing available community and state resources in concert with individual and family needs.

The "elderly" population runs the gamut from the "young old," 55 to 75 years; the "middle old," from 75 to 85 years; and the "old old," 85 years and over.

Elder law as we know it today grew out of the need of older Americans who were living longer, often with chronic illnesses, to access available legal, medical, and custodial care. The Older Americans Act of 1965 (the Act) (4), as amended, established a legal framework within which older Americans would be provided with a range of programs and services designed to assist them to better care for themselves or to be cared for by others. The Act focuses on the areas of income, housing, health, employment, retirement, and community services. As such, it has served as the cornerstone of the development of Elder law as a separate legal discipline.

A threshold question for an Elder law attorney is "Who is the client?" Often, the first person to make contact with the attorney is the adult child of the elder who is the subject of the planning. This distinction is important because the attorney-client relationship is of a fiduciary nature, which means that the attorney owes a duty of undivided loyalty to the client.

Many elders are reluctant to discuss how they really feel in the presence of their children. The Elder law attorney must be attuned to the existence of family dissonance and ensure, if meeting with the elder, that it is clear to all concerned that the elder is the client, not the children. The attorney must be certain that the plan put in place is the plan desired by the elder, and not the elder's children.

If the attorney meets only with the child, or a friend of the elder, then the child or the friend is the attorney's client. The only exception is when the child or friend meets with an attorney while acting in the capacity of attorney-in-fact for the elder under a valid durable power-of-attorney or health care proxy.

ADVANCE DIRECTIVES

Doctrine of Informed Consent

The Doctrine of Informed Consent finds its roots in the 14th Amendment to the United States Constitution's liberty interest and the right to privacy carved out by the Supreme Court, which protects private or personal activity from government interference. The idea of a living will or advance health care directive can trace its history through a body of case law beginning as far back as 1891 (5) that maintains the individual's right to determine what happens to him or her, and to be free of the restraint or interference of others as long as the individual is operating within the parameters of legal authority. Some states have gone a step further in protecting these rights by enacting informed consent statutes.

There are three elements to the Doctrine of Informed Consent: knowledge, volition, and competence. Consent requires disclosure of the risks and benefits of the proposed treatment, the effects of treatment or nontreatment, and who will be providing the treatment. The consent must be given voluntarily, free of coercion or manipulation, and the patient must be competent in order to give the consent. As long as the patient is deemed capable of giving or withholding consent, the patient's wishes must be respected.

In *Cruzan v. Director, Missouri Dept. of Health* (6), the Supreme Court established a constitutional right to refuse medical treatment, and in *Washington v. Glucksberd* (7), the Court provided guidance on the degree of autonomy to be afforded to a terminally ill patient. The right to refuse treatment is not absolute. It may be limited by four state interests:

1. Preserving human life
2. Safeguarding standards and integrity of the medical profession
3. Preventing suicide
4. Protecting innocent parties, such as children and incompetents (7).

The Patient Self-Determination Act

The Patient Self-Determination Act (the PSDA) (8), passed in 1990, and implemented on December 1, 1991, encourages individuals to make choices and decisions in advance regarding the kind of medical care they wish to accept or refuse, prior to becoming incapable of expressing their wishes because of illness. However, caution must be exercised by the patient, or the patient's advocate, when admitted to the hospital or other health care facility that, no document is signed without a clear understanding of its purpose and import.

Competence

Individuals are deemed legally competent when they become majors. Competence is a legal concept and is specific to the task at hand. The burden of proving incompetence rests with the party asserting the claim. We must be competent, in the legal sense, when we execute a health care proxy and/or a living will or either give or withhold permission for treatment. Competency for executing a health care proxy is often defined by the statutes in the jurisdiction where the document is being executed.

Capacity

Capacity is a medical perspective. The four factors that should be assessed when evaluating an individual's capacity to consent to treatment are:

1. understanding—does the individual understand the risks and benefits of treatment or nontreatment;
2. appreciation—does the individual have insight into his or her level of illness and the treatment options;
3. reasoning—is the individual able to manipulate information rationally; and
4. expression—does the individual manifest consistency in his or her choices when it comes to accepting or rejecting treatment options.

The ability to consent to treatment will depend on the complexity of the treatment plan. For example, a risky treatment will require a higher level of competency than a simple treatment that is easy to explain.

Health Care Proxies and Medical Directives

When people execute a health care proxy, they give another person the authority to make health care decisions for them, should they become unable to communicate their wishes. Having a health care proxy in place will help ensure that their wishes will be carried out.

A "medical directive," "living will," or "advance directive" gives direction on what kind of care a person wishes to receive, and includes instruction on beginning or terminating life-sustaining treatment. Forty-six states and the District of Columbia provide authority for both health care proxies and living wills. Massachusetts, Michigan, and New York authorize only health care proxies, and Alaska provides only for living wills (9).

Careful selection of the health care agent is very important. One must be sure to appoint someone who will be able to carry out the individual's wishes, regardless of how he or she feels about the individual's choices.

It is very important for people to have their health care proxy available should they become ill unexpectedly. Their doctor should have a copy and they should discuss its terms with him or her. The U.S. Living Will Registry (10) will electronically store advance directives, organ donor information, and emergency contact information, and will make them available to health care providers across the country, 24 hours a day, through an automated system.

Durable Power-of-Attorney for Finances

A power-of-attorney grants to the "attorney-in-fact" the legal right to act on a person's behalf in financial and business matters. The attorney-in-fact steps into the person's shoes and is obligated to act in the person's best interest, and for the person's benefit. The term "durable" indicates that the power of the agent will continue even after the principal becomes incapacitated.

A power-of-attorney takes effect as soon as it is signed by an individual. However, a "springing" power-of-attorney takes effect only when conditions in the document are met. The usual requirement is that one or more physicians certify in writing that the individual is incapable of handling his or her affairs. People do not give up their rights when they execute a power-of-attorney, but they do bestow concurrent rights on their named attorney-in-fact.

This power can be revoked at any time before they become incapacitated. They merely have to notify their agent in writing. When agent receives the letter, agent can no longer act under the power-of-attorney. It is important to relay to the person who is selected as the agent that he or she cannot be held liable for his or her acts unless the agent knowingly acts improperly or with gross negligence. Also, depending on how the power is written, an individual can have more than one attorney-in-fact, and both parties can be required to act together, or be allowed to act independently. The attorney-in-fact should keep detailed records of his or her actions on a person's behalf, and make sure that his or her personal funds are not commingled with the client's.

GUARDIANSHIP AND SURROGATE DECISION MAKING

Old age and infirmity are not sufficient bases for guardianship. Nor are erratic, idiosyncratic, or irrational behavior sufficient reasons for guardianship. Just because an individual makes bad decisions is not a cause to seek guardianship for that person.

Guardianship is a legal relationship whereby the state Court with the designated jurisdiction gives one person (the guardian) the power to make personal and financial decisions for another (the ward). A guardian may be appointed when the designated Court determines that an individual is unable to care for himself or herself and/or his or her estate by reason of mental illness, mental retardation, or physical incapacity.

Guardianship is appropriate when impaired judgment or capacity poses a major threat to a person's welfare. A medical evaluation by a licensed physician is necessary to establish the proposed ward's condition. However, only a court can determine the need for a guardian.

A person under guardianship suffers substantial deprivation of basic civil liberties, such as the right to consent to medical care, the right to vote, and the right to choose where to live.

A properly executed, durable power-of-attorney can avoid the need for a conservatorship—or guardian for a person's estate. A health care proxy, executed when the individual was competent, can avoid the need for guardianship of the person.

Unless limited by the court, the guardian has total control over the finances and the personal decisions of the ward. This includes deciding where the ward will live, determining how the ward's funds will be spent, and making routine medical decisions for the ward. In cases involving extraordinary medical decisions, such as life-sustaining medical care, the administration of antipsychotic drugs, or commitment to a mental health facility, the guardian must to seek the approval of the court in a separate proceeding.

MEDICARE

Medicare is a federal health insurance program covering acute and postacute care for approximately 42 million elderly and disabled Americans (11). Enacted by Congress in 1965 as Title XVIII of the Social Security Act, it provides coverage for most people over 65 years of age, and some younger people who are disabled, as well as for persons suffering from end-stage renal disease. Medicare now has four parts. Part A provides hospital insurance; Part B provides medical insurance; Part C or Medicare + Choice, now renamed Medicare Advantage (MA), provides hospital and medical coverage through health care plans operated by private businesses; and Medicare Part D is the new prescription drug benefit, aslo provided through private ensurers.

Medicare Part A

Those persons who have accrued 40 or more quarters of employment and are covered by Social Security need not pay a premium for Medicare Part A. The Omnibus Reconciliation Act of 1997 provides certain individuals who not eligible for Social Security or Railroad Retirement benefits with the opportunity to purchase Medicare coverage at reduced premiums. Medicare premiums are recalculated each year.

A benefit period, or "spell of illness," begins the day a patient enters a hospital or a skilled nursing facility (SNF) as an inpatient, and continues through 60 days after discharge or if the patient is admitted to a SNF within 30 days of discharge from the hospital to be treated for the same condition. A benefit period runs for a maximum of 150 days in a hospital, and for a maximum of 100 days in a SNF.

Table 1 shows the Medicare Part A Hospital Insurance benefits for 2005.

Medicare Part B

Unlike Medicare Part A, Medicare Part B charges a monthly premium, which is usually deducted from a participant's Social Security payment. Part B supplements

Table 1 Medicare Part A Hospital Insurance

Service provided	Medicare covers	Individual pays
Hospital inpatient		
Days 1–60	Everything after deductible	Deductible: $912
Days 61–90	Everything after copayment	Copayment: $228/day
60 "Reserve Days"	Everything after copayment	Copayment: $456/day
Reserve days may be used only once in a participant's lifetime		
Beyond 150 days	Nothing	All costs beyond 150 days
Psychiatric inpatient		
Same coverage as other hospital inpatient but with a lifetime limit of 190 days—patient pays all costs after 190 days		
SNF: If daily skilled care needed following a three-day hospital stay		
Days 1–20	Everything	Nothing
Days 21–100	Everything after copayment	Copayment: $114/day
Beyond 100 days	Nothing	Everthing
Home health care	Everything except 20% of medical equipment	20% of approved amount for medical equipment
Hospice: Care for terminal illness	Everything except $5 per prescription and the lesser of 5% or $912 for respite care	Copayment of $5 per prescription; the lesser of 5% or $912 for respite care
Blood: Received during hospital or SNF stay	All after the first three pints	For the first three pints of blood each year

Abbreviation: SNF, skilled nursing facility.

the benefits provided under Part A. The major benefit under Part B is payment for physicians' services. In addition, Part B will cover home health care, durable medical equipment, outpatient physical therapy, and X-ray and diagnostic testing. Home care is also covered under Part B if the participant did not have a hospital stay of three days or more prior to home or SNF services or has exceeded the 100-day limit under Part A. A complete listing of available services under Medicare Part B can be found at the Medicare web site, www.medicare.gov. Details of Medicare Part B are provided in Table 2.

The Balanced Budget Act of 1997 created a law called the "Ban on Balanced Billing" (12). Under this law, in certain states, a physician cannot charge a Medicare participant more for a service than the rate that Medicare allows for the service. The states that have passed these charge-limit laws are Connecticut, Massachusetts, Minnesota, New York, Ohio, Pennsylvania, Rhode Island, and Vermont. This law does not apply to all medical providers.

Medicare deductibles are expected to increase each year by the estimated annual percentage increase in Part B expenditures. In other words, they will be increasing significantly as Part B expenditures increase. In addition, currently all Part B participants pay the same monthly premium for coverage ($78.20 in 2005). Beginning in 2007, the monthly premiums will be based on income, with higher-income seniors paying higher premiums. The percentage increases are shown below in Table 3.

At the age of 65, those who receive Social Security or Railroad Retirement benefits will be automatically enrolled in Medicare Part B. Those not yet 65 years can enroll in Medicare Part B when they sign up for Social Security or Railroad

Table 2 Medicare Part B Medical Insurance

Service provided	Medicare covers	Individual pays
Monthly premium		$78.20 per month
Annual deductible		$110.00 per year
Physician costs	80% of approved amount	20% of approved amount
Outpatient hospital care	80% of approved amount	A maximum of $912
Clinical lab services	Approved amount	Nothing
Medical equipment supplies	80% of approved amount	All other costs
Some preventative services	80 to 100%	20% of approved amount or nothing depending on the service
Mental health services		
Partial hospitalization	Same as psychiatric hospital	See Table 1
Outpatient	50% of approved amount	50% of approved amount

Plus up to an additional 15% of the Medicare approved amount if the doctor or supplier does not accept assignment

Retirement benefits. This initial enrollment period begins three months before the month in which a person turns 65 and ends three months after the month he or she turns 65. It is important to note that eligibility for Medicare starts at the age of 65 regardless of when a person becomes eligible for full Social Security benefits. For those who fail to enroll during the initial enrollment period, the general enrollment period runs from January 1 through March 31 of each year. The premium costs will increase for every 12-month period in which a person could have enrolled but did not. The special enrollment period is available for those who wait to enroll in Medicare because that person or the spouse is still working and has group health plan coverage through a current employer or a union-based plan. The grace period to apply for benefits extends eight months beyond either loss of benefits or termination of employment.

Medicare Advantage

Health Maintenance Organizations have been an option under Medicare since the 1970s. The Balanced Budget Act of 1997 expanded the choices under Medicare+Choice to include Preferred Provider Organization (PPO) Plans, provider-sponsored organizations, private Fee-for-Service plans, and medical savings account plans, along with high deductible insurance plans.

In January 2006, Title I of the Medicare Prescription Drug, Improvement, and Modernization Act (MMA) of 2003 (13) will change the name of the

Table 3 Medicare Part B Premium Rates Beginning in 2007

Participant's share (%)	Income
25	$80,000 or under
35	$80,000–100,000
50	$100,000–$150,000
65	$150,000–$200,000
80	$200,000 and over

Medicare+Choice program to MA and provide incentives to health care programs to contract with the Center for Medicare and Medicaid Services (CMS).

MA consists of private health plans that provide alternatives to the traditional Medicare program. These plans are available in many areas and eliminate the need to purchase a Medigap policy by providing additional benefits not available under Medicare Parts A and B. MA plans include Medicare Managed Care Plans, Medicare PPO plans, Medicare Private Fee-for-Service Plans, and Medicare Specialty Plans. Participants will pay a premium for their MA plan in addition to the Part B premium that they already pay.

As a rule, participants in Medicare+Choice plans were able to enroll in and disenroll from a plan at any time during the year. In 2006, under MA, this option will be limited to once during a six-month period. There are plans to shorten this to three-month periods in the years to come.

Beginning in 2006, there will be 26 MA regions. These regions will be made up of either single states or groups of states, and are designed to maximize the choice to the beneficiaries, particularly in rural areas where a choice in plans has not been historically provided.

In order to participate in a MA plan, one must have Medicare Part A and Part B coverage. MA plans ordinarily provide all Medicare covered benefits. One can explore the available options by going to the My Medicare.gov web site at http://www.medicare.gov/Choices/Overview.asp and clicking on Medicare Personal Plan.

Medicare Part D

In January 2006, Title II of the MMA puts into effect the Medicare Part D prescription drug benefit. The Medicare Part D benefit constitutes a major overhaul of the Medicare statute. Until it is implemented, temporary help is provided through Medicare-approved drug discount cards and transitional assistance for low-income beneficiaries.

To be eligible to enroll in the prescription drug plan (PDP), an individual must:

1. already participate in Medicare Parts A or B;
2. live in the PDP service area; and
3. not be enrolled in another PDP or MA plan that offers a prescription drug program (14).

An individual may also enroll in one of two special MA plans—a health savings account or a private Fee-for-Service plan—if no drug benefit is offered through the particular plan. The initial enrollment period begins November 15, 2005, and runs through May 15, 2006, for those already participating in Medicare and those who become eligible for participation effective from January 2006.

Medicare beneficiaries will have the option of changing plans once a year during the "annual election period" that will run between November 15 and December 31. The election takes effect January 1 of the following year.

Under certain circumstances, an individual may change plans at other times of the year under outlined exceptions to the standard rule. Enrollment in a new plan must take place within 63 days of the termination of the original coverage. If current Medicare beneficiaries fail to enroll in Part D during the initial enrollment period, and they do not have any other source of prescription coverage, they may have to pay a late enrollment penalty. All PDPs must offer a basic drug benefit. PDPs and MAs may also offer additional or "supplemental" coverage (14).

CMS has divided the country into 34 PDP regions and 26 MA regions. At least two PDPs must be offered in each region and at least one of them must not be a MA plan. If two plans are not available, CMS will offer a "fallback" plan offering basic drug coverage (14). Each plan must offer a list of those medications that have a negotiated reduced price, or medications that have received a rebate from the particular pharmaceutical company. If an enrollee purchases drugs from the list, or "formulary," his or her drug costs may be lowered. The availability of Part D coverage does not affect Part B coverage of some classes of drugs, such as those administered in a doctor's office.

Each plan has the freedom to set its own monthly premium. It is estimated by CMS that the monthly premium will average around $37 per month. These premiums may be deducted from the individual's Social Security check or can be paid directly to the plan in which the individual participates. In addition, the premiums may be paid by the enrollee's employer or other employee-based health care plans. If a participant does not receive a Social Security check and does not participate in an employer-sponsored plan, he or she may make the payment directly to CMS, which will then pay the PDP or MA.

The statute mandates that all plans provide basic drug coverage. The deductibles, copayments, and out-of-pocket maximums will be adjusted annually based upon increases in prescription drug costs. In 2006, a beneficiary's out-of-pocket expenses are limited to $3600. Once this limit is reached, the catastrophic benefit limits are activated and an additional $2 to $5 per prescription will be charged. In 2007, the charge will be 5% of the prescription costs. Details of Part D benefits are presented in Table 4.

However, the statute allows individual plans to offer a benefit that is equal to or actuarially equivalent to the basic benefit. As a result, participants may be confronted with different plans with, among other provisions, different premiums, deductibles, and copayments. Purchases from in-network pharmacies or mail-order pharmacies may be less expensive than filling prescriptions at the local pharmacy. Medicare beneficiaries will be confronted with the need to compare the various plans in order to determine which one offers the best deal.

The effect of this program on those Medicare beneficiaries who have lower drug costs is that they will be paying the greatest percentage of their drug costs out of their pocket, with Medicare paying a minimal amount. (See the Kaiser Family Foundation Part D calculator at www.kff.org/medicare/rxdrugscalculator.cfm.).

Medicare and Medicaid Dual Eligibles

Dual eligibles, or dual enrollees, are very low income beneficiaries who are enrolled in both Medicare and Medicaid. Of these, approximately one-third reside in nursing facilities, and a greater percentage suffer from Alzheimer's disease than those covered

Table 4 Basic Medicare Part D Benefit

Drug cost	Participant pays	Medicare pays	Cost to participant
Deductible: $250	$250	Zero	$250
Up to: $2250	25%	75%	$500
Up to: $5100	100%	Zero	$2850
Above $5100	$2 generic or $5 brand names; after 2007, 5%	95%	$3600

by Medicare alone. They are also more likely to have other chronic conditions. With the enactment of the MMA, dual enrollees will be prevented from receiving what is called "wrap around" benefits. That is, if their Medicare drug plan does not cover a specific drug, dual enrollees will not automatically be able to receive coverage from Medicaid. In addition, dual eligibles now rely on Medicaid to pay Medicare premiums and to cover benefits that Medicare does not cover, such as long-term care.

Medicare Part D for Dual Eligibles and Low Income Beneficiaries

The MMA provides for payment of prescription costs for those who are eligible for both Medicare and Medicaid. Potential problems exist if the Medicaid formulary is different from the PDP and MA formularies, resulting in dual eligibles facing difficulties in getting necessary medications.

For low income individuals, the MMA subsidizes the premium, eliminates the deductible, and/or reduces the copayments based upon the income and assets of the individuals and whether or not they also receive Medicaid benefits.

Nursing Home Residents and Medicare Part D

There is much concern at the time of this writing that the new Medicare drug benefit will result in a loss of prescription coverage for thousands of nursing home residents. At present, most nursing home residents have drug coverage through Medicaid. As a result of the Medicare law, those nursing home residents who are "dual eligibles"— that is, eligible for both Medicare and Medicaid—are scheduled to lose their Medicaid drug coverage on January 1, 2006. At that time, Medicare Part D will assume this coverage.

As explained above, a major component of the potential savings from this new program revolves around the beneficiary being able to weigh the different plans being offered in his or her area in order to make sure that the individual enrolls in the plan that best suits the individual's needs. Most nursing home residents are in no condition to make such choices. Many suffer from Alzheimer's disease or some other form of dementia, and many others have other mental impairments, making it impossible for them to make such decisions. Many are facing loss of coverage altogether if the plan in their area chooses not to cover the medication they are receiving. The new law does not cover certain barbiturates and benzodiazepines that are commonly prescribed for nursing home residents for seizure disorders, acute anxiety, panic attacks, and muscle spasms. Even though Medicaid is authorized to cover prescription drugs explicitly excluded under Medicare, not all state Medicaid programs cover all of the drugs.

CMS is tasked with implementing the new law. It has decided to arbitrarily assign nursing home residents and other dual eligibles to a plan from which they can then switch. The dilemma then becomes, what if the pharmacy to which they are assigned is not the same as the one the nursing home contracts with? Who has the authority to choose a plan for an incompetent resident? And what of those nursing home residents who do not receive Medicaid but still need assistance in choosing a plan? There are concerns that many residents will fall through the cracks and not be covered by any plan.

The burden of keeping all of the various plans and drug coverage straight will fall on the nursing homes, which will also be loaded with the task of dealing with numerous providers (as opposed to just one—Medicaid) and trying to sort out the various appeal processes when coverage of a particular drug is denied.

Coordination of Medicare and Medicaid

Coordination between the two programs is difficult for many reasons, not the least of which are differing definitions of "medical necessity," different coverage rules for the same services, and the fact that Medicaid cannot cover a service until all other available methods of payment, including Medicare, have been exhausted.

The coverage rules differ markedly in the areas of community and institutional long-term care. For example, there is a distinct difference between SNF services and nursing facility services. As explained above, Medicare pays for skilled and rehabilitative services in a SNF after three days of hospitalization. Payment is made for a maximum of 100 days. Medicaid pays for nursing and rehabilitative care provided in a nursing facility on an inpatient basis. There is no limit to the number of days of coverage as long as the care is medically necessary, as defined by state statute. This type of care is often referred to as custodial care. Medicaid requires that a share of the cost be covered in part by a portion of the institutionalized individual's monthly income. Medicaid pays the difference.

To be eligible for home care under Medicare, the beneficiary must be considered "homebound." That is, it would take a maximum effort for the individual to leave his or her home and is not something that is done in the ordinary course of the person's day. Nursing and aide services are limited to a maximum of 35 hr/wk. Medicaid home health services must include part-time nursing services, home health aide services, and provision of medical supplies, equipment, and appliances suitable for use in the home. It is up to the individual states, however, to determine the amount of coverage for physical or occupational therapy, speech pathology, and audiology services. Both Medicare and Medicaid home health services must be provided by certified home health agencies (15).

HOSPICE

The Medicare program offers an all-inclusive hospice care benefit. The hospice benefit provides end-of-life care to terminally ill patients and their families, with the emphasis on comfort, compassion, and dignity. The focus is on the person, not the disease and the goal is care and comfort, not cure.

Care is most often provided in the person's home, although it can also be provided in free-standing hospice facilities, hospitals, and even nursing homes. A family member or friend serves as the primary care giver, while the hospice staff visits regularly to make assessments and to provide additional care and services. The hospice staff is on call 24 hr/day, seven days a week. In addition, hospice care can continue after the death of the patient by providing bereavement counseling for the patient's family and loved ones.

The hospice team develops a plan of care focusing on the need for pain management and symptom control. The plan will indicate the medical and support services required, such as nursing and personal care, as well as the medical equipment needed, and tests and procedures and medication necessary for high-quality comfort care.

Hospice is available under Medicare Part A. Those who enroll for hospice care waive the standard Medicare benefits for treatment of terminal illness. There is no deductible or coinsurance payment for hospice care. Participants retain access to all Medicare benefits for conditions unrelated to their terminal illness. A hospice patient can opt out of hospice care at any time.

To qualify for hospice benefits, a person must:

1. have Medicare Part A;
2. be certified by his or her doctor as terminally ill with a life expectancy of six months or less—a beneficiary can receive hospice benefits for two periods of 90 days each and an unlimited number of periods of 60 days each;
3. sign a statement choosing the Medicare Hospice benefit; and
4. enroll in a program.

The hospice benefit is now available to people suffering from Alzheimer's. Because it is more difficult for physicians to make a diagnosis of terminal illness within six months for people suffering from Alzheimer's, owing to the fact that the disease does not progress in the same manner as other illnesses, the CMS, in a program memorandum, stated that the six-month test is a general one and that "medical prognostication is not an exact science" (16). Guidelines have been developed by the National Hospice and Palliative Care Organization to help identify which dementia patients are more likely to have a prognosis of six months or less.

MEDIGAP INSURANCE

Medigap insurance fills in the gaps left by traditional, or original, Medicare. A Medigap policy is the supplemental health insurance sold by private insurance companies, but only interacts with the original Medicare, and not with Medicare + Choice, now MA, or Medicaid. There are currently 10 standardized Medigap plans labeled "A" through "J," Plan A being the most basic, and Plan J, the most comprehensive. Each plan is standardized by federal and state laws. While each plan has a different set of benefits, each one must provide basic, or core, benefits. In addition, all plans with the same letter must offer the same benefits, no matter what state a person resides in. Medigap policies do not cover long-term care, vision or dental care, or unlimited prescription drugs.

The basic benefits include the following:

1. Medicare Part A coinsurance for days 61 through 150 for a hospital stay
2. The cost of 365 extra days of hospital care during the participant's lifetime after Medicare coverage ends
3. Medicare Part B coinsurance or copayment after the annual deductible is met
4. Fifty percent coinsurance for outpatient mental health services
5. Payment for the first three pints of blood used each year.

When comparing the premiums charged by different insurance companies, it is essential that the same policies be compared. People should purchase their Medigap coverage during the "open enrollment" period that begins six months from their 65th birthday if they are enrolled in Medicare Part B. During this period, an insurance company cannot deny them coverage, place conditions on a policy, nor charge them more for a policy because of past or present health problems. If they purchase a policy during the open enrollment period, and have at least six months of previous coverage, the insurance company cannot impose a pre-existing condition waiting period. For assistance in purchasing a Medigap policy, the local State Health Insurance Assistance Program should be contacted. These organizations can be located through the Medicare web site at www.medicare.gov. Click on "Search Tools" and then on "Helpful Contacts."

HIPAA

The HIPAA of 1996 was enacted to protect the portability of insurance for those who move, change or lose their jobs, marry or divorce, or undergo some other qualifying event that would cause a break in their health insurance coverage. In addition, under HIPAA, the Secretary of Health and Human Services (HHS) was required to enact regulations governing the transmission of a person's identifiable health insurance information. The Secretary enacted these regulations, setting the standards and administrative guidelines for privacy and security. Also addressed were penalties for violations. These rules took effect on April 15, 2003. HIPAA clarified previous operating procedures by stating categorically that patient records belong to the patient, except in circumstances where access would affect public welfare. HIPAA also gave health care providers greater discretion as to who may have access to a patient's information and why. These regulations have imposed hurdles to accessing information, which was unintended by the legislation.

Essentially, HIPAA regulations and standards apply to health plans, health care clearing houses, and to any health care provider who transmits health information in electronic form. These groups are called "covered entities." There are many "explanations" as to who or what is or is not, a covered entity, either directly or by association. These nuances create substantial misunderstanding as to the application of the regulations. To be a covered entity, a plan must provide medical care; provide care, services, or supplies; transmit health information from one entity to another; provide physical and mental health services; bill for health services; or be paid for health services. More information on HIPAA can be found on the Web at http://cms.hhs.gov/hipaa.

VETERANS AID AND ATTENDANCE BENEFITS

Aid and Attendance benefits through the Veterans Administration (VA) are an often overlooked benefit available to veterans of the armed services, or their dependents, who served during World Wars I and II, the Korean War, the Vietnam War, or the Persian Gulf War. In order to qualify for this benefit, the veteran or dependent must be totally disabled due to a non-service connected condition, in need of the aid and attendance of another person, and in financial need. The applicant need not be helpless, but it must be shown that he or she needs the regular attendance of another person. For example, a person in an assisted living facility is presumed to be in need of Aid and Attendance.

This benefit provides a monthly payment up to a maximum of $1675. If the applicant's monthly income exceeds this amount, certain items can be deducted from income, including unreimbursed medical expenses paid by the applicant, to assist in qualifying for some portion of the available benefit. Unreimbursed medical expenses include health insurance premiums; medications taken at the direction of a doctor; costs of adult day care centers as long as some medical or nursing service is provided for the disabled; the costs of long-term care and assisted living facilities (ALFs); and the costs of in-home attendants.

The income received from Aid and Attendance benefits is not considered available to the beneficiary in a long-term care facility, when calculating the amount that the resident must pay monthly to the nursing home. It is a way of affording someone in a long-term care setting more than the $60 on average that he or she is allowed to keep each month for personal needs. The local Veteran's Service Office can assist in filing the application through the VA. It may take up to six months to be approved but it will be retroactive to the month of application (17).

MEDICAID

Medicaid is a federally funded, state-run program that provides medical assistance for individuals and families with limited incomes and resources. As Title XIX of the Social Security Act, it delegates authority to HHS to approve the plans submitted by the states. The CMS oversees the operations of the programs within each state. Participation by the states is voluntary, but every state has a Medicaid program, as does the District of Columbia. The costs of the program are shared by the states and the federal government. Programs can vary widely from state to state. The federal statute sets the guidelines, but each state is free to modify those guidelines in developing its program. However, the states are not permitted to institute regulations that are more restrictive than the federal statute allows without receiving permission to do so from HHS.

Today's Americans face the real possibility of seeking long-term care in a nursing home for themselves if they are elders or for a loved one. Long-term care in nursing homes consists mainly of assistance with the tasks of daily living, such as eating, dressing, and bathing. Medicare or private medical insurance does not cover this care. While long-term care insurance policies are available to those who can afford them, the primary financial assistance available to the middle class is Medicaid. Medicaid is a public assistance program with many rules and prerequisites for eligibility.

To qualify for Medicaid benefits, an individual must be both medically and financially eligible. For an individual over 65 years to be deemed medically needy, either in the community or in a long-term care facility, he or she must require assistance with more than one activity of daily living. The six activities of daily living are: eating, bathing, toileting, ambulating, dressing, and transferring from one position to another.

Medicaid eligibility rules and benefits differ for those under and over the age of 65. There are also different rules governing community versus institutional care. The Older Americans Act, responding to the growing number of older people and the diversity of their needs, established the Administration on Aging (AoA) as an agency of HHS. The AoA is an advocate agency for older Americans. The AoA disseminates information and engages in outreach activities in the community to educate older people and their caregivers as to the benefits and services that are available to help them. The nine regional AoA offices provide funding and support to the local Area Agencies on Aging (AAA) in each state. AAAs provide supportive services to those elders within their service areas. They provide access services, such as information and referral, outreach, case management, and transportation. In-home services include homemakers, personal care attendants, meals on wheels, home repair, and rehabilitation. In the community, the AAAs support community centers, congregate meal programs, and support adult day care. They also oversee the safety and well-being of elders through the nursing home ombudsman program, protective services, and health and fitness programs. Local AAAs are an excellent source of information on local available resources. The nationwide toll-free hotline number is 1–800–677–1116 and information on services anywhere in the nation can be obtained by calling.

ASSISTED LIVING AND CONTINUING CARE COMMUNITIES

Two new styles of communal living have emerged over the past several years. Continuing Care Retirement Communities (CCRCs) offer the complete spectrum of senior living. Typically, an individual or a couple will move to a CCRC when they are both still capable of independent living. These facilities require an entrance fee as well as monthly rent and maintenance fees. Some portion of the entry fee is generally returned if the individual moves within a specified period of time, or, when the individual dies, it is returned to his or her estate. Eligibility for new residents is based on their age, financial assets, income level, and physical health and mobility. If a resident's health begins to fail, CCRCs offer assisted living apartments and nursing home long-term care.

ALFs offer private apartments along with services to those who require more assistance than independent living, but not as much as nursing home care. Communal dining is available, as well as aides who provide reminders of when to take medication, or assist with laundry and other chores such as shopping and transportation.

Unlike with nursing homes, there are no benefit programs (with very limited exceptions) that provide assistance for payment in CCRCs and ALFs. Some long-term care insurance policies will provide benefits to a policy owner living in an ALF. Also, unlike nursing homes, both these types of facilities are unregulated, and as a result, consumer protections vary greatly from state to state and facility to facility. No one should move to either type of facility without having an attorney review the contract ahead of time, to ensure that the prospective resident knows exactly what he or she is getting into.

CONCLUSION

As the tide of elders begins to swell in the United States, communities and lawmakers will be forced to face the needs of this increasingly needy population. In addition to ensuring the quality of care in long-term care facilities, more and more states and local communities will come to recognize the need for increasing community-based services, and for providing parity in funding for both institutional and community services.

REFERENCES

1. Federal Interagency Forum on Aging-Related Statistics. Older Americans: Key Indicators of Well-Being. Federal Interagency Forum on Aging-Related Statistics. Washington, D.C.: U.S. Government Printing Office, November, 2004:3.
2. Title XVIII, Social Security Act, 42 U.S.C. Section 1395 et seq.
3. Title XIX, Social Security Act, 42 U.S.C. Section 1901 et seq.
4. 42 U.S.C. Section 3001 et seq., 1965 as amended.

5. Union Pacific Railway Co. v. Botsford, 141 U.S. 250 (1891).
6. Cruzan v. Director, Missouri Department of Health, 497 U.S. 291 (1990).
7. Washington v. Glucksberg, 521 U.S. 702 (1997).
8. Id.
9. 42 C.F.R. Section 489.100 et seq.
10. Advance Health Care Directives: A Handbook for Professionals. American Bar Association, 2002.
11. http://www.uslivingwillregistry.com.
12. The Henry J. Kaiser Family Foundation. Medicare Spending and Financing Fact Sheet—April 2005. Website: www.kff.org.
13. The Balanced Budget Act of 1997; Public Law 105–33, Section 1852: Benefits and Beneficiary Protections.
14. Public Law 108–173.
15. Center For Medicare Education: Prescription Drug Benefits Under Part D of the Medicare Modernization Act—The Genie's Out of the Bottle. Website: www.MedicareEd.org.
16. Id
17. Id.
18. Harry S. Margolis Esq., Kenneth M. Coughlin, eds. The ElderLaw Report: Switch to Medicare Drug Plan Places Nursing Home Residents at Risk; Volume XVI, Number 11, June 2005.
19. Center For Medicare Education: Medicare for People With Alzheimer's Disease. Website: www.MedicareEd.org.
20. The ElderLaw Report: An Overlooked Benefit for Elderly Veterans: "Aid-and-Attendance" Help; Volume XVI, Number 7, February 2005.

7

Acute and Chronic Leukemias in Older Adults

Richard M. Stone
Department of Medicine, Harvard Medical School and Adult Leukemia Program, Department of Adult Oncology, Dana Farber Cancer Institute, Boston, Massachusetts, U.S.A.

INTRODUCTION

In contrast to the solid tumors, hematopoietic neoplasms are generally present diffusely at the outset, therefore demanding systemic therapy. Certain tumors of the hematopoietic system, particularly certain subtypes of the acute and chronic leukemias, despite their widespread nature, respond very well to therapy and are even curable with such a systemic approach. However, there is wide heterogeneity in the pathophysiology and natural history of the four main subtypes of acute and chronic leukemia: acute myeloid leukemia (AML), acute lymphoblastic leukemia (ALL), chronic myeloid leukemia (CML), and chronic lymphocytic leukemia (CLL). The age distribution of these disorders varies widely, with ALL being a disease largely of children, CML of middle-aged adults, and AML and CLL having a median age in the seventh decade of life (1).

An important issue in the acute leukemias is the difference in disease biology amongst younger versus older adults. For example, the incidence of disease-related poor prognostic factors is much higher in both AML and ALL when either disease presents in people over the age of 60, compared with the same disease in younger adults. The reason for these intrinsic age-related differences in biology is not clear. However, because both these conditions are malignant transformations of a hematopoietic stem cell, presumably residing in the bone marrow, some speculation is possible. The most primitive bone marrow stem cells are, of their very nature, long-lived, and must withstand a host of environmental and other insults throughout the person's lifetime. The accumulation of such insults on a genetic level could predispose to leukemia; alternatively, cell senescence that occurs with aging could result in a smaller number of primordial stem cells, each of which is more susceptible to stress and injury, possibly resulting in an increased likelihood of neoplastic transformation. In any event, both biologic and host factors yield a different expectation in biology, natural history, response, and tolerance of therapy in older versus younger adults in the acute and, to a certain degree, the chronic leukemias as well.

The therapeutic approach to these neoplasms also is highly heterogeneous. Curative approaches in the acute leukemias require intensive multiagent chemotherapy, sometimes including hematopoietic stem cell transplants. Given the rigors of these approaches, and the obvious different constitutional makeup of the average younger versus older adult, the safety of administration of such intensive therapy is a major issue in the older age cohort. In the chronic leukemias, which in general are treated much less intensively, the initial approach to treatment in the older versus younger patient is similar. Nonetheless, the inability to perform full hematopoietic stem cell transplant in the older adult is an important issue. Finally, the advent of newer therapies in all of these conditions will call for rethinking of formerly held concepts.

ACUTE MYELOID LEUKEMIA

The therapy of AML in the older adult is a particularly difficult problem (2,3), given the intrinsic degree of disease-resistance and host factors that make the application of standard induction chemotherapy daunting. The median age for AML is 68, so the majority of patients with this condition face a choice between supportive and intensive therapies. More effective and less toxic therapies are clearly needed. Some are in development, yet, for the foreseeable future, induction chemotherapy followed by postremission chemotherapy, although associated with a high rate of serious (including fatal) toxicity and poor overall outcome, will provide the only chance for cure, albeit low, in most patients. Adults under the age of 60 who enroll in cooperative group clinical trials (4–6) achieve remission 70% to 80% of the time when compared to a similarly treated group of older patients who can expect a 45% complete remission rate. The toxic death rate is 20% during induction for older patients, but less than 10% for younger patients. If an older patient does achieve remission, only 20% can expect to be long-term disease-free survivors compared with approximately 40% to 50% in younger adults with the same disease.

What other reasons account for these markedly inferior outcomes when older adults with AML receive chemotherapy? First, there is ample evidence that older adults tolerate intensive chemotherapy less well than do their younger counterparts. Older patients have an increased incidence of comorbid diseases (7), especially vascular disease, which could result in impaired cardiac and renal function, diminishing the ability to withstand the stress of sepsis secondary to myelosuppressive chemotherapy. Second, there is a concomitant decreased ability to clear chemotherapy, potentially resulting in a higher drug level and a longer exposure to potentially toxic agents (8). Older patients are more likely to have prolonged blood count nadirs after exposure to chemotherapy, which may be due in part to a so-called decreased hematopoietic stem cell reserve (9).

Perhaps the most important reason for the older adults' inferior responses to chemotherapy when compared with younger adults is due to the intrinsic disease biology. One thinks of AML in the elderly as a disease that derives from a more proximal stem cell in the hematopoietic hierarchy. Early stem cells require the capacity to be long-lived and therefore need to be able to survive in a stressful environment. The result of this hardiness is an increased resistance to chemotherapy. One mechanism of such resistance is the increased likelihood of expression of genes mediating drug efflux, such as MDR1, MSH2, MRP, and LRP, in cells from older patients with AML (10). One of the most important prognostic factors in AML are the cytogenetics at diagnosis (11). Older adults are much less likely to have cells that display the so-called favorable cytogenetic abnormalities (12) [inversion 16, t(8;21), t(15;17)], which are associated with a high likelihood of cure with chemotherapy. On the other hand, older adults are more likely to have myeloblasts that display the loss of the long arm or all of chromosomes 5 and/or 7, or have complex cytogenetic abnormalities, all typical of prior myelodysplastic syndrome or alkylating agent–induced leukemia. Such chromosomal abnormalities augur for a poor response to chemotherapy in patients of any age. The difficult host and biological factors noted above are thought to account for the disappointing results with chemotherapy in this age cohort across many trials. Since the early 1990s, most large cooperative groups have chosen to place older adults in separate trials, acknowledging the different therapeutic considerations in this age cohort (13–18). Nonetheless, very similar induction chemotherapy is currently used to treat AML patients of all ages. The backbone of induction chemotherapy, designed to reduce the leukemic burden from approximately 10^{12} cells at diagnosis down to a remission level of 10^9 or lower, is three days of anthracycline plus seven days of continuous infusion of cytarabine. Although some older randomized studies suggest that idarubicin might be a superior choice for anthracycline (19,20), the most recent studies suggest that daunorubicin remains the standard (21). The Cancer and Leukemia Group B (CALGB) has fashioned a three-drug induction regimen including daunorubicin, cytarabine, and etoposide, which appears to be associated with response rates similar to those seen with standard $3+7$ (16). A formal comparison of these two regimens has not been performed. One of the major problems with induction chemotherapy is the 15% to 25% early mortality rate. Improvements in supportive care may have lowered this astounding figure over the last decade.

Although there may be uniformity about the use of standard induction chemotherapy in patients who choose an aggressive approach, the optimal postremission therapy dedicated to reducing the leukemic burden from undetectable to compatible with long-term disease-free survival is not clear. The relative success of intensive chemotherapy, particularly high-dose ara-C, in the postremission setting in younger adults does not translate to older adults with AML. The pivotal trial CALGB 8525 that documented the benefits of high-dose ara-C in the postremission setting in younger adults (4) with AML failed to show any improvement in disease-free or overall survival in older age when comparing $3\,g/m^2$ for six doses, $400\,mg/m^2$ for five days, or $100\,mg/m^2$ per day each given for four courses. Based on concerns that it would be difficult to administer four intensive cycles to older adults, CALGB went on to test a modified regimen, including a somewhat lower dose of high-dose ara-C, with mitoxantrone, for two cycles. This was not superior to four cycles of low-dose ara-C (22). There have not been any trials that have documented a superiority for a more intensive versus less intensive approach, although older trials with nontreatment controls (23,24) (at least in younger patients) suggest that at least some postremission therapy should be applied. Such therapy could take the form of a repetition of the induction course for one or two cycles, or modified high-dose ara-C. Those rare older adults with a favorable chromosomal abnormality should probably receive intensive chemotherapy if it is believed tolerable. Nonetheless, the chance for high-dose ara-C-induced neurotoxicity increases with age, particularly in the setting of renal and hepatic dysfunction (25).

The role of nonmyeloablative bone marrow transplantation is currently being intensively explored as a means to achieve a high likelihood of long-term disease control. It is feasible to consolidate an older adult who has achieved remission with a nonmyeloablative approach if a donor, particularly a matched sibling, exists. Although the treatment-related mortality of this approach ranges from 5% to 20%, long-term benefits have yet to be documented. One recent study suggests that nonmyeloablative transplantation is as effective as a full transplant (26). The Southwest Oncology Group is currently performing an important trial in which all patients enrolled on their upfront treatment trial who achieve remission and who have a sibling donor will be allocated to a nonmyeloblative transplant in order to prospectively study the potential influence of this novel approach on the natural history of AML in older adults.

Because of the high toxic death rate in older adults with AML, hematopoietic growth factors that could potentially enhance neutrophil and platelet recovery, and thereby lead to a lower incidence of severe toxicity, have been analyzed. The recent history of hematopoietic growth factors as supportive agents for AML can be characterized as undergoing three stages: concern, promise, and disappointment. There was initial concern about the use of these agents to treat patients with AML and other myeloid malignancies because of the known ability of other growth factors to stimulate leukemic proliferation (27). Receptors for granulocyte colony-stimulating and granulocyte macrophage colony-stimulating factors (GM-CSF) exist on the surface of leukemic cells. In fact, studies in which myeloid growth factors were used to improve the cytopenias associated with myelodysplastic syndrome did show a (usually) transient increase in myeloblasts (28). Nonetheless, the concerns regarding leukemic stimulation were ultimately subsumed by a desire to reduce treatment-related morbidity/mortality in older adults with AML. It was thought that if the period of neutropenia could be shortened by granulocyte colony-stimulating factor (G-CSF) or GM-CSF, then there would be a lower likelihood of infectious deaths, resulting in an improvement in the complete remission rate. At least six large prospective randomized trials (13–15,17,18,29) were completed in older adults with AML to determine if G-CSF or GM-CSF administration could improve the clinical results. Only one of these trials, conducted by the Eastern Cooperative Oncology Group (14), documented an improvement in the complete remission rate, apparently due to a reduction in toxic deaths. Essentially, all trials confirmed a reduction in the duration of neutropenia but failed to show any obvious survival benefit. However, hematopoietic growth factors (HGFs) are safe and there was no evidence of excess leukemia resistance.

The reduction in neutropenic duration could indeed have a clinical benefit regarding earlier hospital discharge and a shorter time on intravenous antibiotics. The results of a large trial in younger adults who were randomized either to receive G-CSF or observation after both induction and postremission therapy suggested a significant reduction in duration of neutropenia and a decrease in the hospitalization rate and duration after consolidation therapy (29). As such, it seems quite justifiable to use G-CSF in the postremission setting as a means to decrease morbidity secondary to chemotherapy, and the use of this agent (perhaps based on economic considerations) during remission induction is optional. The hematopoietic growth factors could have a role in enhancing the response to chemotherapy if used before or during chemotherapy, but this aspect will be discussed subsequently.

THE BASIC DILEMMA: AGGRESSIVE CHEMOTHERAPY OR SUPPORTIVE CARE?

Because of the high toxicity and poor outcome, the chance of upfront mortality is higher than the chance of long-term disease-free survival. Many patients and physicians have questioned the appropriateness of induction chemotherapy in older adults with AML. Fewer than half of all people over the age of 65 with AML receive chemotherapy, and only about a quarter of those above the age of 70 do so (30). Moreover, the results obtained in large cooperative group or small multi-institutional phase II trials may not be generalizable for most patients. Many patients in the community are not being referred to centers where treatment is even possible. Only two clinical trials, both conducted in Europe in the 1980s, tried to address the question of whether aggressive treatment of AML in the elderly upon diagnosis makes sense. The HOVON Cooperative Group randomized patients to immediate induction therapy upon diagnosis versus observation until hematological or clinical instability ensued, whereupon chemotherapy would be administered. A one-month survival advantage accrued to those who received the early chemotherapy, but no quality-of-life measures were assessed in this trial, and there was a high up-front mortality rate (31). A study conducted mainly in France, randomized patients to either low-dose ara-C or standard induction chemotherapy (32). The complete remission rate as well as the chance of survival was significantly higher in those who were given standard dose chemotherapy; however, the up-front mortality was, as expected, much higher and the magnitude of the survival benefit was again measured in weeks. Although these two studies are sometimes used as a justification for chemotherapy in patients who could at least be considered chemotherapy candidates, the quality-of-life cost including hospitalization and up front death of an early aggressive approach is still substantial.

Research regarding how older patients decide to receive aggressive therapy or not is badly needed. Sekeres et al. attempted to begin to answer this question by conducting a survey of patients [AML or high-grade myelodysplastic syndrome (MDS)] who could receive either induction therapy or a nonintensive approach (33). All were seen in a tertiary care center. About half chose induction chemotherapy. The patients who chose induction chemotherapy tended to be younger and had a lower platelet count. Perhaps the most interesting finding from this preliminary study was the fact that patients consistently inflated the chance of cure compared to what their physicians felt was likely and what was documented in the medical record. Secondly, even though multiple therapeutic options were offered to the patients, at least as documented in the physician's notes, patients consistently stated that they were not offered options about therapy and that their care was directed by their physician. Clearly, efforts to promote communication to this cohort of patients are badly needed. At the moment, we are particularly bereft of nonintensive approaches that are potentially efficacious.

NOVEL APPROACHES

Although the precise molecular pathogenesis of most leukemias in older adults has not been elucidated, there is an increased understanding about certain genetic and biological aspects of these diseases, which could be exploited therapeutically. Although a detailed discussion of experimental therapies in AML is beyond the scope of this treatise, it is relevant to cover certain of the more promising approaches. As mentioned earlier, HGFs have been used to stimulate AML blasts to enter the cell cycle, thereupon making them potentially susceptible to S-phase specific agents such as ara-C. This so-called priming approach has been tested and, except in one notable recent trial in younger adults with AML (34), has not been successful (14).

Based largely on the success of imatinib's ability to inhibit bcr-abl in CML, mutated c-Kit in gastrointestinal stromal cell tumors, and activated platelet-derived growth factor receptor alpha in the hypereosinophilic syndrome, the search for a similar tyrosine kinase inhibitor for AML has proceeded rapidly. Blasts from about 30% of patients with AML can be shown to harbor a mutation in the FLT3 membrane receptor tyrosine kinase (35). These mutations are usually manifested by a repeat of between 3 and sometimes greater than 33 amino acids in the juxtamembrane region [so-called internal tandem duplication (ITD)]. About 5% of patients with AML have an activating point mutation in the so-called activation loop in the C-terminal portion of the protein. These mutations, particularly the ITD, confer an adverse prognosis (36). Constructs containing activated FLT3 can transform factor-dependent cell lines (37). Expression in hematopoietic stem cells can lead to a fatal myeloproliferative disorder in a murine model. Several drugs that inhibit activated FLT3 and have promise based on preclinical studies are now being developed for clinical use (38–41) in patients whose AML has a FLT3 mutation. Although these agents have biological activity, the likelihood of a single agent causing complete remissions in advanced leukemia is low. The current trend in the development of these agents is to combine them with chemotherapy (42).

Another type of signal transduction inhibitor was originally designed to disrupt the function of activated *ras*, thought to be an important gene in causing leukemogenesis. This class of agents, known as the farnesyl transferase inhibitors, takes advantage of the fact that the *ras* protooncogene protein requires a post-translation modification in which a lipid moiety (farnesyl group) is added prior to membrane anchoring and activation. While it is now not believed that these drugs exert their mechanism of action via inhibition of activated *ras*, members of this class of drugs do have an activity in myelodysplastic syndromes and AML. Based on Phase I results in which the farnesyl transferase inhibitor tipifarnib showed activity in advanced leukemia (43), (and despite disappointing results in a Phase II trial in a large number of relapsed patients) (44), a recent Phase II trial (45) suggests that there may be a role for this agent in untreated, poor prognosis older adults with AML. Most of the patients in the Phase II trial were between the ages 65 to 75 with a prior history of myelodsyplastic syndrome, or were aged above 75. Of the 140 patients with these characteristics, 15% achieved a remission, with an early death rate of 12%, suggesting that oral therapy with tipifarnib might be a reasonable alternative to chemotherapy in a selected group of patients. A Phase III trial comparing supportive care to tipifarnib in patients over the age of 70 with AML is currently being conducted in Europe.

ACUTE LYMPHOBLASTIC LEUKEMIA

Age is a critically important prognostic factor in patients with ALL (46). One of the great success stories of chemotherapy is the 80% to 90% cure rate that is achieved now when children with ALL receive multiagent chemotherapy, including induction, central nervous system prophylaxis, intensification, and prolonged maintenance therapy. To date, the results have been nowhere near as favorable in adults, with a 30% to 40% cure rate expected in those between the ages of 18 to 60 and a 10% to 20% cure rate and a 10% long-term disease-free survival rate expected in those over the age of 60 (47–50). One of the most important reasons for the inferior outcome with age is the increased incidence of Philadelphia chromosome-positive ALL, which represents a proximal stem cell mutation that is incurable with chemotherapy, and requires consolidation of remission with an allogeneic transplant to achieve a reasonable chance of long-term disease control (51). Preliminary studies with chemotherapy in combination with imatinib (52) provide some hope but no certainty that some adults with Philadelphia chromosome ALL might enjoy long-term disease-free survival without an allogeneic stem cell transplant. A recent study suggests that older adults treated with a combination of chemotherapy and imatinib, especially if chemotherapy and imatinib are given concurrently as opposed to sequentially, can achieve a high remission rate (53); whether or not this will translate into long-term disease control remains unclear.

Because of the relative rarity of ALL in patients over the age of 60, there have been no large trials dedicated solely to the treatment of this patient cohort. However, several lessons can be gleaned from large perspective randomized trials of therapeutic interventions in ALL in adults (which include patients of all adult ages). First, adults over the age of 60 rarely can tolerate the intense induction approach that is routinely administered to younger adults. In older patients, the dose of cyclophosphamide had to be reduced, and importantly, the duration of steroid exposure was truncated from 28 days to 7 days because of a high rate of fatal sepsis. Secondly, the use of G-CSF, if given as a supportive measure during induction, ameliorates prolonged neutropenia and reduces the incidence of infectious death (51). Third, even with the maximally tolerated dose-induction therapy, aggressive postremission intensification, cranial prophylaxis, and prolonged maintenance, long-term disease survival is unusual (10% to 20%) in those older adults who do achieve remission.

CHRONIC MYELOID LEUKEMIA

Historically, age has not played a major role in therapeutic decision-making for patients with CML because of both the relatively long natural history of the disease, as well as the tolerability of available therapies. Although CML is not generally a disease of older adults, the incidence is appreciable in this age cohort. The recent paramount success of targeted therapy (54,55) with the orally available small molecule imatinib has caused a major change in the therapeutic landscape of CML; the impact of this change on age-related issues is still being discerned. Nonetheless, the higher response rate and durability of responses with the use of imatinib has decreased the reliance on allogeneic bone marrow transplant as a therapeutic modality in CML, potentially brightening the outlook for older patients with this disease.

CML, a disease pathophysiologically dependent on an activation of the abl tyrosine kinase by virtue of its fusion to bcr sequences [a consequence of the Philadelphia translocation: t(9;22)], has at least two, and usually three, distinct phases. Patients almost always present in the so-called chronic or stable phase characterized by an often asymptomatic elevation of the white blood cell count with a left-shifted differential including basophilia and thrombocytosis, and splenomegaly. Although, sometimes, significant constitutional symptoms can be associated with this phase, most patients can live relatively normal lives for the four to eight years (even pre-imatinib), before transforming to a more aggressive course. Without allogeneic transplant (or possibly long-term imatinib therapy in some cases), CML inevitably transforms into a preterminal blast phase, characterized by the appearance of immature hematopoietic elements that are identical to acute leukemia, generally of myeloid lineage but occasionally other hematopoietic lineages. The blast phase is often preceded by a so-called accelerated phase characterized by worsening constitutional symptoms and an increasing splenomegaly, and a less stable hematologic picture. The duration of the stable phase can be estimated in a given patient based on disease features at presentation. The presence of significant thrombocytosis, basophilia, peripheral blasts, and/or splenomegaly generally heralds a shorter time in stable phase and a more aggressive clinical course (56,57). Older patients are more likely to experience a shorter time in stable phase than younger patients with CML.

Before the advent of interferon, the first agent clearly shown to prolong the natural history of CML (58), therapy was mainly palliative with the use of oral cytotoxic agents to control blood counts and any constitutional symptoms. Patients with an available donor and who were deemed young enough (generally below age 40) to undergo aggressive therapy were referred within the first year of diagnosis for an allogeneic transplant (59). Because major durable responses were relatively rare with the use of interferon and/or interferon plus cytarabine (60), allogeneic transplant remained the mainstay of therapy for patients up until the fifth decade of life. Interferon, although helpful in some patients, was poorly tolerated, especially in older patients, due to flu-like symptoms, fatigue, and high incidence of psychiatric problems (61).

The therapeutic algorithm has clearly changed now that imatinib, when given to newly diagnosed patients, produces an 80% likelihood of major cytogenetic remissions (of which 75% are complete responses). Such a high response rate as well as the initial apparent durability, albeit with limited follow-up, has yielded an evolution in the treatment algorithm for CML. Moreover, recent reports of responses to novel tyrosine kinase inhibitors in patients who have exhibited clinical and genetic resistance to imatinib (61,62) suggest that even more reliance will be placed on medical, as opposed to transplant, therapy of this disease. In addition, reduced intensity conditioning transplants can be applied more readily in older adults, even those aged up to 75, and show promise for the long-term control of CML (63). The use of imatinib has led to the relegation of allogeneic bone marrow transplant to a younger (perhaps than age 30) population in which one cannot rely on a long-term response to imatinib.

Therefore, for the older adult who presents with CML, it seems relatively straightforward that imatinib should be the initial treatment of choice. The likelihood of response to imatinib appears independent of patient age. Whether or not side effects of imatinib such as diarrhea, muscles cramps, or fluid retention, are more likely in the older person is not clear. Significant issues regarding the treatment of older adults with CML still remain. First, while the initial starting dose of imatinib is 400 mg a day, there are data that a higher dose (800 mg) might lead to a faster and more likely response (64). Side effect considerations argue against the routine use of a high dose of imatinib, particularly in older patients, until such data clearly show that higher doses lead to longer survival. Second, imatinib rarely eradicates molecular evidence of disease, even when used early in the natural history; disease resistance can emerge, often due to the acquisition of novel ATP binding site mutations (65) that prevent imatinib's action. Such data suggests that it might be wise to develop adjunctive therapy to yield a more profound response early on in a patient's disease course. Such therapy could include the use of additional agents such as interferon, cytarabine, or the aforementioned novel bcr-abl inhibitors. Finally, given the ability of CML to respond to immunologically based therapies such as adoptive immunotherapy after postallogeneic transplant relapse (66), it is reasonable to hope that this type of approach could "clean-up" the minimal residual disease after initial response to imatinib. Immunological therapies could potentially have an appeal for older adults if toxicity is minimized. At this time, reduced conditioning transplants represent the most active immunotherapy potentially useful in this age cohort, but more specific and less toxic approaches such as peptide vaccines (67) could be interesting to develop clinically.

CHRONIC LYMPHOCYTIC LEUKEMIA

Perhaps because CLL is a disease usually seen in older adults and because the biology of the disease, unlike AML, is not obviously age-dependent, the therapeutic strategy for older adults with CLL is similar to that for the relatively younger adults with the same disease. CLL is more aptly thought of as a lymphoproliferative neoplasm than as "leukemia" (68,69). The malignant cell in CLL is a CD5-positive B cell generally with weak surface immunoglobin expression. Disease features include ubiquitous bone marrow involvement that may or may not have an effect on the hemoglobin and the platelet count, and a significant leukocytosis with benign appearing lymphocytes. Immune disregulation is common with up to 50% of patients exhibiting either autoimmune hemolytic anemia and/or autoimmune thrombocytopenia. At least 50% of patients with CLL have a suppression of normal immunoglobulin production leading to hypergammaglobulenemia with an increased incidence of infections due to encapsulated microorganisms. Nonetheless, many patients with CLL present in an asymptomatic fashion with either a high white blood cell count and/or lymph node enlargement, and can be followed expectantly.

Prognosis in CML depends on the stage of the disease at presentation. Rai et al. (70) and Binet et al. (71) are long-used staging classifications that relegate patients into one of several prognostic groups. Patients with an asymptomatic elevation of the white blood cell count with or without minimal lymphadenopathy are a group with median survival not terribly different from that in age-matched controls. A second group with prominent lymphadenopathy and/or splenomegaly has an intermediate prognosis with a five- to eight-year median survival. Finally, a group of patients who exhibit nonautoimmune anemia or thrombocytopenia have an inferior prognosis with a median survival of several years. Recently, more biologically based prognostic factors have been developed. The expression of the Zap-70 (72) protein, CD38 (73) positivity on immunophenotypic analysis, and particularly the presence of unmutated immunoglobulin genes (74) have each been associated with a relatively poor response to chemotherapy. Although it is often difficult to perform standard karyotypic analysis on CLL cells due to their low-growth fraction, the use of fluorescent in situ hybridization (FISH; interphase cytogenetics) has made it possible to assign different prognostic categories to specific chromosomal abnormalities (75). For example, abnormalities of the long-arm of chromosome 14 are associated with a relatively favorable prognosis, whereas abnormalities of the short-arm chromosome 17, with an inferior outcome.

In the future, it is possible that clinically quiescent but biologically aggressive CLL might be treated in the presymptomatic stage. At present, the indications for treatment (as opposed to observation) of patients with CLL rest on the development of clinical symptoms. Such problems are either due to accumulation of CLL cells in lymph nodes and spleen causing intolerable lymphadenopathy or painful splenomegaly, or due to the effect of CLL on bone marrow production of red cells and/or platelets. To date, early and/or aggressive treatment of presymptomatic CLL has not been associated with a survival benefit. In fact, the disease is not currently considered curable. Even the use of high-dose chemotherapy with autologous stem cell rescue (76,77) or allogeneic transplant (78) (standard or nonmyeloablative) has not been conclusively shown to improve survival. One of the major reasons for the difficulty in showing that transplantation is a superior therapeutic strategy in CLL is the long natural history even in nontransplanted patients and the intrinsic selection bias of patients going on nonrandomized limited-institution transplant studies.

Treatment options for symptomatic patients with CLL are expanding rapidly. In general, treatments are adequately tolerated in all age groups, such that there are no markedly different treatment considerations in older adults when compared to younger adults, major comorbid illness not withstanding. Historically, patients were treated with an oral alkylating agent, such as chlorambucil, often in combination with steroids. A large randomized trial comparing chlorambucil to fludarabine suggested that the response rate to fludarabine was much greater (60% compared to 7%) (79), although there was no survival advantage. This nucleoside analogue has supplanted oral alkylating agent therapy as a first-line treatment for CLL. However, fludarabine requires daily administration for five days approximately every four weeks, which is certainly logistically challenging for many older adults. Secondly, fludarabine is a potent inhibitor of T-cells, which can predispose patients to opportunate infections (80). Thirdly, occasionally via an uncertain mechanism of immune disregulation, fludarabine can engender autoimmune thrombocytopenia or anemia (81). While the anti-CD20 monoclonal (82) antibody rituximab has limited single agent activity in CLL (perhaps because of the relatively muted expression of CD20 in most cases of CLL), several recent studies have shown that rituximab in combination with fludarabine yields a high response rate (83,84). A study conducted by the CALGB (82) suggests that when fludarabine and rituximab are given simultaneously, remission rates in the 60% range can be expected. Fludarabine is now available in oral form, which could aid the applicability of this agent in older adults (85). Even more impressively, when fludarabine, cyclophosphamide, and rituximab are given together, CR rates of 71% have been reported with median survival of at least 92 months. Another antibody, alemtuzamab, (Campath^{TM}) has major activity in patients with CLL that has relapsed after initial therapy (86). Because alemtuzumab kills lymphoid cells that express CD52, which is ubiquitously expressed, this is a potent immunosuppressive agent and should be used with caution in patients of all ages, particularly older adults. Studies are underway to determine the feasibility of using alemtuzumab earlier in the disease course, in combination or in sequence with fludarabine and rituximab.

REFERENCES

1. Heath C, Wiernik PH, Canellos GP, et al. Epidemiology and Hereditary Aspects of Acute Leukemia. 3rd ed. New York: Churchill-Livingston, 1996.
2. Sekeres MA, Stone RM. The challenge of acute myeloid leukemia in older patients. Curr Opin Oncol 2002; 14:24–30.
3. Estey EH. How I treat older patients with AML. Blood 2000; 96:1670–1673.
4. Mayer RJ, Davis RB, Schiffer CA, et al. Intensive postremission chemotherapy in adults with acute myeloid leukemia. Cancer and Leukemia Group B [see comment]. N Engl J Med 1994; 331:896–903.
5. Rees JK, Gray RG, Swirsky D, Hayhoe FG. Principal results of the Medical Research Council's 8th acute myeloid leukaemia trial. Lancet 1986; 2:1236–1241.
6. Cassileth PA, Lynch E, Hines JD, et al. Varying intensity of postremission therapy in acute myeloid leukemia. Blood 1992; 79:1924–1930.

7. Beghe C, Balducci L. Biological basis of cancer in the older person. Cancer Treat Res 2005; 124:189–221.
8. Lichtman SM. Chemotherapy in the elderly. Semin Oncol 2004; 31:160–174.
9. Balducci L, Hardy CL, Lyman GH. Hemopoiesis and aging. Cancer Treat Res 2005; 124:109–134.
10. Leith CP, Kopecky KJ, Godwin J, et al. Acute myeloid leukemia in the elderly: assessment of multidrug resistance (MDR1) and cytogenetics distinguishes biologic subgroups with remarkably distinct responses to standard chemotherapy. A Southwest Oncology Group study. Blood 1997; 89:3323–3329.
11. Grimwade D, Walker H, Oliver F, et al. The importance of diagnostic cytogenetics on outcome in AML: analysis of 1,612 patients entered into the MRC AML 10 trial. The Medical Research Council Adult and Children's Leukaemia Working Parties [see comment]. Blood 1998; 92:2322–2333.
12. Grimwade D, Walker H, Harrison G, et al. The predictive value of hierarchical cytogenetic classification in older adults with acute myeloid leukemia (AML): analysis of 1065 patients entered into the United Kingdom Medical Research Council AML11 trial. Blood 2001; 98:1312–1320.
13. Stone RM, Berg DT, George SL, et al. Granulocyte-macrophage colony-stimulating factor after initial chemotherapy for elderly patients with primary acute myelogenous leukemia. Cancer and Leukemia Group B [see comment]. N Engl J Med 1995; 332:1671–1677.
14. Rowe JM, Andersen JW, Mazza JJ, et al. A randomized placebo-controlled phase III study of granulocyte-macrophage colony-stimulating factor in adult patients (>55 to 70 years of age) with acute myelogenous leukemia: a study of the Eastern Cooperative Oncology Group (E1490). Blood 1995; 86:457–462.
15. Rowe J, Neuberg D, Friedenberg W, et al. A phase III study of three induction regimens and of priming with GM-CSF in older adults with acute myeloid leukemia: a trial by the Eastern Cooperative Oncology Group. Blood 2004; 103:479 485.
16. Baer MR, George SL, Dodge RK, et al. Phase 3 study of the multidrug resistance modulator PSC-833 in previously untreated patients 60 years of age and older with acute myeloid leukemia: Cancer and Leukemia Group B Study 9720. Blood 2002; 100:1224–1232.
17. Godwin JE, Kopecky KJ, Head DR, et al. A double-blind placebo-controlled trial of granulocyte colony-stimulating factor in elderly patients with previously untreated acute myeloid leukemia: a Southwest Oncology Group study (9031). Blood 1998; 91:3607–3615.
18. Lowenberg B, Suciu S, Archimbaud E, et al. Use of recombinant GM-CSF during and after remission induction chemotherapy in patients aged 61 years and older with acute myeloid leukemia: final report of AML-11, a phase III randomized study of the Leukemia Cooperative Group of European Organisation for the Research and Treatment of Cancer and the Dutch Belgian Hemato-Oncology Cooperative Group. Blood 1997; 90:2952–2961.
19. Wiernik PH, Banks PL, Case DC Jr., et al. Cytarabine plus idarubicin or daunorubicin as induction and consolidation therapy for previously untreated adult patients with acute myeloid leukemia. Blood 1992; 79:313–319.
20. Reiffers J, Huguet F, Stoppa AM, et al. A prospective randomized trial of idarubicin vs daunorubicin in combination chemotherapy for acute myelogenous leukemia of the age group 55 to 75. Leukemia 1996; 10:389–395.
21. Anderson JE, Kopecky KJ, Willman CL, et al. Outcome after induction chemotherapy for older patients with acute myeloid leukemia is not improved with mitoxantrone and etoposide compared to cytarabine and daunorubicin: a Southwest Oncology Group study. Blood 2002; 100:3869–3876.
22. Stone R, Berg D, Geroge S, et al. Post-remission therapy in older patients with de novo acute myeloid leukemia: a randomized trial comparing mitoxantrone and intermediate-dose cytarabine with standard-dose cytarabine. Blood 2001; 98:548–553.

23. Cassileth PA, Begg CB, Bennett JM, et al. A randomized study of the efficacy of consolidation therapy in adult acute nonlymphocytic leukemia. Blood 1984; 63:843–847.
24. Bloomfield C. Postremission therapy in acute myeloid leukemia. J Clin Oncol 1985; 3:1570–1572.
25. Rubin EH, Andersen JW, Berg DT, Schiffer CA, Mayer RJ, Stone RM. Risk factors for high-dose cytarabine neurotoxicity: an analysis of a Cancer and Leukemia Group B trial in patients with acute myeloid leukemia. J Clin Oncol 1992; 10:948–953.
26. Alyea EP, Kim HT, Ho V, et al. Comparative outcome of nonmyeloablative and myeloablative allogeneic hematopoietic cell transplantation for patients older than 50 years of age. Blood 2005; 105:1810–1814.
27. Vallenga E, Ostapovicz D, O'Rourke B, Griffin JD. Effects of recombinant IL-3, GM-CSF and G-CSF on proliferation of leukemic clonogenic cells in short-term and long-term cultures. Leukemia 1987; 1:584–589.
28. Herman F, Lindemann A, Klein H, et al. Effect of recombinant human GM-CSF in patients with myelodysplastic syndromes with excess blasts. Leukemia 1989; 3: 335–378.
29. Heil G, Hoelzer D, Sanz MA, et al. A randomized, double-blind, placebo-controlled, phase III study of filgrastim in remission induction and consolidation therapy for adults with de novo acute myeloid leukemia. The International Acute Myeloid Leukemia Study Group. Blood 1997; 90:4710–4718.
30. Menzin J, Lang K, Earle CC, Kerney D, Mallick R. The outcomes and costs of acute myeloid leukemia among the elderly. Arch Intern Med 2002; 162:1597–1603.
31. Lowenberg B, Zittoun R, Kerkhofs H, et al. On the value of intensive remission-induction chemotherapy in elderly patients of 65+ years with acute myeloid leukemia: a randomized phase III study of the European Organization for Research and Treatment of Cancer Leukemia Group [see comment]. J Clin Oncol 1989; 7:1268–1274.
32. Tilly H, Castaigne S, Bordessoule D, et al. Low-dose cytarabine versus intensive chemotherapy in the treatment of acute nonlymphocytic leukemia in the elderly. J Clin Oncol 1990; 8:272–279.
33. Sekeres MA, Stone RM, Zahrieh D, et al. Decision-making and quality of life in older adults with acute myeloid leukemia or advanced myelodysplastic syndrome. Leukemia 2004; 18:809–816.
34. Lowenberg B, van Putten W, Theobald M, et al. Effect of priming with granulocyte colony-stimulating factor on the outcome of chemotherapy for acute myeloid leukemia [see comment]. N Engl J Med 2003; 349:743–752.
35. Gilliland DG, Griffin JD. The roles of FLT3 in hematopoiesis and leukemia. Blood 2002; 100:1532–1542.
36. Kottaridis PD, Gale RE, Frew ME, et al. The presence of a FLT3 internal tandem duplication in patients with acute myeloid leukemia (AML) adds important prognostic information to cytogenetic risk group and response to the first cycle of chemotherapy: analysis of 854 patients from the United Kingdom Medical Research Council AML 10 and 12 trials. Blood 2001; 98:1752–1759.
37. Weisberg E, Boulton C, Kelly LM, et al. Inhibition of mutant FLT3 receptors in leukemia cells by the small molecule tyrosine kinase inhibitor PKC412. Cancer Cell 2002; 1:433–443.
38. Kelly LM, Yu JC, Boulton CL, et al. CT53518, a novel selective FLT3 antagonist for the treatment of acute myelogenous leukemia (AML). Cancer Cell 2002; 1:421–432.
39. Stone RM, DeAngelo DJ, Klimek V, et al. Patients with acute myeloid leukemia and an activating mutation in FLT3 respond to a small-molecule FLT3 tyrosine kinase inhibitor, PKC412. Blood 2005; 105:54–60.
40. Smith BD, Levis M, Beran M, et al. Single-agent CEP-701, a novel FLT3 inhibitor, shows biologic and clinical activity in patients with relapsed or refractory acute myeloid leukemia. Blood 2004; 103:3669–3676.

41. De Angelo DJ, Stone R, Heaney ML, et al. Phase II evaluation of the tyrosine kinase inhibitor MLN518 in patients with acute myeloid leukemia (AML) bearing a FLT3 internal tandem duplication (ITD) mutation. Blood 2004; 104:496a.

42. Giles F, Schiffer C, Kantarjian H, et al. Phase I study of PKC412 and oral FLT3 kinase inhibitor in sequential and concomitant combinations with daunorubicin and cytarabine (DAA) induction and high-dose cytarabine (HDAra-C) consolidation in newly diagnosed patients with AML. Blood 2004; 104:78a [262].

43. Karp JE, Lancet JE, Kaufmann SH, et al. Clinical and biologic activity of the farnesyltransferase inhibitor R115777 in adults with refractory and relapsed acute leukemias: a phase 1 clinical-laboratory correlative trial. Blood 2001; 97:3361–3369.

44. Harousseau JL, Reiffers J, Lowenberg J, et al. Zarnestra (R115777) in patients with relapsed and refractory acute myelogenous leukemia (AML): results of a multicenter phase II study. Blood 2003; 102:176a [614].

45. Lancet J, Gotlieb J, Gojo I, et al. Tipifarnib (Zarnestra™) in previously untreated poor-risk AML of the elderly: updated results of a multicenter phase II trial. Blood 2004; 104:[149a].

46. Faderl S, Jeha S, Kantarjian HM. The biology and therapy of adult acute lymphoblastic leukemia. Cancer 2003; 98:1337–1354.

47. Silverman LB, Gelber RD, Dalton VK, et al. Improved outcome for children with acute lymphoblastic leukemia: results of Dana-Farber Consortium Protocol 91–01. Blood 2001; 97:1211–1218.

48. Larson RA, Dodge RK, Burns CP, et al. A five-drug remission induction regimen with intensive consolidation for adults with acute lymphoblastic leukemia: Cancer and Leukemia Group B Study 8811. Blood 1995; 85:2025–2037.

49. Kantarjian HM, O'Brien S, Smith TL, et al. Results of treatment with hyper-CVAD, a dose-intensive regimen, in adult acute lymphocytic leukemia. J Clin Oncol 2000; 18:547–561.

50. Larson RA, Dodge RK, Linker CA, et al. A randomized controlled trial of filgrastim during remission induction and consolidation chemotherapy for adults with acute lymphoblastic leukemia: CALGB study 9111. Blood 1998; 92:1556–1564.

51. Dombret H, Gabert J, Boiron JM, et al. Outcome of treatment in adults with Philadelphia chromosome-positive acute lymphoblastic leukemia—results of the prospective multicenter LALA-94 trial. Blood 2002; 100:2357–2366.

52. Thomas DA, Faderl S, Cortes J, et al. Treatment of Philadelphia chromosome-positive acute lymphocytic leukemia with hyper-CVAD and imatinib mesylate. Blood 2004; 103:4396–4407.

53. Ottmann OG, Wassmann B, Pfeifer H, et al. Imatinib given concurrently with induction chemotherapy is superior to imatinib subsequent to induction and consolidation in newly diagnosed Philadelphia-positive acute lymphoblastic leukemia (PH+ALL). Blood 2004; 104:197a.

54. Deininger MW, Holyoake TL. Can we afford to let sleeping dogs lie? [comment]. Blood 2005; 105:1840–1841.

55. O'Brien SG, Guilhot F, Larson RA, et al. Imatinib compared with interferon and low-dose cytarabine for newly diagnosed chronic-phase chronic myeloid leukemia [see comment]. N Engl J Med 2003; 348:994–1004.

56. Sokal JE, Baccarani M, Russo D, et al. Staging and prognosis in chronic myelogenous leukemia. Semin Hematol 1988; 25:49–61.

57. Hasford J, Pfirrmann M, Hehlmann R, et al. A new prognostic score for survival of patients with chronic myeloid leukemia treated with interferon alfa. Writing Committee for the Collaborative CML Prognostic Factors Project Group. J Natl Cancer Inst 1998; 90:850–858.

58. Anonymous. Interferon alfa-2a as compared with conventional chemotherapy for the treatment of chronic myeloid leukemia. The Italian Cooperative Study Group on Chronic Myeloid Leukemia [see comment]. N Engl J Med 1994; 330:820–825.

59. Goldman JB, Druker BJ. Chronic myeloid leukemia: current treatment options. Blood 2001; 98:2039–2042.
60. Guilhot F, Chastang C, Michallet M, et al. Interferon alfa-2b combined with cytarabine versus interferon alone in chronic myelogenous leukemia. French Chronic Myeloid Leukemia Study Group [see comment]. N Engl J Med 1997; 337:223–229.
61. Giles F, Kantarjian H, Wassmann B, et al. A phase I/II study of AMN107, a novel aminopyrimidine inhibitor of Bcr-Abl, on a continuous daily dosing schedule in adult patients(pts) with imatinib-resistant advanced phase chronic myeloid leukemia (CML) or relapsed/refractory Philadelphia chromosome (Ph+) acute lymphocytic leukemia (ALL). Blood 2004; 104:10a[22].
62. Sawyers CL, Shah NP, Kantarjian HM, et al. Hematologic and cytogenetic responses in imatinib-resistant chronic phase chronic myeloid leukemia patients treated with the dual SRC/ABL kinase inhibitor BMS-354825: results from a phase I dose escalation study. Blood 2004; 104:4a[1].
63. Or R, Shapira MY, Resnick I, et al. Nonmyeloablative allogeneic stem cell transplantation for the treatment of chronic myeloid leukemia in first chronic phase [see comment]. Blood 2003; 101:441–445.
64. Kantarjian H, Talpaz M, O'Brien S, et al. High-dose imatinib mesylate therapy in newly diagnosed Philadelphia chromosome-positive chronic phase chronic myeloid leukemia. Blood 2004; 103:2873–2878.
65. Gorre ME, Mohammed M, Ellwood K, et al. Clinical resistance to STI-571 cancer therapy caused by BCR-ABL gene mutation or amplification [comment]. Science 2001; 293:876–880.
66. Giralt S, Hester J, Huh Y, et al. CD8-depleted donor lymphocyte infusion as treatment for relapsed chronic myelogenous leukemia after allogeneic bone marrow transplantation. Blood 1995; 86:4337–4343.
67. Cathcart K, Pinilla-Ibarz J, Korontsvit T, et al. A multivalent bcr-abl fusion peptide vaccination trial in patients with chronic myeloid leukemia. Blood 2004; 103:1037–1042.
68. Byrd JC, Stilgenbauer S, Flinn IW. Chronic lymphocytic leukemia. Hematology 2004:163–183.
69. Chiorazzi N, Rai KR, Ferrarini M. Chronic lymphocytic leukemia. N Engl J Med 2005; 352:804–815.
70. Rai KR, Sawitsky A, Cronkite EP, et al. Clinical staging of chronic lymphocytic leukemia. Blood 1975; 46:219–234.
71. Binet JL, Auguier A, Dighiero G. A new prognostic classification of chronic lymphocytic leukemia derived from a multivariate survival analysis. Cancer 1981; 48:198–206.
72. Rassenti LZ, Huynh L, Toy TL, et al. ZAP-70 compared with immunoglobulin heavy-chain gene mutation status as a predictor of disease progression in chronic lymphocytic leukemia [see comment]. N Engl J Med 2004; 351:893–901.
73. Ibrahim S, Keating M, Do KA, et al. CD38 expression as an important prognostic factor in B-cell chronic lymphocytic leukemia [see comment]. Blood 2001; 98:181–186.
74. Hamblin TJ, Orchard JA, Ibbotson RE, et al. CD38 expression and immunoglobulin variable region mutations are independent prognostic variables in chronic lymphocytic leukemia, but CD38 expression may vary during the course of the disease [see comment]. Blood 2002; 99:1023–1029.
75. Gozzetti A, Crupi R, Tozzuoli D. The use of fluorescence in situ hybridization (FISH) in chronic lymphocytic leukemia (CLL). Hematology 2004; 9:11–15.
76. Leporrier M, Chevret S, Cazin B, et al. Randomized comparison of fludarabine, CAP, and ChOP in 938 previously untreated stage B and C chronic lymphocytic leukemia patients. Blood 2001; 98:2319–2325.
77. Dreger P, Montserrat E. Autologous and allogeneic stem cell transplantation for chronic lymphocytic leukemia. Leukemia 2002; 16:985–992.

78. Doney KC, Chauncey TR, Applebaum FR. Allogeneic related-donor hemetopoietic stem cell transplantation for treatment of chronic lymphocytic leukemia bone marrow transplantation. 2002; 29:817–823.

79. Rai KR, Peterson BL, Appelbaum FR, et al. Fludarabine compared with chlorambucil as primary therapy for chronic lymphocytic leukemia [see comment]. N Engl J Med 2000; 343:1750–1757.

80. Perkins JG, Flynn JM, Howard RS, et al. Frequency and type of serious infections in fludarabine-refractory B-cell chronic lymphocytic leukemia and small lymphocytic lymphoma: implications for clinical trials in this patient population. Cancer 2002; 94:2033–2039.

81. Weiss RB, Freiman J, Kweder SL, et al. Hemolytic anemia after fludarabine therapy for chronic lymphocytic leukemia [see comment]. J Clin Oncol 1998; 16:1885–1889.

82. Rossi JF, van Hoof A, de Boeck K, et al. Efficacy and safety of oral fludarabine phosphate in previously untreated patients with chronic lymphocytic leukemia. J Clin Oncol 2004; 22:1260–1267.

83. Byrd JC, Peterson BL, Morrison VA, et al. Randomized phase 2 study of fludarabine with concurrent versus sequential treatment with rituximab in symptomatic, untreated patients with B-cell chronic lymphocytic leukemia: results from Cancer and Leukemia Group B 9712 (CALGB 9712)[see comment]. Blood 2003; 101:6–14.

84. Schulz H, Klein SK, Rehwald U, et al. Phase 2 study of a combined immunochemotherapy using rituximab and fludarabine in patients with chronic lymphocytic leukemia. Blood 2002; 100:3115–3120.

85. Lin TS, Grever MR, Byrd JC. Changing the way we think about chronic lymphocytic leukemia. J Clin Oncol 2005; 23:4009–4012.

86. Keating MJ, Flinn I, Jain V, et al. Therapeutic role of alemtuzumab (Campath-1H) in patients who have failed fludarabine: results of a large international study. Blood 2002; 99:3554–3561.

8

Multiple Myeloma and Plasma Cell Dyscrasias

Jonathan E. Kolitz
Don Monti Division of Oncology/Division of Hematology, North Shore University Hospital, Manhasset, New York, U.S.A.

Stuart M. Lichtman
Memorial Sloan-Kettering Cancer Center, Commack, New York, U.S.A.

Sam Mazj
Hematopoietic Stem Cell Transplantation, Stanford University Medical Center, Stanford, California, U.S.A.

INTRODUCTION

The plasma cell dyscrasias are characterized by the presence of a monoclonal serum immunoglobulin, bone marrow infiltration with clonally derived plasma cells and/or plasmacytoid lymphocytes, and variable end-organ involvement principally affecting hematopoiesis, the skeletal system, and renal function. A wide spectrum of disorders are included in this category, including Waldenstrom's macroglobulinema (1) and amyloidosis (2). These diseases range from indolent diseases such as monoclonal gammopathy of uncertain significance (MGUS) (3) and smoldering myeloma (SM) (4) to plasma cell leukemia, an aggressive, often rapidly fatal disease (5).

Multiple myeloma (MM) is a malignancy of monoclonal plasma cells. It principally affects older patients, with a median age at presentation of nearly 70 years (6). Data from the Surveillance, Epidemiology, and End Results program, last updated in 2002, show a slight male predominance and an approximately twofold increased incidence in African-Americans. The number of expected new cases in 2003 was projected to be 14,600, with 10,900 deaths recorded in 2002. Whether or not the incidence of the disease is increasing has been disputed (7). Exposure to benzene and ionizing radiation has been implicated in causing the disease, although the etiology is mostly unknown (8).

MONOCLONAL GAMMOPATHY OF UNCERTAIN SIGNIFICANCE

For a diagnosis of MGUS, patients must have less than 10% plasma cells in the marrow, absence of end-organ involvement, minimal or no urinary light chain excretion, and an M-spike of level lower than that accepted or observed in myeloma (9). As in overt myeloma, clonal chromosomal abnormalities occur in MGUS (10). MGUS is found in approximately 3% of persons older than 70 years. The probability of development of myeloma has been most strongly associated with the level of the M-spike at diagnosis (3). At 20 years, 16% of patients presenting with an M-spike less than or equal to 0.5 g/dL will progress, as compared with 49% of patients presenting with levels ≥2.5 g/dL. The cumulative likelihood of progression to myeloma among all patients with MGUS increases over time from 12% at 10 years to 30% at 25 years, with an overall annual incidence of about 1% per year. Other than the level of the diagnostic M-spike, no reliable predictors of progression have been identified, including background suppression of the uninvolved immunoglobulins, light chain excretion, and the beta-2 microglobulin level. The predictive value of determining the kappa/lambda ratio of free serum light chains is being validated (11). Because there is no evidence that the risk of progression decreases or disappears with time, lifelong monitoring is suggested.

SOLITARY PLASMACYTOMA

Solitary plasmacytoma is characterized by the presence of medullary or extramedullary tumor consisting of monoclonal plasma cells. In addition, skeletal films must show no additional lytic lesions and a bone marrow must contain no evidence of MM. The immunofixation of the serum and concentrated urine often shows no M-protein. Therapy of the solitary lesion often results in disappearance of the M-protein. Tumoricidal irradiation (4000 to 5000 cGy) is the treatment of choice. Overt MM develops in approximately 50% of patients with solitary plasmacytoma. Progression occurs most often within three years (12). Extramedullary plasmacytomas appear to have a better prognosis following radiotherapy than solitary bone plasmacytomas, with about 70% of patients cured with radiotherapy (13). Aneuploidy appears to be more prevalent in bone as compared with extramedullary plasmacytomas (14).

AMYLOIDOSIS

Amyloidosis is an uncommon disease characterized by the accumulation in vital organs of misfolded, fibrillar proteins (2). When associated with plasma cell diseases, the misfolded proteins are monoclonal immunoglobulin lambda light chains and the condition is termed "AL amyloidosis." It can occur in 12% to 15% of patients with MM. The clinical features include the nephrotic syndrome, cardiomyopathy, heptomegaly, macroglossia, neuropathy, carpal tunnel syndrome, and periorbital purpura (15). Treatments have included colchicines with and without melphalan and prednisone (MP), high-dose dexamethasone with and without α interferon, and autologous stem cell transplantation (ASCT). A Phase III trial has shown that therapy with MP results in objective responses and improved overall survival (OS) (median 18 vs. 8.5 months) as compared with colchicine in patients with primary amyloidosis (16). Promising early data using high-dose dexamethasone induction followed by dexamethasone and α interferon maintenance show that 24% of patients achieved complete remission and 45% had improvement in end-organ function. The median OS in that study was 31 months (17). Selected patients may benefit from ASCT (18). In the relapsed setting, responses have been achieved using thalidomide and dexamethasone, albeit with significant toxicity, including a 26% incidence of symptomatic bradycardia (19).

INDOLENT MM

About 5% to 15% of patients meet marrow diagnostic criteria for myeloma but have relatively quiescent disease associated with low tumor burden. Generally, such patients do not have renal disease or significant bone disease and anemia. This presentation has been called indolent myeloma or SM (20).

It is recommended that chemotherapy not be instituted until there is a significant risk of complications. This is particularly true of elderly patients with significant comorbidities. An analysis of 101 consecutive, asymptomatic patients identified risk factors for progression. Serum IgG M-spike greater than 3.0 g/dL, immunoglobin (Ig) A protein type, and significant Bence Jones proteinuria affected outcomes. The presence of two or more of these features signified high-risk disease with early progression (median 17 months), whereas the absence of any variable was associated with prolonged stability (median 95 months) (21).

Patients with indolent or smoldering disease are best served by careful monitoring. Patients with indolent disease can respond to thalidomide, but whether such early therapy impacts on the disease's ultimate evolution remains to be determined (22). With the possible exception of bisphosphonate therapy, therapy directed against MM is not generally advisable for treatment of smoldering or indolent myeloma outside of a clinical trial setting.

MULTIPLE MYELOMA

MM is a malignancy of monoclonal plasma cells that accounts for 10% of all hematologic cancers. Almost 40% of patients in one large series were over age 70 when diagnosed (23). The five-year survival rate for all patients had been approximately 25% to 30% until the advent of newer, targeted therapies and the wide application of ASCT. Median survival is now extending beyond five to seven years, especially among patients who are sensitive to therapy (24).

Findings that suggest the diagnosis include lytic bone lesions, anemia, azotemia, and hypercalcemia (23). The biological basis for the skeletal and hematologic effects of progressive MM is being increasingly defined (25). Clinical manifestations and diagnostic studies are outlined in Tables 1 and 2.

A simple and powerful three-stage system has been devised, based solely on measurements of serum albumin and β_2 microglobulin (26). As this International Staging System (ISS) undergoes prospective use, it may replace the more cumbersome Durie-Salmon system (Table 3) (27).

Prognostic factors in MM include renal function, serum calcium, β_2 microglobulin, and C-reactive protein, plasma cell labeling index, serum interleukin (IL)-6 and soluble IL-6 receptor levels, lactate dehydrogenase, performance status, and cytogenetics (28,29). Deletion of 13q has been associated with poor prognosis (30).

Therapy of Symptomatic Myeloma

A partial list of treatment regimens for MM is outlined in Table 4. Historically, MM has been treated with single (usually melphalan) or multiple alkylating agents combined with prednisone. Other regimens have used combinations of alkylating agents, vincristine and doxorubicin, or a regimen of continuous infusion vincristine and

Table 1 Clinical Manifestations of MM

System	Manifestation
Skeletal	Bone pain, fractures of the vertebrae or ribs, lytic lesions in 70% at diagnosis
Hematopoietic	Normocytic, normochromic anemia present in 60% of patients at diagnosis
Endocrine	20% of newly diagnosed patients have hypercalcemia (>11.5 mg/dL) secondary to bone destruction
Renal	20% of patients present with renal insufficiency and another 20% develop it during the course of their illness. Bence Jones proteinuria is the most common cause; amyloidosis, hypercalcemia or light chain deposition may also contribute
Infections	Patients with myeloma develop bacterial infections; recently gram-negative organisms have been the most common pathogens, surpassing the gram-positive organisms

Abbreviation: MM, multiple myeloma.

Table 2 Diagnostic Methods in the Plasma Cell Dyscrasias

Modality	Comment
CBC	Peripheral smear may reveal Rouleaux formation, rarely circulating plasma cells
Serum calcium, creatinine, BUN, calcium, phosphate	Renal insufficiency and hypercalcemia are urgent indications for initiation of therapy
Serum immunoprotein studies	Immunofixation, quantitative immunoglobulins; quantitative serum light chains important in light chain or nonsecretory disease
Serum β_2 microglobulin and C-reactive protein	Prognostic indicators
Bone marrow aspirate and biopsy	MGUS usually associated with <10% plasma cells; myeloma can be diagnosed with 10–30% or >30% plasma cells depending on presence of minor criteria
Cytogenetics and FISH	Important to identify poor prognostic groups, especially del (13q)
24 hr urine	Measure total protein, creatinine, quantitative light chain excretion, Bence Jones protein and immunofixation
Skeletal survey	Long bones, skull, ribs, spine, and pelvis
MRI	Assessment of symptomatic areas; for complete assessment in suspected solitary plasmacytoma
PET and bone scan	Not used routinely; may be of value in selected patients to ensure early disease, especially in solitary plasmacytomas

Abbreviations: MGUS, monoclonal gammopathy of uncertain significance; FISH, fluoresence in situ hybridization; MRI, magnetic resonance imaging; PET, positron emission tomography.

Table 3 New International Staging System

Stage	Criteria	Median survival (mos)
I	Serum β_2 microglobulin $<3.5\,mg/L$	62
	Serum albumin $\geq 3.5\,g/dL$	
II	Not stage I or III	44
III	Serum β_2-microglobulin $\geq 5.5\,mg/L$	29

There are two categories for stage II: serum β_2-microglobuling $<3.5\,mg/L$ and serum albumin $<3.5\,g/dL$; or serum β_2-microglobulin 3.5 to $<5.5\,mg/L$ irrespective of the serum albumin level.
Source: From Ref. 26.

doxorubicin combined with high-dose dexamethasone [vincristine, adriamycin, dexamethasone (VAD) regimen], or dexamethasone as a single agent. Median event-free survival and OS of 18 and 33 months, respectively, were observed in 1555 chemotherapy-naïve patients with MM treated within the Southwest Oncology Group, using a variety of alkylator and/or doxorubicin-based regimens (35). Of note, survival did not differ between responding and nonresponding patients, with only patients progressing on therapy having inferior outcomes. A Phase III comparison of MP versus a multiple alkylator regimen (the M2) in untreated MM showed that the M2 induced a significantly higher response rate and remission duration, although survival advantages appeared marginal (31).

The VAD regimen has been used extensively, particularly prior to ASCT in patients. The cumbersome nature of this regimen may be at least partly outweighed in older patients by the reduced cardiotoxicity associated with infusional anthracycline therapy. No randomized data exist, however, demonstrating significant increased efficacy for VAD as compared with alkylator-based regimens or with therapies using bolus administration of doxorubicin and vincristine in untreated patients. The bulk of the VAD regimen's antimyeloma activity may be derived from the high-dose dexamethasone (32).

Table 4 Treatment Regimens for MM

Regimen	Schedule (wks)
Thalidomide/dexamethasone: thalidomide 200 mg po qhs and dexamethasone 40 mg po on days 1–4, 9–12, 17–20	4
High-dose dexamethasone 40 mg/day po on days 1–4; 9–12; 17–20; consider alternating with four weeks of two pulses	4
VAD: vincristine (0.4 0 mg/day i.v.) + doxorubicin ($9\,mg/m^2$/day i.v.) by continuous infusion on days 1–4 and dexamethasone 40 mg/day po on days 1–4, 9–12, 17–20	4
BLTD: Biaxin 500 mg po bid, thalidomide 100–200 mg po qhs daily, dexamethasone 40 mg po once/weekly	4
MP: melphalan (8–$9\,mg/m^2$/day po) + prednisone (100 mg/day po) days 1–4	4–6
VBMCP (M2): vincristine 0.03 mg/kg i.v. day 1; BCNU 0.5 mg/kg i.v. day 1; melphalan 0.25 mg/kg po days 1–4; cyclophosphamide 10 mg/kg i.v. day 1; prednisone 1 mg/kg po days 1–7 and 0.5 mg/kg days 8–14	6

Abbreviation: MM, multiple myeloma.
Source: From Refs. 31–34.

A liposomal formulation of daunorubicin (DaunoXome, DNX) and a pegylated liposomal doxorubicin (Doxil, Caelyx) have been studied in combination with vincristine and standard as well as reduced doses of dexamethasone. Doxil can safely replace doxorubicin when combined with i.v. bolus vincristine and standard or reduced dose of dexamethasone, resulting in a variant of VAD with equivalent efficacy and reduced toxicities (36).

The introduction of thalidomide as an effective treatment for MM has considerably affected management strategies. Thalidomide is an orally available agent with protean antiangiogenic, anti-inflammatory, and immunomodulatory properties (37). Reports of significant antitumor activity in relapsed and refractory MM (38) have rapidly led to Phase III testing. The Eastern Cooperative Oncology Group (ECOG) compared thalidomide plus dexamethasone against dexamethasone alone in newly diagnosed MM. An interim analysis showed that the thalidomide arm was associated with a significantly higher (80% vs. 53%, $P = 0.0023$) response rate (33). A retrospective analysis of untreated patients given thalidomide and dexamethasone or VAD prior to ASCT has shown a significantly higher response to the thalidomide-containing regimen (76% vs. 52%, $P = 0.0004$) (39).

Thalidomide, while not myelosuppressive, can cause peripheral neuropathy, thrombophlebitis, constipation, and sedation. In the ECOG trial, the incidence of thromboembolic complications was 16% among patients receiving thalidomide versus only 3% in patients treated with dexamethasone alone. The most effective way to prevent thrombophlebitis in patients treated with thalidomide-based therapies is not clear. Low-molecular-weight heparin prophylaxis may be especially effective (40). Thalidomide doses above 200 mg daily are difficult to tolerate, especially by older patients who are susceptible to the central nervous system depressive effects of the drug as well as to the gastrointestinal toxicities and peripheral neuropathy. Combination regimens, such as thalidomide and dexamethasone, limit the thalidomide dose to 200 mg daily. BLT-D is another regimen that uses lower doses of thalidomide (100–200 mg/day) in combination with dexamethasone, given once a week along with clarithromycin, an agent that may potentiate the effect of glucocorticoids (34). Combination therapy with melphalan, prednisone and thalidomide is being investigated and may also prove active and tolerable in elderly patients (41).

Derivatives of thalidomide with more potent immunomodulatory properties and different toxicity profiles (ImiDs) are undergoing development. CC-4047 (Actimid, Celgene) (42) and CC-5013 (Lenalidomide, Celgene) (43) are both orally available and active in relapsed/refractory MM, including patients who have previously received thalidomide. These agents are more myelosuppressive and have less neurologic and gastrointestinal toxicities than thalidomide.

Therapy targeting the proteasome has shown promise in untreated and relapsed/refractory MM. Bortezomib (Velcade, Millenium) is an i.v. proteasome inhibitor that has been shown to be superior to dexamethasone with respect to incidence of major response (38% vs. 18%, $P < 0.001$), progression-free survival (PFS), and OS in a 669-patient Phase III trial (44). The median age in that trial was 62. A subset analysis of patients from that trial, aged 65 or older, demonstrated similar findings favoring bortezomib (45).

Arsenic trioxide is another agent with proapoptic and antiangiogenic properties, which has been undergoing evaluation in the treatment of MM. Early data suggest antitumor activity and acceptable toxicity in relapsed/refractory patients (46), which may be enhanced with ascorbic-acid-mediated depletion of intracellular glutathione levels (47). New agents undergoing evaluation in MM are outlined in Table 5.

Table 5 New Agents for the Treatment of MM

Agent	Mechanisms of action	Development
Lenalidomide	Proapoptotic; effects on microenvironment including inhibition of cell adhesion, angiogenesis, and cytokine production	Phase III
ATO	Like lenalidomide; immunomodulatory effects on natural killer and cytotoxic T cells	Phase II/III
Oblimersen	Antisense inhibition of bcl-2 RNA translation; proapoptotic	Phase III
PTK787	Inhibition of VEGF	Phase II
Tipifarnib, Lonafarnib	Farnesyl transferase and ras inhibition	Phase II
SAHA	Histone deacetylase inhibition, induces apoptosis	Phase I
Geldanamycin	hsp90 inhibitor; may help overcome bortezomib resistance	Phase I

Abbreviations: ATO, arsenic trioxide; hsp90, heat shock protein 90; MM, multiple myeloma; SAIIA, suberoylanilidehydroxamic acid; VEGF, vascular endothelial growth factor.
Source: From Refs. 48,49.

Maintenance strategies in responding patients following initial chemotherapy, with or without ASCT, have been studied using various agents, including low-dose α interferon, steroids, and thalidomide. In a group of 261 older patients (median age 69) in a plateau phase of response following treatment with MP, low-dose α interferon prolonged PFS but not OS without adversely affecting quality of life (50). Alternate-day treatment with 50 mg of prednisone favorably affected PFS and OS among patients previously responsive to VAD-based regimens (51). Ongoing trials are focusing on studying the value of thalidomide as a maintenance therapy (52).

Transplantation in the Therapy of Myeloma

ASCT has been compared with conventional chemotherapy for treatment of MM in randomized trials. Studies with the longest follow-up intervals indicate that single (53,54) or tandem (double) (55) transplants offer significant advantages over chemotherapy alone with respect to RFS and OS in patients up to age 65. Among factors most likely to adversely affect outcomes are chromosome 13 deletions, serum β_2 microglobulin levels, and time to transplant (56).

The role of matched sibling donor or unrelated allogeneic transplantation using reduced-intensity, nonmyeloablative conditioning regimens in MM is being evaluated. Early data suggest that such approaches are feasible, associated with significant one-year therapy-related mortality (TRM, 22%) and appear not to benefit heavily pretreated or chemoresistant patients (57). Preliminary data from a trial in which "genetic randomization" was used to compare tandem autografts with an autograft followed by a reduced-intensity transplant given only to those patients with human leucocyte antigen (HLA)–matched sibling donors, have yet to show significant differences (58). That study was open only to patients with adverse prognostic features, and included patients up to age 65. Clear clinical benefit, with superior RFS and OS overriding an expected increase in TRM, will have to be established before such a strategy will be routinely used in older patients.

The Effect of Age in the Therapy of Myeloma

Many studies that indicate that age is a poor prognostic indicator are community-based and may have accepted patients with poor performance scores and increased comorbidity. In some trials from tertiary centers, in which patient selection may have been more restrictive, no effect of age was noted (6). Age tends to be identified as an adverse factor in univariate but not in multivariate analyses (28). The presentation of active MM does not vary with age (59). Median survivals of patients older and younger than 65 years have been compared according to ISS stage. Outcomes did favor younger patients, with median survivals of 69 versus 47 months (Stage I), 50 versus 37 months (Stage II), and 33 versus 24 months (Stage III) (26). A report of 425 uniformly treated patients older than 65 years validated the ISS and suggested that a high plasma cell proliferation index is associated with especially poor outcomes in advanced-stage patients (60).

A retrospective analysis consisting of 57 of 225 patients over 60 years of age who underwent an autotransplant after peripheral stem cell mobilization showed no difference in either the median number of CD^{34+} cells collected or the time to engraftment (61). A retrospective analysis using transplant registry data demonstrated that outcomes among 110 transplanted patients aged 60 or older were similar to those in 382 younger patients. The older patients' 100-day and one-year mortality (5% and 8%) did not differ from that observed in the younger patients (6% and 9%) (62). Advanced age should not be considered a major obstacle to active treatment. Older patients with symptomatic MM tolerate chemotherapy and should be offered treatment.

Ancillary Therapies in MM

Skeletal complications are a serious problem in this disease. Osteoporosis, pain, and fracture are devastating complications. These complications are caused by soluble factors that stimulate osteoclasts to resorb bone. In addition to approved bisphosphonates such as zoledronic acid, the system of osteoclast activation involving osteoprotegerin—receptor activator of nuclear factor kB and its ligand—is undergoing pharmacologic manipulations in new trials that may lead to better treatments aimed at impeding bone loss (63).

Bone destruction is a common cause of morbidity in MM. Bisphosphonates are a class of agents that have been shown in a variety of studies to reduce bony complications associated with this disease (64). There are toxicities associated with this therapy, including renal insufficiency and osteonecrosis of the jaw (ONJ). Published literature suggests that renal function deterioration occurs in 8.8% to 15.2% of patients at recommended dose of 4 mg infused intravenously over 15 minutes.

Zoledronic acid and pamidronate disodium are indicated for the treatment of patients with MM. In clinical trials, the risk for renal function deterioration was significantly increased in patients who received zoledronic acid over five minutes compared to patients who received the same dose over 15 minutes. In addition, the risk for renal function deterioration and renal failure was significantly increased in patients who received a dose of 8 mg, even when given over 15 minutes. While this risk is reduced with the 4 mg dose administered over 15 minutes, deterioration in renal function can still occur. Risk factors for the deterioration of renal function include elevated baseline creatinine and multiple cycles of bisphosphonate treatment. Zoledronate is not recommended in patients with severe renal impairment. Dose modification based on creatinine clearance is now recommended.

In a nonrandomized retrospective analysis of 293 patients, 12% of patients developed renal dysfunction associated with bisphosphonate use. The incidence of renal toxicity was more prominent in the elderly group (>80 years old) with use of bisphosphonates. Increase in serum creatinine was observed in 20% of the elderly group when compared to other age groups (11%). Renal dysfunction occurs in all age groups with use of bisphosphonates. The elderly may be particularly susceptible due to a higher incidence of renal insufficiency. They may require closer monitoring of renal function with the use of bisphosphonates and frequent dose adjustments (65).

ONJ has been reported in patients with cancer receiving treatment including use of bisphosphonates, chemotherapy, and/or corticosteroid therapy. The majority of reported cases have been associated with dental procedures such as tooth extraction. A dental examination with appropriate preventive dentistry should be considered prior to treatment with bisphosphonates in patients with concomitant risk factors. While on treatment, these patients should avoid invasive dental procedures if possible. No data are available as to whether discontinuation of bisphosphonate therapy reduces the risk of ONJ in patients requiring dental procedures (66).

Routine use of bisphosphonates, particularly in patients with indolent disease without evidence of osteopenia, should be undertaken cautiously, however, taking into account uncommon but potentially serious nephrotoxic effects (67), as well as the growing appreciation of the risk of development of avascular necrosis of the jaw (68).

Surgical interventions, such as vertebroplasty or kyphoplasty, can help improve the functional status of severely affected patients with compression fractures (69). Myeloid and erythroid colony-stimulating factors have been widely used to reduce disease- and therapy-related infectious complications and anemia. Patients who receive high-dose dexamethasone may benefit from pneumocystis prophylaxis with trimethoprim–sulfamethazole.

REFERENCES

1. Dimopoulos MA, Kyle RA, Anagnostopoulos A, et al. Diagnosis and management of Waldenstrom's macroglobulinemia. J Clin Oncol 2005; 23:1564–1577.
2. Merlini G, Bellotti V. Molecular mechanisms of amyloidosis. N Engl J Med 2003; 349: 583–596.
3. Kyle RA, Therneau TM, Rajkumar SV, et al. A long-term study of prognosis in monoclonal gammopathy of undetermined significance. N Engl J Med 2002; 346:564–569.
4. Rosinol L, Blade J, Esteve J, et al. Smoldering multiple myeloma: natural history and recognition of an evolving type. Br J Haematol 2003; 123:631–636.
5. Saccaro S, Fonseca R, Veillon DM, et al. Primary plasma cell leukemia: report of 17 new cases treated with autologous or allogeneic stem-cell transplantation and review of the literature. Am J Hematol 2005; 78:288–294.
6. Gautier M, Cohen HJ. Multiple myeloma in the elderly. J Am Geriatr Soc 1994; 42:653–664.
7. Kyle RA, Therneau TM, Rajkumar SV, et al. Incidence of multiple myeloma in Olmsted County, Minnesota: trend over 6 decades. Cancer 2004; 101:2667–2674.

8. Riedel DA, Pottern LM. The epidemiology of multiple myeloma. Hematol Oncol Clin North Am 1992; 6:225–247.
9. Criteria for the classification of monoclonal gammopathies, multiple myeloma and related disorders: a report of the International Myeloma Working Group. Br J Haematol 2003; 121:749–757.
10. Rasillo A, Tabernero MD, Sanchez ML, et al. Fluorescence in situ hybridization analysis of aneuploidization patterns in monoclonal gammopathy of undetermined significance versus multiple myeloma and plasma cell leukemia. Cancer 2003; 97:601–609.
11. Rajkumar SV, Kyle RA, Therneau TM, et al. Serum free light chain ratio is an independent risk factor for progression in monoclonal gammopathy of undetermined significance (MGUS). Blood 2005; 3:1038.
12. Kyle RA. Monoclonal gammopathy of undetermined significance and solitary plasmacytoma. Implications for progression to overt multiple myeloma. Hematol Oncol Clin North Am 1997; 11:71–87.
13. Chao MW, Gibbs P, Wirth A, et al. Radiotherapy in the management of solitary extramedullary plasmacytoma. Intern Med J 2005; 35:211–215.
14. Guida M, Casamassima A, Abbate I, et al. Solitary plasmacytoma of bone and extramedullary plasmacytoma: two different nosological entities? Tumori 1994; 80:370–377.
15. Kyle RA, Gertz MA. Primary systemic amyloidosis: clinical and laboratory features in 474 cases. Semin Hematol 1995; 32:45–59.
16. Kyle RA, Gertz MA, Greipp PR, et al. A trial of three regimens for primary amyloidosis: colchicine alone, melphalan and prednisone, and melphalan, prednisone, and colchicine. N Engl J Med 1997; 336:1202–1207.
17. Dhodapkar MV, Hussein MA, Rasmussen E, et al. Clinical efficacy of high-dose dexamethasone with maintenance dexamethasone/alpha interferon in patients with primary systemic amyloidosis: results of United States Intergroup Trial Southwest Oncology Group (SWOG) S9628. Blood 2004; 104:3520–3526.
18. Seldin DC, Anderson JJ, Sanchorawala V, et al. Improvement in quality of life of patients with AL amyloidosis treated with high-dose melphalan and autologous stem cell transplantation. Blood 2004; 104:1888–1893.
19. Palladini G, Perfetti V, Perlini S, et al. The combination of thalidomide and intermediate-dose dexamethasone is an effective but toxic treatment for patients with primary amyloidosis (AL). Blood 2005; 105:2949–2951.
20. Greipp PR. Smoldering, asymptomatic stage 1, and indolent myeloma. Curr Treat Options Oncol 2000; 1:119–126.
21. Weber DM, Dimopoulos MA, Moulopoulos LA, et al. Prognostic features of asymptomatic multiple myeloma. Br J Haematol 1997; 97:810–814.
22. Rajkumar SV. Thalidomide in newly diagnosed multiple myeloma and overview of experience in smoldering/indolent disease. Semin Hematol 2003; 40:17–22.
23. Kyle RA, Gertz MA, Witzig TE, et al. Review of 1027 patients with newly diagnosed multiple myeloma. Mayo Clin Proc 2003; 78:21–33.
24. Alvares CL, Davies FE, Horton C, et al. Long-term outcomes of previously untreated myeloma patients: responses to induction chemotherapy and high-dose melphalan incorporated within a risk stratification model can help to direct the use of novel treatments. Br J Haematol 2005; 129:607–614.
25. Barille-Nion S, Barlogie B, Bataille R, et al. Advances in biology and therapy of multiple myeloma. Hematology 2003:248–278.
26. Greipp PR, San Miguel J, Durie BGM, et al. International staging system for multiple myeloma. J Clin Oncol 2005; 4:242.
27. Durie BG, Salmon SE. A clinical staging system for multiple myeloma. Correlation of measured myeloma cell mass with presenting clinical features, response to treatment, and survival. Cancer 1975; 36:842–854.
28. Kyle RA. Prognostic factors in multiple myeloma. Stem Cells 1995; 2(suppl 13):56–63.

29. Tricot G, Sawyer JR, Jagannath S, et al. Unique role of cytogenetics in the prognosis of patients with myeloma receiving high-dose therapy and autotransplants. J Clin Oncol 1997; 15:2659–2666.

30. Fonseca R, Harrington D, Oken MM, et al. Biological and prognostic significance of interphase fluorescence in situ hybridization detection of chromosome 13 abnormalities ({Delta}13) in multiple myeloma: an Eastern Cooperative Oncology Group Study. Cancer Res 2002; 62:715–720.

31. Oken MM, Harrington DP, Abramson N, et al. Comparison of melphalan and prednisone with vincristine, carmustine, melphalan, cyclophosphamide, and prednisone in the treatment of multiple myeloma: results of Eastern Cooperative Oncology Group Study E2479. Cancer 1997; 79:1561–1567.

32. Kumar S, Lacy MQ, Dispenzieri A, et al. Single agent dexamethasone for pre-stem cell transplant induction therapy for multiple myeloma. Bone Marrow Transplant 2004; 34:485–490.

33. Rajkumar S, Blood E, Vesole DH, et al. A randomised phase III trial of thalidomide plus dexamethasone versus dexamethasone in newly diagnosed multiple myeloma (E1A00): a trial conducted by the Eastern Cooperative Oncology Group. Proc Am Soc Clin Oncol 2004:558.

34. Coleman M, Leonard J, Lyons L, et al. BLT-D [clarithromycin (Biaxin), low-dose thalidomide, and dexamethasone] for the treatment of myeloma and Waldenstrom's macroglobulinemia. Leuk Lymphoma 2002; 43:1777–1782.

35. Durie BGM, Jacobson J, Barlogie B, et al. Magnitude of response with myeloma frontline therapy does not predict outcome: importance of time to progression in Southwest Oncology Group Chemotherapy Trials. J Clin Oncol 2004; 22:1857–1863.

36. Hussein MA, Anderson KC. Role of liposomal anthracyclines in the treatment of multiple myeloma. Semin Oncol 2004; 31:147–160.

37. Franks ME, Macpherson GR, Figg WD. Thalidomide. Lancet 2004; 363:1802–1811.

38. Barlogie B, Desikan R, Eddlemon P, et al. Extended survival in advanced and refractory multiple myeloma after single-agent thalidomide: identification of prognostic factors in a phase 2 study of 169 patients. Blood 2001; 98:492–494.

39. Cavo M, Zamagni E, Tosi P, et al. Superiority of thalidomide and dexamethasone over vincristine-doxorubicin-dexamethasone (VAD) as primary therapy in preparation for autologous transplantation for multiple myeloma. Blood 2005; 2:522.

40. Zangari M, Barlogie B, Anaissie E, et al. Deep vein thrombosis in patients with multiple myeloma treated with thalidomide and chemotherapy: effects of prophylactic and therapeutic anticoagulation. Br J Haematol 2004; 126:715–721.

41. Antonio P, Sara B, Pellegrino M, et al. Oral melphalan, prednisone and thalidomide for multiple myeloma. Blood (ASH Annual Meeting Abstracts) 2005; 106:779.

42. Schey SA, Fields P, Bartlett JB, et al. Phase I study of an immunomodulatory thalidomide analog, CC-4047, in relapsed or refractory multiple myeloma. J Clin Oncol 2004; 22:3269–3276.

43. Richardson PG, Schlossman RL, Weller E, et al. Immunomodulatory drug CC-5013 overcomes drug resistance and is well tolerated in patients with relapsed multiple myeloma. Blood 2002; 100:3063–3067.

44. Richardson PG, Sonneveld P, Schuster MW, et al. Bortezomib or high-dose dexamethasone for relapsed multiple myeloma. N Engl J Med 2005; 352:2487–2498.

45. Richardson P, Sonneveld P, Schuster MW, et al. Safety and efficacy of bortezomib in high-risk and elderly patients with relapsed myeloma. Proc Am Soc Clin Oncol 2005; 23:6533.

46. Hussein MA, Saleh M, Ravandi F, et al. Phase 2 study of arsenic trioxide in patients with relapsed or refractory multiple myeloma. Br J Haematol 2004; 125:470–476.

47. Bahlis NJ, McCafferty-Grad J, Jordan-McMurry I, et al. Feasibility and correlates of arsenic trioxide combined with ascorbic acid-mediated depletion of intracellular glutathione for the treatment of relapsed/refractory multiple myeloma. Clin Cancer Res 2002; 8:3658–3668.

48. Chanan-Khan AAN, Hohl RJ, et al. Randomized multicenter phase 3 trial of high-dose dexamethasone (dex) with or without oblimersen sodium (G3139; Bcl-2 antisense; genasense) for patients with advanced multiple myeloma (MM). Blood 2004:104.

49. Harousseau JL, Shaughnessy J Jr, Richardson P. Multiple myeloma. Hematology 2004; 2004:237–256.

50. Schaar CG, Kluin-Nelemans HC, te Marvelde C, et al. Interferon-{alpha} as maintenance therapy in patients with multiple myeloma. Ann Oncol 2005; 16:634–639.

51. Berenson JR, Crowley JJ, Grogan TM, et al. Maintenance therapy with alternate-day prednisone improves survival in multiple myeloma patients. Blood 2002; 99:3163–3168.

52. Stewart AK, Chen CI, Howson-Jan K, et al. Results of a multicenter randomized phase II trial of thalidomide and prednisone maintenance therapy for multiple myeloma after autologous stem cell transplant. Clin Cancer Res 2004; 10:8170–8176.

53. Attal M, Harousseau JL, Stoppa AM, et al. A prospective, randomized trial of autologous bone marrow transplantation and chemotherapy in multiple myeloma. N Engl J Med 1996; 335:91–97.

54. Child JA, Morgan GJ, Davies FE, et al. High-dose chemotherapy with hematopoietic stem-cell rescue for multiple myeloma. N Engl J Med 2003; 348:1875–1883.

55. Attal M, Harousseau JL, Facon T, et al. Single versus double autologous stem-cell transplantation for multiple myeloma. N Engl J Med 2003; 349:2495–2502.

56. Tricot G, Spencer T, Sawyer J, et al. Predicting long-term (> or = 5 years) event-free survival in multiple myeloma patients following planned tandem autotransplants. Br J Haematol 2002; 116:211–217.

57. Crawley C, Lalancette M, Szydlo R, et al. Outcomes for reduced-intensity allogeneic transplantation for multiple myeloma: an analysis of prognostic factors from the Chronic Leukaemia Working Party of the EBMT. Blood 2005; 105:4532–4539.

58. Moreau P, Garban F, Facon T, et al. Preliminary results of IFM9903 and IFM9904 protocols comparing autologous followed by miniallotransplantation and double autologous transplantation in high-risk de novo multiple myeloma. Blood 2003; 102:43a.

59. Blade J, Munoz M, Fontanillas M, et al. Treatment of multiple myeloma in elderly people: long-term results in 178 patients. Age Ageing 1996; 25:357–361.

60. Garcia-Sanz R, Gonzalez-Fraile MI, Mateo G, et al. Proliferative activity of plasma cells is the most relevant prognostic factor in elderly multiple myeloma patients. Int J Cancer 2004; 112:884–889.

61. Guba SC, Vesole DH, Jagannath S, et al. Peripheral stem cell mobilization and engraftment in patients over age 60. Bone Marrow Transplant 1997; 20:1–3.

62. Reece DE, Bredeson C, Perez WS, et al. Autologous stem cell transplantation in multiple myeloma patients <60 vs.>/=60 years of age. Bone Marrow Transplant 2003; 32: 1135–1143.

63. Lipton A. New therapeutic agents for the treatment of bone diseases. Expert Opin Biol Ther 2005; 5:817–832.

64. Rosen LS, Gordon D, Tchekmedyian S, et al. Zoledronic acid versus placebo in the treatment of skeletal metastases in patients with lung cancer and other solid tumors: a phase III, double-blind, randomized trial—the Zoledronic Acid Lung Cancer and Other Solid Tumors Study Group. J Clin Oncol 2003; 21:3150–3157.

65. Mazj S, Lichtman SM. Renal dysfunction associated with bisphosphonate use: retrospective analysis of 293 patients with respect to age and other clinical characteristics. Proc Am Soc Clin Oncol 2004; 23:8039a.

66. Ruggiero SL, Mehrotra B, Rosenberg TJ, et al. Osteonecrosis of the jaws associated with the use of bisphosphonates: a review of 63 cases. J Oral Maxillofac Surg 2004; 62:527–534.

67. Markowitz GS, Fine PL, Stack JI, et al. Toxic acute tubular necrosis following treatment with zoledronate (Zometa). Kidney Int 2003; 64:281–289.

68. Marx RE. Pamidronate (Aredia) and zoledronate (Zometa) induced avascular necrosis of the jaws: a growing epidemic. J Oral Maxillofac Surg 2003; 61:1115–1117.

69. Lane JM, Hong R, Koob J, et al. Kyphoplasty enhances function and structural alignment in multiple myeloma. Clin Orthop Relat Res 2004:49–53.

9

Lymphoma

Nirish S. Shah, William B. Ershler, and Dan L. Longo
Clinical Research Branch, National Institute on Aging, Harbor Hospital, National Institutes of Health, Baltimore, Maryland, U.S.A.

BACKGROUND

Many forms of lymphoma occur commonly in older adults. In general, the principles of diagnosis and management of lymphoid malignancies are not influenced by patient age. Certain issues may require special attention, but as with other malignancies, with appropriate attention to physiological details, intelligent treatment decisions are likely to result in improved quality of life and survival in older patients with lymphoma.

Many older patients will be challenged by compromised function of various organ systems. For example, declining liver function limits drug metabolism and declining renal function impairs drug excretion. Also, organs with decreased functional reserve are more susceptible to chemotherapy- or radiotherapy-induced injury. Furthermore, age-reduced bone marrow capacity may result in prolonged treatment–induced cytopenias with a consequent greater risk of neutropenic fevers and sepsis. However, it should be borne in mind that not all individuals age at the same rate, and within an individual, different organ systems may preserve function better than others over the years. Thus, it is difficult to generalize treatment strategies based upon age itself, and much wiser, albeit more cumbersome, to individualize treatment based upon a comprehensive assessment of physical function and a thoughtful analysis of those cognitive, social, and affective factors that assume increasing importance with age.

Based on a preconceived and often inaccurate notion that the elderly are "poor risk," many are treated with suboptimal doses of drugs or receive regimens with one or more of the component drugs omitted, or treatment is arbitrarily delayed. There may also be a bias against treatment based upon a lack of knowledge of age-adjusted life expectancy (Table 1) (1).

Currently, we do not have validated measures of physiologic reserve. Thus, optimal management of the older lymphoma patient requires good clinical judgment. Thoughtful and compassionate care administered on a case-by-case basis is likely to be met with success both in enhancing survival and in improving quality of life.

Table 1 Life Expectancy in the Elderly According to the Health Status

Age (yr)	Life expectancy (yr) according to health status		
	Healthy	Average	Sick
65	20	18.5	9.7
70	15.8	14.8	8.6
75	12.1	11.5	7.3
80	8.8	8.4	5.9
85	6.1	5.9	4.5

Source: From Ref. 1.

EPIDEMIOLOGY

According to the National Cancer Institute SEER estimates (2), 62,250 new cases of lymphoma occurred in 2004, of which the majority were non-Hodgkin's lymphoma (NHL). During the same year, there were 19,410 and 1320 deaths from non-Hodgkin's and Hodgkin's lymphoma, respectively. On a population basis, NHL is noted in 19 per 100,000 people each year.

NHL occurs more commonly in whites than blacks (19.7 per 100,000 and 14.7 per 100,000 in 2001) and more commonly in males than females (1.48:1). It is a disease of older people, with over half of the new cases occurring in patients aged 60 years and over and 38% of cases occurring in patients over the age of 70 years. The age-adjusted incidence rate is 9.7 per 100,000 in those younger than 65 compared to 86.5 per 100,000 for those over 65 years of age. For those over age 75, the incidence rates are over 100 per 100,000. Hodgkin's disease (HD) is less frequent in the elderly, with only 20% of all cases appearing in those over 60 years.

The incidence of the NHL in the United States increased at a rate of 3% to 4% per annum between 1930 and 1990 but has apparently stabilized since.

CLASSIFICATION

Lymphoid malignancies include acute and chronic lymphocytic leukemia (CLL), HD, and NHL, as well as disorders of the plasma cells, including multiple myeloma. Leukemia and myeloma are described elsewhere in this volume. NHLs are a heterogeneous group of malignancies of various cellular lineages and their classification has evolved over the past several decades. Currently, the World Health Organization classification system has gained popularity among clinicians and pathologists (Table 2).

INITIAL EVALUATION AND STAGING

In addition to a careful clinical examination, a complete blood count and assessment of serum chemistries and sedimentation rate are important first steps in adequately staging a patient. A CT scan of the chest, abdomen, and pelvis is warranted to delineate the spread of the disease. These tests, coupled with a bone marrow biopsy, would suffice as a primary evaluation. Patients with NHL should also have assessment of serum lactic dehydrogenase (LDH) and beta-2 microglobulin levels. The Ann Arbor staging classification is utilized for both Hodgkin's as well as NHL (Table 3).

Table 2 WHO Classification of Lymphoid Malignancies

B-cell	T-cell	HD
Precursor B-cell neoplasm	Precursor T-cell neoplasm	Nodular lymphocyte–predominant HD
Precursor B lymphoblastic leukemia/lymphoma (precursor B-cell acute lymphoblastic leukemia)	Precursor T lymphoblastic lymphoma/leukemia (precursor T-cell acute lymphoblastic leukemia)	
Mature (peripheral) B-cell neoplasms	Mature (peripheral) T-cell neoplasms	Classic HD
B-cell chronic lymphocytic leukemia/small lymphocytic lymphoma	T-cell prolymphocytic leukemia	Nodular sclerosis HD
		Lymphocyte-rich HD
		Mixed-cellularity HD
B-cell prolymphocytic leukemia	T-cell granular lymphocytic leukemia	Lymphocyte-depletion HD
Lymphoplasmacytic lymphoma	Aggressive NK cell leukemia	
Splenic marginal zone B-cell lymphoma (± villous lymphocytes)	Adult T-cell lymphoma/leukemia (HTLV-I+)	
Hairy cell leukemia	Extranodal NK/T-cell lymphoma, nasal type	
Plasma cell myeloma/plasmacytoma	Enteropathy-type T-cell lymphoma	
Extranodal marginal zone B-cell lymphoma of MALT type	Hepatosplenic γδ T-cell lymphoma	
Mantle cell lymphoma	Subcutaneous panniculitis-like T-cell lymphoma	
Follicular lymphoma	Mycosis fungoides/Sezary syndrome	
Nodal marginal zone B-cell lymphoma (± monocytoid B-cells)	Anaplastic large cell lymphoma, primary cutaneous type	
Diffuse large B-cell lymphoma	Peripheral T-cell lymphoma (NOS)	
Burkitt's lymphoma/Burkitt cell leukemia	Angioimmunoblastic T-cell lymphoma	
	Anaplastic large cell lymphoma, primary systemic type	

Abbreviations: HTLV, human T-cell lymphotropic virus; MALT, mucosa-associated lymphoid tissue; NK, natural killer; NOS, not otherwise specified; WHO, World Health Organization; HD, Hodgkin's disease.
Source: From Ref. 3.

Table 3 Ann Arbor Staging System for Lymphoma

Stage	Definition
I	Involvement of a single lymph node region or lymphoid structure (e.g., spleen, thymus, and Waldeyer's ring)
II	Involvement of two or more lymph node regions on the same side of the diaphragm (the mediastinum is a single site; hilar lymph nodes should be considered "lateralized" and, when involved on both sides, constitute stage II disease)
III	Involvement of lymph node regions or lymphoid structures on both sides of the diaphragm
III_1	Subdiaphragmatic involvement limited to spleen, splenic hilar nodes, celiac nodes, or portal nodes
III_2	Subdiaphragmatic involvement includes para-aortic, iliac, or mesenteric nodes plus structures in III_1
IV	Involvement of extranodal site(s) beyond that designated as "E" More than one extranodal deposit at any location Any involvement of liver or bone marrow
A	No symptoms
B	Unexplained weight loss of >10% of the body weight during the six months before staging investigation Unexplained, persistent, or recurrent fever with temperatures >38°C during the previous month Recurrent drenching night sweats during the previous month
E	Localized, solitary involvement of extralymphatic tissue, excluding liver and bone marrow

Source: From Ref. 3.

NON-HODGKIN'S LYMPHOMA

Based on the natural history of the disease, NHLs can be divided into aggressive and indolent variants (Table 4). The aggressive lymphomas, if untreated, can progress rapidly and lead to shortened survival in a few months, whereas indolent lymphomas have a long course extending for years during which, for some patients, no treatment is required.

AGGRESSIVE NHL

Clinical Presentation and Prognosis

The most frequent lymphoma in the elderly is diffuse large B-cell lymphoma (DLCL). The elderly are more likely to have localized disease or an extranodal presentation and less likely to have bulky disease compared to the young (4). The elderly are more likely to have small lymphocytic lymphoma (SLL), immunocytoma, and mantle cell lymphoma (MCL), while they are less likely to have follicular lymphoma (FL) compared to the young. However, poor functional status as well as bone marrow involvement is seen more frequently in the old (5). Clinical presentation of selected NHLs is outlined in Table 5 (3). Very highly aggressive lymphomas, such as Burkitt's lymphoma and lymphoblastic lymphoma do not occur very commonly in the elderly.

Age is an important prognostic factor for NHL. Age is an independent negative risk factor for survival for patients with lymphoma and is an integral component of the International Prognostic Index (IPI) for aggressive NHL (Table 6) (6).

Table 4 NHL According to Clinical Course of the Tumor

B-cell tumors	T-cell tumors
Indolent tumors	
Follicular lymphoma	Mycosis fungoides
Splenic marginal zone lymphoma	
MALT lymphoma	T-cell large granular lymphocytic
Plasmacytoma/multiple myeloma	leukemia
Lymphoplasmacytic lymphoma	
Small lymphocytic lymphoma/CLL	
B-cell prolymphocytic leukemia	
Hairy cell leukemia	
Aggressive tumors	
Diffuse large B-cell lymphoma	Peripheral T-cell lymphoma
Mantle cell lymphoma	Anaplastic large T-cell/null cell
Precursor B lymphoblastic leukemia/lymphoma	lymphoma
Burkitt's lymphoma/leukemia	Adult T-cell leukemia/lymphoma
	T-cell prolymphocytic leukemia

Abbreviations: CLL, chronic lymphocytic leukemia; NHL, non-Hodgkin's lymphoma; MALT, mucosa-associated lymphoid tissue.

Complete remission (CR) rates decrease from 68% in patients younger than 35 years to 45% in the oldest group (3). This results in lower overall and five-year disease-free survivals in the elderly. However, it is worth mentioning that once a CR is achieved, it is as durable in the aged as in the young. In fact, more deaths occurred in older patients due to causes other than lymphoma. Elderly patients frequently receive less intensive therapy and this may contribute to the reduced CR rates and shorter survival.

The IPI is an accurate tool for assessing the prognosis of patients with aggressive NHL. IPI is composed of five components—age, Ann Arbor stage of the disease, serum LDH, performance status, and number of extranodal sites. In the elderly, an age-adjusted IPI (this index excludes age and extranodal sites) carries the same accuracy. While IPI is accurate in prognosticating the aggressive lymphomas, a newly described FL International Prognostic Index (FLIPI) is an accurate prognostic indicator for the indolent lymphomas (7). FLIPI also has five components: age, hemoglobin, serum LDH, involved nodal sites, and stage (Table 7). A comparison of both prognostic indices is given in Table 8.

Management

Localized disease

DLCL is the commonest of all NHLs, accounting for about 40% of all cases. The disease is most frequently disseminated at the time of diagnosis with only 20% presenting in stage IA or IIA.

Current treatment for localized DLCL is typically combined radiation therapy and chemotherapy because this approach yields superior results compared to either modality alone (8–10). A large Southwest Oncology Group Phase III Trial with 401 participants demonstrated superiority of three cycles of CHOP[a] therapy combined

---

[a] CHOP: cyclophosphamide, doxorubicin, vincristine, prednisone.

Table 5 Clinical Features of Selected NHLs

Disease	Median age (yr)	Frequency in children	Male (%)	Stage I/II vs. III/IV (%)	B symptoms (%)	Bone marrow involvement (%)	Gastrointestinal tract involvement (%)	% Surviving 5 yr
B-cell CLL/SLL	65	Rare	53	9 vs. 91	33	72	3	51
Mantle cell lymphoma	63	Rare	74	20 vs. 80	28	64	9	27
Extranodal marginal zone B-cell lymphoma of MALT type	60	Rare	48	67 vs. 33	19	14	50	74
Follicular lymphoma	59	Rare	42	33 vs. 67	28	42	4	72
Diffuse large B-cell lymphoma	64	~25% of childhood NHL	55	54 vs. 46	33	16	18	46
Burkitt's lymphoma	31	~30% of childhood NHL	89	62 vs. 38	22	33	11	45
Precursor T-cell lymphoblastic lymphoma	28	~40% of childhood NHL	64	11 vs. 89	21	50	4	26
Anaplastic large T/null cell lymphoma	34	Common	69	51 vs. 49	53	13	9	77
Peripheral T-cell NHL	61	~5% of childhood NHL	55	20 vs. 80	50	36	15	25

Abbreviations: CLL, chronic lymphocytic leukemia; SLL, small lymphocytic lymphoma; MALT, mucosa-associated lymphoid tissue; NHL, non-Hodgkin's lymphoma.
Source: From Ref. 5.

Table 6 IPI for NHL

Clinical risk factors

IPI
1 Age $\geq$ 60 yr
2 Serum lactate dehydrogenase levels elevated
3 Performance status $\geq$2 (ECOG) or $\leq$70 (Karnofsky)
4 Ann Arbor stage III or IV
5 More than one site of extranodal involvement

Age-adjusted IPI
1 Serum lactate dehydrogenase levels elevated
2 Performance status $\geq$2 (ECOG) or $\leq$70 (Karnofsky)
3 Ann Arbor stage III or IV

Note: Patients are assigned a number for each risk factor they have
IPI
0,1 factors = low risk 35% of cases; five-year survival, 73%.
2 factors = low-intermediate risk 27% of cases; five-year survival, 51%.
3 factors = high-intermediate risk 22% of cases; five-year survival, 43%.
4,5 factors = high risk 16% of cases; five-year survival, 26%.
Age-adjusted IPI (age $\geq$60)
0 factors = low risk, five-year survival, 56%.
1 factor = low-intermediate risk, five-year survival, 44%.
2 factors = high-intermediate risk, five-year survival, 37%.
3 factors = high risk, five-year survival, 21%.
Abbreviations: IPI, International Prognostic Index; NHL, non-Hodgkin's lymphoma.
Source: From Ref. 6.

with involved-field radiation therapy (40–55 Gy) when compared to eight cycles of CHOP alone in terms of five-year progression-free (77% vs. 64%) and overall survival (82% vs. 72%) (9). Addition of rituximab to CHOP improves outcomes in advanced stage disease (see below), but it has not been tested in patients with localized disease. Use of radiation therapy alone in limited stage aggressive disease is associated with worse outcomes. A Japanese retrospective study showed five-year OS[b] and DFS[c] of 33% and 31% in 81 patients over 70 years of age who had stage I and II NHL and were unfit for chemotherapy. All the patients were treated with radiotherapy only (primary site + immediate adjacent site) (11).

A recent trial showed chemotherapy with adriamycin, cyclophosphamide, vincristine, bleomycin, and prednisone (ACVBP) regimen, which includes bleomycin and higher doses of doxorubicin and cyclophosphamide, to be superior to CHOP chemotherapy followed by radiation therapy in terms of event-free and overall survival in younger individuals (12). The ACVBP regimen was followed by sequential maintenance chemotherapy by methotrexate, etoposide, ifosfamide, and cytarabine. The intense ACVBP therapy is more toxic, resulting in almost twice as many treatment-related deaths in "poor risk" elderly patients with advanced disease (13). It remains to be seen if such an aggressive regimen is more appropriate in older people with localized disease, and whether the addition of radiotherapy or monoclonal antibodies has any impact on the outcomes.

---

[b] OS: overall survival.
[c] DFS: disease-free survival.

Table 7   Follicular Lymphoma International Prognostic Index

	Indicator		
1 Age $\geq$ 60 years			
2 Hemoglobin $<$ 12 g/dL			
3 LDH $>$ normal			
4 Involved nodal sites $>$ 4			
5 Ann Arbor stage III or IV			
No. of indicators present	FLIPI	5-year OS	10-year OS
0, 1	Low	90	70
2	Intermediate	77	50
3 or more	High	50	35

Abbreviations: FLIPI, follicular lymphoma International Prognostic Index; LDH, lactic dehydrogenase.
Source: From Ref. 7.

Advanced stage disease

The majority of patients with DLCL present with advanced stage disease. There remains significant concern over the use of aggressive combination chemotherapy in the elderly. An older person with lymphoma is more likely to present with poor performance status, limited functional organ reserve, and polypharmacy (taking numerous medications). The older patient presents management challenges that are further complicated by social beliefs, variations in the support system, and the physician's views on appropriateness of an aggressive therapy.

In a retrospective analysis by Dixon et al. (14), older patients were found to have a lower CR rate and shorter OS when treated with CHOP, with or without bleomycin, compared to younger patients. However, the chemotherapy dose was decreased by 50% or more in the elderly. A subgroup analysis of 23 elderly patients who received full dose treatment revealed a similar rate and duration of CR compared to the younger group. However, the OS was still significantly less. This reduced survival may be due to causes of death other than lymphoma (15). This notion was supported by Vose et al. in a group of 157 patients of whom 112 were over 60 years of age. They found no significant difference in CR rate between the young and old treated with CAPBOP (cyclophosphamide, doxorubicin, procarbazine, bleomycin, vincristine, and prednisone). However, there was a significant difference between the two groups in five-year overall survival (62% vs. 34%). This difference in survival was secondary to deaths unrelated to lymphoma (16). It was also noted that almost 25% of the elderly were given suboptimal therapy based on their chronological age despite having a good performance status (17).

CHOP combination chemotherapy was first utilized in the treatment of NHL in the early 1970s. Since then, many second and third generation combinations have been examined in clinical trials, including MACOP-B[d], m-BACOD[e], and

---

[d] MACOP-B: methotrexate, doxorubicin, cyclophosphamide, vincristine, prednisone, and bleomycin.

[e] m-BACOD: low-dose methotrexate, doxorubicin, cyclophosphamide, vincristine, dexamethasone, and bleomycin.

ProMACE/CytaBOM[f]. However, until recently, CHOP was the standard of care for aggressive NHL (see below). A four-arm randomized clinical study failed to prove the superiority of second and third generation combinations (18).

Doxorubicin-induced cardiotoxicity remains a significant concern regarding the use of the CHOP regimen and thus, various regimens substituting mitoxantrone for doxorubicin [CNOP[g] (17,19–21) and VMP[h] (22)] have been tested. However, these regimens have proven to be less efficacious than CHOP.

There has been recent interest in administration of CHOP chemotherapy at a more frequent interval than every three weeks (23,24). Administered on a two-week schedule, CHOP has been shown to be both safe and effective, resulting in better remission rates as well as disease-free and overall survival. However, when used in the intensive schedule, an increase in hematologic toxicity is anticipated and growth factor support is recommended. Clinical trials evaluating biweekly CHOP regimen plus rituximab are currently underway. The role of these dose-intense regimens in elderly patients needs to be established by prospective randomized trial, because hematological toxicity might preclude widespread application.

The major adverse consequence of many lymphoma treatment regimens applied to older patients is bone marrow toxicity and resulting cytopenias. Growth factor trials either specifically focused upon the elderly or in post hoc subgroup analysis have demonstrated only a limited advantage to their prophylactic use. Although most have shown a decrease in the occurrence and duration of post-treatment neutropenia associated with fewer episodes of febrile neutropenia, colony-stimulating factors have failed to demonstrate a significant increase in CR rate or survival (19,25,26).

Biologic therapy, however, has made its way into the mainstream of lymphoma therapy. Rituximab, a chimeric antibody to the CD20 cell surface antigen found on most B-cells, was shown, when administered with CHOP, to be superior to CHOP alone, with increases in CR rate (76% vs. 63%) and two-year OS (70% vs. 57%) (27). This trial was specifically conducted in patients over 60 years of age. A very promising aspect about rituximab was the absence of increased toxicity when used in combination with chemotherapy (28).

Summary

CHOP+rituximab is the new standard of care for the elderly patient with lymphoma. Doxorubicin is a critical component of treatment and should not be withheld arbitrarily simply on the basis of age.

In a patient with evidence of CHF[i], alternatives to CHOP including CNOP (mitoxantrone substituted for doxorubicin) may be administered; however, these treatments are likely to provide inferior results. ProMACE/CytaBOM may be effective in the elderly and it uses much lower doses of doxorubicin than those in CHOP. Hematopoietic growth factors decrease febrile neutropenia, rate of severe infection, and hospitalizations, but have not been shown to improve the CR rate or OS.

---

[f] ProMACE-CytaBOM: prednisone, doxorubicin, cyclophosphamide, and etoposide, followed by cytarabine, bleomycin, vincristine, and methotrexate.

[g] CNOP: mitoxantrone substituted for doxorubicin in CHOP.

[h] VMP: etoposide, mitoxantrone, and prednimustine.

[i] CHF: congestive heart failure.

INDOLENT NHL

By far the commonest indolent NHL is FL, which can be seen in three histological grades (I–III) based on the relative number of large cells. The grade I and II FLs are indolent in behavior, whereas grade III FL has a clinical course that is most often considered aggressive. The indolent lymphoma group also includes marginal zone lymphoma (MZL), prolymphocytic leukemia, and lymphoplasmacytoid lymphoma. For indolent lymphoma, the median survival is typically 7 to 10 years. However, to date, no cure exists for advanced stage indolent lymphomas.

Small-cell lymphocytic lymphoma is the tissue-based counterpart of CLL and the treatment for SLL is similar to that for CLL. Similarly, lymphoplasmacytoid lymphoma is closely related to multiple myeloma and Waldenstrom's macroglobulinemia.

Prognostic Indicators

The prognostic model used for the aggressive NHL also reflects prognosis for patients with indolent lymphomas. However, few patients with FL have high or high-intermediate IPI risks. As described previously, a new FLIPI has been proposed (7). This model is compared to the IPI in Table 8 and it predicts programs with a more even distribution of patients in various risk groups.

Management

Limited Stage Disease

About 15% of the patients present with limited stage disease. Indolent lymphomas are possibly curable when discovered early and radiation therapy is administered with curative intent. However, relapses as late as 13 years after treatment have been observed (29).

When treated with involved-field radiation therapy alone, a 10-year disease-free survival of 28% to 53% and OS of 52% to 79% have been reported (30–33). Seymour et al. (29) described a prospective trial of a large group of early stage patients treated with involved-field radiation therapy in combination with 10 cycles of COP-B (cyclophosphamide, vincristine, prednisone, and bleomycin) or CHOP-B (doxorubicin added for relatively aggressive disease). At 10 years of follow-up, OS was of 83% and 10-year relapse-free survival (RFS) was 76%. Patients over 60 years of age had slightly less favorable outcomes (OS 75% and RFS 64% at 10 years). Although the results are very promising, there was no direct comparison to radiation

Table 8 Comparison of IPI and FLIPI

	IPI	FLIPI
1	Age $\geq$ 60	Age $\geq$ 60
2	Ann Arbor stage III or IV	Ann Arbor stage III or IV
3	Serum LDH > normal	Serum LDH > normal
4	More than one extranodal site involvement	More than four nodal sites involvement
5	Performance status >2 (ECOG) or <70 (Karnofsky)	Hemoglobin <12 g/dL

Abbreviations: FLIPI, follicular lymphoma International Prognostic Index; IPI, International Prognostic Index; LDH, lactic dehydrogenase; ECOG, Eastern Cooperative Oncology Group.

therapy alone in this study. A clinical trial comparing radiation therapy to combined modality therapy is currently underway.

Advanced Stage Disease

About 85% of patients present with advanced disease, yet the disease may remain indolent for years (median survival between 6 and 12 years). Although amenable to chemotherapy, relapse generally occurs between 2.5 and 4 years. Once relapsed, the disease responds to chemotherapy, but the response rates and duration decrease with each relapse. Disease transformation to a more aggressive variant with predominance of large cells is a frequent terminal event. After transformation, the disease behaves as an aggressive lymphoma (DLCL) and the prognosis is poor. However, some patients may respond to aggressive therapy. The rate of histological progression seems to be unaffected by treatment; about 7% of patients undergo progression to aggressive lymphomas annually and by the time of death nearly all patients with FL have experienced histologic progression.

Patients with stage III and IV indolent lymphoma are a therapeutic challenge because no curative treatment is currently available. Treatments range from single-agent chemotherapy to combination chemotherapy to biological agents including interferon-alpha and rituximab or a combination of chemotherapy and biological therapy. Radiation therapy and radioimmunotherapy (radiolabeled monoclonal antibodies) are also active in the disease. Furthermore, for selected patients, some have advocated observation alone, whereas, in contrast, others have advocated a role for bone marrow transplant. Despite the wide array of treatment options, there has been no treatment or combination of treatments that has been proven to significantly increase overall survival.

Because of the indolent course of the disease, an initial period of "watchful waiting" is very appealing, especially in the elderly (unless the patient has localized disease). In prospective trials, no difference has been demonstrated between observation and early chemotherapy. However, it should be noted that the CR rates and duration of the remissions are longer in the group treated initially compared with the observation groups. This apparent advantage has not, however, resulted in a survival advantage for the early treatment population. Using this strategy, the median time to initiation of chemotherapy is two to three years. Of note, about one-fifth of the patients in observation protocol remain free of an indication to begin chemotherapy at 10 years. In a long-term follow-up of a large prospective U.K. trial on indolent NHL, 19% of patients who did not receive any treatment were alive at 10 years. However, in a subset of patients over age 75 ($n = 20$), 40% were alive for the same duration without requiring any therapeutic intervention (34). If one is to choose the watchful waiting approach, careful patient selection is essential. The presence of B symptoms, peripheral blood cytopenia, kidney or liver involvement,or any life-endangering organ involvement require a more immediate treatment.

Various combinations of chemotherapy have been attempted. No regimen is superior to the others with regard to survival advantage.

A single-agent oral alkylating agent such as chlorambucil or cyclophosphamide may be an attractive choice in the elderly because of ease of administration and relatively low toxicity. When used alone, this therapy results in response rates of 60% to 80% with about half of all patients achieving a complete response.

Combination chemotherapy with cyclophosphamide, vincristine, and prednisone (CVP) is also effective and may result in slightly higher CR of 60% to 70%. The addition of an anthracycline has not been shown to provide useful benefit (35,36). Although chemotherapy has definite benefit, no specific regimen has proven superior with regard to overall survival. In fact, Peterson et al. (36) showed that CHOP-B was no better than single-agent chlorambucil.

Fludarabine, a purine nucleoside analogue, is also an active agent used in the treatment of indolent lymphoma. Used alone, it can induce remissions in about 60% to 80% of all treatment-naive patients (although less CR is observed). Addition of an anthracycline to fludarabine does not lead to any clinical advantage (37). Combination of fludarabine with other active agents such as mitoxantrone (38) and dexamethasone results in a high response rate of over 90%. This regimen was shown to be equivalent to a more complicated and more toxic alternating drug regimen (39).

In relapsed patients, chemotherapy may still be used to induce remission. Fludarabine remains an attractive agent inducing remission in half of relapsed patients. When combined with cyclophosphamide and mitoxantrone, the response is increased appreciably.

As mentioned, no data exist proving superiority of one modality of treatment over another with regard to survival (35). Combination chemotherapy prolongs the progression-free survival. However, this advantage is balanced by the inherent risks of chemotherapy toxicity and its effect on quality of life—factors that are particularly relevant for older lymphoma patients.

The use of interferon for treatment of indolent lymphoma remains controversial (35,40). A meta-analysis demonstrated its usefulness as a maintenance therapy in patients pretreated with aggressive combination chemotherapy, who had responded to the therapy. It was shown that the DFS was increased with addition of interferon alpha as a maintenance agent. However, the data are not conclusive. In 2000, Fisher et al. showed in a large randomized trial no benefit to maintenance therapy with interferon alpha (41). Interferon may be successful at keeping the lymphoma out of sight, but its use has not consistently extended overall survival.

When used in previously untreated patients, rituximab produces response in 47% to 73% of patients with up to 37% achieving a CR. Moreover, when combined with combination chemotherapy, rituximab has shown an excellent overall response rate (100%) and CR rate (87%) (42). The median time to progression is 83.5 months. Similar responses are seen when rituximab is combined with CNOP (cyclophosphamide, mitoxantrone, vincristine, and prednisone) producing OR[j] of 90% and CR rate of 70% (43). A recent U.K. trial published in abstract form, reports that when combined with CVP, R-CVP yields better overall response rates (81% vs. 57%), CR rate (40% vs. 10%), and time to treatment failure (median 27 months vs. 7 months) than CVP alone (44). However, it must be noted that CVP alone has never performed as poorly in prior studies. With regard to long-term survival, there are currently no conclusive data. However, long-term follow-up of a well-conducted randomized trial comparing combination chemotherapy with and without rituximab needs to be done to examine whether a survival advantage is seen with chemoimmunotherapy.

Rituximab is also active in relapsed patients with indolent NHL. When used in this setting, rituximab with fludarabine, cyclophosphamide, and mitoxantrone

---

[j] OR: overall response rate.

(FCM) induces responses in over three-fourths of patients and about a third of all patients achieve CR.

Initial results have shown a survival advantage in the rituximab-FCM arm. Once again, with regard to overall survival, it will take an analysis of long-term data on a large number of patients to determine if the addition of rituximab offers an advantage (45,46).

Results of the use of rituximab as a maintenance therapy were recently published (47). In this trial, previously treated patients who had progression of the disease were treated with rituximab monotherapy. Patients showing objective response to rituximab monotherapy were further evaluated. Addition of rituximab as a maintenance therapy every six months resulted in a longer progression-free survival (31 months) compared to no maintenance therapy (7.4 months). However, the patients not receiving maintenance therapy with rituximab received rituximab at the time of disease progression, and the median duration of rituximab benefit (defined by cumulative period of objective response to rituximab therapy at any time or a stable disease lasting more than six months after rituximab administration) in this group was 27 months, which was statistically not different from 31 months in the maintenance therapy. The role of rituximab maintenance is not yet well established and further studies are needed.

Two new agents have recently been approved by the Food and Drug Administration for use in the treatment of rituximab-refractory indolent NHL—Yttrium-90–conjugated ibritumomab and Iodine-131–conjugated tositumomab. Both are targeted to CD20 and both have demonstrated activity in rituximab-resistant FL. They produce responses in about two-thirds to three-fourths of patients (48,49). I^{131} tositumomab is also effective as a single agent in previously untreated patients with over 90% OR and 75% CR (50). However, use of these agents as a primary therapy requires further randomized studies. No evidence suggests that these agents are curative when used alone.

Even with aggressive therapy, such as high-dose chemotherapy with autologous bone marrow or stem cell transplant, overall survival has not been demonstrably prolonged (51,52). In fact, in older patients with marginal functional reserve, the preparatory regimen for stem cell transplant may be prohibitively toxic. Thus, enthusiasm for such an aggressive approach has been slow to develop. However, in well-selected elderly patients, effective transplant strategies have been implemented. Depending on the condition of the patient, autologous stem cell transplants can be safely used in patients at least up to 70 years of age.

Summary

No curative treatment exists for advanced stage indolent lymphomas. In carefully selected patients, a watch and wait approach may be appropriate. Various therapies are effective in inducing remission. Once achieved, the remission is maintained for a longer time with more effective therapy and with maintenance therapy, but no documented changes have been shown so far in overall survival.

The role of interferon alpha is still debatable. Rituximab and radiolabeled antibodies to CD20 are exciting new additions showing an increased CR rate and DFS at a short follow-up. We need longer follow-up data to see their effects on survival.

If a patient in good physical health is judged to be able to withstand high-dose chemotherapy, stem cell transplant may be a viable option in the setting of relapsed disease.

MARGINAL ZONE LYMPHOMA

MZL and mantle cell lymphoma (MCL) occur with high frequency in the elderly. Together, they account for between 5% and 10% of all lymphomas.

The MZLs are considered indolent with a behavior similar to that of FL. Various subtypes of MZL exist, including nodal MZL, splenic MZL, and extranodal MZL. Extranodal MZL includes lymphoma of the mucosa-associated lymphoid tissue (MALT) (extranodal MZL of MALT type). Nodal MZL has an indolent natural history and, like FL, may undergo histologic progression to DLCL. MZL of MALT type is often initiated through chronic antigenic stimulation.

MALT lymphoma commonly presents in the stomach, although it may involve other extranodal sites including orbit, intestine, thyroid, lung, breast, salivary gland, urinary bladder, kidney, and CNS.

Etiologic association has been made of bacterium *Helicobacter pylori* with gastric MALT lymphoma. It has been proposed that *H. pylori* infection of the stomach results in chronic gastritis thereby activating the underlying lymphoid tissue and ultimately leading to a monoclonal proliferation of B-cells, which in turn may lead to development of gastric MALT. Strains of *H. pylori* expressing CagA protein seem to play a role in the pathogenesis of the lymphoma. Antibodies to CagA protein were present in 95% of patients with lymphoma compared with 67% of patients with *H. pylori* gastritis without lymphoma (53).

However, when gastritis develops in autoimmune conditions like pernicious anemia, such increase in incidence of MALT lymphoma has not been observed. The reason for this may be the type and location of the gastritis. In autoimmune gastritis, also called type A gastritis, there is predominant involvement of the gastric fundus and body whereas with type B gastritis commonly seen with *H. pylori* infection, the antrum is initially involved, which spares the intrinsic factor-producing parietal cells. Intrinsic factor may be a host-related factor that promotes the inflammatory process that leads to subsequent monoclonal proliferation of B-cells and lymphoma.

Gastric MALT lymphoma usually presents with symptoms of dyspepsia, i.e. heartburn and epigastic pain. This disease is usually localized when diagnosed. Treatment of *H. pylori* results in remission of the disease in about 50% of cases. The development of CR may take several months after the completion of triple antibiotic therapy for the *H. pylori*. The patients who show CR almost always have a flat superficial primary lesion (54). Lymphoma that has progressed beyond the superficial layer of the mucosa responds less favorably to antibiotics alone, though such tumors may have a very good response with local radiation therapy.

Treatment with combination chemotherapy using COP (cyclophosphamide, vincristine, and prednisone) with involved-field radiation leads to cure in almost all patients with early stage MALT lymphoma (29). Once the disease spreads to lymph nodes, it behaves in a manner analogous to FL although there is some suggestion that at this point the prognosis may not be as favorable (55). Gastric MALT lymphoma that progresses to aggressive DLCL should be treated like de novo DLCL at other sites.

The MALT lymphomas in other sites are also linked to chronic infections and inflammatory conditions (Table 9). Some of the infectious agents include *Chlamydia psittaci*, *Borrelia burgdorferi*, and *Campylobacter jejuni*, which are associated with MALT lymphoma in ocular adnexa, skin, and small intestine, respectively. Similarly, chronic inflammation of Hashimoto's thyroiditis is linked to thyroid MALT lymphoma (56).

Splenic MZL is responsible for about one-fourth of low-grade B-cell tumors affecting the spleen. Hepatitis C infection is associated with this lymphoma.

Table 9 Etiologic Relationship of Chronic Inflammation and Infections with MALT in Various Locations

Causative agent/condition	Site of MALT lymphoma
Helicobacter pylori	Stomach
Campylobacter jejuni	Small intestine
Borrelia burgdorferi	Skin
Chlamydia psittaci	Ocular adnexal tissue
Hashimoto's disease	Thyroid gland
Sjogren's disease	Salivary glands

Abbreviation: MALT, mucosa-associated lymphoid tissue.

Splenectomy is effective therapy and so is the treatment of the underlying hepatitis C infection. However, a poor response to alkylating agents is seen with this subgroup.

Both nodal MZL and splenic MZL can transform to aggressive large cell lymphoma, conferring a poor prognosis.

MANTLE CELL LYMPHOMA

Berard described an entity called malignant lymphoma, lymphocytic type, showing intermediate grade of differentiation, in the late 1970s. Further research in histology, immunology, and cytogenetics led to the discovery that this entity of lymphoma arose from the mantle zone of the lymph nodes and the name MCL was made popular in the early 1980s (57,58).

MCL is a B lymphoid malignancy with CD5 positivity and overexpression of cyclin-D1. It comprises approximately 5% to 8% of all lymphomas. With a median age of 63 years, it is commonly seen in the elderly.

MCL commonly involves spleen, bone marrow, Waldeyer's ring, and gastrointestinal tract and it has been associated with lymphomatous polyposis (59).

MCL shares some clinical characteristics with both indolent and aggressive lymphoma. Like the aggressive lymphomas, MCL has a shorter median survival (3–4 years) but, like the indolent lymphomas the disease appears incurable with the treatment available at this time (60).

Three types of MCL exist based on the histological characteristics. Of the three, the diffuse type of MCL has the poorest life expectancy (16 months) compared with blastic and nodular types for which the median survival is in the range of 50 to 55 months (61).

Few prospective studies have been reported regarding treatment of MCL. Treatment with COP and CHOP seems to yield similar results with total response rate of 80% to 90% and CR rate in about half of all patients. However, the durability of the response remains very poor, with a median RFS in the range of one year (61,62).

Fludarabine has been shown to be effective in the treatment of MCL with overall response rates of up to 60% (37). Regardless of the initial treatment used, it appears that nearly all patients relapse. Response to second-line therapy is generally less satisfactory with fewer and less durable remissions.

New evidence has emerged demonstrating the usefulness of combining rituximab with chemotherapy, although when used alone as a single agent, rituximab has limited activity. Use of FCM together with rituximab seems very promising in relapsed or refractory patients. In a recent trial of 40 patients with MCL with over three-fourths of patients over the age of 60 years, there was an overall response in more than half of the patients with higher CR (29%) and two-year OS (65%) with R-FCM compared to FCM alone (0% and 35%, respectively) (46). Similarly, Lenz et al. showed that combination of CHOP and rituximab resulted in higher total response rates and CR rates (94% and 34%) compared to CHOP alone (75% and 7%) and prolonged time to treatment failure (21 months vs. 14 months). However, no survival advantage was noted with addition of rituximab (63).

In an effort to obtain longer disease-free and overall survivals, autologous stem cell transplantation has been attempted after high-dose chemotherapy. However, as with the case for indolent lymphomas, limited bone marrow reserve and associated susceptibility to infections prohibit the stem cell transplant in elderly patients with comorbid illness.

HODGKIN'S LYMPHOMA

Epidemiology

Seven thousand, eight hundred and eighty new cases of Hodgkin's lymphoma occurred in the United States in the year 2004. There were 1320 deaths due to the disease that year (2). Hodgkin's lymphoma occurs more commonly in males; male to female ratio is 1.2:1. Unlike NHL, only 20% of all cases occur in persons over 60 years of age (64,65). Hodgkin's lymphoma is described as a disease having a bimodal age distribution, with the first spike in disease incidence in the second and third decade and the second spike in the sixth and seventh decade of life. Whether these peaks reflect distinct disease entities with similar histologic manifestations has not been resolved.

Clinical Presentation

Hodgkin's lymphoma is histologically classified into classical HD and nodular lymphocyte predominance HD. The classical HD is further divided into lymphocyte-rich, nodular sclerosis, mixed cellularity, and lymphocyte depletion subtypes. In young adults, nodular sclerosis is the commonest histology. On the other hand, the elderly have a higher prevalence of mixed cellularity HD (65–67). It has also been suggested that many cases of the HD in elderly may actually represent NHLs that were difficult to diagnose accurately before the advent of newer genetic and immunologic techniques (68).

Unlike NHL, where the disease is pathologically similar in the young and the old patients, Hodgkin's lymphoma in the elderly has quite different clinical characteristics. This is manifested by the difference in histological type, difference in cytogenetic markers, and association with Epstein–Barr virus (EBV). Positivity of EBV DNA in the Reed–Sternberg cell of the older patients seems to be correlated with worse prognosis in population-based studies. However, in the case of the young, the opposite seems to be the case (65,69).

Prognosis

Compared to the survival in younger patients, survival in the elderly patients with HD is decreased. Various causes for this diminished survival have been proposed: more aggressive disease, different histological type, poor outcomes with EBV positivity, and, probably more importantly, coexisting frailty. A population-based study showed 56% of HD patients over the age of 60 years had at least one comorbid illness, and this was significantly associated with lower frequency of chemotherapy administration (70). Also, as with other malignancies, there is a seeming unwillingness on the part of treating physicians to manage these patients aggressively (71). Older patients more often receive suboptimal dosages of chemotherapy. Also, deaths in this age group due to causes unrelated to the lymphoma or its treatment result in lower overall survivals, and so the comparisons of overall survival should be done with age-matched survival statistics. One uncontrolled trial also found a higher incidence of treatment-related secondary malignancies in the elderly (67).

A population-based study showed five-year disease-specific survival of 100% and 52% in early stage HD in ages 60 to 69 years and age 70 years and over, respectively. In the same study, the five-year disease-specific survival for advanced disease was found to be only 36% and 14%, respectively (65).

Several clinical indicators seem to influence outcomes in HD. These include age over 45 years, low serum albumin <4 g, low hemoglobin <10.5 g/dL, stage IV disease, leukocytosis (>15,000), and lymphopenia (<600). However, the international collaborative study defining these prognostic factors included patients only up to the age of 65 years. Thus, it is not defined whether age >65 years is associated with a poorer outcome (72).

Management

In last four decades, progress in therapeutics has made Hodgkin's lymphoma a curable disease in about 85% of patients. The treatment of the early stages of disease had classically been extended-field radiation therapy, although a third of all patients relapsed (73). However, most of the relapses are amenable to salvage treatment and this group of patients enjoy an overall long-term survival of approximately 90%. The mortality seen in this group has been linked with premature coronary artery disease and development of secondary malignancies related to the use of radiation therapy. Tumors of solid organs occur after 5 to 10 years, with risk increasing over a prolonged period ranging to decades. The secondary malignancies continue to show up in long-term follow-up of initial curative treatment trials. No plateau in risk is evident in series of patients followed up to 30 years. The incidence of fatal myocardial infarction is increased threefold in patients treated with mediastinal radiation.

These life-threatening toxicities have led to an alternate management approach seeking to minimize the radiation therapy in treatment of the early stage disease. One may want to argue that the long-term complications of radiation therapy should not be a concern in elderly patients, as they have a limited life expectancy. However, physicians may underestimate life expectancy. As pointed out in Table 1, even at older ages, patients may have a longer survival than might be expected.

There is an increasing tendency to treat early stage disease patients with a short course of chemotherapy and involved-field radiation therapy. While combined modality approaches have a very small increase in disease-free survival, overall survival is not increased compared to chemotherapy alone, both because of effective salvage therapy and late radiation therapy–related deaths. A randomized study has shown that ABVD[k] alone is as effective as ABVD plus radiation therapy for early stage HD (74).

---

[k] ABVD: doxorubicin, bleomycin, vinblastine, dacarbazine.

An appropriate treatment for elderly patients of all stages is six cycles of ABVD therapy alone. However, it should be noted that there is a definite role of radiation therapy in the treatment of HD. The two main indications for radiation therapy are the presence of bulky tumor (>10 cm in diameter or >1/3 of the thorax in case of mediastinal disease) (75) or the occurrence of a partial response to the chemotherapeutic regimen. Addition of radiation to involved fields in these settings can help achieve durable complete remissions.

Various trials including ABVD and MOPP[l] in an alternating or hybrid regimen have failed to show superiority of either regimen to ABVD alone (76). Some regimens (e.g., BEACOPP[m]) may be too toxic for routine use in the elderly. A recent trial in elderly patients showed 21% therapy-related deaths with BEACOPP therapy (76). Stanford V[n] has the disadvantage of employing radiation therapy in all patients. Radiation therapy should be restricted to the subset of patients who receive it for optimal outcome, as discussed above.

There is a natural concern about using ABVD combination in the elderly, especially when they have a pre-existing cardiac, renal, pulmonary, or hepatic comorbidity. However, ad hoc reduction or modification in the treatment should be avoided. It should also be noted that the drugs in their recommended dose schedule are unlikely to produce permanent damage. In a patient with multiple comorbidities, full doses of medications should be given on the first day and, depending on the outcomes, appropriate dose adjustment should be done in response to actually encountered toxicities, rather than blindly altering the drugs in anticipation of toxicity.

In the case of relapsed disease, various options are available, depending on the initial modality of the treatment. If a patient relapses following radiation therapy alone, the patient remains sensitive to the combination chemotherapy. However, a relapse in a patient initially treated with chemotherapy would require high-dose chemotherapy with autologous stem cell transplant. In general, 30% to 65% of patients receiving high-dose therapy achieve long-term freedom from relapse, although results of this therapy in the elderly have not been systematically studied.

THE ELDERLY LYMPHOMA PATIENT

The use of hemopoietic growth factors has not improved survival, but there is clear evidence that neutropenia, infectious complications, and hospital stays are reduced as a consequence of their use. Thus, the use of G-CSF[o] should be considered when using myelosuppressive chemotherapy (77–79). Similarly, use of erythropoietin to maintain hemoglobin levels at or above 12 g/dL improves quality of life and may enhance treatment response (78,80,81).

Devising the optimal therapeutic approach to an elderly patient is oftentimes difficult. It is important to leave behind the commonly held underestimates of life

---

[l] MOPP: mechlorethamine, vincristine, procarbazine, prednisone.

[m] BEACOPP: bleomycin, etoposide, doxorubicin, cyclophosphamide, vincristine, procarbazine, and prednisone.

[n] Stanford V: doxorubicin, vinblastine, mechlorethamine, vincristine, bleomycin, etoposide, and prednisone combined with radiation to bulky lymph node sites, 5 cm or more in diameter.

[o] G-CSF: granulocyte colony-stimulating factor.

expectancy and drug tolerability in this age group because these have been shown to be incorrect when appropriate assessment of organ function and comorbidities is considered (14).

A useful approach is to individualize treatment. Yet, such an approach without careful consideration runs the risk of ad hoc dose reduction. To provide more objective basis, treatment may be administered based upon some form of comprehensive geriatric assessment (CGA). Typically, CGA consists of assessment of activity of daily living (ADL), instrumental activity of daily living (IADL), coexisting depression, social support, comorbid illness, and geriatric syndromes.

Based on CGA, patients can be divided in three groups (82–84). The first group, G_1, is the group of healthy elderly. These patients are functionally independent, have no serious comorbid illness, and are free from geriatric syndromes. The second group, G_2, consists of the patients who are partially dependent on their ADL or IADL and have up to two moderately severe comorbid conditions. Finally, frail elderly make up the third group, G_3. Those individuals who are dependent on more than one ADL, have three or more comorbidities, or have more than one geriatric syndrome are considered frail. Age over 85 should not be considered a strict criterion for frailty.

The G_1 patients are very similar to younger patients and no treatment modification is usually required. The frail patients are at the highest risk for treatment toxicity and palliative treatment is more likely to be the optimal treatment plan (82,83,85). However, it is the second group of patients who need the most attention. Treatment individualization is recommended based on associated conditions and physiologic parameters.

While interpreting the various parameters of CGA, the following should be kept in mind. The presence of a disease does not automatically disqualify a patient from receiving life-saving treatment. Rather, severity of the disease should be taken into account. For example, the presence of high blood pressure is not the same as having hypertensive cardiomyopathy, and anthracycline-containing therapy should not be withheld. Similarly, prednisone should not be withheld in a diabetic as long as the resulting hyperglycemia can be controlled. A pilot study based on principles of CGA is underway by Bernardi et al. in elderly patients with aggressive NHL (86). This nonblinded study included patients over age of 70 years. After excluding frail individuals, patients underwent individualized chemotherapy based on functional status (ADL and IADL), major organ system functions, and coexisting medical conditions. At one-year follow-up of this study, assessed patients ($n = 19$) had 90% overall response, with 79% complete response. Long-term follow-up is yet to be seen.

FUTURE DIRECTIONS

There are limitations in our current understanding of lymphomas in the elderly. It is important to determine why age is a prognostic factor in lymphoma. Is the disease different in the elderly? Is the response to therapy different in the elderly? Do toxicities or comorbid illnesses prevent the use of therapy delivered in optimal doses and schedule? The elderly should be included in clinical trials, and efforts to assess the ability of the CGA to measure physiologic reserve should be undertaken. The day is eagerly anticipated when we can rationally individualize management to optimize antitumor effects and minimize toxicity.

REFERENCES

1. Extermann M, Balducci L, Lyman GH. What threshold for adjuvant therapy in older breast cancer patients? J Clin Oncol 2000; 18:1709–1717.
2. Non-Hodgkin's lymphoma *Cancer Statistics Review*: SEER database from the National Cancer Institute.
3. Armitage JO, Longo DL. Malignancies of the lymphoid cells. In: Kasper DL, Braunwald E, Fauci AS, Hauser SL, Longo DL, Jameson JL, eds. Harrison's Principles of Internal Medicine. 16th edition. New York: McGraw-Hill, 2005.
4. d'Amore F, Brincker H, Christensen BE, et al. Non-Hodgkin's lymphoma in the elderly. A study of 602 patients aged 70 or older from a Danish population-based registry. The Danish LYEO-Study Group. Ann Oncol 1992; 3:379–386.
5. Effect of age on the characteristics and clinical behavior of non-Hodgkin's lymphoma patients. The Non-Hodgkin's Lymphoma Classification Project. Ann Oncol 1997; 8: 973–978.
6. A predictive model for aggressive non-Hodgkin's lymphoma. The International Non-Hodgkin's Lymphoma Prognostic Factors Project. N Engl J Med 1993; 329: 987–994.
7. Solal-Celigny P, Roy P, Colombat P, et al. Follicular lymphoma International Prognostic Index. Blood 2004; 104:1258–1265.
8. Tsang RW, Gospodarowicz MK. Management of localized (stage I and II) clinically aggressive lymphomas. Ann Hematol 2001; 80(suppl 3):B66–B72.
9. Miller TP, Dahlberg S, Cassady JR, et al. Chemotherapy alone compared with chemotherapy plus radiotherapy for localized intermediate- and high-grade non-Hodgkin's lymphoma. N Engl J Med 1998; 339:21–26.
10. Aviles A, Delgado S, Ruiz H, de la Torre A, Guzman R, Talavera A. Treatment of non-Hodgkin's lymphoma of Waldeyer's ring: radiotherapy versus chemotherapy versus combined therapy. Eur J Cancer B Oral Oncol 1996; 32B:19–23.
11. Wylie JP, Cowan RA, Deakin DP. The role of radiotherapy in the treatment of localised intermediate and high grade non-Hodgkin's lymphoma in elderly patients. Radiother Oncol 1998; 49:9–14.
12. Reyes F, Lepage E, Ganem G, et al. ACVBP versus CHOP plus radiotherapy for localized aggressive lymphoma. N Engl J Med 2005; 352:1197–1205.
13. Tilly H, Lepage E, Coiffier B, et al. Intensive conventional chemotherapy (ACVBP regimen) compared with standard CHOP for poor-prognosis aggressive non-Hodgkin lymphoma. Blood 2003; 102:4284–4289.
14. Dixon DO, Neilan B, Jones SE, et al. Effect of age on therapeutic outcome in advanced diffuse histiocytic lymphoma: the Southwest Oncology Group experience. J Clin Oncol 1986; 4:295–305.
15. Bordonaro R, Fratino L, Serraino D. Treatment of non-Hodgkin's lymphomas in elderly patients. Clin Lymphoma 2004; 5:37–44.
16. Vose JM, Armitage JO, Weisenburger DD, et al. The importance of age in survival of patients treated with chemotherapy for aggressive non-Hodgkin's lymphoma. J Clin Oncol 1988; 6:1838–1844.
17. Peters FP, Lalisang RI, Fickers MM, et al. Treatment of elderly patients with intermediate- and high-grade non-Hodgkin's lymphoma: a retrospective population-based study. Ann Hematol 2001; 80:155–159.
18. Fisher RI, Gaynor E, Dahlberg S, et al. Comparision of standard regimen (CHOP) with three intensive chemotherapy regimens for advanced non Hodgkin's lymphoma. N Engl J Med 1993; 328:1002–1006.
19. Osby E, Hagberg H, Kvaloy S, et al. CHOP is superior to CNOP in elderly patients with aggressive lymphoma while outcome is unaffected by filgrastim treatment: results of a Nordic Lymphoma Group randomized trial. Blood 2003; 101:3840–3848.

20. Sonneveld P, de Ridder M, van der Lelie H, et al. Comparison of doxorubicin and mitoxantrone in the treatment of elderly patients with advanced diffuse non-Hodgkin's lymphoma using CHOP versus CNOP chemotherapy. J Clin Oncol 1995; 13:2530–2539.
21. Pangalis GA, Vassilakopoulos TP, Michalis E, et al. A randomized trial comparing intensified CNOP vs. CHOP in patients with aggressive non-Hodgkin's lymphoma. Leuk Lymphoma 2003; 44:635–644.
22. Tirelli U, Errante D, Van Glabbeke M, et al. CHOP is the standard regimen in patients > or = 70 years of age with intermediate-grade and high-grade non-Hodgkin's lymphoma: results of a randomized study of the European Organization for Research and Treatment of Cancer Lymphoma Cooperative Study Group. J Clin Oncol 1998; 16: 27–34.
23. Pfreundschuh M, Trumper L, Kloess M, et al. Two-weekly or 3-weekly CHOP chemotherapy with or without etoposide for the treatment of elderly patients with aggressive lymphomas: results of the NHL-B2 trial of the DSHNHL. Blood 2004; 104:634–641.
24. Wunderlich A, Kloess M, Reiser M, et al. Practicability and acute haematological toxicity of 2- and 3-weekly CHOP and CHOEP chemotherapy for aggressive non-Hodgkin's lymphoma: results from the NHL-B trial of the German High-Grade Non-Hodgkin's Lymphoma Study Group (DSHNHL). Ann Oncol 2003; 14:881–893.
25. Doorduijn JK, van der Holt B, van Imhoff GW, et al. CHOP compared with CHOP plus granulocyte colony-stimulating factor in elderly patients with aggressive non-Hodgkin's lymphoma. J Clin Oncol 2003; 21:3041–3050.
26. Hackshaw A, Sweetenham J, Knight A. Are prophylactic hematopoietic growth factors of value in the management if patients with aggressive non-Hodgkin's lymphoma? Br J Cancer 2004; 90:1302–1305.
27. Coiffier B, Lepage EBJ, Herbrecht R, et al. CHOP chemotherapy plus rituximab compared with CHOP alone in elderly patients with diffuse large-B-cell lymphoma. N Engl J Med 2002; 346:235–242.
28. Coiffier B. Immunochemotherapy: the new standard in aggressive non-Hodgkin's lymphoma in the elderly. Semin Oncol 2003; 30:21–27.
29. Seymour JF, Pro B, Fuller LM, et al. Long-term follow-up of a prospective study of combined modality therapy for stage I-II indolent non-Hodgkin's lymphoma. J Clin Oncol 2003; 21:2115–2122.
30. Pendlebury S, el Awadi M, Ashley S, Brada M, Horwich A. Radiotherapy results in early stage low grade nodal non-Hodgkin's lymphoma. Radiother Oncol 1995; 36:167–171.
31. Wilder RB, Jones D, Tucker SL, et al. Long-term results with radiotherapy for stage I-II follicular lymphomas. Int J Radiat Oncol Biol Phys 2001; 51:1219–1227.
32. McLaughlin P, Fuller L, Redman J, et al. Stage I-II low-grade lymphomas: a prospective trial of combination chemotherapy and radiotherapy. Ann Oncol 1991; 2(suppl 2): 137–140.
33. A clinical evaluation of the International Lymphoma Study Group classification of non-Hodgkin's lymphoma. The Non-Hodgkin's Lymphoma Classification Project. Blood 1997; 89:3909–3918.
34. Ardeshna KM, Smith P, Norton A, et al. Long-term effect of a watch and wait policy versus immediate systemic treatment for asymptomatic advanced-stage non-Hodgkin lymphoma: a randomised controlled trial. Lancet 2003; 362:516–522.
35. Baldini L, Brugiatelli M, Luminari S, et al. Treatment of indolent B-cell nonfollicular lymphomas: final results of the LL01 randomized trial of the Gruppo Italiano per lo Studio dei Linfomi. J Clin Oncol 2003; 21:1459–1465.
36. Peterson BA, Petroni GR, Frizzera G, et al. Prolonged single-agent versus combination chemotherapy in indolent follicular lymphomas: a study of the Cancer and Leukemia Group B. J Clin Oncol 2003; 21:5–15.
37. Zinzani PL, Magagnoli M, Moretti L, et al. Randomized trial of fludarabine versus fludarabine and idarubicin as frontline treatment in patients with indolent or mantle-cell lymphoma. J Clin Oncol 2000; 18:773–779.

38. Zinzani PL, Magagnoli M, Bendandi M, et al. Efficacy of fludarabine and mitoxantrone (FN) combination regimen in untreated indolent non-Hodgkin's lymphomas. Ann Oncol 2000; 11:363–365.
39. Tsimberidou AM, McLaughlin P, Younes A, et al. Fludarabine, mitoxantrone, dexamethasone (FND) compared with an alternating triple therapy (ATT) regimen in patients with stage IV indolent lymphoma. Blood 2002; 100:4351–4357.
40. Cheson BD. The curious case of the baffling biological. J Clin Oncol 2000; 18:2007–2009.
41. Fisher RI, Dana BW, LeBlanc M, et al. Interferon alpha consolidation after intensive chemotherapy does not prolong the progression-free survival of patients with low-grade non-Hodgkin's lymphoma: results of the Southwest Oncology Group randomized phase III study 8809. J Clin Oncol 2000; 18:2010–2016.
42. Czuczman MS, Weaver R, Alkuzweny B, Berlfein J, Grillo-Lopez AJ. Prolonged clinical and molecular remission in patients with low-grade or follicular non-Hodgkin's lymphoma treated with rituximab plus CHOP chemotherapy: 9-year follow-up. J Clin Oncol 2004; 22:4711–4716.
43. Economopoulos T, Fountzilas G, Pavlidis N, et al. Rituximab in combination with CNOP chemotherapy in patients with previously untreated indolent non-Hodgkin's lymphoma. Hematol J 2003; 4:110–115.
44. Marcus R, Imrie K, Belch A, et al. An international multi-centre, randomized, open-lable, phase III trial comparing rituximab added to CVP chemotherapy to CVP chemotherapy alone in untreated stage III/IV follicular non-Hodgkin's lymphoma (Abstract). Blood 2003; 102:28a.
45. Forstpointner R, Hanel A, Repp R, et al. Increased response rate with rituximab in relapsed and refractory follicular and mantle cell lymphomas—results of a prospective randomized study of the German Low-Grade Lymphoma Study Group. Dtsch Med Wochenschr 2002; 127:2253–2258.
46. Forstpointner R, Dreyling M, Repp R, et al. The addition of rituximab to a combination of fludarabine, cyclophosphamide, mitoxantrone (FCM) significantly increases the response rate and prolongs survival as compared with FCM alone in patients with relapsed and refractory follicular and mantle cell lymphomas: results of a prospective randomized study of the German Low-Grade Lymphoma Study Group. Blood 2004; 104:3064–3071.
47. Hainsworth JD, Litchy S, Shaffer DW, Lackey VL, Grimaldi M, Greco FA. Maximizing therapeutic benefit of rituximab: maintenance therapy versus re-treatment at progression in patients with indolent non-Hodgkin's lymphoma—a randomized phase II trial of the Minnie Pearl Cancer Research Network. J Clin Oncol 2005; 23:1088–1095.
48. Witzig TE, Flinn IW, Gordon LI, et al. Treatment with ibritumomab tiuxetan radioimmunotherapy in patients with rituximab-refractory follicular non-Hodgkin's lymphoma. J Clin Oncol 2002; 20:3262–3269.
49. Kaminski MS, Zelenetz AD, Press OW, et al. Pivotal study of iodine I 131 tositumomab for chemotherapy-refractory low-grade or transformed low-grade B-cell non-Hodgkin's lymphomas. J Clin Oncol 2001; 19:3918–3928.
50. Kaminski MS, Tuck M, Estes J, et al. 131I-tositumomab therapy as initial treatment for follicular lymphoma. N Engl J Med 2005; 352:441–449.
51. Johnston LJ, Stockerl-Goldstein KE, Hu WW, et al. Toxicity of high-dose sequential chemotherapy and purged autologous hematopoietic cell transplantation precludes its use in refractory/recurrent non-Hodgkin's lymphoma. Biol Blood Marrow Transplant 2000; 6:555–562.
52. Freedman AS, Gribben JG, Neuberg D, et al. High-dose therapy and autologous bone marrow transplantation in patients with follicular lymphoma during first remission. Blood 1996; 88:2780–2786.

53. Eck M, Schmausser B, Haas R, Greiner A, Czub S, Muller-Hermelink HK. MALT-type lymphoma of the stomach is associated with *Helicobacter pylori* strains expressing the CagA protein. Gastroenterology 1997; 112:1482–1486.

54. Schechter NR, Portlock CS, Yahalom J. Treatment of mucosa-associated lymphoid tissue lymphoma of the stomach with radiation alone. J Clin Oncol 1998; 16:1916–1921.

55. Fisher RI, Dahlberg S, Nathwani BN, Banks PM, Miller TP, Grogan TM. A clinical analysis of two indolent lymphoma entities: mantle cell lymphoma and marginal zone lymphoma (including the mucosa-associated lymphoid tissue and monocytoid B-cell sub-categories): a Southwest Oncology Group study. Blood 1995; 85:1075–1082.

56. Jaffe ES. Common threads of mucosa-associated lymphoid tissue lymphoma pathogenesis: from infection to translocation. J Natl Cancer Inst 2004; 96:571–573.

57. Jaffe ES, Bookman MA, Longo DL. Lymphocytic lymphoma of intermediate differentiation—mantle zone lymphoma: a distinct subtype of B-cell lymphoma. Hum Pathol 1987; 18:877–880.

58. Bookman MA, Lardelli P, Jaffe ES, Duffey PL, Longo DL. Lymphocytic lymphoma of intermediate differentiation: morphologic, immunophenotypic, and prognostic factors. J Natl Cancer Inst 1990; 82:742–748.

59. O'Briain DS, Kennedy MJ, Daly PA, et al. Multiple lymphomatous polyposis of the gastrointestinal tract. A clinicopathologically distinctive form of non-Hodgkin's lymphoma of B-cell centrocytic type. Am J Surg Pathol 1989; 13:691–699.

60. Leonard JP, Schattner EJ, Coleman M. Biology and management of mantle cell lymphoma. Curr Opin Oncol 2001; 13:342–347.

61. Weisenburger DD, Vose JM, Greiner TC, et al. Mantle cell lymphoma. A clinicopathologic study of 68 cases from the Nebraska Lymphoma Study Group. Am J Hematol 2000; 64:190–196.

62. Meusers P, Engelhard M, Bartels H, et al. Multicentre randomized therapeutic trial for advanced centrocytic lymphoma: anthracycline does not improve the prognosis. Hematol Oncol 1989; 7:365–380.

63. Lenz G, Dreyling M, Hoster E, et al. Immunochemotherapy with rituximab and cyclophosphamide, doxorubicin, vincristine, and prednisone significantly improves response and time to treatment failure, but not long-term outcome in patients with previously untreated mantle cell lymphoma: results of a prospective randomized trial of the German Low Grade Lymphoma Study Group (GLSG). J Clin Oncol 2005; 23:1984–1992.

64. Kennedy BJ, Loeb V Jr, Peterson VM, Donegan WL, Natarajan N, Mettlin C. National survey of patterns of care for Hodgkin's disease. Cancer 1985; 56:2547–2556.

65. Stark GL, Wood KM, Jack F, Angus B, Proctor SJ, Taylor PR. Hodgkin's disease in the elderly: a population-based study. Br J Haematol 2002; 119:432–440.

66. Eghbali H, Hoerni-Simon G, de Mascarel I, Durand M, Chauvergne J, Hoerni B. Hodgkin's disease in the elderly. A series of 30 patients aged older than 70 years. Cancer 1984; 53:2191–2193.

67. Bosi A, Ponticelli P, Casini C, et al. Clinical data and therapeutic approach in elderly patients with Hodgkin's disease. Haematologica 1989; 74:463–473.

68. Westin EH, Longo DL. Lymphoma and myeloma in older patients. Semin Oncol 2004; 31:198–205.

69. Gandhi MK, Tellam JT, Khanna R. Epstein–Barr virus-associated Hodgkin's lymphoma. Br J Haematol 2004; 125:267–281.

70. van Spronsen DJ, Janssen-Heijnen ML, Breed WP, Coebergh JW. Prevalence of co-morbidity and its relationship to treatment among unselected patients with Hodgkin's disease and non-Hodgkin's lymphoma, 1993–1996. Ann Hematol 1999; 78:315–319.

71. Specht L, Nissen NI. Hodgkin's disease and age. Eur J Haematol 1989; 43:127–135.

72. Hasenclever D, Diehl V. A prognostic score for advanced Hodgkin's disease. International Prognostic Factors Project on Advanced Hodgkin's Disease. N Engl J Med 1998; 339:1506–1514.

73. Zijlstra JM, Dressel AJ, Mens JW, et al. Radiation therapy in early stage Hodgkin's disease: long-term results and adverse effects. Hematol J 2002; 3:179–184.

74. Rueda A, Alba E, Ribelles N, Sevilla I, Ruiz I, Miramon J. Six cycles of ABVD in the treatment of stage I and II Hodgkin's lymphoma: a pilot study. J Clin Oncol 1997; 15:1118–1122.

75. Fabian CJ, Mansfield CM, Dahlberg S, et al. Low-dose involved field radiation after chemotherapy in advanced Hodgkin disease. A Southwest Oncology Group randomized study. Ann Intern Med 1994; 120:903–912.

76. Diehl V, Thomas RK, Re D. Part II: Hodgkin's lymphoma—diagnosis and treatment. Lancet Oncol 2004; 5:19–26.

77. Balducci L, Extermann M. Cancer chemotherapy in the older patient: what the medical oncologist needs to know. Cancer 1997; 80:1317–1322.

78. Balducci L, Yates J. General guidelines for the management of older patients with cancer. Oncology (Huntingt) 2000; 14:221–227.

79. Repetto L, Carreca I, Maraninchi D, Aapro M, Calabresi P, Balducci L. Use of growth factors in the elderly patient with cancer: a report from the Second International Society for Geriatric Oncology (SIOG) 2001 Meeting. Crit Rev Oncol Hematol 2003; 45:123–128.

80. Littlewood TJ. The impact of hemoglobin levels on treatment outcomes in patients with cancer. Semin Oncol 2001; 28:49–53.

81. Littlewood TJ, Bajetta E, Nortier JW, Vercammen E, Rapoport B. Effects of epoetin alfa on hematologic parameters and quality of life in cancer patients receiving nonplatinum chemotherapy: results of a randomized, double-blind, placebo-controlled trial. J Clin Oncol 2001; 19:2865–2874.

82. Maartense E, Kluin-Nelemans HC, Noordijk EM. Non-Hodgkin's lymphoma in the elderly. A review with emphasis on elderly patients, geriatric assessment, and future perspectives. Ann Hematol 2003; 82:661–670.

83. Balducci L. The geriatric cancer patient: equal benefit from equal treatment. Cancer Control 2001; 8:1–25; quiz 27–28.

84. Zagonel V. Importance of a comprehensive geriatric assessment in older cancer patients. Eur J Cancer 2001; 37(suppl 7):S229–S233.

85. Balducci L. Geriatric oncology: challenges for the new century. Eur J Cancer 2000; 36:1741–1754.

86. Bernardi D, Milan I, Balzarotti M, Spina M, Santoro A, Tirelli U. Comprehensive geriatric evaluation in elderly patients with lymphoma: feasibility of a patient-tailored treatment plan. J Clin Oncol 2003; 21:754; author reply 755.

10

Breast Cancer

Pearl H. Seo
Duke University Medical Center and Veterans Affairs Medical Center, Durham, North Carolina, U.S.A.

Gretchen G. Kimmick
Duke University Medical Center, Durham, North Carolina, U.S.A.

INTRODUCTION

As the foremost cancer diagnosis and the second leading cause of cancer-related death in women in the United States, breast cancer is greatly feared. Incidence rates continue to increase, though at a slower rate than in previous years, possibly reflecting the increased use of hormone replacement therapy or increased prevalence of obesity, or both (1). In 2005, breast cancer is expected to account for 32% (211,240) of all new cancer cases among women (2). Fortunately, disease-related mortality decreased from 1990 to 2001, with an annual decrease of 2.3% ($P > 0.05$) (2).

Incidence of and mortality from breast cancer increase with increasing age (3–8). The probability of developing breast cancer is 1 in 207, from birth to the age of 39, 1 in 24 between the ages of 40 and 59, and one in seven between the ages of 60 and 79 (2). Over time, incidence rates continue to rise for women over the age of 50, a trend not seen in younger age groups (5). Unfortunately, 10-year survival in women with node-positive disease is worse for older women too: 49% for women aged 46 to 50 versus 35% for women older than 75 years; $P < 0.001$ (9). This difference was not, however, seen for women with node-negative disease. Historically, the higher mortality rate was explained by "less than standard" treatment.

The guiding principles of breast cancer management are early detection, aggressive local therapy to prevent recurrence of breast cancer at the primary site, and systemic therapy to prolong survival by preventing the development or slowing down the progression of metastatic disease. Less aggressive management of breast cancer in older women is widely reported. Older women were less likely to be screened (10,11), more frequently diagnosed at advanced stage (8,12,13), more likely to have nonstandard initial therapy, and less likely to participate in clinical trials (8,14–19). Current research is directed at increasing the number of older women who have screening mammography, increasing breast cancer awareness, specifically defining the utility of surgical, medical, and radiation approaches to breast cancer in older women, and exploring methods to increase participation of older women in clinical trials.

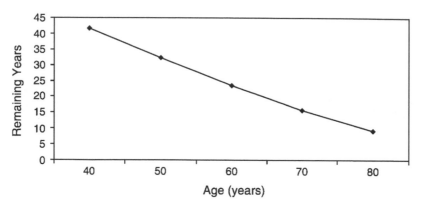

Figure 1 Remaining life years. *Source*: From Ref. 20.

The United States' geriatric population is also growing. More of the U.S. population is reaching older ages as a result of reduced death rates in all age groups (Fig. 1). The probability of surviving to an older age, and therefore, a longer life expectancy, is expected at all ages now, compared to in the past. Compared to 1980, when persons aged 65 and older represented 11.3% of the total population, it is projected that in 2030, one in five Americans, or 20%, will be over 65 years old (21). Almost half of all newly diagnosed breast cancers in the United States occur in women over the age of 65 (8). If incidence rates remain stable, by 2030, two-thirds of patients with breast cancer will be 65 years old or older (22), and by 2050, the total number of breast cancer cases will double (23).

Although not unique to older individuals, chronic disease is more common with advancing age. Almost 80% of people over the age of 65 have at least one chronic disease, and approximately one-third have three or more chronic diseases (24). This is important for two reasons: first, the choice of therapy is influenced by the presence of coexisting diseases that may increase complications; second, in clinical trials, the best measure of success of cancer treatment is overall survival, which may be limited by coexisting illness, making the benefit of therapy difficult to evaluate.

Because older women with breast cancer are likely to suffer from more than one illness, and the risk of death increases as the number of major comorbid conditions increases, it is important to identify the specific cause of death in assessing the impact of breast cancer treatment on survival. Attempts have been made to develop a "comorbidity index" to assess the risk of dying from specific concurrent conditions among women diagnosed with breast cancer (25–28). Interestingly, Satariano et al. found that even after adjusting for other confounding factors, women with two or more comorbidities are two times more likely than those without comorbid conditions to die from breast cancer (29). In a second study conducted by Satariano and Ragland, the effect of comorbidity and breast cancer stage on three-year survival in women with primary breast cancer was examined (24). This longitudinal observational study of 936 women aged 40 to 84 found that women with three or more comorbid conditions had a 20-fold higher rate of mortality from causes other than breast cancer. The effect of comorbidity was independent of age, disease stage, tumor size, histologic tumor type, type of treatment, race, and social and behavioral factors. Houterman et al. examined the effect of age and serious comorbid conditions on treatment decisions, the occurrence of serious complications within one year after diagnosis, and survival in 527 breast cancer patients, of which 373 patients were

40 to 69 years old and 154 patients were aged 70 and older (25). Neither treatment choice nor the number of complications was related to comorbidity. In multivariate analysis, the severity of concomitant illness was significantly associated with survival, such that on comparing women with low or moderate and high severity of concomitant disease to those with no comorbidity, the hazard ratios for death were 2.43 (95% CI 1.27–4.66) and 2.87 (95% CI 1.40–5.90), respectively, for those younger than 70 years and 1.63 (95% CI 0.58–4.59) and 2.97 (95% CI 1.12–7.86), respectively, for those aged 70 and older. In women with breast cancer, therefore, comorbidity level is positively associated with disease-specific and overall mortality.

The main goals of breast cancer therapy are to prolong survival and to improve the quality of remaining survival. The life expectancy of older women is frequently viewed as limited, but is actually substantial (Fig. 1). An otherwise healthy woman who lives to be 70 years old is expected to live another 15.7 years and an 80-year-old woman, 9.3 years.

STAGING AND PROGNOSTIC INDICATORS

Breast cancer stage is directly related to risk of recurrence and to survival (Fig. 2). Staging, as described by the American Joint Committee for Cancer (AJCC) guidelines (31), is useful in all patients for determination of prognosis and for making treatment-related decisions. The AJCC breast cancer staging criteria categorize the extent of malignancy according to the size of the primary tumor (T), the nodal involvement (N), and the occurrence of metastases (M) (Table 1).

Tumor size (the largest diameter of the invasive component) and the extent of nodal involvement (number of axillary nodes removed and number positive) are determined from the specimen pathology. For the extent of nodal involvement to reflect the prognosis accurately, sentinel lymph node mapping and sampling should be done or at least six nodes should be examined in a standard axillary dissection specimen. The pathology report should also include: histological type and tumor grade; assessment of tumor necrosis, vascular invasion, lymphatic invasion, and skin involvement; percentages of ductal carcinoma in situ (DCIS) and invasive carcinoma in the primary tumor; and immunohistochemical analyses of estrogen receptor (ER) and progesterone receptor (PR) and human epidermal growth factor receptor-2 (HER-2/*neu*, c-erbB2) in the primary tumor. Other markers, such as tumor DNA content and S-phase activity by flow cytometry, Mib-1 or Ki-67, oncogene expression, such

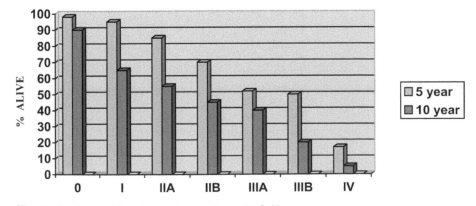

Figure 2 Survival by stage. *Source*: From Ref. 30.

Table 1 AJCC Staging Criteria for Breast Cancer

Symbol (TNM system)	Meaning
Primary tumor (T)	
TX	Primary tumor cannot be assessed
T0	No evidence of primary tumor
Tis	Carcinoma in situ; intraductal carcinoma, lobular carcinoma in situ, or Paget's disease of the nipple with no tumor
T1	Tumor ≤ 2 cm in greatest dimension
	T1a ≤ 0.5 cm in greatest dimension
	T1b >0.5 cm but not >1 cm in greatest dimension
	T1c >1 cm but not >2 cm in greatest dimension
T2	Tumor >2 cm but not >5 cm in greatest dimension
T3	Tumor >5 cm in greatest dimension
T4	Tumor of any size with direct extension to chest wall or skin (includes inflammatory carcinoma)
Regional lymph nodes (N)	
NX	Regional lymph nodes cannot be assessed (e.g., previously removed)
N0	No regional lymph-node metastases
N1	Metastasis to movable ipsilateral axillary nodes
N2	Metastases to ipsilateral axillary nodes fixed to one another or to other structures
	N2a: Metastasis in ipsilateral axillary lymph nodes fixed to one another (matted) or to other structures
	N2b: Metastasis only in clinically apparent ipsilateral internal mammary nodes and in the absence of clinically evident axillary lymph node metastasis
N3	Metastases to ipsilateral internal mammary lymph nodes
Distant metastasis (M)	
MX	Presence of distant metastasis cannot be assessed
M0	No evidence of distant metastasis
M1	Distant metastases (including metastases to ipsilateral supraclavicular lymph nodes)
Clinical stage	
0	Tis, N0, M0
1	T1, N0, M0
IIA	T0, N1, M0
	T1, N1, M0
	T2, N0, M0
IIB	T2, N1, M0
	T3, N0, M0
IIIA	T0 or T1, N2, M0
	T2, N2, M0
	T3, N1 or N2, M0
IIIB	T4, any N, M0
	Any T, N3, M0
IV	Any T, any N, MI

Abbreviations: AJCC, American Joint Committee for Cancer; TNM, primary tumor nodal involvement metastasis.
Source: From Ref. 31.

as other epidermal growth factor receptors, and protease activity, such as cathepsin-D, can also be determined from paraffin sections and may be useful prognostically.

Preoperative evaluation includes complete history and physical examination, mammography, chest radiograph, complete blood count, and serum chemistries (with liver function tests and calcium). These studies are helpful in determining the presence of comorbid illness in addition to finding metastases. Bilateral mammography should be performed on all patients to evaluate both the ipsilateral and contralateral breast for other nonpalpable lesions. Asymptomatic patients with an unremarkable preliminary evaluation require no further staging procedures. Skeletal surveys, radionuclide bone scanning, and computerized tomographic scanning of the brain, chest, abdomen, and pelvis are unnecessary in asymptomatic patients with normal physical findings and initial blood work. The use of tumor markers, such as the carcinoembryonic antigen and mucin antigens (CA15–3 and CA27.29), in patient management is controversial and not recommended on a routine basis.

Infiltrating ductal carcinoma (IDC) is the most common histological breast tumor type in older women, and it accounts for 75% to 80% of cases (8). Risk of invasive lobular cancer (ILC) appears to be higher among users of hormone replacement therapy (32), and a retrospective cohort study found that survival rates are better and appear to be improving over time for ILC patients, compared to IDC patients (33). Aggressive tumor types, medullary carcinoma and inflammatory cancer, may be less frequent, and indolent histologies, colloid and papillary carcinoma, may be more common in older women than in younger women (34,35). These are uncommon histologies, however, representing less than 10% of mammary carcinomas.

The pattern of prognostic markers seen in breast cancers in older women indicate that breast tumors in this population may be slower growing, more differentiated, and more hormone-responsive. Tumors in older patients more frequently have markers indicating slower cell proliferation: lower thymidine-^{3}H labeling indices; higher frequency of diploid tumors; and lower histologic grade (36–41). They are more frequently, moderately to well differentiated (34,42). Genetic alterations in tumor cells generally reflect less aggressive histology, including normal p53 expression and absence of expression of epidermal growth factor receptor one and c-erbB2 (HER-2/*neu*) (36,37). Breast cancers in postmenopausal women are more likely to express hormone receptors (39,43–45).

Despite this, survival is similar in older and younger women with localized and regional stages of breast cancer, and, paradoxically, older women fare worse with metastatic disease (3,8,46). This may be explained by the pattern of hormone receptor expression. Tumors in older women are more often ER positive/PR negative and, therefore, carry a worse prognosis than ER-positive/PR-positive tumors (47). Honma et al. reported that breast cancers in women older than age 85 are less frequently PR positive and more frequently androgen-receptor positive (48). They noted that the ER-alpha/PR status of tumors in older women was distinctly different than that of premenopausal women. These authors postulated that this pattern of hormone receptor expression was related to the extremely low endogenous ER levels in very old women, and that androgen and androgen receptor may play significant roles in the pathogenesis of breast carcinomas in this age group. Quong et al. explored the relationship of ER expression and the expression of ER-inducible genes, such as the PR receptor, and age-dependent markers of oxidative stress (49). Their findings support the hypotheses that dysregulated ER expression underlies the age-specific increase in breast cancer incidence after age 50 and that oxidative stress and loss of ER-inducible PR expression in ER-positive tumors leads to higher-risk ER-positive/PR-negative breast cancers with aging.

Summary of staging and prognostic indicators: Adequate staging predicts recurrence and should include preoperative complete history and physical examination, bilateral mammography, chest radiograph, complete blood count, and serum chemistries, including liver function tests and calcium; followed by removal of the primary tumor and clinical assessment of or sampling of the axillary nodes. Further work-up is based on results of these tests. The tumor pathology report should include notation regarding invasive tumor size, presence and number of involved lymph nodes and the number of lymph nodes examined, tumor type, tumor grade, presence or absence of lymphovascular invasion, ER and PR assays, and c-erbB2 (HER-2/*neu*) analysis.

PREVENTION AND DIAGNOSIS

Prevention

Risk factors for breast cancer include older age, white race, family history of breast cancer, history of benign breast hyperplasia, radiation exposure, early menarche, late age at birth of first child, late menopause, obesity, taller stature, oral contraceptive use, postmenopausal estrogen replacement therapy, and alcohol use (50,51). Primary prevention of breast cancer would require modification of known predisposing factors. Types of diet, lifestyle, and nutritional supplements are being investigated to determine their influence in controlling risk (e.g., obesity) or conferring protection against uncontrollable factors (e.g., aging and race).

Diet is a potentially modifiable risk factor. The prospective Malmo Cancer and Diet Cohort (Malmo, Sweden) analysis of postmenopausal women revealed that a high-fiber diet was associated with a 42% lower risk of breast cancer, with a high-fiber, low-fat diet convening the lowest risk (52). There was no association with any specific plant or grain food group. When specifically focusing on fruits and vegetables, results from the Pooling Project of Prospective Studies of Diet and Cancer and the five-year follow-up of the European Prospective Investigation into Cancer and Nutrition trials showed no relationship between the amount of fruit and vegetable consumption and breast cancer incidence (53,54). Both of these large studies included pre- and postmenopausal women. Polyphenol compounds found in phytoestrogens such as soy and in green tea have been examined to explain the decreased incidence of breast cancer in Asian women. In the Los Angeles Asian Breast Cancer Study, there was an inverse relationship between soy intake and green tea intake and breast cancer (55,56). However, questions remain on the timing of such dietary habits (i.e., prepubertal soy intake), amount, and whether genetic factors, such as tea–polyphenol metabolism, come into play (57,58).

Many people also hope that vitamin supplements, because of their availability, will decrease breast cancer risk. Antioxidants such as vitamins A, C, and E have been taken for presumed protective effects with rather limited evidence (59,60). In a large international, randomized, double blind, placebo control trial of vitamin E 400 IU to placebo, Heart Outcomes Prevention Evaluation showed that vitamin E supplementation, after a median seven years, did not influence cancer incidence or cardiovascular events. Perhaps more reflective of the elderly population, this trial required subjects to have cardiovascular disease or diabetes as comorbid illness, but only 25% of subjects were women, which could have affected the breast cancer outcome (61). High level of folate ingestion has not clearly shown to be beneficial except when alcohol is also consumed. In the Nurses Health Study, high plasma folate did not show a statistical benefit in breast cancer incidence, except in women drinking at least one drink per day [relative risk (RR) 0.11], compared to nondrinkers (RR 0.72) (62). A similar interaction with alcohol was found in the Iowa Women's Health Study. Postmenopausal women with low folate ingestion and any alcohol use were at a 40% increased risk for breast cancer. In postmenopausal women with a family history of breast cancer, lower folate levels and alcohol use were independent risk factors. Only with high folate ingestion and alcohol abstinence was there no elevated risk (63).

Risk of and mortality from breast cancer is also related to increased weight, particularly being overweight. In the Nurses' Health Study, increased waist circumference was significantly associated with postmenopausal breast cancer after adjustment for other breast cancer–risk factors (RR 1.34), which was highest in women who never used hormone replacement therapy (RR 1.83) (64). Controlling for age and other risk factor–related death, the Cancer Prevention Study II of the American Cancer Society evaluating 495,477 women for 16 years showed 34% increased mortality from breast cancer with body mass index (BMI) 25 to 30, which doubled at BMI >40 (65).

Exercise has been shown to decrease this risk, both by decreasing body mass and through possible alterations in estrone metabolism (66,67). In a study conducted with 74,171 postmenopausal women aged 50 to 79, McTiernan et al. revealed that regular strenuous physical activity at age 35 conveyed 14% decreased risk of breast cancer at five years of follow-up. Further analysis showed that moderate exercise (1.25–2.5 hours of brisk walking weekly) had the greatest impact, but, interestingly, in the thinner women. Whether the strenuousness of the exercise and the current or lifetime physical activity influence risk remains under study.

Overall, diet and lifestyle modification in elderly women may attenuate breast cancer risk. More importantly, these generally "healthy" habits are also beneficial to known, common, competing mortality risks of cardiovascular disease, diabetes, and cerebrovascular disease. Use of selective estrogen receptor modulators (SERMs), which are known to be effective in the treatment of breast cancer, have proven efficacy in decreasing incidence of breast cancer.

There have been four breast cancer prevention trials comparing tamoxifen and placebo (68–71). The largest of these trials, the National Surgical Adjuvant Breast and Bowel Project Prevention trial (NSABP P1), showed a dramatic 50% reduction in the incidence of invasive and noninvasive breast cancer in women taking tamoxifen (68). All women aged 60 and older were eligible to participate, regardless of other risk factors. Yet, only 30% of trial participants were older than 60 years, and 6% were older than 70 years. These impressive results must be tempered with caution, because tamoxifen use was not associated with decreased mortality, and was associated with a statistically significant increase in risk of endometrial cancer and thromboembolic events in postmenopausal women. Based on the strength of these results, five years of tamoxifen is approved in the United States for prevention of breast cancer in high-risk postmenopausal women. Similarly, at 50 months' median follow-up, the International Breast Cancer Intervention Study-I (IBIS) showed a 32% reduction in incident breast cancers for women taking tamoxifen, but noted a significant increase in thromboembolic events and in deaths from all causes in the tamoxifen group (71). Increases in mortality were seen from cancers other than breast cancer, pulmonary emboli, other vascular causes, and cardiac deaths. The Royal Marsden and Italian Trials did not show the same degree of benefit from tamoxifen, but participants were at overall lower risk for breast cancer and dropout rates were high.

A meta-analysis of the four breast cancer prevention trials, with NSABP P1 and updated data from the three European trials, showed an overall reduction in breast cancer incidence of 38% (72). Of note, the reduction was in only ER-positive breast cancers, with no effect on ER-negative breast cancers. In addition, rates of endometrial cancer and venous thromboembolic events increased in all the tamoxifen prevention trials. No effect on breast cancer mortality has yet been proven.

Overall, in the prevention trials, the absolute breast cancer risk reduction was less than 2 per 100 patients (73). The decision to use tamoxifen in the preventive setting requires that one carefully weighs the risks and benefits. Gail et al. created a model of breast cancer risk assessment using the Breast Cancer Detection Demonstration Project information (74). This analysis incorporates age, age at menarche, age at first live birth, previous biopsies, and first-degree relatives with breast cancer; it is available on the National Cancer Institute's website. Simple and easy to use, the model calculates a woman's risk of breast cancer in five years and up to the age of 90. The risks of same-aged women without breast cancer–risk factors are also presented, enabling comparison. Table 2 shows the minimal five-year risk of invasive breast cancer for the benefit of preventive tamoxifen to exceed the risks in the general population, using data on toxicity from the NSABP P1 trial (75). For example, the Gail model five-year risk of invasive breast cancer for a 72-year-old woman with an intact uterus must be 7% or more in order for the benefits of tamoxifen to outweigh its risks. Of course, the Gail model is just a starting point, because it does not incorporate other known breast cancer–risk factors, pathology of previous biopsies, and genetic mutations, and is more reliable for Caucasian women than other ethnic groups.

Hoping to improve the therapeutic index of treatment, another SERM, raloxifene (raloxifene hydrochloride), has been studied. Used for the prevention and treatment of osteoporosis, raloxifene has estrogen antagonistic effects on breast tissue, while lacking estrogen agonist effects on the uterus (76). The multiple outcomes of raloxifene evaluation (MORE) trial was a multicenter, randomized, double-blind placebo controlled trial of postmenopausal women with osteoporosis and showed that with four years of raloxifene, there was a 72% risk reduction of invasive ER-positive breast cancer (76,77). There was an increased risk of thromboembolic events that persisted in the raloxifene extension trial, Continuing Outcomes Relevant to Evista (CORE), which continued the randomization of raloxifene or placebo for another four years. Invasive breast cancers were decreased by 59%. Although not statistically significant, thromboembolic events remained elevated, which confers some worry because subjects with limited clotting risk were selected. A head-to-head prevention trial comparing tamoxifen and raloxifene [NSABP P2, the Study of Tamoxifen and Raloxifene (STAR)] in women at high risk for breast cancer has finished accrual in November 2004 (78).

Table 2 Minimal Five-Year Risk of Invasive Breast Cancer (from Gail Model of Risk Assessment) for Tamoxifen's Benefit to Exceed Risk in the General Population, by Age

	Age (years)				
	35–39	40–49	50–59	60–69	70–79
Uterus intact	1.5	1.5	4.0	>7.0	>7.0
No uterus	1.5	1.5	1.5	3.5	6.0

Source: From Ref. 75.

Nonsteroidal anti-inflammatory drugs (NSAIDs), such as aspirin and ibuprofen, may decrease the risk of breast cancer. Population-based case–control studies (Long Island Breast Cancer Study Project, North Carolina Breast Cancer and Carcinoma In-situ Study, and the prospective Women's Health Initiative Observational Study) showed risk reduction ranging from 20% to 60% of mostly ER-positive tumors (79–81). More investigation is necessary to determine the dose, frequency, duration, and safety of NSAID use for chemoprevention.

A family history of breast cancer, implying a genetic defect, may be important in 6% to 19% of all cases of breast cancer (82,83). Genetic predisposition is particularly important in early-onset breast cancer, diagnosed before the age of 50, but is probably not a major factor in the geriatric population. BRCA1, the first gene found to be related to breast cancer, is located on chromosome 17q, and accounts for approximately 2% to 3% of breast cancers and 16% to 45% of familial breast cancers; it portends an increased risk for both breast cancer and ovarian cancers (84–86). Women who are carriers for BRCA1 and have a strong family history of breast cancer are estimated to have an 85% lifetime risk for developing breast cancer; 51% will develop breast cancer by the time they are 50 years old, and 87% by the age of 70 (87,88). Women with BRCA1 who live to the age of 70 have a cumulative risk of 65% for bilateral breast cancers.

Another gene, BRCA2, is located on chromosome 13q (89). Linkage studies suggest that 35% of high-risk families may have BRCA2 gene mutations (88). BRCA2 may be more important in postmenopausal cases of breast cancer. The lifetime breast cancer risk for BRCA2 mutation carriers in families where breast cancer is common is estimated to be 85%. In women who have BRCA1 or BRCA2 mutations, but not necessarily a strong family history of breast cancer, the estimated risk of breast cancer is lower—only 56% by the age of 70 (86). There are probably many modifying factors, including genetic, hormonal, and environmental, that determine whether a genetic mutation will lead to cancer.

Summary of breast cancer prevention: Give consideration to the use of preventive tamoxifen in women whose risk of breast cancer outweighs the risk of complications, based on the Gail Model tool. General good health recommendations include a well-balanced diet, i.e., a high-fiber, low-fat diet, weight control to maintain ideal BMI ($22–24\,\mathrm{kg/m^2}$), and exercise.

Screening

Secondary prevention of breast cancer involves screening mammography and breast physical examination. Promotion of these two measures of early detection has reduced breast cancer–related mortality. Maximal benefit occurs in younger women aged 50 to 59, where the use of mammography and breast physical examination biennially reduced mortality by 60% over three to seven years, and the use of mammography alone reduced mortality by 40% (90).

Direct evidence of effectiveness among older women is limited to two Swedish randomized trials that included women up to age 70 and 74 (91,92). Both of these trials reported RR reductions of 28% to 32% in mortality among women who were 65 to 74 years old (93,94). However, when subgrouped, most of the benefit was in the younger age group, 65 to 69 years old, with nonsignificant benefit in women who were 70 to 74 years old (94).

With age, the breast changes from a dense glandular organ to a less dense, smaller organ containing more fat. This change in architecture increases the contrast between normal and abnormal breast tissue, making it easier to find malignancies by mammography in older women. In a large prospective study of 329,495 women in the National Cancer Institute's Breast Cancer Surveillance Consortium, the sensitivity of mammography in detecting breast cancer improved with age. In women aged 60 to 69, 70 to 79, and 80 to 89, mammographic sensitivity was 73.3%, 81.4%, and 86.1%, respectively. Specificity remained high in all three age groups, at 93% to 94% (95).

Faulk et al. compared age-specific screening results in 10,915 women older than 65 years (old) and 21,226 women aged 50 to 64 (young), who were referred by a physician for mammography (96). The overall rate of abnormal interpretations was 5% in both young and old age groups. Older women were twice as likely to have abnormal screening findings judged to be suspicious for malignancy (10% vs. 5%, $P =$ NS), and were also more likely to have abnormalities judged to be characteristic of malignancy (4% vs. 1%, $P =$ NS). The number of breast cancer cases among abnormal screening interpretations [positive predictive value (PPV)], the number of malignancies among biopsies prompted by screening (biopsy yield), and the number of women with cancer per 1000 examinations (cancer detection rate), were all higher in the older subgroup (Table 3). Showing similar results, a 2002 study of 167,211 screening mammograms in British Columbia revealed equivalent rates of abnormalities on mammograms in women aged 70 and older compared to women who were 40 to 69 years old, with the former having increased cancer diagnoses (97).

Breast cancers diagnosed by mammogram are of a smaller size and in an earlier stage than those found by other means. Randolph and colleagues evaluated 12,038 Medicare beneficiaries aged 69 and older who were diagnosed with breast cancer in 1995–1996. Older women ($\geq$75 years) who did not undergo mammography screening had larger tumors when compared to younger women (69–74 years) (27.9 mm vs. 23.8 mm, $P < 0.001$). When women participated in annual screening in the two years prior to diagnosis, tumor size decreased in both age groups, and the size difference noted with advanced age was eliminated (15.1 mm vs. 15.0 mm, $P > 0.2$) (98). This was true for disease stage as well. In women who did not participate in screening, 56% of the older group and 47% of the younger presented with greater than stage IIA disease ($P < 0.001$). This difference declined with screening to 26% of the older and 28% of the younger group having higher stage with screening ($P > 0.2$).

Nearly all North American organizations (i.e., U.S. Preventive Services Task Force, The Canadian Task Force on Preventive Health, and American Cancer Society) support annual mammography screening, starting at variable ages (40 or 50) without a delineated stopping age. The decision to screen older women is complicated by considerations of increased comorbidity and reduced life expectancy. To evaluate the cost–benefit ratio of breast cancer screening (clinical examinations

Table 3 PPV, Biopsy Yield, and Cancer Detection Rate Among Younger and Older Women

Age (years)	PPV (%)	Biopsy yield (%)	Cancer detection rate[a]
50–64	12	40	5.7
65+	20	56	9.2

[a]Number of women with cancer per 1000 examinations.
Abbreviation: PPV, positive predictive value.
Source: From Ref. 96.

and mammography) in women older than 65 years, with and without comorbid conditions, Mandelblatt et al. used a decision analysis model (99). In this report, early detection of breast cancer by screening yielded increases in life expectancy for all older women despite age and coexisting medical conditions, although the magnitude of benefit decreased with increasing age.

McPherson et al. evaluated 5186 women aged 65 to 101 who were diagnosed with breast cancer by mammography, and found that mammographic diagnosis extended a survival benefit in breast cancer mortality except in those women with severe comorbidities (100). Mandelblatt et al. performed a cost effectiveness–analysis of screening and found that, on average, extending biennial screening to age 75 or 80 would cost $34,000 to $88,000 (2002 U.S. Dollars) per life year gained, when compared to stopping screening at age 65 (101). In general, it is recommended that screening in older women be individualized, with discontinuation of screening mammography when life expectancy is less than five years (which includes any woman older than the age of 85), or when severe comorbidities or functional limitations are present (102,103).

Biennial screening mammography became a Medicare covered benefit in 1991, changing to an annual benefit in 1999. Mammography rates were initially low but have improved. In a study of 10,000 female Medicare beneficiaries in Michigan aged 65 or older in 1993, 43% did not have a mammogram in the five-year study period, but those who did averaged 2.8 mammograms (104). In a 1996–2000 study reporting mammography use by women aged 50 to 90 participating in the Health and Retirement Study and Asset and Health Dynamics among the Oldest Old studies, 80% of 64-year-olds had mammograms, with this rate declining to 40% by the age of 85 to 90 (105). This finding is corroborated in a study of 882 women aged 80 and older responding to the 2000 National Health Interview Survey, where approximately 51% had a screening mammogram in the previous two years (106). Factors influencing receipt of mammogram included higher education, being married, higher income, healthy habits (nonsmokers, regular vigorous exercise), having more physicians involved in care (especially obstetricians and gynecologists), fewer inpatient admissions, and younger age (104,105,107).

Summary of screening recommendations: We recommend annual screening mammography and physician breast exam in all women aged 85 and younger, who are functioning well and are in good health.

Diagnosis

Any palpable breast mass in a postmenopausal woman requires biopsy. Mammography may be helpful in characterizing the mass and/or finding other suspicious areas; however, mammography may not image palpable lesions in as many as 20% of patients (108). The majority of palpable masses in older women are malignant. Fine-needle aspiration (FNA) biopsy is a highly reliable method of tissue diagnosis. If the FNA is negative or inconclusive, unless the mass proves to be a cyst and resolves after aspiration, further biopsy through repeat FNA or excision is necessary. For patients who have a mass that is characteristic of malignancy, detected on either physical examination or mammography, initial surgical removal of the lesion through lumpectomy or mastectomy with axillary evaluation may be preferable to a two-stage procedure involving an FNA or excisional biopsy followed by definitive surgery.

Mammographically detected breast lesions also require biopsy. If these are nonpalpable, either stereotactic or needle-localized biopsy is necessary. Stereotactic large-core needle biopsy is now widely accepted as a reliable method of providing a histological diagnosis for mammographically detected suspicious and indeterminate breast lesions (109–111). This technique is relatively noninvasive and allows pathological evaluation of a mammographic abnormality. Needle-localization biopsy allows for removal of the abnormal lesion for tissue diagnosis. For some patients, after careful discussion, follow-up physical examination and repeat mammography of the lesion in several months is appropriate. For most patients, however, the fear of breast cancer and the possibility that even a low-risk lesion may prove to be malignant is a compelling motive for lesion biopsy or excision.

Summary of diagnostic recommendations: A diagrammatic approach to a breast abnormality in an older woman is provided in Figure 3.

BREAST CARCINOMA IN SITU

The common morphologies of breast carcinoma in situ are ductal and lobular. Surveillance, Epidemiology, and End Results (SEER) cancer registries data from 1980 to 2001 show a 7.2-fold increase in incidence (35 in 100,000 to 59 in 100,000) of DCIS among women aged 30 and older, with the greatest increase in women aged 50 to 69, an increase attributed to increased widespread mammographic screening (112). In the time period corresponding to when Medicare insured mammograms, 1992 to 2001, DCIS incidence rates approximately doubled in women aged 60 to 69, 70 to 79, and 80 or older.

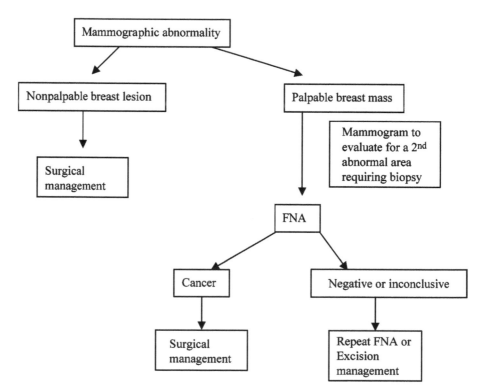

Figure 3 Approach to a suspicious breast lesion in an older woman. *Abbreviation*: FNA, fine needle aspirate.

The vast majority of DCIS is diagnosed after finding mammographic abnormalities of microcalcifications and/or soft-tissue densities, largely without clinical findings (113). DCIS is considered a precursor lesion and part of a spectrum of changes starting from atypical hyperplasia and leading to invasive disease (114,115). The natural history of DCIS is extrapolated from earlier case series studies of women whose biopsies were initially misdiagnosed as benign breast disease and were later reclassified as DCIS. The larger of these studies reported that 14% to 32% of women develop invasive cancer in 15 to 30 years (116,117).

The goal of treating DCIS is to prevent the recurrence of both in situ and invasive disease. Historically, DCIS was treated with mastectomy, which cured almost all patients. There are no randomized trials comparing mastectomy to breast-conserving surgery or lumpectomy. In a meta-analysis, recurrence rates after mastectomy and lumpectomy were 1.4% and 8.9%, respectively (118). However, there is no difference in survival, with 1% to 2% rates of 10-year breast cancer–mortality in DCIS patients, regardless of treatment (119).

After breast-conserving surgery, recurrence is nearly all ipsilateral, with half in situ and half invasive disease. Findings from three randomized control trials of lumpectomy versus lumpectomy plus radiation [NSABP B17, European Organization for Research and Treatment of Cancer (EORTC) 10853, and UK DCIS Trial] show recurrence rates of 14% to 32% (120–122). Recurrence risk is reduced by half when radiation therapy (RT) is given after lumpectomy. Of note, the majority of the subjects in these studies were 50 to 65 years old. Thus, the treatment recommendation for DCIS is breast-conserving surgery with radiotherapy unless contraindicated. Axillary dissection finds metastases in less than 1.5% of patients and is generally not recommended (123).

It has been suggested that lumpectomy alone, without local RT, may be appropriate for patients with low grade lesions less than 2.0 to 2.5 cm in diameter, with generous (>1 cm) margins of normal tissue surrounding the in-situ component (124). The recently closed European Cooperative Oncology Group (ECOG E-5194) randomized trial of lumpectomy alone should offer more conclusive results.

The addition of tamoxifen to lumpectomy and RT was studied in two trials: NSABP B24 and UK DCIS Trial (121,125). The addition of tamoxifen reduced the recurrence rate in the NSABP B24 study only, specifically in ER-positive DCIS. There was no survival benefit in either study. Side effects, such as endometrial cancer and stroke, were seen with tamoxifen.

The incidence of lobular carcinoma in situ (LCIS) is far less than DCIS, although the true incidence is hard to determine because of its lack of clinical and mammographic signs. It is usually an incidental finding after breast biopsy performed for another reason. There has been a steady increase in incidence in postmenopausal women, largely due to increased mammographic screening. During 1992–2001, the incidence of LCIS in the SEER registries increased for every age group. There was a 1.6-fold increase in 60- to 69-year-old women, a 1.4-fold in 70- to 79-year-old women, and a 3.0-fold increase in women aged 80 or older, corresponding to an absolute increase of 5 in 100,000 to 8 in 100,000 women aged 50 and older (126).

LCIS occurs bilaterally in 25% to 35% of patients and is considered to generally increase the risk of invasive disease, including contralateral breast cancers. In a study of the Connecticut Tumor Registry, women diagnosed with LCIS were 2.6 times more likely to have a contralateral breast cancer diagnosed within the following six months than women diagnosed with DCIS (127). The diagnosis of LCIS, therefore, serves as marker of subsequent risk of breast cancer. Treatment options range from observation to bilateral mastectomy (128). However, the current recommendation is close follow-up of these patients without aggressive surgery.

Summary of breast carcinoma in situ: For DCIS that is less than 2.5 cm in diameter, either mastectomy or lumpectomy followed by radiation are acceptable options. For larger size lesions, mastectomy is preferred. Axillary assessment is not necessary. Tamoxifen may be considered to decrease the risk of ipsilateral tumor recurrence in women treated with lumpectomy and RT, who have hormone receptor–positive lesions. LCIS is an indicator of increased risk; complete excision is not necessary. Tamoxifen may be considered to decrease risk of future breast cancer.

MANAGEMENT OF NONMETASTATIC BREAST CANCER

Local Therapy of Breast Cancer: Surgery and RT

Breast Surgery

Modified radical mastectomy (MRM) with axillary dissection and lumpectomy with axillary dissection followed by local radiation are the accepted local treatments for early breast cancer. Long-term follow-up and an overview of randomized trials show equivalent survival for the two modalities with local recurrence rates generally less than 8% (129,130). The choice of surgical treatment is made after consultation between the patient, surgeon, and radiation oncologist. Indications for mastectomy include tumor size too large to allow acceptable cosmetic result after lumpectomy, tumor involvement of muscle or skin, and contraindications to radiation.

Breast surgery is a low-risk operative procedure. Healthy older people tolerate surgery well with perioperative risk determined by the presence and severity of comorbid illnesses (131). Operative mortality is generally in the range of 1% to 2% (132,133).

Historically, however, older women are less likely than younger women to have breast-conserving surgery. In 1991, Lazovich et al. reported that the likelihood of breast-conserving surgery decreases with increasing age (134). Unfortunately, age continues to bias surgical treatment. In a study examining the adherence to practice guidelines at M.D. Anderson Cancer Center from 1997 to 2002, older age was associated with the lack of definitive surgery, either mastectomy or lumpectomy (135).

Wide excision of the primary tumor alone in older women has resulted in local control rates ranging from 71% to 97% (136–138). In general, these results are inferior to other treatments such as lumpectomy and breast radiation, especially in younger women.

Studies have shown that body image is important to women of any age, and body image is linked to improved quality of life, adjustment to breast cancer diagnosis, and mental health (139–141). However, in older women, other factors such as the need to curtail the number of trips to the hospital due to limited mobility or access to transportation may steer the treatment recommendation and preference toward mastectomy. Overall, including the older women in the treatment decision and adhering to their preferences is a key component to improved treatment acceptance and quality of life.

Axillary Assessment

The role of axillary dissection in older women with small breast tumors is under scrutiny. Axillary dissection is regarded primarily as a staging procedure and secondarily as a form of locoregional control. Traditionally, this was performed with removal of level I and II axillary lymph nodes. Lymphatic mapping with sentinel node biopsy has become an acceptable, widely used procedure with less morbidity; however, its success depends on technical issues (the surgeon's experience, tracer used, etc.), and long-term outcome results compared with axillary dissection are not yet available (142,143).

Major complications of the axillary dissection procedure are infrequent, and include injury or thrombosis of the axillary vein and injury to the motor nerves of the axilla. However, there is significant morbidity both in the short and long term. In women undergoing breast-conserving surgery, axillary dissection makes both general anesthesia and hospitalization necessary, whereas lumpectomy alone is an outpatient procedure that can be done using local anesthetics. Other potential problems associated with axillary dissection include seroma formation, shoulder dysfunction, anesthesia in intercostobrachial nerve distribution, lymphedema of the arm, increased breast edema, and arm or shoulder pain (144–146).

Lymphedema is particularly troubling. Its incidence is reported to range from 1.5% to 62.5% (132). This wide range is probably a reflection of the fact that lymphedema is not life threatening, is usually mild, rarely limits functions, and is not uniformly reported. In older women in whom mobility and use of the upper extremities may already be a concern due to arthritis or other comorbid illness, lymphedema and the pain associated with axillary dissection may severely restrict motion and functional capacity.

Axillary evaluation through lymphatic mapping with sentinel node biopsy is a significantly less morbid procedure (143–145). Sentinel node biopsy is a standard alternative for women with early-stage, clinically node-negative breast cancer. The sentinel node identification rates are best when both blue dye and radioactive colloid or albumin is used (147). When the dye is used, there is risk of allergic reaction to it. Axillary dissection is necessary in the presence of clinically palpable lymph nodes and in cases where there is a positive sentinel node.

It has been suggested that axillary dissection be foregone in certain subgroups of women with small primary breast cancers. Physical examination may assist in predicting nodal involvement, but false-negative (27–32%) and false-positive rates (25–31%) are high (148). In women with very small tumors (<1 cm), axillary node involvement has been found in 12% to 37%. Factors influencing axillary nodal involvement are the presence of lymphovascular invasion, tumor palpability, higher nuclear grade, and tumor size (149,150).

Some investigators suggest that older women do not require axillary lymph node dissection because the knowledge gained does not influence systemic adjuvant treatment choice (151–154). Martelli et al. evaluated 671 women aged 70 and older who underwent breast surgery with or without axillary dissection. All women received tamoxifen after their surgery. Axillary evaluation did not improve distant metastases or survival, and axillary recurrence occurred at a low rate of 6% in 10 years of follow-up (155).

Adjuvant RT

RT decreases ipsilateral breast recurrence after lumpectomy, and it is the standard of care. In a randomized study with 12 years of follow-up, Fisher et al. demonstrated that the rate of local failure after lumpectomy with negative margins decreased from 35% to 10% by the addition of postoperative irradiation, with the majority of local recurrences observed in the first five years (156).

Breast radiation is well tolerated in older women. Wyckoff et al. found a comparable number of treatment interruptions, overall duration of treatment and frequency of cutaneous and hematological toxicity in women aged 65 and older who underwent conservative surgery and radiation compared to the younger patients (157). Kantorowitz et al. reviewed the outcome in patients treated with segmental mastectomy, with or without radiation, and confirmed the benefit and tolerability of radiation. Toxicities such as breast and arm edema, pneumonitis, pulmonary fibrosis, and myositis were modest. Cosmesis was acceptable (136). A more recent study of 196 women aged 70 or older showed only five of them as having problems of arm mobility and lymphedema after radiation treatment (158).

However, the schedule and duration of adjuvant breast radiation may be an obstacle for older patients. One approach to this problem has been changing RT schedules. Accelerated hypofractionated radiotherapy delivers larger daily doses of radiation in a three-week period and has shown equivalent low rate of local recurrence compared to the standard radiation schedule (159).

Another approach is to use partial breast irradiation. This approach stems from the observation that the majority of breast recurrences are found in the 1 to 2 cm area of the original cancer. On limiting the area of breast tissue irradiated, the delivery dose can be accelerated as well, thereby reducing the entire duration of treatment to four to five days. There are several techniques that have been developed, including three-dimensional conformal external beam radiotherapy, multicatheter interstitial brachytherapy, and balloon catheter brachytherapy. Intraoperative radiotherapy is another treatment technique that is the ultimate in treatment acceleration, by delivering one large fraction at the time of surgical excision. All are promising new treatment options; however, the body of evidence needs to be more robust in the areas of appropriate patient selection, clinical criteria, and toxicity for each modality for all women. Randomized control studies are currently underway.

Recent results lend credence to another treatment option for hormone receptor–positive, stage I breast cancer in older women: tamoxifen only after lumpectomy without RT. Hughes et al. randomized 636 women aged 70 and older with stage I (tumors 2 cm or less, and clinically negative axillary nodes), ER-positive breast cancer into two groups: lumpectomy, radiation and tamoxifen or lumpectomy and tamoxifen. There was no difference in distant metastases or five-year overall survival. The only significant finding was a difference in local or regional recurrence: 1% with radiation compared to 4% without radiation. A better quality of life, improved cosmesis, and less adverse events favored the tamoxifen only group (160).

In women with ER-negative cancers, radiation is recommended to decrease recurrence risk. Additionally, chest wall radiation is used after mastectomy in high-risk patients, large tumors and axillary lymph node involvement, with resulting decreased incidence of systemic metastases and prolonged survival (161).

Summary of local therapy recommendations: Healthy older women who are eligible for breast-conserving surgery should be offered the choice between mastectomy and breast-conserving surgery. We recommend that axillary dissection and/or sentinel node biopsy be discussed in the context of the clinical presentation, and, in most cases, to gain prognostic information. In patients in whom its result will not alter the systemic adjuvant therapy offered, it is reasonable to omit axillary assessment. In women aged more than 70 with hormone receptor–positive, stage I breast cancer, it is reasonable to offer lumpectomy followed by adjuvant hormonal therapy, and omit RT. Older women with tumors larger than 2 cm should receive adjuvant radiation after lumpectomy. Adjuvant radiation should also be given after mastectomy in cases where the tumor is large (5 cm or larger) and when there are four or more involved axillary lymph nodes.

Primary Hormonal Therapy

In patients whose tumors are large or in whom the immediate risks of surgical intervention may outweigh the benefits, primary hormonal therapy is useful. In those with hormone receptor–positive, advanced, but localized tumors (T3 or T4 tumors), neoadjuvant hormonal therapy, with an aromatase inhibitor or tamoxifen, is an excellent option and may decrease the extent of surgery needed or obviate the need for surgery. In those with serious comorbid conditions or frailty, oral hormonal therapy may be a reasonable alternative to surgery.

Neoadjuvant hormonal therapy is highly effective for hormone receptor–positive breast cancers (162). Although cytotoxic chemotherapy has been more extensively studied in the neoadjuvant setting, hormonal therapy is very effective for tumors expressing hormone receptors and is considerably less toxic. Aromatase inhibitors are currently the most effective agents, with up to 30% greater response rates compared to tamoxifen and breast-conserving surgery more often possible in those initially deemed ineligible (162,163). In these studies, differences in response rates between aromatase inhibitors and tamoxifen were particularly notable in tumors that were HER-2/*neu* positive and ER positive (88% vs. 21%, $P = 0.0004$) (162).

In older women who suffer considerable comorbidity or frailty, or who refuse surgical intervention, primary treatment with a hormonal agent may be useful. In one study, 79 of 302 patients aged 70 or older received tamoxifen as first-line treatment, 61% because of comorbidity and 11% by patient choice (164). Local control, however, is an issue (165). Retrospective series and prospective trials demonstrate that tamoxifen alone is the least effective single modality for local control in patients with operable breast cancer. Response rates range from 28% to 100%, with one-third to two-thirds of patients developing progressive local disease and necessitating salvage therapy with radiotherapy or surgery (Table 4) (168,169,173, 178–181,183,185–193).

Long-term results of randomized trials regarding this issue are now appearing. Two important randomized trials by the EORTC were published in 2003 (168,169). The first compared MRM to tamoxifen as sole initial therapy for operable breast cancer in women aged 70 and older (168). At 10-year median follow-up, progression (29% vs. 68%, logrank $P < 0.0001$) and local progression (11% vs. 92%, logrank $P < 0.0001$) were more common with tamoxifen alone; overall survival was similar in the two groups (73% vs. 61%). The other was a randomized trial of standard surgery, defined as MRM, versus less extensive surgery, wide local excision (WLE), and tamoxifen (T) (169). At a median follow-up of approximately 10 years, there were significantly more locoregional relapses in the WLE-T group (26% vs. 16%), but more distant metastases in the MRM group (28% vs. 13%). Survival rates were similar (72% vs. 69%). The Italian Group for Research on Endocrine Therapy in the elderly trial reported inferior results, at median follow-up of 80 months, using tamoxifen alone versus adjuvant tamoxifen after surgery (183). Local progression was more common in the tamoxifen arm, 45% versus 11%. The Cancer Research Campaign updated their trial of tamoxifen alone versus optimal surgery plus tamoxifen, now with a median follow-up of 12.7 years (184). This study also reported more relapses (56.1% vs. 24.9%) and more deaths (30% vs. 19%) in the group receiving

Table 4 Outcomes of Local Treatment of Early Stage Breast Cancer in Older Women[a]

	Overall survival	Disease-free survival	Breast recurrence	References
Modified radical mastectomy	82–85% at five years	83–95% at five years	1–30%[b] at five years	(129,166,167)
	28–28% at 10 years	33% at 10 years	11–33% at 10 years	(168,169)
Lumpectomy and radiation	65–90% at five years	85% at five years	1–13% at five years	(170,171)
	50–77% at 10 years	79–90% at 10 years		
Radiation and tamoxifen	87% at three years	72% at three years	14% at three years	(172)
	31% at 10 years	24% at 10 years	26% at 10 years	(169)
Wide excision and tamoxifen	64–75% at five years	46–92% at 5 years	3–32%	(166,167, 173–176)
Wide excision alone	69% at five years	85% at five years	3–19%	(136,138,177)
	30–41% at nine years			
Tamoxifen alone	47–80% at two years	NA	30–60%	(135,173, 178–182)
	47–59% at five years		64% at five years	(183)
	39% at 6.6 years	20% at 6.6 years	47% at 6.6 years	(168)
	28–42% at 10 years	33% at 10 years	62% at 10 years	(184)

NA, not applicable
[a]Data for overall and disease-free survivals were pooled from the references given.
[b]Breast, chest wall, and regional lymph node recurrences.

tamoxifen alone. From these trials, we can conclude that using tamoxifen alone is an inadequate treatment; both local control and survival are adversely affected when surgery is omitted from primary therapy. We should resort to using hormonal agents alone only when life expectancy is severely limited.

The combination of tamoxifen and hypofractionated once-weekly radiation (6.5 Gy per fraction for a total of five fractions to the breast and seven to the tumor bed) is also an option for older women unable or unwilling to have surgery (194). Local control was achieved in 81% for T1 and 96% for T2 tumors at three years. Overall and disease-free survival at three years was comparable to other treatment approaches.

Summary of primary hormonal therapy: The strategy of primary hormonal therapy may be useful in older women with large, unresectable cancer, those unable to undergo surgery due to comorbid illness, those in whom life expectancy is limited to months rather than years, or those who refuse surgery. Primary hormonal therapy is associated with a good initial response in hormone receptor–positive tumors, but an unacceptable local control over time. In addition, giving weekly, as opposed to daily, radiation treatments, is more convenient for frail older people and has been proven to be effective in early-stage breast cancer.

Systemic Adjuvant Therapy

After initial management with mastectomy or lumpectomy followed by RT, women with stage I and stage II breast cancer have a 10-year risk of recurrence of 25% to 30% and 50% to 90%, respectively (195). Breast cancer recurrence is, therefore, a major concern. In older women with breast cancer metastatic to axillary lymph nodes, breast cancer–related deaths are more common than deaths due to other non-malignant disease (24). In two large adjuvant trials of tamoxifen therapy in older patients with node-positive breast cancer, only 10% to 20% of patients died of causes unrelated to breast cancer (196,197).

Current management guidelines recommend that adjuvant systemic treatment be considered for any woman with an invasive breast cancer measuring >1 cm in size (198–200). The 2005-updated meta-analysis of adjuvant therapy trials by the Early Breast Cancer Trialists' Collabotative Group (EBCTCG) with 15-year survival data clearly shows benefit of tamoxifen and chemotherapy in improving relapse-free and overall survival in women with early-stage breast cancer (201).

Adjuvant Hormonal Therapy

Adjuvant therapy for hormone receptor–positive breast cancer in women over the age of 70 invariably includes hormonal manipulation. The comprehensive meta-analysis of adjuvant therapy trials by the EBCTCG showed that postmenopausal patients treated with tamoxifen had a significantly lower risk of tumor recurrence and death, when compared to those randomized to observation alone (201). The ratio of annual event rates for recurrence and mortality in women with hormone receptor–positive breast cancer using five years of tamoxifen versus those not using tamoxifen were: 0.66 [standard error (SE) 0.05] and 0.76 (SE 0.07) for those aged 50 to 59; 0.54 (SE 0.05) and 0.65 (SE 0.06) for those aged 60 to 69; and 0.49 (SE 0.12) and 0.63 (SE 0.15) for those aged 70 and older. The proportional benefits in terms of breast cancer relapse and mortality were similar for women with node-negative and node-positive tumors, and the benefit of five years of tamoxifen was evident beyond five years of active therapy. Only patients with ER-positive tumors benefited from tamoxifen, as did women with unrecorded ER status; women with tumors devoid of ER receptor derived no benefit from tamoxifen therapy regardless of age.

The aromatase inhibitors, anastrozole, letrozole, and exemestane, are proving their use in the adjuvant setting: anastrozole compared to tamoxifen, letrozole compared to placebo after five years of adjuvant tamoxifen, and exemestane for two to three years after tamoxifen compared to tamoxifen alone, to complete a five-year course of adjuvant hormonal therapy (202–204). Based on results of the ATAC (Anastrozole versus Tamoxifen Against the Combination) trial, anastrozole was approved for adjuvant treatment in breast cancer (202). In the ATAC trial, anastrozole was more effective than tamoxifen in decreasing the recurrence of breast cancer at a median follow-up of 60 months. A placebo-controlled study that compared stopping tamoxifen after five years to changing treatment to letrozole for another five years was stopped early when less recurrence was seen at a median follow-up of 2.4 years (204). The estimated four-year, disease-free survival (including local or metastatic recurrences or new contralateral breast cancers) from the time of switching treatment was 93% in the group treated with letrozole compared to 87% in the group treated with placebo. Letrozole decreased the hazard of recurrence by approximately half, regardless of nodal status, though the absolute benefit for those at low risk is very small. The difference in survival between groups was not statistically significant. A third trial studied five years of tamoxifen versus two to three years of tamoxifen followed by exemestane for the rest of the five-year course (203). At a median follow-up of 30.6 months, there was a 32% reduction in recurrence in women who switched to exemestane; the overall survival was not yet statistically different. The most recent consensus statement regarding the use of aromatase inhibitors as adjuvant therapy for postmenopausal women supports the use of these agents in the adjuvant setting, either as initial therapy or after initial treatment with tamoxifen (205).

The choice of initial hormonal adjuvant therapy can be based on risks and benefits of tamoxifen versus the aromatase inhibitors. Almost 30 years of experience with tamoxifen makes our knowledge regarding its therapeutic profile immense. Tamoxifen decreases risk of breast cancer recurrence and death, decreases risk of cancer in the opposite breast, decreases loss of bone mineral or osteoporosis, and decreases cholesterol and the chance of fatal heart attack; side effects of tamoxifen include menopausal symptoms, gynecological symptoms, endometrial changes, eye changes, and liver changes, and increased risk of endometrial and gastrointestinal cancers, stroke, and blood clots (206,207). Like tamoxifen, the aromatase inhibitors are associated with symptoms of estrogen deprivation; they may cause slightly fewer hot flashes, however, and more arthritis, arthralgias, and myalgia and a loss in bone mineral density compared to tamoxifen or placebo (202–204). As a group, aromatase inhibitors do not increase the risk of endometrial cancer, vaginal bleeding and discharge, thrombotic events, and cerebrovascular events, as is seen with tamoxifen. In older patients with a history of thromboembolism or those who cannot tolerate tamoxifen, aromatase inhibitors are certainly indicated for women with hormone receptor–positive tumors, if adjuvant hormonal therapy is planned.

There is also mounting evidence that hormone receptor–positive tumors overexpressing HER-2/*neu* (c-erbB2) do not gain as large a benefit from, and may be relatively resistant to, tamoxifen (162,208–211). Twenty-year results of a prospective trial of adjuvant tamoxifen versus no tamoxifen found that women with HER-2/*neu* overexpressing breast cancers gain less benefit from tamoxifen than those with HER-2/*neu* normal breast cancers (212). Tamoxifen had no benefit on survival (HR 1.09, 95% CI 0.63–1.87) in HER-2/*neu* positive tumors; whereas, in negative tumors, it was beneficial (HR 0.59, 95% CI 0.4–0.87). An aromatase inhibitor, therefore, could be considered to be optimal endocrine therapy for postmenopausal women with hormone receptor–positive and HER-2/*neu* overexpressing breast cancers.

Adjuvant hormonal therapy, therefore, should be considered for all women with hormone receptor–positive breast cancer, and every effort should be made to encourage compliance with at least a five-year course of therapy (212). Older women, especially those over the age of 80, may be at a particularly high risk for undertreatment (213,214). Education regarding the tremendous benefit of adjuvant hormonal therapy is also necessary to increase compliance (212,215). Undertreatment with adjuvant hormonal therapy may put older breast cancer patients at risk for recurrence and death.

Adjuvant hormonal therapy recommendations: Adjuvant hormonal therapy should be discussed with all older women who have hormone receptor–positive breast cancer. Due to lower toxicity and lower recurrence and death rates with aromatase inhibitors compared to tamoxifen, aromatase inhibitors are the preferred adjuvant hormonal agents for many postmenopausal women with nonmetastatic breast cancer.

Adjuvant Chemotherapy

Combination chemotherapy in stage II, premenopausal and postmenopausal (<70 years old) patients, with or without lymph node involvement, improves relapse-free and overall survival (201,216). The addition of chemotherapy to the management of breast cancer in older women has not yielded results as impressive as that in premenopausal women. In the report of the 2000 EBCTCG meta-analysis, the ratio of annual death rates for women receiving adjuvant chemotherapy compared to no chemotherapy was 0.91 (SE 0.04) in women aged 60 to 69 compared to 0.70 (SE 0.05) in women aged 40 to 49 (201). Many of the breast cancer adjuvant trials included in the meta-analysis excluded women over the age of 70 (217–221). Within the meta-analysis of polychemotherapy trials, however, there were few women older than 70 years and very few older than 80 years (201). For women aged 70 and older, the ratio of annual events and deaths for those receiving chemotherapy and those not receiving chemotherapy was 0.88 (SE 0.11) and 0.87 (SE 0.12). This is the first EBCTCG report to show significant improvement in relapse and death rates from chemotherapy in women over the age of 70. Consensus guidelines recommend that chemotherapy be considered for older women with node-positive breast cancer and hormone receptor–negative breast cancers (199).

Older age predicts a decline in recommendation to deliver adjuvant chemotherapy (222–224), but may also predict use of arbitrarily lower doses of chemotherapy. Lower doses may partially explain the lower effectiveness of chemotherapy in postmenopausal women (225,226). Muss et al. reported an analysis of data from four randomized Cancer and Leukemia Group B (CALGB) trials of adjuvant chemotherapy in 6489 node-positive patients, of whom 159 were aged 70 or older (227). Patients receiving more treatment [higher chemotherapy doses or anthracyclines in addition to cyclophosphamide methotrexate and 5-fluorouracil (CMF)-type regimens, or taxanes in addition to doxorubicin and cyclophosphamide (AC)] had superior relapse-free and overall survival compared to those receiving less treatment. The difference was especially pronounced in patients aged 65 and older, where the reduction in hazard of failure and death attributed to more chemotherapy compared to less was 42% and 27%; comparatively reduction in hazard of failure and death were 20% and 16% for women aged 51 to 64 and 18% and 17% for women age 50 or less. However, older patients also experienced more treatment-related mortality (1.5% vs. 0.2–0.7%). Healthy older women with metastatic breast cancer, however, tolerate standard chemotherapy regimens as well as younger women (228,229). One study of doxorubicin-containing adjuvant regimens showed similar tolerability in patients aged 65 and older compared to those 50 to 69 years old (230). When used in older women, therefore, doses of adjuvant chemotherapy agents should be optimized.

The value of chemotherapy, when added to hormonal therapy in postmenopausal women with stage II, ER-positive breast cancers remains controversial; several trials suggest no benefit compared to tamoxifen alone (217,231,232), whereas other reports suggest a role for chemotherapy in addition to tamoxifen (217,233,234). Although prospective trials have addressed the use of adjuvant chemotherapy when added to tamoxifen in postmenopausal women, no such trial has addressed the issue specifically in women over the age of 70. Because the value of adjuvant chemotherapy decreases with increasing age, trials are needed to determine the effect of adjuvant chemotherapy when added to hormonal therapy on relapse-free survival, overall survival, and quality of life. For now, with mounting evidence showing that treatment according to consensus recommendations leads to improved survival, older women with the risk of recurrence high enough to justify chemotherapy should be offered treatment (235).

Summary of adjuvant chemotherapy recommendations: The risks and benefits of adjuvant chemotherapy in older women should be carefully weighed. If eligible for a clinical trial, this should be offered as the preferred option. As discussed above, there are several acceptable options for adjuvant chemotherapy regimens. The choice of regimen should be made based on efficacy and toxicity profile.

Follow-Up After Treatment of Early Breast Cancer

After completion of primary management of early breast cancer, follow-up is required to monitor for tumor recurrence and toxicities of treatment. With regard to monitoring for tumor recurrence, although there is no evidence that close follow-up results in improved overall survival, the detection of early skin or lymph-node (soft tissue) recurrence may result in more effective palliation (236). Extensive laboratory and radiological procedures are available for detection of metastatic disease, but trials indicate that a brief, focused history, and a limited physical examination (skin, chest, breast, and abdominal examination) detects more than 75% of metastases (237,238). Mammography is an exception and should be performed on a yearly basis to detect new primary lesions because a history of breast cancer is a risk factor for another breast cancer. Moreover, follow-up visits provide an opportunity for patients to express concerns and for physicians to give reassurance. With regard to monitoring for toxicity of treatment, particular attention should be paid to older women. In a study assessing the quality of life and psychosocial adjustment in the 15 months after breast cancer diagnosis in women over the age of 65, significant deterioration in self-reported physical functioning was found in women with more comorbid conditions and those who received chemotherapy (239). Higher comorbidity level was also associated with a decline in mental health scores.

Because of the growing concern over health care costs, many organizations are formulating guidelines for follow-up. The American Society of Clinical Oncology guidelines are presented in Table 5 (103). In addition to mammograms and follow-up visits with the oncologist and the gynecologist, patients should be educated about the symptoms of breast cancer recurrence, so that these are reported and evaluated promptly. Regular visits with primary care physician is also recommended for general health maintenance, because older persons are at risk of other health issues (240).

Summary of follow-up recommendations: See Table 5.

Table 5 Follow-Ups of Women with Early Breast Cancer After Diagnosis and Initial Treatment

	Frequency of examination during intervals after diagnosis		
	0–3 yr	3–5 yr	5+ yr
History/physical exam	Every 3–6 mo	Every 6–12 mo	Yearly
Breast self-exam	Monthly	Monthly	Monthly
Mammograms	Yearly	Yearly	Yearly
Gynecological exams	Yearly	Yearly	Yearly
Other	PRN	PRN	PRN

PRN = as required.
Abbreviation: PRN, pro re nata.
Source: From Ref. 103.

METASTATIC BREAST CANCER

Once metastatic, breast cancer is rarely curable. Palliation of symptoms and optimization of the quality of life are the major goals of therapy. Hormonal therapy, because of its low toxicity, is recommended for first-line therapy in metastatic breast cancer, regardless of hormone receptor status, unless the disease is rapidly progressive or there is major visceral organ dysfunction.

As initial therapy, hormonal therapy elicits complete and partial responses in 30% to 40% of unselected patients, with response durations averaging about one year. Half of those with ER-positive breast tumors respond (241). The recommended sequence of endocrine therapy is as follows: aromatase inhibitor → tamoxifen or fulvestrant → megestrol acetate → estrogens or corticosteroids. Patients who have demonstrated responsiveness to a previous hormonal agent are most likely to respond to subsequent agents.

Initial response rates are generally higher with chemotherapy than with endocrine therapy. Eventual survival, however, is not significantly influenced by initial treatment choice (242). This was also true in a randomized trial comparing tamoxifen versus chemotherapy (CMF) as initial therapy for metastatic breast cancer in women older than 65 years, of whom 15–16% had ER-negative breast cancer, in this study, the response rate to CMF was 31%, whether it was initial treatment or given after progression occurred on tamoxifen. In another trial comparing chemotherapy, chemotherapy plus tamoxifen, and tamoxifen alone, response rates were 45%, 51%, and 22%, respectively (244). Both trials found higher initial response rates to the chemotherapy, but similar survival for all groups.

Chemotherapy is generally offered to those patients with progressive metastatic breast cancer whose tumors have demonstrated resistance to endocrine therapy. Healthy older women with metastatic breast cancer treated with standard chemotherapy have response rates and toxicity profiles similar to those of younger women (228,229). Chemotherapy-related myelosuppression is more common in older patients, although its duration and severity have not resulted in major differences in bleeding or in mortality related to neutropenia and infection (228,245,246). In patients with solid tumors treated with palliative doses of chemotherapy, severe nonhematologic toxicity is similar for both young and old (228). Gelman and Taylor treated 92 patients, aged 65 to 90, with a CMF regimen, modifying the methotrexate dosage based on creatinine clearance (247). Response rates were substantially lower for these patients compared to a younger cohort treated with CMF, but duration of response, time to failure, and survival were all longer in the older women. In a retrospective analysis of women treated with chemotherapy on state-of-the-art research protocols, Christman and colleagues showed no difference in response, time to failure, or survival for older women compared to younger patients (245).

The anthracyclines and taxanes are considered to be the most effective agents against breast cancer. Cardiac toxicity related to anthracyclines is more common in older people (248). Dexrazoxane (Zenicard^{TM}), a cardioprotective agent, may be useful in ameliorating anthracycline-induced cardiotoxicity (249–251). Mitoxantrone is less cardiotoxic and has efficacy similar to doxorubicin; it is a reasonable alternative in older women (252,253). Overall tolerability of doxorubicin-based chemotherapy has been retrospectively studied in older women (≥65 years) versus younger women (<65 years) (254). Records of 1011 women (252 aged 50–54, 254 aged 55–59, 261 aged 60–64, 158 aged 54–69, 64 aged 70–74, 21 aged 75–79, and one over the age of 80) were reviewed. On comparing women less than 65 years old with those aged 65 or older, response rates were higher in younger women ($P = 0.001$), but overall survival times were similar ($P = 0.06$). Dose intensity was comparable between the two groups ($P = 0.49$). Neutropenic fevers occurred with equal frequency (16%), but fever was more common in women aged 65 or older (12% vs. 17%, $P = 0.05$).

Paclitaxel (255,256) and docetaxel (257,258) are also very effective in metastatic breast cancer. Paclitaxel can be used at similar dose intensities in older and younger women (259).

Another potentially useful chemotherapeutic agent is vinorelbine, which requires weekly administration, but, other than hematologic toxicity, is generally well tolerated (260,261). Sorio et al. examined the pharmacokinetics and tolerance of vinorelbine (30 mg/m^2 i.v. on days one and eight every three weeks) in 25 women who were older than 65 years with metastatic breast cancer (262). The systemic clearance rate was large (mean 23.4 l/kg), and the terminal half-life was long (mean 26.2 hours), which were all similar to parameters previously noted in younger women. Tolerance was also acceptable, with only 37% experiencing severe neutropenia. Of 20 evaluable patients, there were six partial responses. Vogel et al. reported a similar study of 56 women aged 60 and older getting weekly vinorelbine as first-line chemotherapy for metastatic breast cancer (263). Doses were delayed during the first course in 71% of patients. Objective response rate was 38%, and there were two (4%) complete responses. At least one episode of grade three to four granulocytopenia occurred in 45 patients (80%), and six developed fever in the setting of neutropenia. Likewise, in a retrospective review of 24 women aged 70 and older receiving single-agent vinorelbine at 30 mg/m^2 days one and eight every three weeks, the main toxicity was hematologic, and the response rate was 37.5% (264).

Combination therapy with vinorelbine (25 mg/m^2 on days 1 and 8) and gemcitabine (1000 mg/m^2 on days one and eight) on a 21-day cycle was also studied in older patients (265). In 34 patients over the age of 65, this combination had significant activity. The overall response rate was 53%, and a complete response was obtained in five patients (15%). Grade three to four neutropenia occurred in only seven cases (20%), none with febrile neutropenia.

Capecitabine, an oral 5-fluorouracil prodrug, is an excellent option in older patients who prefer oral chemotherapy. It is effective and well tolerated in older women, though starting at lower initial doses than that used in younger patients is suggested. This is particularly true in the setting of mild to moderate renal impairment or hyperbilirubinemia. In one prospective study, 73 patients aged 65 and older received single agent capecitabine, initially at 1250 mg/m^2, twice daily for 14 of every 21 days (266). Due to two toxic deaths in the first 30 patients, the starting dose was reduced to 1000 mg/m^2 twice daily. This dose was well tolerated (grade three or four diarrhea, nausea, fatigue in <10%), and the response rate was 37%. Trastuzumab, a humanized antibody to HER-2/neu, may also be effective in older women with HER-2/neu-positive tumors.

In metastatic disease, RT can be very useful to relieve bone pain, treat isolated metastatic lesions in other sites, and treat intracranial metastases or spinal cord compression. There is very little information about the use of RT for metastatic breast cancer in older women. Extrapolation of data in adjuvant setting implies that it is useful with minimal excess toxicity. Clearly, if RT is indicated because of intracranial metastases or bone pain, the benefits of therapy outweigh the possible risks.

In a study evaluating relationships between physician and cancer patient survival estimates, patients' perceived quality of life, care preferences, and outcomes, and how they vary across middle-aged (45–64) and older (≥65) patient groups, fewer older patients preferred cardiopulmonary resuscitation (CPR) or life-prolonging treatments (267). Aggressive care was not related to prolonged life in either group. Preference to extend life was related to a patient's estimate for survival, but was not associated with physician prognostic estimate or with perceived quality of life. Perceived quality of life was not associated with care preferences in older patients, whereas in middle-aged patients, perceived poor quality of life was associated with less preference for CPR.

Summary of metastatic breast cancer recommendations: Due to its excellent therapeutic index, we recommend hormonal therapy for initial treatment for metastatic breast cancer in all patients, regardless of hormone receptor status. Sequential hormonal therapy should be used as long as a response to previous hormonal agents is seen. When the disease becomes resistant to hormonal therapy, or in cases where the disease is causing life-threatening symptoms, we recommend the use of chemotherapy.

CONCLUSIONS AND RECOMMENDATIONS

Breast cancer in older women is a major national health concern. Over 50% of breast cancers are diagnosed in women older than 65 years, a quickly growing segment of our population. Healthy older women should be offered state-of-the-art screening and treatment for breast cancer. This includes mammography, surgery, RT, and adjuvant therapy for early-stage tumors. Clinical trials focusing on the role of adjuvant treatment in older women with breast cancer are of paramount importance. In older women with comorbid conditions or frailty that may limit survival or jeopardize surgical or other treatment outcomes, primary treatment with hormonal agents or adjuvant therapy with hormonal therapy alone after surgery may be warranted. Outside of the clinical trials setting, metastatic disease should be treated similarly in all age groups.

REFERENCES

1. Ghafoor A, Jemal A, Ward E, et al. Trends in breast cancer by race and ethnicity. CA Cancer J Clin 2003; 53:342–355.
2. Jemal A, Murray T, Ward E, et al. Cancer statistics, 2005. CA Cancer J Clin 2005; 55:10–30.
3. Adami HO, Malker B, Holmberg L, et al. The relation between survival and age at diagnosis in breast cancer. N Engl J Med 1986; 315:559–563.
4. Kessler LG. The relationship between age and incidence of breast cancer. Population and screening program data. Cancer 1992; 69:1896–1903.
5. Ries LAG, Eisner MP, Kosary CL, et al. SEER Cancer Statistics Review, 1975–2001, http://seer.cancer.gov/csr/1975_2001/. Bethesda, MD: National Cancer Institute, 2004.
6. Services USDoHaH: Health United States 1996–97 and Injury Chartbook. DHHS Publication No. (PHS) 97–1232, 1997.
7. Statistics USNCfH: Vital statistics of the United States, US Census Bureau, 2001.
8. Yancik R, Ries LG, Yates JW. Breast cancer in aging women. A population-based study of contrasts in stage, surgery, and survival. Cancer 1989; 63:976–981.
9. Holli K, Isola J. Effect of age on the survival of breast cancer patients. Eur J Cancer 1997; 33:425–428.
10. Brown JT, Hulka BS. Screening mammography in the elderly: a case–control study. J Gen Intern Med 1988; 3:126–131.

11. Robie PW. Cancer screening in the elderly. J Am Geriatr Soc 1989; 37:888–893.
12. Allen C, Cox EB, Manton KG, et al. Breast cancer in the elderly. Current patterns of care. J Am Geriatr Soc 1986; 34:637–642.
13. Rosen PP, Lesser ML, Kinne DW. Breast carcinoma at the extremes of age: a comparison of patients younger than 35 years and older than 75 years. J Surg Oncol 1985; 28:90–96.
14. Bergman L, Dekker G, van Leeuwen FE, et al. The effect of age on treatment choice and survival in elderly breast cancer patients. Cancer 1991; 67:2227–2234.
15. Bouchardy C, Rapiti E, Fioretta G, et al. Undertreatment strongly decreases prognosis of breast cancer in elderly women. J Clin Oncol 2003; 21:3580–3587.
16. Greenfield S, Blanco DM, Elashoff RM, et al. Patterns of care related to age of breast cancer patients. JAMA 1987; 257:2766–2770.
17. Kimmick GG, Peterson BL, Kornblith AB, et al. Improving accrual of older persons to cancer treatment trials: a randomized trial comparing an educational intervention with standard information: CALGB 360001. J Clin Oncol 2005; 23:2201–2207.
18. Mor V, Masterson-Allen S, Goldberg RJ, et al. Relationship between age at diagnosis and treatments received by cancer patients. J Am Geriatr Soc 1985; 33:585–589.
19. Silliman RA, Guadagnoli E, Weitberg AB, et al. Age as a predictor of diagnostic and initial treatment intensity in newly diagnosed breast cancer patients. J Gerontol 1989; 44:M46–M50.
20. Department of Health and Human Services NCfHS: National Vital Statistics Report. web: www.dhhs.gov 52, 2003.
21. Yancik R. Cancer burden in the aged: an epidemiologic and demographic overview. Cancer 1997; 80:1273–1283.
22. Stewart JA, Foster RS Jr. Breast cancer and aging. Semin Oncol 1989; 16:41–50.
23. Edwards BK, Howe HL, Ries LA, et al. Annual report to the nation on the status of cancer, 1973–1999, featuring implications of age and aging on U.S. cancer burden. Cancer 2002; 94:2766–2792.
24. Satariano WA, Ragland DR. The effect of comorbidity on 3-year survival of women with primary breast cancer. Ann Intern Med 1994; 120:104–110.
25. Houterman S, Janssen-Heijnen ML, Verheij CD, et al. Comorbidity has negligible impact on treatment and complications but influences survival in breast cancer patients. Br J Cancer 2004; 90:2332–2337.
26. Klabunde CN, Warren JL, Legler JM. Assessing comorbidity using claims data: an overview. Med Care 2002; 40:IV-26–35.
27. Lash TL, Thwin SS, Horton NJ, et al. Multiple informants: a new method to assess breast cancer patients' comorbidity. Am J Epidemiol 2003; 157:249–257.
28. Satariano WA. Aging, comorbidity, and breast cancer survival: an epidemiologic view. Adv Exp Med Biol 1993; 330:1–11.
29. Satariano WA, Ragheb NE, Dupuis MA, et al. Comorbidity in Older Women with Breast Cancer: An Epidemiologic Approach, Cancer in the Elderly: Approaches to Early Detection and Treatment. New York: Springer, 1989:71.
30. Chap LI, Barshy SH, Bassett LW, et al. Breast Cancer: Natural History and Pretreatment Assessment, Cancer Treatment. Philadelphia, PA: W.B. Saunders Company, 2001:507.
31. Singletary SE, Allred C, Ashley P, et al. Revision of the American Joint Committee on Cancer staging system for breast cancer. J Clin Oncol 2002; 20:3628–3636.
32. Li CI, Malone KE, Porter PL, et al. Reproductive and anthropometric factors in relation to the risk of lobular and ductal breast carcinoma among women 65–79 years of age. Int J Cancer 2003; 107:647–651.
33. Li CI, Moe RE, Daling JR. Risk of mortality by histologic type of breast cancer among women aged 50 to 79 years. Arch Intern Med 2003; 163:2149–2153.
34. Schaefer G, Rosen PP, Lesser ML, et al. Breast carcinoma in elderly women: pathology, prognosis, and survival. Pathol Annu 1984; 19 Pt 1:195–219.

35. Schottenfeld D, Robbins GF. Breast cancer in elderly women. Geriatrics 1971; 26: 121–131.
36. Diab SG, Elledge RM, Clark GM. Tumor characteristics and clinical outcome of elderly women with breast cancer. J Natl Cancer Inst 2000; 92:550–556.
37. Eppenberger-Castori S, Moore DH Jr, Thor AD, et al. Age-associated biomarker profiles of human breast cancer. Int J Biochem Cell Biol 2002; 34:1318–1330.
38. Gentili C, Sanfilippo O, Silvestrini R. Cell proliferation and its relationship to clinical features and relapse in breast cancers. Cancer 1981; 48:974–979.
39. Lyman GH, Lyman S, Balducci L, et al. Age and the risk of breast cancer recurrence. Cancer Control 1996; 3:421–427.
40. Meyer JS, Hixon B. Advanced stage and early relapse of breast carcinomas associated with high thymidine labeling indices. Cancer Res 1979; 39:4042–4047.
41. Taylor IW, Musgrove EA, Friedlander ML, et al. The influence of age on the DNA ploidy levels of breast tumours. Eur J Cancer Clin Oncol 1983; 19:623–628.
42. Henderson IC. Biologic variations of tumors. Cancer 1992; 69:1888–1895.
43. Daidone MG, Coradini D, Martelli G, et al. Primary breast cancer in elderly women: biological profile and relation with clinical outcome. Crit Rev Oncol Hematol 2003; 45:313–325.
44. McCarty KS Jr, Silva JS, Cox EB, et al. Relationship of age and menopausal status to estrogen receptor content in primary carcinoma of the breast. Ann Surg 1983; 197: 123–127.
45. von Rosen A, Gardelin A, Auer G. Assessment of malignancy potential in mammary carcinoma in elderly patients. Am J Clin Oncol 1987; 10:61–64.
46. Ugnat AM, Xie L, Morriss J, et al. Survival of women with breast cancer in Ottawa, Canada: variation with age, stage, histology, grade and treatment. Br J Cancer 2004; 90:1138–1143.
47. Lamy PJ, Pujol P, Thezenas S, et al. Progesterone receptor quantification as a strong prognostic determinant in postmenopausal breast cancer women under tamoxifen therapy. Breast Cancer Res Treat 2002; 76:65–71.
48. Honma N, Sakamoto G, Akiyama F, et al. Breast carcinoma in women over the age of 85: distinct histological pattern and androgen, oestrogen, and progesterone receptor status. Histopathology 2003; 42:120–127.
49. Quong J, Eppenberger-Castori S, Moore D 3rd, et al. Age-dependent changes in breast cancer hormone receptors and oxidant stress markers. Breast Cancer Res Treat 2002; 76:221–236.
50. Harris JR, Lippman ME, Veronesi U, et al. Breast cancer (1). N Engl J Med 1992; 327:319–328.
51. Sweeney C, Blair CK, Anderson KE, et al. Risk factors for breast cancer in elderly women. Am J Epidemiol 2004; 160:868–875.
52. Mattisson I, Wirfalt E, Johansson U, et al. Intakes of plant foods, fibre and fat and risk of breast cancer—a prospective study in the Malmo Diet and Cancer Cohort. Br J Cancer 2004; 90:122–127.
53. Smith-Warner SA, Spiegelman D, Yaun SS, et al. Intake of fruits and vegetables and risk of breast cancer: a pooled analysis of cohort studies. JAMA 2001; 285: 769–776.
54. van Gils CH, Peeters PH, Bueno-de-Mesquita HB, et al. Consumption of vegetables and fruits and risk of breast cancer. JAMA 2005; 293:183–193.
55. Wu AH, Yu MC, Tseng CC, et al. Green tea and risk of breast cancer in Asian Americans. Int J Cancer 2003; 106:574–579.
56. Wu AH, Yu MC, Tseng CC, et al. Plasma isoflavone levels versus self-reported soy isoflavone levels in Asian-American women in Los Angeles County. Carcinogenesis 2004; 25:77–81.
57. Limer JL, Speirs V. Phyto-oestrogens and breast cancer chemoprevention. Breast Cancer Res 2004; 6:119–127.

58. Wu AH, Tseng CC, Van Den Berg D, et al. Tea intake, COMT genotype, and breast cancer in Asian-American women. Cancer Res 2003; 63:7526–7529.

59. Hulten K, Van Kappel AL, Winkvist A, et al. Carotenoids, alpha-tocopherols, and retinol in plasma and breast cancer risk in northern Sweden. Cancer Causes Control 2001; 12:529–537.

60. Nissen SB, Tjonneland A, Stripp C, et al. Intake of vitamins A, C, and E from diet and supplements and breast cancer in postmenopausal women. Cancer Causes Control 2003; 14:695–704.

61. Lonn E, Bosch J, Yusuf S, et al. Effects of long-term vitamin E supplementation on cardiovascular events and cancer: a randomized controlled trial. JAMA 2005; 293:1338–1347.

62. Zhang SM, Willett WC, Selhub J, et al. Plasma folate, vitamin B6, vitamin B12, homocysteine, and risk of breast cancer. J Natl Cancer Inst 2003; 95:373–380.

63. Sellers TA, Grabrick DM, Vierkant RA, et al. Does folate intake decrease risk of postmenopausal breast cancer among women with a family history? Cancer Causes Control 2004; 15:113–120.

64. Huang Z, Willett WC, Colditz GA, et al. Waist circumference, waist:hip ratio, and risk of breast cancer in the Nurses' Health Study. Am J Epidemiol 1999; 150:1316–1324.

65. Calle EE, Rodriguez C, Walker-Thurmond K, et al. Overweight, obesity, and mortality from cancer in a prospectively studied cohort of U.S. adults. N Engl J Med 2003; 348:1625–1638.

66. Matthews CE, Fowke JH, Dai Q, et al. Physical activity, body size, and estrogen metabolism in women. Cancer Causes Control 2004; 15:473–481.

67. McTiernan A, Kooperberg C, White E, et al. Recreational physical activity and the risk of breast cancer in postmenopausal women: the Women's Health Initiative Cohort Study. JAMA 2003; 290:1331–1336.

68. Fisher B, Costantino JP, Wickerham DL, et al. Tamoxifen for prevention of breast cancer: report of the National surgical adjuvant breast and bowel project P-1 Study. J Natl Cancer Inst 1998; 90:1371–1388.

69. Powles TJ. The Royal Marsden Hospital (RMH) trial: key points and remaining questions. Ann N Y Acad Sci 2001; 949:109–112.

70. Veronesi U, Maisonneuve P, Sacchini V, et al. Tamoxifen for breast cancer among hysterectomised women. Lancet 2002; 359:1122–1124.

71. Cuzick J, Forbes J, Edwards R, et al. First results from the International Breast Cancer Intervention Study (IBIS-I): a randomised prevention trial. Lancet 2002; 360:817–824.

72. Cuzick J, Powles T, Veronesi U, et al. Overview of the main outcomes in breast-cancer prevention trials. Lancet 2003; 361:296–300.

73. Chlebowski RT, Col N, Winer EP, et al. American Society of Clinical Oncology technology assessment of pharmacologic interventions for breast cancer risk reduction including tamoxifen, raloxifene, and aromatase inhibition. J Clin Oncol 2002; 20:3328–3343.

74. Gail MH, Brinton LA, Byar DP, et al. Projecting individualized probabilities of developing breast cancer for white females who are being examined annually. J Natl Cancer Inst 1989; 81:1879–1886.

75. Gail MH, Costantino JP, Bryant J, et al. Weighing the risks and benefits of tamoxifen treatment for preventing breast cancer. J Natl Cancer Inst 1999; 91:1829–1846.

76. Cummings SR, Eckert S, Krueger KA, et al. The effect of raloxifene on risk of breast cancer in postmenopausal women: results from the MORE randomized trial. Multiple Outcomes of Raloxifene Evaluation. JAMA 1999; 281:2189–2197.

77. Cauley JA, Norton L, Lippman ME, et al. Continued breast cancer risk reduction in postmenopausal women treated with raloxifene: 4-year results from the MORE trial. Multiple outcomes of raloxifene evaluation. Breast Cancer Res Treat 2001; 65:125–134.

78. Vogel VG, Costantino JP, Wickerham DL, et al. National Surgical Adjuvant Breast and Bowel Project update: prevention trials and endocrine therapy of ductal carcinoma in situ. Clin Cancer Res 2003; 9:495S–501S.

79. Harris RE, Chlebowski RT, Jackson RD, et al. Breast cancer and nonsteroidal anti-inflammatory drugs: prospective results from the Women's Health Initiative. Cancer Res 2003; 63:6096–6101.

80. Moorman PG, Grubber JM, Millikan RC, et al. Association between non-steroidal anti-inflammatory drugs (NSAIDs) and invasive breast cancer and carcinoma in situ of the breast. Cancer Causes Control 2003; 14:915–922.

81. Terry MB, Gammon MD, Zhang FF, et al. Association of frequency and duration of aspirin use and hormone receptor status with breast cancer risk. JAMA 2004; 291:2433–2440.

82. Colditz GA, Willett WC, Hunter DJ, et al. Family history, age, and risk of breast cancer. Prospective data from the Nurses' Health Study. JAMA 1993; 270:338–343.

83. Slattery ML, Kerber RA. A comprehensive evaluation of family history and breast cancer risk. The Utah Population Database. JAMA 1993; 270:1563–1568.

84. Couch FJ, DeShano ML, Blackwood MA, et al. BRCA1 mutations in women attending clinics that evaluate the risk of breast cancer. N Engl J Med 1997; 336:1409.

85. Miki Y, Swensen J, Shattuck-Eidens D, et al. A strong candidate for the breast and ovarian cancer susceptibility gene BRCA1. Science 1994; 266:66.

86. Struewing JP, Hartge P, Wacholder S, et al. The risk of cancer associated with specific mutations of BRCA1 and BRCA2 among Ashkenazi Jews. N Engl J Med 1997; 336:1401.

87. Easton DF, Bishop DT, Ford D, et al. Genetic linkage analysis in familial breast and ovarian cancer: results from 214 families. Am J Hum Genet 1993; 52:678.

88. Weber BL, Garber JE. Familial breast cancer: recent advances. Cedar Knolls, NJ: Lippman-Raven Healthcare, 1997.

89. Wooster R, Neuhausen SL, Mangion J, et al. Localization of a breast cancer susceptibility gene, BRCA2, to chromosome 13q12–13. Science 1994; 265:2088.

90. Rimer BK, Harris JR, Lippman ME, et al. Breast Cancer Screening, Diseases of the Breast. Philadelphia, J.B.: Lippincott Company, 1996:307.

91. Andersson I, Aspegren K, Janzon L, et al. Mammographic screening and mortality from breast cancer: the Malmo mammographic screening trial. BMJ 1988; 297:943–948.

92. Tabar L, Vitak B, Chen HH, et al. The Swedish Two-County Trial twenty years later. Updated mortality results and new insights from long-term follow-up. Radiol Clin North Am 2000; 38:625–651.

93. Chen HH, Tabar L, Fagerberg G, et al. Effect of breast cancer screening after age 65. J Med Screen 1995; 2:10–14.

94. Nystrom L, Andersson I, Bjurstam N, et al. Long-term effects of mammography screening: updated overview of the Swedish randomised trials. Lancet 2002; 359:909–919.

95. Carney PA, Miglioretti DL, Yankaskas BC, et al. Individual and combined effects of age, breast density, and hormone replacement therapy use on the accuracy of screening mammography. Ann Intern Med 2003; 138:168–175.

96. Faulk RM, Sickles EA, Sollitto RA, et al. Clinical efficacy of mammographic screening in the elderly. Radiology 1995; 194:193.

97. Kan L, Olivotto IA, Warren Burhenne LJ, et al. Standardized abnormal interpretation and cancer detection ratios to assess reading volume and reader performance in a breast screening program. Radiology 2000; 215:563–567.

98. Randolph WM, Goodwin JS, Mahnken JD, et al. Regular mammography use is associated with elimination of age-related disparities in size and stage of breast cancer at diagnosis. Ann Intern Med 2002; 137:783–790.

99. Mandelblatt JS, Wheat ME, Monane M, et al. Breast cancer screening for elderly women with and without comorbid conditions. A decision analysis model. Ann Intern Med 1992; 116:722–730.

100. McPherson CP, Swenson KK, Lee MW. The effects of mammographic detection and comorbidity on the survival of older women with breast cancer. J Am Geriatr Soc 2002; 50:1061–1068.

101. Mandelblatt J, Saha S, Teutsch S, et al. The cost-effectiveness of screening mammography beyond age 65 years: a systematic review for the U.S. Preventive Services Task Force. Ann Intern Med 2003; 139:835–842.

102. Screening for breast cancer: recommendations and rationale. Ann Intern Med 2002; 137:344–346.

103. Smith RA, Saslow D, Sawyer KA, et al. American Cancer Society guidelines for breast cancer screening: update 2003. CA Cancer J Clin 2003; 53:141–169.

104. Van Harrison R, Janz NK, Wolfe RA, et al. Characteristics of primary care physicians and their practices associated with mammography rates for older women. Cancer 2003; 98:1811–1821.

105. Ostbye T, Greenberg GN, Taylor DH Jr, et al. Screening mammography and Pap tests among older American women 1996–2000: results from the Health and Retirement Study (HRS) and Asset and Health Dynamics Among the Oldest Old (AHEAD). Ann Fam Med 2003; 1:209–217.

106. Schonberg MA, McCarthy EP, Davis RB, et al. Breast cancer screening in women aged 80 and older: results from a national survey. J Am Geriatr Soc 2004; 52:1688–1695.

107. Harrison RV, Janz NK, Wolfe RA, et al. 5-year mammography rates and associated factors for older women. Cancer 2003; 97:1147–1155.

108. Donegan WL. Evaluation of a palpable breast mass. N Engl J Med 1992; 327:937.

109. Bassett L, Winchester DP, Caplan RB, et al. Stereotactic core-needle biopsy of the breast: a report of the Joint Task Force of the American College of Radiology, American College of Surgeons, and College of American Pathologists. CA Cancer J Clinic 1997; 47:171.

110. Parker SH, Burbank F, Jackman RJ, et al. Percutaneous large-core breast biopsy: a multi-institutional study. Radiology 1994; 193:359.

111. Parker SH, Lovin JD, Jobe WE, et al. Nonpalpable breast lesions: stereotactic automated large-core biopsies. Radiology 1991; 180:403.

112. Li CI, Daling JR, Malone KE. Age-specific incidence rates of in situ breast carcinomas by histologic type, 1980 to 2001. Cancer Epidemiol Biomarkers Prev 2005; 14:1008–1011.

113. Stomper PC, Connolly JL, Meyer JE, et al. Clinically occult ductal carcinoma in situ detected with mammography: analysis of 100 cases with radiologic–pathologic correlation. Radiology 1989; 172:235–241.

114. Allred DC, Mohsin SK, Fuqua SA. Histological and biological evolution of human premalignant breast disease. Endocr Relat Cancer 2001; 8:47–61.

115. Lakhani SR. The transition from hyperplasia to invasive carcinoma of the breast. J Pathol 1999; 187:272–278.

116. Eusebi V, Feudale E, Foschini MP, et al. Long-term follow-up of in situ carcinoma of the breast. Semin Diagn Pathol 1994; 11:223–235.

117. Page DL, Dupont WD, Rogers LW, et al. Continued local recurrence of carcinoma 15–25 years after a diagnosis of low grade ductal carcinoma in situ of the breast treated only by biopsy. Cancer 1995; 76:1197–1200.

118. Boyages J, Delaney G, Taylor R. Predictors of local recurrence after treatment of ductal carcinoma in situ: a meta-analysis. Cancer 1999; 85:616–628.

119. Ernster VL, Barclay J, Kerlikowske K, et al. Mortality among women with ductal carcinoma in situ of the breast in the population-based surveillance, epidemiology and end results program. Arch Intern Med 2000; 160:953–958.

120. Fisher B, Dignam J, Wolmark N, et al. Lumpectomy and radiation therapy for the treatment of intraductal breast cancer: findings from National Surgical Adjuvant Breast and Bowel Project B-17. J Clin Oncol 1998; 16:441–452.

121. Houghton J, George WD, Cuzick J, et al. Radiotherapy and tamoxifen in women with completely excised ductal carcinoma in situ of the breast in the UK, Australia, and New Zealand: randomised controlled trial. Lancet 2003; 362:95–102.

122. Julien JP, Bijker N, Fentiman IS, et al. Radiotherapy in breast-conserving treatment for ductal carcinoma in situ: first results of the EORTC randomised phase III trial 10853.

EORTC Breast Cancer Cooperative Group and EORTC Radiotherapy Group. Lancet 2000; 355:528–533.

123. Leonard GD, Swain SM. Ductal carcinoma in situ, complexities and challenges. J Natl Cancer Inst 2004; 96:906–920.

124. Schwartz GF. The role of excision and surveillance alone in subclinical DCIS of the breast. Oncology 1994; 8:21.

125. Fisher B, Dignam J, Wolmark N, et al. Tamoxifen in treatment of intraductal breast cancer: National Surgical Adjuvant Breast and Bowel Project B-24 randomised controlled trial. Lancet 1999; 353:1993–2000.

126. Rawal R, Lorenzo Bermejo J, Hemminki K. Risk of subsequent invasive breast carcinoma after in situ breast carcinoma in a population covered by national mammographic screening. Br J Cancer 2005; 92:162–166.

127. Claus EB, Stowe M, Carter D, et al. The risk of a contralateral breast cancer among women diagnosed with ductal and lobular breast carcinoma in situ: data from the Connecticut Tumor Registry. Breast 2003; 12:451–456.

128. Osborne MP, Hoda SA. Current management of lobular carcinoma in situ of the breast. Oncology 1994; 8:45.

129. Fisher B, Anderson S, Bryant J, et al. Twenty-year follow-up of a randomized trial comparing total mastectomy, lumpectomy, and lumpectomy plus irradiation for the treatment of invasive breast cancer. N Engl J Med 2002; 347:1233–1241.

130. Fisher B, Jeong JH, Anderson S, et al. Twenty-five-year follow-up of a randomized trial comparing radical mastectomy, total mastectomy, and total mastectomy followed by irradiation. N Engl J Med 2002; 347:567–575.

131. Samain E, Schauvliege F, Deval B, et al. Anesthesia for breast cancer surgery in the elderly. Crit Rev Oncol Hematol 2003; 46:115–120.

132. Morrow M. Breast disease in elderly women. Surg Clin North Am 1994; 74:145–161.

133. Svastics E, Sulyok Z, Besznyak I. Treatment of breast cancer in women older than 70 years. J Surg Oncol 1989; 41:19–21.

134. Lazovich DA, White E, Thomas DB, et al. Underutilization of breast-conserving surgery and radiation therapy among women with stage I or II breast cancer. JAMA 1991; 266:3433–3438.

135. Giordano SH, Hortobagyi GN, Kau SW, et al. Breast cancer treatment guidelines in older women. J Clin Oncol 2005; 23:783–791.

136. Kantorowitz DA, Poulter CA, Sischy B, et al. Treatment of breast cancer among elderly women with segmental mastectomy or segmental mastectomy plus postoperative radiotherapy. Int J Radiat Oncol Biol Phys 1988; 15:263–270.

137. Reed MW, Morrison JM. Wide local excision as the sole primary treatment in elderly patients with carcinoma of the breast. Br J Surg 1989; 76:898–900.

138. Veronesi U, Costa A. Conservative surgery in breast cancer. Ann N Y Acad Sci 1993; 698:212–218.

139. Fallowfield LJ, Hall A, Maguire P, et al. Psychological effects of being offered choice of surgery for breast cancer. BMJ 1994; 309:448.

140. Figueiredo MI, Cullen J, Hwang YT, et al. Breast cancer treatment in older women: does getting what you want improve your long-term body image and mental health? J Clin Oncol 2004; 22:4002–4009.

141. de Haes JC, Curran D, Aaronson NK, et al. Quality of life in breast cancer patients aged over 70 years, participating in the EORTC 10850 randomised clinical trial. Eur J Cancer 2003; 39:945–951.

142. Senn HJ, Thurlimann B, Goldhirsch A, et al. Comments on the St. Gallen Consensus 2003 on the Primary Therapy of Early Breast Cancer. Breast 2003; 12:569–582.

143. Veronesi U, Paganelli G, Viale G, et al. A randomized comparison of sentinel-node biopsy with routine axillary dissection in breast cancer. N Engl J Med 2003; 349: 546–553.

144. Peintinger F, Reitsamer R, Stranzl H, et al. Comparison of quality of life and arm complaints after axillary lymph node dissection versus sentinel lymph node biopsy in breast cancer patients. Br J Cancer 2003; 89:648–652.

145. Gosselink R, Rouffaer L, Vanhelden P, et al. Recovery of upper limb function after axillary dissection. J Surg Oncol 2003; 83:204–211.

146. Mandelblatt JS, Edge SB, Meropol NJ, et al. Predictors of long-term outcomes in older breast cancer survivors: perceptions versus patterns of care. J Clin Oncol 2003; 21: 855–863.

147. Motomura K, Inaji H, Komoike Y, et al. Combination technique is superior to dye alone in identification of the sentinel node in breast cancer patients. J Surg Oncol 2001; 76:95–99.

148. Harris L, Swain SM. The role of primary chemotherapy in early breast cancer. Semin Oncol 1996; 23:31–42.

149. Barth A, Craig PH, Silverstein MJ. Predictors of axillary lymph node metastases in patients with T1 breast carcinoma. Cancer 1997; 79:1918.

150. Fein DA, Fowble BL, Hanlon AL, et al. Identification of women with T1–T2 breast cancer at low risk of positive axillary nodes. J Surg Oncol 1997; 65:34.

151. Feigelson BJ, Acosta JA, Feigelson HS, et al. T1 breast carcinoma in women 70 years of age and older may not require axillary lymph node dissection. Am J Surg 1996; 172: 487–489; discussion 489–490.

152. Haffty BG, Ward B, Pathare P, et al. Reappraisal of the role of axillary lymph node dissection in the conservative treatment of breast cancer. J Clin Oncol 1997; 15:691–700.

153. Naslund E, Fernstad R, Ekman S, et al. Breast cancer in women over 75 years: is axillary dissection always necessary? Eur J Surg 1996; 162:867–871.

154. Truong PT, Bernstein V, Wai E, et al. Age-related variations in the use of axillary dissection: a survival analysis of 8038 women with T1–T2 breast cancer. Int J Radiat Oncol Biol Phys 2002; 54:794–803.

155. Martelli G, Miceli R, De Palo G, et al. Is axillary lymph node dissection necessary in elderly patients with breast carcinoma who have a clinically uninvolved axilla? Cancer 2003; 97:1156–1163.

156. Fisher B, Anderson S, Redmond CK, et al. Reanalysis and results after 12 years of follow-up in a randomized clinical trial comparing total mastectomy with lumpectomy with or without irradiation in the treatment of breast cancer. N Engl J Med 1995; 333:1456–1461.

157. Wyckoff J, Greenberg H, Sanderson R, et al. Breast irradiation in the older woman: a toxicity study. J Am Geriatr Soc 1994; 42:150–152.

158. Cutuli B, Aristei C, Martin C, et al. Breast-conserving therapy for stage I–II breast cancer in elderly women. Int J Radiat Oncol Biol Phys 2004; 60:71–76.

159. Whelan T, MacKenzie R, Julian J, et al. Randomized trial of breast irradiation schedules after lumpectomy for women with lymph node-negative breast cancer. J Natl Cancer Inst 2002; 94:1143–1150.

160. Hughes KS, Schnaper LA, Berry D, et al. Lumpectomy plus tamoxifen with or without irradiation in women 70 years of age or older with early breast cancer. N Engl J Med 2004; 351:971–977.

161. Arriagada R, Rutqvist LE, Mattsson A, et al. Adequate locoregional treatment for early breast cancer may prevent secondary dissemination. J Clin Oncol 1995; 13: 2869–2878.

162. Ellis MJ, Coop A, Singh B, et al. Letrozole is more effective neoadjuvant endocrine therapy than tamoxifen for ErbB-1- and/or ErbB-2-positive, estrogen receptor-positive primary breast cancer: evidence from a phase III randomized trial. J Clin Oncol 2001; 19:3808–3816.

163. Smith IE. Letrozole versus tamoxifen in the treatment of advanced breast cancer and as neoadjuvant therapy. J Steroid Biochem Mol Biol 2003; 86:289–293.

164. Hooper SB, Hill AD, Kennedy S, et al. Tamoxifen as the primary treatment in elderly patients with breast cancer. Ir J Med Sci 2002; 171:28–30.

165. Fowble B. An assessment of treatment options for breast conservation in the elderly woman with early stage breast cancer. Int J Radiat Oncol Biol Phys 1995; 31:1015–1017.

166. von Rueden DG, Sessions SC. Alternative therapy for elderly patients with breast cancer. Am Surg 1994; 60:72–78.

167. van Zyl JA, Muller AG. Tumour excision plus continuous tamoxifen compared with modified radical mastectomy in patients over 70 years of age with operable breast cancer. J Surg Oncol 1995; 59:151–154.

168. Fentiman IS, Christiaens MR, Paridaens R, et al. Treatment of operable breast cancer in the elderly: a randomised clinical trial EORTC 10851 comparing tamoxifen alone with modified radical mastectomy. Eur J Cancer 2003; 39:309–316.

169. Fentiman IS, van Zijl J, Karydas I, et al. Treatment of operable breast cancer in the elderly: a randomised clinical trial EORTC 10850 comparing modified radical mastectomy with tumorectomy plus tamoxifen. Eur J Cancer 2003; 39:300–308.

170. Solin LJ, Recht A, Fourquet A, et al. Ten-year results of breast-conserving surgery and definitive irradiation for intraductal carcinoma (ductal carcinoma in situ) of the breast. Cancer 1991; 68:2337–2344.

171. Wazer DE, Erban JK, Robert NJ, et al. Breast conservation in elderly women for clinically negative axillary lymph nodes without axillary dissection. Cancer 1994; 74: 878–883.

172. Maher M, Campana F, Mosseri V, et al. Breast cancer in elderly women: a retrospective analysis of combined treatment with tamoxifen and once-weekly irradiation. Int J Radiat Oncol Biol Phys 1995; 31:783–789.

173. Bates T, Riley DL, Houghton J, et al. Breast cancer in elderly women: a Cancer Research Campaign trial comparing treatment with tamoxifen and optimal surgery with tamoxifen alone. The Elderly Breast Cancer Working Party. Br J Surg 1991; 78: 591–594.

174. Dunser M, Haussler B, Fuchs H, et al. Tumorectomy plus tamoxifen for the treatment of breast cancer in the elderly. Eur J Surg Oncol 1993; 19:529–531.

175. Martelli G, Moglia D, Boracchi P, et al. Surgical resection plus tamoxifen as treatment of breast cancer in elderly patients: a retrospective study. Eur J Cancer 1993; 29A:2080–2082.

176. Odendaal Jde V, Apffelstaedt JP. Limited surgery and tamoxifen in the treatment of elderly breast cancer patients. World J Surg 2003; 27:125–129.

177. Clark RM, McCulloch PB, Levine MN, et al. Randomized clinical trial to assess the effectiveness of breast irradiation following lumpectomy and axillary dissection for node-negative breast cancer. J Natl Cancer Inst 1992; 84:683–689.

178. Akhtar SS, Allan SG, Rodger A, et al. A 10-year experience of tamoxifen as primary treatment of breast cancer in 100 elderly and frail patients. Eur J Surg Oncol 1991; 17:30–35.

179. Gazet JC, Markopoulos C, Ford HT, et al. Prospective randomised trial of tamoxifen versus surgery in elderly patients with breast cancer. Lancet 1988; 1:679–681.

180. Horobin JM, Preece PE, Dewar JA, et al. Long-term follow-up of elderly patients with locoregional breast cancer treated with tamoxifen only. Br J Surg 1991; 78:213–217.

181. Robertson JF, Ellis IO, Elston CW, et al. Mastectomy or tamoxifen as initial therapy for operable breast cancer in elderly patients: 5-year follow-up. Eur J Cancer 1992; 28A:908–910.

182. Gazet JC, Ford HT, Coombes RC, et al. Prospective randomized trial of tamoxifen versus surgery in elderly patients with breast cancer. Eur J Surg Oncol 1994; 20:207–214.

183. Mustacchi G, Ceccherini R, Milani S, et al. Tamoxifen alone versus adjuvant tamoxifen for operable breast cancer of the elderly: long-term results of the phase III randomized controlled multicenter GRETA trial. Ann Oncol 2003; 14:414–420.

184. Fennessy M, Bates T, MacRae K, et al. Late follow-up of a randomized trial of surgery plus tamoxifen versus tamoxifen alone in women aged over 70 years with operable breast cancer. Br J Surg 2004; 91:699–704.
185. Allan SG, Rodger A, Smyth JF, et al. Tamoxifen as primary treatment of breast cancer in elderly or frail patients: a practical management. Br Med J (Clin Res Ed) 1985; 290:358.
186. Bergman L, van Dongen JA, van Ooijen B, et al. Should tamoxifen be a primary treatment choice for elderly breast cancer patients with locoregional disease? Breast Cancer Res Treat 1995; 34:77–83.
187. Ciatto S, Bartoli D, Iossa A, et al. Response of primary breast cancer to tamoxifen alone in elderly women. Tumori 1991; 77:328–330.
188. Ciatto S, Cirillo A, Confortini M, et al. Tamoxifen as primary treatment of breast cancer in elderly patients. Neoplasma 1996; 43:43–45.
189. Mustacchi G, Milani S, Pluchinotta A, et al. Tamoxifen or surgery plus tamoxifen as primary treatment for elderly patients with operable breast cancer: The G.R.E.T.A. Trial. Group for Research on Endocrine Therapy in the Elderly. Anticancer Res 1994; 14:2197–2200.
190. Preece PE, Wood RA, Mackie CR, et al. Tamoxifen as initial sole treatment of localised breast cancer in elderly women: a pilot study. Br Med J (Clin Res Ed) 1982; 284: 869–870.
191. Robertson JF, Todd JH, Ellis IO, et al. Comparison of mastectomy with tamoxifen for treating elderly patients with operable breast cancer. BMJ 1988; 297:511–514.
192. van Dalsen AD, de Vries JE. Treatment of breast cancer in elderly patients. J Surg Oncol 1995; 60:80–82.
193. Salmon RJ, Remvikos Y, Campana F, et al. Neo adjuvant Tamoxifen in post menopausal patients with operable breast cancer. Eur J Surg Oncol 2003; 29:831–834.
194. Rostom AY, Pradhan DG, White WF. Once weekly irradiation in breast cancer. Int J Radiat Oncol Biol Phys 1987; 13:551–555.
195. Hellman S, Harris JR, Harris JR, et al. Natural History of Breast Cancer, Diseases of the Breast. Philadelphia: Lippincott Williams & Wilkins, 2000:407.
196. Castiglione M, Gelber RD, Goldhirsch A. Adjuvant systemic therapy for breast cancer in the elderly: competing causes of mortality. International Breast Cancer Study Group. J Clin Oncol 1990; 8:519–526.
197. Cummings FJ, Gray R, Tormey DC, et al. Adjuvant tamoxifen versus placebo in elderly women with node-positive breast cancer: long-term follow-up and causes of death. J Clin Oncol 1993; 11:29–35.
198. Aapro MS. Adjuvant therapy of primary breast cancer: a review of key findings from the 7th International Conference, St. Gallen, February 2001. Oncologist 2001; 6:376–385.
199. Carlson RW, Edge SB, Theriault RL. NCCN: breast cancer. Cancer Control 2001; 8:54–61.
200. Adjuvant Therapy for Breast Cancer. NIH Consensus Statement, 2000; 17:1.
201. Effects of chemotherapy and hormonal therapy for early breast cancer on recurrence and 15-year survival: an overview of the randomised trials. Lancet 2005; 365:1687–1717.
202. Baum M, Budzar AU, Cuzick J, et al. Anastrozole alone or in combination with tamoxifen versus tamoxifen alone for adjuvant treatment of postmenopausal women with early breast cancer: first results of the ATAC randomised trial. Lancet 2002; 359: 2131–2139.
203. Coombes RC, Hall E, Gibson LJ, et al. A randomized trial of exemestane after two to three years of tamoxifen therapy in postmenopausal women with primary breast cancer. N Engl J Med 2004; 350:1081–1092.
204. Goss PE, Ingle JN, Martino S, et al. A randomized trial of letrozole in postmenopausal women after five years of tamoxifen therapy for early-stage breast cancer. N Engl J Med 2003; 349:1793–1802.

205. Winer EP, Hudis C, Burstein HJ, et al. American Society of Clinical Oncology technology assessment on the use of aromatase inhibitors as adjuvant therapy for postmenopausal women with hormone receptor-positive breast cancer: status report 2004. J Clin Oncol 2005; 23:619–629.

206. Braithwaite RS, Chlebowski RT, Lau J, et al. Meta-analysis of vascular and neoplastic events associated with tamoxifen. J Gen Intern Med 2003; 18:937–947.

207. Dignam JJ, Fisher B. Occurrence of stroke with tamoxifen in NSABP B-24. Lancet 2000; 355:848–849.

208. Muss HB, Thor AD, Berry DA, et al. c-erbB-2 expression and response to adjuvant therapy in women with node-positive early breast cancer. N Engl J Med 1994; 330:1260–1266.

209. Wright C, Nicholson S, Angus B, et al. Relationship between c-erbB-2 protein product expression and response to endocrine therapy in advanced breast cancer. Br J Cancer 1992; 65:118–121.

210. Houston SJ, Plunkett TA, Barnes DM, et al. Overexpression of c-erbB2 is an independent marker of resistance to endocrine therapy in advanced breast cancer. Br J Cancer 1999; 79:1220–1226.

211. Jukkola A, Bloigu R, Soini Y, et al. c-erbB-2 positivity is a factor for poor prognosis in breast cancer and poor response to hormonal or chemotherapy treatment in advanced disease. Eur J Cancer 2001; 37:347–354.

212. Demissie S, Silliman RA, Lash TL. Adjuvant tamoxifen: predictors of use, side effects, and discontinuation in older women. J Clin Oncol 2001; 19:322–328.

213. Blackman SB, Lash TL, Fink AK, et al. Advanced age and adjuvant tamoxifen prescription in early-stage breast carcinoma patients. Cancer 2002; 95:2465–2472.

214. Silliman RA, Guadagnoli E, Rakowski W, et al. Adjuvant tamoxifen prescription in women 65 years and older with primary breast cancer. J Clin Oncol 2002; 20:2680–2688.

215. Fink AK, Gurwitz J, Rakowski W, et al. Patient beliefs and tamoxifen discontinuance in older women with estrogen receptor–positive breast cancer. J Clin Oncol 2004; 22:3309–3315.

216. Fisher B, Jeong JH, Bryant J, et al. Treatment of lymph-node-negative, oestrogen-receptor-positive breast cancer: long-term findings from National Surgical Adjuvant Breast and Bowel Project randomised clinical trials. Lancet 2004; 364:858–868.

217. Boccardo F, Rubagotti A, Amoroso D, et al. Chemotherapy versus tamoxifen versus chemotherapy plus tamoxifen in node-positive, oestrogen-receptor positive breast cancer patients. An update at 7 years of the 1st GROCTA (Breast Cancer Adjuvant Chemo-Hormone Therapy Cooperative Group) trial. Eur J Cancer 1992; 28:673–680.

218. Bonadonna G, Valagussa P, Brambilla C, et al. Primary chemotherapy in operable breast cancer: eight-year experience at the Milan Cancer Institute. J Clin Oncol 1998; 16:93–100.

219. Fisher B, Dignam J, Wolmark N, et al. Tamoxifen and chemotherapy for lymph node-negative, estrogen receptor-positive breast cancer. J Natl Cancer Inst 1997; 89:1673–1682.

220. Fisher B, Redmond C, Legault-Poisson S, et al. Postoperative chemotherapy and tamoxifen compared with tamoxifen alone in the treatment of positive-node breast cancer patients aged 50 years and older with tumors responsive to tamoxifen: results from the National Surgical Adjuvant Breast and Bowel Project B-16. J Clin Oncol 1990; 8:1005–1018.

221. Taylor SGt, Knuiman MW, Sleeper LA, et al. Six-year results of the Eastern Cooperative Oncology Group trial of observation versus CMFP versus CMFPT in postmenopausal patients with node-positive breast cancer. J Clin Oncol 1989; 7:879–889.

222. DeMichele A, Putt M, Zhang Y, et al. Older age predicts a decline in adjuvant chemotherapy recommendations for patients with breast carcinoma: evidence from a tertiary care cohort of chemotherapy-eligible patients. Cancer 2003; 97:2150–2159.

223. Singh R, Hellman S, Heimann R. The natural history of breast carcinoma in the elderly: implications for screening and treatment. Cancer 2004; 100:1807–1813.

224. Woodard S, Nadella PC, Kotur L, et al. Older women with breast carcinoma are less likely to receive adjuvant chemotherapy: evidence of possible age bias? Cancer 2003; 98:1141–1149.

225. Henderson IC, Hayes DF, Gelman R. Dose–response in the treatment of breast cancer: a critical review. J Clin Oncol 1988; 6:1501–1515.

226. Hryniuk WM, Levine MN, Levin L. Analysis of dose intensity for chemotherapy in early (stage II) and advanced breast cancer. NCI Monogr 1986:87–94.

227. Muss HB, Woolf S, Berry D, et al. Adjuvant chemotherapy in older and younger women with lymph node-positive breast cancer. JAMA 2005; 293:1073–1081.

228. Begg CB, Cohen JL, Ellerton J. Are the elderly predisposed to toxicity from cancer chemotherapy? An investigation using data from the Eastern Cooperative Oncology Group. Cancer Clin Trials 1980; 3:369–374.

229. Christman K, Muss HB, Case LD, et al. Chemotherapy of metastatic breast cancer in the elderly. The Piedmont Oncology Association experience [see comment]. JAMA 1992; 268:57–62.

230. Muss H, Cooper MR, Hoen H, et al. Adjuvant chemotherapy in older women with node positive breast cancer: The Piedmont Oncology Association experience. Proc Am Soc Clin Oncol 1992; 11:12x.

231. Endocrine responsiveness and tailoring adjuvant therapy for postmenopausal lymph node-negative breast cancer: a randomized trial. J Natl Cancer Inst 2002; 94: 1054–1065.

232. Pritchard KI, Paterson AH, Fine S, et al. Randomized trial of cyclophosphamide, methotrexate, and fluorouracil chemotherapy added to tamoxifen as adjuvant therapy in postmenopausal women with node-positive estrogen and/or progesterone receptor-positive breast cancer: a report of the National Cancer Institute of Canada Clinical Trials Group. Breast Cancer Site Group. J Clin Oncol 1997; 15:2302–2311.

233. Fisher B, Redmond C, Fisher ER, et al. Systemic adjuvant therapy in treatment of primary operable breast cancer: National Surgical Adjuvant Breast and Bowel Project experience. NCI Monogr 1986; 1:35–43.

234. Effectiveness of adjuvant chemotherapy in combination with tamoxifen for node-positive postmenopausal breast cancer patients. International Breast Cancer Study Group. J Clin Oncol 1997; 15:1385–1394.

235. Hebert-Croteau N, Brisson J, Latreille J, et al. Compliance with consensus recommendations for systemic therapy is associated with improved survival of women with node-negative breast cancer. J Clin Oncol 2004; 22:3685–3693.

236. de Bock GH, Bonnema J, van der Hage J, et al. Effectiveness of routine visits and routine tests in detecting isolated locoregional recurrences after treatment for early-stage invasive breast cancer: a meta-analysis and systematic review. J Clin Oncol 2004; 22:4010–4018.

237. Impact of follow-up testing on survival and health-related quality of life in breast cancer patients. A multicenter randomized controlled trial. The GIVIO Investigators. JAMA 1994; 271:1587–1592.

238. Palli D, Russo A, Saieva C, et al. Intensive vs. clinical follow-up after treatment of primary breast cancer: 10-year update of a randomized trial. National Research Council Project on Breast Cancer Follow-up. JAMA 1999; 281:1586.

239. Ganz PA, Guadagnoli E, Landrum MB, et al. Breast cancer in older women: quality of life and psychosocial adjustment in the 15 months after diagnosis. J Clin Oncol 2003; 21:4027–4033.

240. Earle CC, Burstein HJ, Winer EP, et al. Quality of non-breast cancer health maintenance among elderly breast cancer survivors. J Clin Oncol 2003; 21:1447–1451.

241. Kimmick GG, Muss HB. Endocrine therapy in metastatic breast cancer. Cancer Treat Res 1998; 94:231–254.

242. Kiang DT, Gay J, Goldman A, et al. A randomized trial of chemotherapy and hormonal therapy in advanced breast cancer. N Engl J Med 1985; 313:1241–1246.
243. Taylor SGt, Gelman RS, Falkson G, et al. Combination chemotherapy compared to tamoxifen as initial therapy for stage IV breast cancer in elderly women. Ann Intern Med 1986; 104:455–461.
244. A randomized trial in postmenopausal patients with advanced breast cancer comparing endocrine and cytotoxic therapy given sequentially or in combination. The Australian and New Zealand Breast Cancer Trials Group, Clinical Oncological Society of Australia. J Clin Oncol 1986; 4:186–193.
245. Christman K, Muss HB, Case LD, et al. The relationship of age to treatment response in women with advanced breast cancer: The Piedmont Oncology Association (POA) experience. Proc Am Soc Clin Oncol 1991; 10:85.
246. Begg CB, Elson PJ, Carbone PP, et al. A Study of Excess Hematologic Toxicity in Elderly Patients Treated on Chemotherapy Protocols, Cancer in the Elderly: Approaches to Early Detection and Management. New York, NY: Springer-Verlag, 1989:149.
247. Gelman RS, Taylor SGt. Cyclophosphamide, methotrexate, and 5-fluorouracil chemotherapy in women more than 65 years old with advanced breast cancer: the elimination of age trends in toxicity by using doses based on creatinine clearance. J Clin Oncol 1984; 2:1404–1413.
248. Von Hoff DD, Layard MW, Basa P, et al. Risk factors for doxorubicin-induced congestive heart failure. Ann Intern Med 1979; 91:710–717.
249. Schuchter LM, Hensley ML, Meropol NJ, et al. 2002 update of recommendations for the use of chemotherapy and radiotherapy protectants: clinical practice guidelines of the American Society of Clinical Oncology. J Clin Oncol 2002; 20:2895–2903.
250. Swain SM, Whaley FS, Gerber MC, et al. Delayed administration of dexrazoxane provides cardioprotection for patients with advanced breast cancer treated with doxorubicin-containing therapy. J Clin Oncol 1997; 15:1333–1340.
251. Swain SM, Whaley FS, Gerber MC, et al. Cardioprotection with dexrazoxane for doxorubicin-containing therapy in advanced breast cancer. J Clin Oncol 1997; 15:1318–1332.
252. Benjamin RS. Rationale for the use of mitoxantrone in the older patient: cardiac toxicity. Semin Oncol 1995; 22:11–13.
253. Hainsworth JD. The use of mitoxantrone in the treatment of breast cancer. Semin Oncol 1995; 22:17–20.
254. Ibrahim NK, Frye DK, Buzdar AU, et al. Doxorubicin-based chemotherapy in elderly patients with metastatic breast cancer. Tolerance and outcome. Arch Intern Med 1996; 156:882–888.
255. Gianni L, Capri G, Munzone E, et al. Paclitaxel (Taxol) efficacy in patients with advanced breast cancer resistant to anthracyclines. Semin Oncol 1994; 21:29–33.
256. Holmes FA, Walters RS, Theriault RL, et al. Phase II trial of Taxol, an active drug in the treatment of metastatic breast cancer. J Natl Cancer Inst 1991; 83:1797–1805.
257. Ravdin PM, Burris HA 3rd, Cook G, et al. Phase II trial of docetaxel in advanced anthracycline-resistant or anthracenedione-resistant breast cancer. J Clin Oncol 1995; 13:2879–2885.
258. Valero V, Holmes FA, Walters RS, et al. Phase II trial of docetaxel: a new, highly effective antineoplastic agent in the management of patients with anthracycline-resistant metastatic breast cancer. J Clin Oncol 1995; 13:2886–2894.
259. Bicher A, Sarosy G, Kohn E, et al. Age does not influence Taxol dose intensity in recurrent carcinoma of the ovary. Cancer 1993; 71:594–600.
260. Marty M, Extra JM, Dieras V, et al. A review of the antitumour activity of vinorelbine in breast cancer. Drugs 1992; 44(suppl 4):29–35; discussion 66–69.
261. Weber BL, Vogel C, Jones S, et al. Intravenous vinorelbine as first-line and second-line therapy in advanced breast cancer. J Clin Oncol 1995; 13:2722–2730.

262. Sorio R, Robieux I, Galligioni E, et al. Pharmacokinetics and tolerance of vinorelbine in elderly patients with metastatic breast cancer. Eur J Cancer 1997; 33:301–303.
263. Vogel C, O'Rourke M, Winer E, et al. Vinorelbine as first-line chemotherapy for advanced breast cancer in women 60 years of age or older. Ann Oncol 1999; 10:397–402.
264. Rossi A, Gridelli C, Gebbia V, et al. Single agent vinorelbine as first-line chemotherapy in elderly patients with advanced breast cancer. Anticancer Res 2003; 23:1657–1664.
265. Dinota A, Bilancia D, Romano R, et al. Biweekly administration of gemcitabine and vinorelbine as first line therapy in elderly advanced breast cancer. Breast Cancer Res Treat 2005; 89:1–3.
266. Bajetta E, Procopio G, Celio L, et al. Safety and efficacy of two different doses of capecitabine in the treatment of advanced breast cancer in older women. J Clin Oncol 2005; 23:2155–2161.
267. Rose JH, O'Toole EE, Dawson NV, et al. Perspectives, preferences, care practices, and outcomes among older and middle-aged patients with late-stage cancer. J Clin Oncol 2004; 22:4907–4917.

11

Lung Cancer in the Elderly

Sabrina M. Witherby and Steven M. Grunberg
University of Vermont, Vermont Cancer Center, Burlington, Vermont, U.S.A.

INTRODUCTION

Lung cancer holds a unique but contradictory position among the solid tumors. Although not the most common tumor in terms of incidence or prevalence, the tendency toward a more advanced stage at presentation as well as the short median survival (MS) of patients with this tumor has made lung cancer a particularly lethal problem. In fact, lung cancer has long been the leading cause of cancer death in men, and, since 1987, has also been the leading cause of cancer death in women. Although the incidence of lung cancer is stable in women and decreasing in men, it remains the number one cause of cancer-related mortality in men older than 40 and in women older than 60 years in the United States. With the growth and aging of the population, both the relative and total numbers of elderly patients with lung cancer are expected to rise significantly (1).

EPIDEMIOLOGY AND SCREENING

Lung cancer is predominantly related to chemical carcinogen exposure and has an extended period between first exposure and development of the tumor. Approaches to this tumor (including efforts directed at prevention, detection, and treatment) are therefore by necessity directed at different age groups. Most cases of lung cancer are related to smoking, and most chronic smokers began smoking before reaching adulthood. Efforts for prevention, including increased education and increased taxation (to reduce the affordability of cigarettes), are primarily directed at the young adult and preadult populations. Smoking cessation programs, which may include both pharmacological and behavioral interventions, are then aimed at the young adult and adult populations. However, since the appearance of lung cancer itself is directly related to carcinogen exposure, as expressed in the combined intensity and duration of smoking (pack-years), lung cancer screening, detection, and treatment become greater considerations as the population increases in age. In fact, more than half the patients diagnosed with lung cancer are more than 65 years of age (2).

Although the increased incidence of lung cancer in the elderly might therefore appear to be the natural end point of a continuum, certain features of lung cancer as observed in the older population might be important in terms of detection and treatment. Over the past several decades, adenocarcinoma has become the most common form of lung cancer. Historically, elderly patients have had a higher incidence of squamous carcinoma, which was more often centrally located and associated with a better performance status (1,2). O'Rourke et al. reviewed a database of 22,874 lung cancer cases present in a centralized registry. Lung cancer was localized at the time of diagnosis in only 15.3% of patients less than 55 years of age, but was localized in 25.4% of patients over 74 years of age. Kuo et al. studied 160 Taiwanese lung cancer patients older than 80 years and 60 patients younger than 40 years (3). The most common presenting symptom in the elderly was cough, followed by dyspnea, hemoptysis, chest pain, no symptoms, and finally weight loss. Most elderly patients presented with Stage III or Stage IV disease (35.9% and 32.1%), and adenocarcinoma was more frequently seen than squamous cell carcinoma. Montella et al. studied 1035 lung cancer patients and found no difference in the stage of disease, histology, and performance status at diagnosis in elderly patients when compared to their younger counterparts (4).

Other factors such as diet have been considered as possible contributors to the genesis of lung cancer. Shibata et al. (5) followed 5080 elderly male subjects for eight years and found a reduced risk of lung cancer for subjects with a high consumption of beta-carotene. A strong inverse relationship was found between dietary beta-carotene and smoking status, but the dietary factor did not have an independent effect on lung cancer incidence when adjusted for smoking. Later data from the Beta Carotene and Retinol Efficacy Trial (CARET) trial have confirmed that beta-carotene use is associated with higher cancer risk in smokers, although the increased risk may be limited to women (6,7).

Since squamous cell carcinoma has a predictably strong correlation with smoking, this factor deserves to be further examined. Hoffman et al. (7) noted a 30% to 50% decrease in the risk of developing lung cancer in subjects smoking filtered cigarettes as compared to nonfiltered cigarettes which has been contested in a later study by Brook et al. (8) Theoretically, the incidence of squamous cell carcinoma in the present elderly population could be explained by the fact that these patients began smoking before the introduction of filtered cigarettes and therefore had a more intense carcinogen exposure. If this particular facet of smoking behavior is indeed critical, then the frequent observation of squamous cell carcinoma of the lung in the elderly population should persist at least through the early decades of the 21st century. On the other hand, if the incidence of squamous cell lung cancer in the elderly population merely reflects the fact that older patients have smoked for a longer period of time and therefore generally have a greater overall (pack-year) exposure, then the increased incidence of squamous cell carcinoma in this population will continue and will not be modified by the present cigarette type or composition.

Screening using either chest radiograph or sputum cytology is generally not considered of value in lung cancer. The large-scale lung cancer detection trials sponsored by the National Cancer Institute (NCI) in the 1970s at Johns Hopkins University in Baltimore, MD (10), Memorial Sloan-Kettering Cancer Center in New York City (11), and the Mayo Clinic in Rochester, Minnesota (12), documented an increase in benchmark survival but not an increase in overall survival, and they therefore are considered to reflect lead-time bias and length-related sampling. However, screening for lung cancer in the elderly might be more effective than in younger patients because the risk of developing lung cancer in this population is higher. The risk of developing lung cancer at less than 40 years of age is 0.03%, for 40 to 59 years the risk is 1.06% in men and 0.81% in women, and from 60 to 79 years the risk is 5.75% in men (1 in 17) and 3.91% in women (1 in 26) (1).

This target population can be further enriched by the consideration of pulmonary function tests and pulmonary symptomatology. DeMaria and Cohen (10) noted that dyspnea (a central symptom) is more common in an elderly population with lung cancer, whereas chest pain (a peripheral symptom) tends to be seen in a younger population. Identification of dyspnea as a particularly important symptom would also support the observation that abnormal spirometry (reduced airflow) is a stronger predictor of development of lung cancer than either pack-years of smoking exposure or age (11). Petty has therefore suggested an algorithm in which smokers with abnormal spirometry and symptoms of cough, wheeze, or dyspnea are considered to be a high-risk group more appropriate for intensive lung cancer screening (12).

A systematic review by Humphrey for the U.S. Preventative Task Force, however, examined studies up to 2003 and found little clear evidence to recommend screening in any particular population. The few randomized and case control studies evaluated by them were not limited to an older population. Most were 45 years of age and older, and some did have an upper age limit. Most studies were for screening with chest X-rays. They showed the detection of lung cancer at an earlier stage in the screened population, but there was limited information on the relationship between screening and mortality. Given the lack of clear evidence, further testing should be done in the elderly population. Hopefully the results of the multicenter screening study for prostate, lung, ovarian and colorectal cancers will be empowered to provide further information on the efficacy of screening an elderly cohort.

In addition to chest radiography, screening computed tomographies and sputum cytology may be of use in the elderly. The value of induced sputum cytology has been emphasized by Jack et al. (13), who noted a 58% sensitivity and 100% specificity for induced sputum cytology in the detection of lung cancer in an older population.

TREATMENT

Surgery

Surgical resection is the recommended therapy for patients with Stage I-III non-small-cell lung cancer (NSCLC). However, surgery is not offered to the elderly as frequently, nor are the elderly as frequently enrolled in trials, making it difficult to fully assess what treatment is most appropriate. Major limitations for the use of surgery in the general population include the infrequency in detecting lung cancer at a localized stage [only approximately one-fourth of lung cancer cases are detected while still resectable (14,15)] and that the main environmental risk factor for lung cancer (smoking) also induces both cardiovascular and pulmonary comorbid conditions that independently increase the risk of surgery.

Smith et al., using data from the Virginia Cancer Registry (1985–1989) and Medicare claims records, found that the elderly are still much less likely to be offered surgery as initial therapy (16). In reviewing 2812 cases, the use of surgery as all or part of the initial therapy was found to decrease from 44% in patients aged 65 to 69 years to 6% in those over 85 years. This did not represent increased use of radiotherapy as a less aggressive alternative for primary treatment of lung cancer but rather the tendency to give no therapy at all. Patients receiving no therapy increased from 11% in the 65- to 69-year age group to 52.3% in patients over 85 years of age, whereas the use of radiotherapy alone as primary therapy remained at a relatively constant frequency throughout all the age groups considered. This decreased use of surgery is confirmed in several recent studies, including a 2004 review of Surveillance, Epidemiology and End Results (SEER) data from 1996, in patients with Stages I and II disease by Potosky et al., where lobectomy or pneumonectomy is the recommended treatment. This study showed that 75% of patients under 50 years of age received appropriate surgical resection; this percentage dropped for every five-year increase in age, and only 32% of patients between 75 and 94 years of age were resected as recommended (some patients received limited operations, radiotherapy alone, or no treatment) (14,17–19).

O'Connell et al., using data from the SEER from 1988 to 1997, showed that surgical resection of nine types of localized cancers was considerably less common in the elderly. Data on 200,360 patients with local-stage breast, esophageal, stomach, pancreatic, colon, and rectal cancers, sarcoma, and NSCLC were reviewed, and in all cancer types except breast, colon, and rectal cancers there were statistically significant decreases in "cancer-directed surgery" as age increased. This was particularly marked in NSCLC. Across all ages, surgery was used in 66.9% of patients. The odds ratio of receiving surgery starts to decline after age 60. The highest use of surgery, occurs in people between the ages of 45 and 49 with an odds ratio of 1.66. Between the ages of 60 and 64 the odds ratio drops to 0.55. It drops steadily thereafter: 0.45 from 65 to 69; 0.36 from 70 to 74; 0.23 from 75 to 79; 0.10 from 80 to 84; 0.04 from 85 to 89; and 0.02 from 90 years and older. The P values for patients under 60 years of age are not statistically significant, but are between 0.031 and < 0.0001 thereafter. The SEER database did not include information on the number and severity of comorbidities. O'Connell, however, notes that the reason for not undergoing surgery was similar for patients "refusing" ($<13.1\%$) and "contraindicated" ($<21.5\%$) across tumor types, but in cancers where the elderly were less likely to receive surgery, the rate of surgery being "not recommended" was increased (e.g., lung cancer, 17.1%). There is a trend for age to be the strongest predictor of surgery being "not recommended," which becomes statistically significant across cancer types at the age range 75 to 79 years. It is difficult to ascertain how appropriate this decrease in surgery is without further information on patients' situations and comorbidities. The authors recommend that greater emphasis and future studies focus on preoperative evaluation and assessment of comorbidities rather than age.

The question, therefore, remains as to why the elderly are less likely to be offered surgery as primary therapy. The argument that curative surgery would not make a difference in overall survival due to the limited life expectancy of elderly patients must be rejected, because the average survival of older adults exceeds the average survival of patients with uncontrolled cancer (20). Comorbid conditions do tend to increase with age and might therefore increase the risk of surgery. Increasing comorbidity and increasing age, however, are not necessarily synonymous. These two factors must be separated to identify patient populations where surgery can be safely and successfully performed regardless of advancing age. The best place to evaluate this would be in surgical trials. A recent review of surgical study enrollment across three major U.S. surgical trial groups showed lower rates of inclusion for elderly patients, including enrollment for lung cancer trials. Although 68.1% of lung cancer patients were over 64, the American College of Surgeons Oncology Group studies averaged 53.4% elderly patients, and the Southwest Oncology Group (SWOG) averaged 39% elderly patients. Data from NCI studies were difficult to evaluate as age was broken down into patients younger than 50 years, 50 years and 50 years and older, with the latter comprising 91% of patients.

It is likely that fewer older patients are treated with surgical resection based on early surgical studies showing increased perioperative morbidity and mortality in the older population. More recent studies, however, have shown equal outcomes for the elderly. A possible explanation for this difference is that earlier studies used univariate analysis, as opposed to multivariate analysis, which did not allow them to tease out the effect of age from that of comorbidity, as well as improvements in surgical techniques, selection of patients, and perioperative care.

In a study of 500 patients reported in 1983 by Ginsberg et al., postoperative mortality rates were as much as six times higher in patients over 70 years of age compared to patients under 60 years of age, by univariate analysis (21). Whittle et al. reviewed Medicare data on 1290 patients who underwent surgical resection for lung cancer between 1983 and 1985 (22). The perioperative death rate in this group was 7.4%, with a one-year survival of 69% and a two-year survival of 54%. Subset analysis, however, revealed an increased perioperative death rate and decreased one- and two-year survival in older patients, as well as in male patients and patients undergoing pneumonectomy. In 1987, Sherman and Guidot reviewed 139 cases of patients undergoing lung resection (23). Older patients ($\geq$70 years) had a poorer pulmonary function and more serious comorbidities, and their operative mortality was 9.4% compared to 4.0% in the younger group. No statistically significant difference in postoperative complications, hospital stay, or actuarial survival was found. Cardiopulmonary status was considered to be the most important predictive factor for successful surgery. Damhuis and Schutte reviewed 7899 cases of lung cancer between 1984 and 1992 to determine resection rate and 30-day postoperative mortality. Resection was more likely to be performed in patients under 70 years of age (26%) than those over 70 years of age (14%), and pneumonectomies were performed in 27% of the patients over 70 years of age as compared to 37% of the patients under 70 years of age. Multivariate analysis revealed a significant risk due to both increased age and increased extent of surgery, with a trend to increased perioperative mortality rising with age, from 1.4% in patients under 60 years of age to 3.5% in patients between 60 and 69 years of age, and 4.0% in those over 69 years of age ($P = 0.06$). This trend toward increased mortality for older patients was not considered to be striking, and the risk was considered to be acceptable for the types of surgery performed (24).

The majority of the surgical literature suggests that comorbid conditions rather than age are the deciding factors as to whether surgical resection should be offered to patients with lung cancer. Knott-Craig et al. (25) pointed out that the mortality rate for aggressive lung resection in a general population can run from 3% to 6%, whereas notable morbidity may be seen in 15% to 30% of the population. By comparison, their results of 4.8% mortality and 17.9% morbidity in 41 patients over 70 years of age are quite reasonable. Namikawa et al. (26) reviewed the records of 128 patients over 75 years of age undergoing pulmonary resection for lung cancer. Perioperative (30-day) mortality in this group was only 2.3%. An increase in the death rate two to six months later was attributed to non-cancer-related causes. Breyer et al. (27) reviewed 218 thoracotomies (166 for lung cancer) and noted a death rate of 3% and a complication rate of 34%. However, complications were related to the amount of lung removed, congestive heart failure, and prior lung surgery, with age and sex not considered to be significant factors. Roxburgh et al. (28) summarized a series of 370 patients referred for terminal lung cancer, 179 of whom were operable. Hospital mortality was increased in older (more than 70 years) patients compared to younger patients, with a rate of 4.7% compared to 1.9% for patients undergoing lobectomy and 9.1% compared to 6.2% for patients undergoing pneumonectomy. However, two- and four-year survival rates adjusted for stage were equivalent between the two groups, and surgery was considered to be an acceptable primary therapy. Ishida et al. (29) reviewed 185 cases of patients over 70 years of age undergoing resection for lung cancer. Operative mortality was 3%, and the five-year survival was 48%. Pulmonary complications were predicted by poor presurgical pulmonary function tests and by smoking history in both younger and older groups. Careful evaluation of pulmonary function tests for obstructive or restrictive defects was suggested as being the main factor in determining whether aggressive surgery would be feasible. Cangemi et al. (30) reported a similar postoperative death rate for older and younger patients (4.8% vs. 3%), whereas Jie et al. (31) reviewed 920 cases of NSCLC who under went surgery between 1969 and 1985, and noted no difference in survival based either on tumor histology or on age. Santambrogio et al. (32) reported a prospective series of patients with Stage I or II NSCLC who were treated between 1986 and 1991. There were 519 patients, of whom 54 were over the age of 70. Operative morbidity was only slightly worse in the older group (7.4% vs. 6.9%), as was operative mortality (5.5% vs. 1.3%). Two- and five-year survival for Stage I patients were comparable between groups. van Rens et al. reviewed postoperative survival in 2263 patients who had resection of Stages I, II, and IIIA lung cancer between 1970 and 1992. They found that patients over 65 years of age had a worse overall survival (38% vs. 44%, $P = 0.001$), but survival curves did not differ until four years. This caused them to suggest that increased morbidity was likely due to comorbidities, not lung cancer, and that aggressive surgical treatment in appropriately selected elderly patients was warranted (33).

Octogenarians might be considered to be at particular risk due to increased comorbidity. However, several series have not supported this idea. Shirakusa et al. (34) reported 32 patients over the age of 80 years, of whom 21 underwent lobectomy and three, pneumonectomy. There were no perioperative deaths (within 30 days), whereas the five-year survival for Stage I patients was 79%, and the five-year survival for Stage II patients was 31%. These investigators concluded that the surgical decision should be based on the stage of disease and cardiopulmonary status, rather than age. Pagni et al. (35) reported 54 octogenarians who underwent lung surgery. A lesser but appropriate resection (42 lobectomies and 1 pneumonectomy) was favored, and 3.7% operative mortality and 11% major complications were reported. Survival for all 52 patients discharged from hospital was 86% at one year, 62% at three years, and 42% at five years. For the 39 patients with Stage I disease, the one-year survival was 97%, three-year survival was 78%, and five-year survival was 57%. An aggressive surgical approach (short of pneumonectomy) was therefore suggested for healthy octogenarian patients with Stage I disease. Shimamoto reported on the subset of 34 octogenarians resected for lung cancer from a larger review of all patients resected between 1957 and 1996. He noted that overall survival was comparable among younger and older patients. Many older patients had a more limited resection, due to presence of one or more comorbidities. However, these patients (12/34) had better five-year survival and quality of life (36). Birim et al. reviewed both perioperative and overall survival in 126 patients over the age of 70. They found that the operative mortality (3.2%) was in the same range as that for their younger patients. There was an increase in postoperative morbidity; however, the only risk factor for major complications among these elderly patients was a Charlson comorbidity index score of 3 to 4. Overall survival was worse in patients who smoked and had chronic obstructive pulmonary disease or more advanced pathological stage (IIIA and IIIB), but was not affected by type of resection, histology, sex, forced expiratory volume in the second one, cardiac disease, or Charlson comorbidity index. Over time, survival rates approached those of the general population. The authors concluded that if a strict selection protocol is followed, the perioperative morbidity and mortality of resection for NSCLC will be acceptable, and long-term survival rates will be good.

In addition to careful assessment of comorbidities, several authors recommend a comprehensive geriatric assessment as an important component of preoperative evaluation (37,38). Fukuse et al. did a prospective study of thoracic surgery in 120 patients over the age of 59 years (range: 60–84 years, 89 of whom had lung cancer) who were preoperatively evaluated with comprehensive geriatric assessment. They found that postoperative complications were increased in patients with dependent Activities of Daily Livings (ADLs) as measured by the Barthel index, which was also found to be more predictive than was performance status [by Eastern Cooperative Oncology Group (ECOG) or Karnofsky scales]. They found that dementia, as assessed on a Mini-Mental Status Examination (MMSE), was predictive of postoperative mortality (56% vs. 14%), especially transient postoperative delirium. They recommend that a comprehensive geriatric assessment with the Barthel index and MMSE be added to cardiopulmonary functional assessment in preoperative assessment of elderly patients.

Newer techniques and more aggressive postoperative management can also contribute to improved survival. Knott-Craig et al. (25) described a perioperative protocol for patients undergoing resection for lung cancer that included preoperative digitalis, subcutaneous heparin, veno-occlusive stockings, and aggressive pulmonary toilet. This program resulted in a mortality rate of 4.8% and a morbidity rate of 17.9% in 41 patients over 70 years of age. Francini et al. have suggested that quantitative perfusion lung scan can be used to accurately predict postoperative performance status in patients with compromised pulmonary status preoperatively and thereby allow surgery to be done more safely with better postoperative outcome (39). Roviaro et al., Knott-Craig et al., and Koren et al. have also suggested the value of limited access (video-assisted thoracoscopic) surgery for some patients, particularly those with small peripheral lesions who might not be able to tolerate lobectomy. The use of this procedure might also decrease postoperative pain and improve the speed of surgical recovery. The long-term efficacy of thoracoscopic resection as opposed to formal lobectomy remains to be determined (25,41,42).

Adjuvant Chemotherapy

Several recent, large, multicenter, randomized, placebo-controlled trials have demonstrated a benefit for adjuvant chemotherapy after resection of NSCLC. However, data specifically on the effects of chemotherapy in the elderly are limited. Hotta et al. reviewed outcomes of 5716 patients in 11 randomized trials of adjuvant chemotherapy published from 2000 to 2004 (43). Cisplatin-based and Uracil–Tegafur regimens provided a survival benefit, but these studies were not stratified by age. Arriagada et al. reported a multicenter trial of patients with resected NSCLC and demonstrated benefit of adjuvant chemotherapy with cisplatin-based treatment (44). This study randomized 1867 patients with Stage I-III NSCLC to several different regimens of cisplatin-based adjuvant chemotherapy (including etoposide, vinorelbine, vinblastine, or vindesine) versus placebo. An early stopping rule was invoked when improved survival of patients in the adjuvant chemotherapy arm (five-year survival, 44.5% vs. 40.4%, $P = \;< 0.03$) and an absolute increase in survival of 4.1% were observed. The median patient age was 64 years with a range of 18 to 77 years, and one-quarter of the patients were older than 64 years (496/1867). Among patients aged 65 years and above, there was a 44.1% overall survival in the chemotherapy group (147 deaths out of 263 patients) and 45.3% overall survival in the control group (127 deaths out of 233 patients), which was not statistically significant (interaction $P = 0.46$, trend $P = 0.26$). A second randomized trial of adjuvant therapy with Uracil and Tegafur (UFT) was reported by Kato et al. (45). This study was limited to patients with Stage I, fully resected adenocarcinoma of whom 999 were randomized to UFT or placebo. The five-year survival rate was improved in the UFT as opposed to placebo cohort (88% vs. 85%, $P = 0.047$). Forty-three percent (430/999) of the patients randomized were older than 64 years (range: 45–75 years). The hazard ratio (HR) for death was higher in the older cohort (2.02, $P < 0.001$, multivariate analysis). There was a nonsignificant trend to a decreased HR for death in patients receiving UFT ($P = 0.72$, specific numbers of deaths not available) (46). An additional study of adjuvant therapy with paclitaxel and carboplatin in 344 patients with resected T2N0M0, Stage I non-small-cell carcinoma was recently reported by the Cancer and Leukemia Group B (46,47) survival (HR: 0.69, $P = 0.035$) and lung cancer mortality (HR: 0.51, $P = 0.018$). The current data on adjuvant chemotherapy support improved survival with cisplatin and Uracil–Tegafur–based therapy for all ages, although data on the elderly are quite limited. Stratification for age as well as trials of adjuvant therapy specifically in the elderly population would provide additional insight.

Radiation Therapy

Radiation therapy continues to be widely used for the treatment of NSCLC and can be used with either a palliative intent or for potential cure. It is also used in combination with chemotherapy for both advanced NSCLC and for small-cell lung cancer. Smith et al. found that radiotherapy was the most commonly used primary treatment for NSCLC in patients aged 65 to 69 years and older and was used with a similar frequency (40–50%) in all the older groups (13). Radiotherapy also tends to be used for patients considered medically inoperable (whether due to cardiopulmonary status, age, or simple refusal to undergo surgery).

Definitive Radiotherapy

In the past 10 years numerous studies have shown that curative doses of thoracic radiation therapy are effective and tolerable in the elderly population. Graham et al. analyzed the outcome of 103 patients with Stage I or II NSCLC and a median age of 67 years (48). Survival of patients who received palliative radiotherapy was similar to that of patients who received no therapy at all. Selected patients who received radiotherapy with a curative intent ("definitive radiotherapy") had a two-year survival of 35% and a five-year survival of 14%. Age greater than 70 years was not a significant factor in predicting survival although weight loss, tumor size, and time–dose factor were significant. Noordijk et al. reviewed 50 inoperable patients with Stage I NSCLC, 40 of whom were over 70 years of age (49). Treatment with radiotherapy to a dose of 60 Gy resulted in a response rate of 90%, with a complete response rate of 50% for tumors less than 4 cm in size. Survival was dependent on tumor size but not on age and was similar to that of 86 patients over 70 years of age who had undergone surgery as primary treatment at the same hospital. It was therefore concluded that radiotherapy was a good alternative for patients with tumors less than 4 cm in size.

Several additional series have shown similar results. Furuta et al. (50) treated 32 patients over the age of 75 with Stage I or II NSCLC using definitive radiotherapy (at least 60 Gy). The mean age of patients in this series was 79 years, with 11 patients over 80 years of age. No acute complications were seen that were specific to radiotherapy. The two-year survival was 57%, and the five-year survival was 36%. Most deaths in this series were due to heart disease rather than cancer (7/11 deaths). Gava et al. reviewed 196 patients with lung cancer who were over 70 years of age, 182 of whom received radiotherapy. Of this group, 109 (60%) received radical radiotherapy, whereas 73 (40%) received palliative therapy. The full course of planned radiotherapy was completed by 163 patients (91%). Relief of symptoms of lung cancer was noted in approximately 80%, and quality of life remained stable after treatment, emphasizing the feasibility of radiotherapy in this age group (51). Hayakawa et al. retrospectively reviewed a series of 303 patients with medically inoperable or surgically unresectable NSCLC treated with definitive radiotherapy ($\geq$60 Gy). In this series, 97 patients were 75 years of age or older. These patients were subdivided into two groups, 67 patients aged from 75 to 79 years and 30 patients aged 80 years and older. The two- and five-year survival rates decreased with age, but not to a statistically significant extent (two- and five-year survival for those of age < 75 years were 36% and 12%, respectively, for those of age 75 to 79 years, 32% and 13%, respectively, and for those of age 80 years or older, 28% and 4%, respectively). The performance status of older patients decreased more than younger patients, but overall treatment at full doses was generally well tolerated (52).

Questions concerning radiotherapy dose and concomitant use of radiotherapy and chemotherapy have also been examined. Lonardi et al. (53) reported 71 patients who were at least 70 years of age and who received immediate radiotherapy for symptomatic relief. Half of the patients received more than 50 Gy and half less than 50 Gy. The higher dose group had a superior MS (seven months vs. four months) as well as a superior six-month survival (48% vs. 39%) and 12-month survival (32% vs. 11%). Toxicity was mild with good palliation of both pain and hemoptysis. It was therefore emphasized that patients should receive a higher dose radiotherapy if possible because of the equivalent tolerance and improved outcome. Atagi et al. (54) used a combination of carboplatin and radiotherapy (50–60 Gy over five weeks) in 29 patients with NSCLC and a median age of 79. There was one complete and 14 partial responses (total response rate, 54%). The major toxicity was hematologic, but treatment was tolerable in all patients, again emphasizing the feasibility of such combined therapy even in an elderly patient population. Pignon et al. (55) reviewed survival and toxicity in 1208 patients who received thoracic radiation with curative intent in six separate EORTC trials. Toxicities were compared in the age groups younger than 65 years, 65 to 69 years, and older than 69 years, and only weight loss was increased in the older groups. There was no significant difference in rates of nausea, dyspnea, weakness, esophagitis, or deterioration in performance status by age ($P=0.1$, for toxicity > grade 2).

Complications of Radiotherapy

The use of cranial radiotherapy has raised some special concerns. Catell et al. reported 23 patients over 80 years of age and who received 30 Gy in 10 fractions for brain metastases from either small-cell or NSCLC (56). The full course of therapy was completed by 19 of these patients, and MS was 10 weeks. Poor prognostic factors included a Karnofsky performance status of < 70 and multiple brain metastases. In patients with good performance status, the mean survival (15 weeks) was comparable to that of the younger patients. Cranial radiotherapy for lung cancer in elderly patients was considered to provide benefits equivalent to that in younger patients. However, several series reporting long-term follow-up after cranial radiotherapy have raised questions concerning the possibility of neuropsychiatric deterioration. Laaksonen et al. reported an elderly male with small-cell lung cancer who underwent cranial radiotherapy after two years of interferon treatment and developed a reversible dementia-like syndrome (57). Long-term follow-up of the NCI Navy series of patients who received prophylactic cranial radiotherapy for small-cell lung cancer has also shown a steady and measurable decrease in neuropsychiatric function for many years following therapy. Follow-up of 14 of these patients at six years showed continued, gradual deterioration of neuropsychiatric function (58,59). Other possible contributing etiologic factors in these patients could include a worsening of pre-existing arteriosclerotic vascular disease or a late chemotherapy effect. Cull et al. studied 52 patients who had received prophylactic cranial radiation. Although most were well and had a performance status of 0 or 1 and normal neurological examinations, only 19% had normal (age-adjusted) neuropsychometric testing (60). Gregor et al. (61) randomized 314 patients with small-cell lung cancer after complete induction treatment to three arms; initially, the two prophylactic cranial irradiation arms received 36 Gy in 18 daily fractions and 24 Gy in 12 daily fractions, which was later changed to 30 Gy in 10 daily fractions or 8 Gy in one fraction, with a third arm receiving no radiation treatment. Cranial irradiation significantly reduced the development of brain metastases [HR: 0.44, confidence interval (CI): 0.29–0.27] and was associated with a nonsignificant increase in overall survival. There was no difference in postprocedure quality of life and cognitive function in groups who received cranial irradiation and those who did not. However, all groups showed deterioration in quality of life and cognitive function from pretreatment baseline, which worsened at 6 and 12 months after treatment.

When radiotherapy is used as primary therapy for lung cancer, the question of radiation pneumonitis also arises. Koga et al. reviewed the incidence and severity of radiation pneumonitis in 62 patients with lung cancer (33 below 70 years and 29 above 70 years) receiving 1.5 to 2.0 Gy per day for three to five weeks. The incidence of radiation pneumonitis was found to be proportional to field size and radiation dose in both younger and older patients. Severe radiation pneumonitis tended to be more common in older patients regardless of body size or chemotherapy administered (62).

Pallative Radiotherapy

The palliative effect of radiotherapy has been well documented by Numico et al. (63) in advanced NSCLC patients. Their meta-analysis suggested that hypofractionated schedules were most effective for symptom relief, while higher doses were more effective when measuring survival and local disease control. Overall, radiation reduced chest pain and hemoptysis is 60–80% of patients, and dyspnea and cough in 50–70% patients. However, the optimal dose and timing of radiotherapy for symptom control in an elderly population have not been specifically defined. Although cranial irradiation using whole brain or stercotactic techniques has had good palliative effect in patients with symptomatic brain metastases, this benefit has not been confirmed in the elderly population.

Chemotherapy

The use of chemotherapy in lung cancer has developed over the last several decades. In limited-disease small-cell lung cancer, chemotherapy and radiation will result in an extremely high response rate, an increase in survival, and some cures. Even in extensive-disease small-cell lung cancer, a high response rate to chemotherapy and an increase in survival will be achieved. Recent advances in the chemotherapy of NSCLC have also produced high response rates and a modest increase in survival. However, aggressive systemic therapy is accompanied by the potential for significant toxicity, and careful consideration must be given to the question of whether the benefits outweigh the risks for patients with significant comorbid disease.

The same arguments apply to the elderly. If expected natural survival exceeds expected survival with advanced lung cancer, then therapy that can increase survival with an acceptable level of toxicity and the maintenance of a good quality of life is reasonable. However, one must often take into consideration quantitatively and qualitatively greater levels of comorbid disease. In small-cell lung cancer, the large number of active agents allows the design of numerous highly active combination chemotherapy regimens. Thus, regimens can be selected that will avoid corresponding comorbid disease (i.e., selection of non-nephrotoxic agents for the patient with renal insufficiency or noncardiotoxic agents for the patient with coronary artery disease). Until recently, the limited number of active agents in NSCLC did not allow such flexibility. However, the introduction of several newer families of chemotherapeutic agents (taxanes, topoisomerase I inhibitors, and nucleoside analogues), as well as the development of new chemoprotective agents, now allows the design of regimens following similar principles.

Chemotherapy in Small-Cell Lung Cancer

Reports concerning the effect of age on response and survival in small-cell lung cancer are somewhat contradictory. Albain et al. analyzed the SWOG database of 2580 patients participating in 10 small-cell lung cancer trials between 1976 and 1988, to identify significant prognostic factors and prognostic groups. Age greater than 70 years was found to be a negative prognostic factor for patients with limited disease, but not extensive disease (64). Osterlind et al. (65), using a database of 874 patients, found advanced age to have a borderline negative prognostic effect in extensive disease. Siu et al. (66) reviewed relative outcomes of 80 patients 70 years of age or older among 608 patients with limited-disease small-cell lung cancer who participated in two NCI of Canada studies of combined chemotherapy and radiation. Age was a significant adverse factor in univariate, but not in multivariate, analysis of overall survival (because advanced age correlated with increased dose omissions). The older patients had a comparable MS (13 months vs. 15 months) but increased treatment-related death (5% vs. 2%) (52). Similar results were found in subgroup analyses of other phase III trials by Paccagnella and Favaretto (67) and Yuen et al. (68). Ashley et al., analyzing 674 patients with small-cell lung cancer, found that the response rate was proportional to performance status, but not age, in both univariate and multivariate analyses. Survival was highly dependent on the stage and performance status in both univariate and multivariate analyses, with advanced age having a negative effect ($P = 0.03$) in the multivariate analysis (69). Shepherd et al. (70) examined the effect of advanced age on survival in small-cell lung cancer by analyzing the outcome of 123 patients over 70 years of age divided into three subgroups by age (70–74, 75–80) and >80 years). Survival was not affected by increasing age. On the other hand, Nou (71), examining a database of 345 patients receiving chemotherapy and radiotherapy for small-cell lung cancer, noted a significant effect of both stage and age on survival in multivariate analysis. However, survival was only marginally decreased in patients aged 70 to 75. In spite of increased toxicity, aggressive chemotherapy could therefore still be recommended for this group. It would appear that although there is a trend toward advanced age being a negative prognostic factor for survival in small-cell lung cancer, age often has a marginal effect when compared with stage of disease and performance status. Withholding chemotherapy for small-cell lung cancer strictly because of age, particularly in the patient with a good performance status and limited disease, is not advisable.

The potential for increased toxicity when older patients are treated with chemotherapy is a matter of concern. Both Oshita et al. (72), using a cisplatin-based regimen in patients over 75 years old, and Findlay et al. (73), using an intensive combination of cyclophosphamide, doxorubicin, and vincristine in patients over 70 years old, felt that the level of toxicity (particularly myelosuppression) observed was greater than anticipated. Kelly et al. (74), using a database of 96 patients treated with combination chemotherapy, including vinca alkaloids, noted peripheral neuropathy to be more common in patients over 65 years old. These observations may be due to a generalized decrease in organ function reserve with advancing age. However, differences in the pharmacology of the agents involved must also be considered. Lind et al. (75) reported an increase in volume of distribution and elimination half-life of ifosfamide with advancing age. Teramoto et al. (76) noted that older patients had a greater decrease in oxygen-free radicals, which could be correlated with a decreased, postcisplatin absolute granulocyte count. Because the mechanism of action of many chemotherapeutic agents depends on free radicals, both efficacy and toxicity could potentially be influenced. The effect of age on the pharmacokinetics and pharmacodynamics of chemotherapeutic agents is an area that deserves further investigation.

With the availability of an increasing number of chemotherapeutic agents, several regimens have been adapted for use against small-cell lung cancer in the elderly, with the specific purpose of decreasing toxicity. These have included the single agent etoposide, both orally and intravenously, platinum and etoposide combinations, and multidrug regimens.

Single agent etoposide was a standard treatment for elderly patients in the late 1980s and early 1990s. Several phase II trials of oral etoposide in patients over 70 years of age and patients with poor prognostic factors found good overall response and a modest side-effect profile (77,78). These preliminary results were not substantiated in a phase III trial performed by the Medical Research Council Lung Cancer Working Party (79). Three hundred and thirty-nine patients with poor performance status were randomized to oral etoposide, versus etoposide/vincristine or cyclophosphamide, adriamycin, and vincristine (CAV). The study was stopped when interim analysis showed worse response rate (45% vs. 51%), MS (130 days vs. 183 days), and HR for survival (HR: 1.35, $P = 0.03$) in patients receiving oral etoposide, as well as increased hematological toxicity. A second phase III trial in both elderly and poor performance status patients was also stopped early. One hundred and fifty-five patients were randomized to oral etoposide versus etoposide/cisplatin alternating with CAV. The overall response rate (32.9% vs. 36.3%, $P < 0.01$), MS (4.8 months vs. 5.9 months, $P < 0.05$), and progression-free survival (3.6 months vs. 5.6 months, $P < 0.001$), and a trend to inferior overall survival, were found with oral etoposide alone. Although there was increased nausea and vomiting in the combination chemotherapy arm, symptoms and quality of life were otherwise similar between both groups (80).

One of the most widely used chemotherapy combinations for small-cell lung cancer is etoposide and carboplatin. Carboplatin is considered to be a less toxic alternative to cisplatin, with myelosuppression supplanting the neurotoxicity, nephrotoxicity, and emetogenicity of the parent compound. The etoposide/carboplatin combination given on a q2 week or q3 week basis has been found to be active and extremely well tolerated in patients over 70 years of age by several investigators (81–85). However, Shibata et al. (86), Evans et al. (87), and Raghavan et al. (88) all noted a high level of myelosuppression. Okamoto (84) and Carney (89) have specifically tested an etoposide/carboplatin regimen with the carboplatin dose based on the Calvert formula and found good efficacy and tolerability in phase II trials.

If carboplatin/etoposide is not an appropriate choice, several other regimens have been tested in phase II trials. Westeel treated 41 patients aged 70 years and older with cisplatin, doxorubicin, vincristine, and etoposide (PAVE), with or without thoracic radiation, and found the MS of 11 months to be comparable with studies of etoposide/carboplatin. The side effects of PAVE were comparable to that seen in younger patients except for increased emesis (82,84,90). Neubauer treated 66 patients who were 70 years of age or older with a poor performance status with paclitaxel/carboplatin. All of these patients had extensive stage disease, and the MS of 7.2 months was also considered comparable with other treatment regimens (92). Grunberg treated 57 patients with poor-prognosis extensive disease (performance status 2 or serum albumin < 3.5 g/dL) with a 14-day regimen of oral etoposide and oral cyclophosphamide. The MS was five months in those patients who received 50 mg once a day of each drug and seven months in those who received 50 mg twice a day of each drug. Significant granulocytopenia could be predicted based on a single serum etoposide level on day 2, allowing early dose adjustment if necessary (92).

Low-dose polychemotherapy regimens have been designed to attempt to decrease toxicity in elderly patients and poor-prognosis patients. Phase III trials of several of these regimens have failed to show decreased toxicity, but these regimens have had clearly decreased efficacy. These trials included a comparison of etoposide/vincristine with etoposide, vincristine, methotrexate, and cyclophosphamide, half-dose CAV alternating with carboplatin/etoposide versus full dose, and cyclophosphamide/etoposide/vincristine given for symptomatic disease versus the same regimen on a scheduled basis (93–95).

There is an important role for improved supportive care in elderly patients, given the decreased efficacy of low-dose regimens but increased toxicity of full-dose regimens. Ardizzoni et al. enrolled 95 patients over 70 years of age into a phase II trial of carboplatin/etoposide given as low-dose therapy versus high dose plus lenograstim growth factor support. The response rate was improved with full dose (69% vs. 39%), but despite growth factor support the full-dose therapy had a higher rate of myelotoxicity (0% vs. 12%) (96).

Although combined chemotherapy and radiotherapy is the standard of care in younger patients with limited-disease small-cell lung cancer, the role of combined modality therapy in older patients has been questioned. A meta-analysis of 2140 patients with limited-disease small-cell lung cancer in 13 randomized trials of chemoradiation versus chemotherapy alone showed an overall 5.4% increase in three-year survival. Stratification by age showed benefit in younger patients and a trend against benefit in older patients. Patients under 55 years of age had a relative risk of death of 0.72 (CI: 0.56–0.93) versus relative risk of death of 1.07 (CI: 0.70–1.64) in patients above 70 years (97). Conversely, although fewer elderly patients completed irradiation, a retrospective analysis of two phase III trials by the NCI of Canada evaluating different schedules of chemoradiation revealed no statistical differences in response rate, overall survival, and toxicity in 88 patients of 70 years of age and older compared to younger patients (98). Yuen et al. compared the response of 50 patients who were 70 years of age and older enrolled in a phase III trial of carboplatin/etoposide with radiotherapy either once or twice daily (total dose of 45 Gy) (intergroup trial: 0096). A trend toward worse response rates (80% vs. 88%, $P = 0.11$), event-free survival at five years (16% vs. 19%, $P = 0.18$), and overall survival at five years (16% vs. 22%, $P = 0.05$) in the elderly subset was observed. It was postulated that much of this was due to increased morbidity in the first six months, particularly increased hematologic toxicity in the elderly (grade 4–5 hematological toxicity, 84% vs. 61%, $P \leq 0.01$). Despite the improved survival of younger patients, response was considered to be comparable, and the authors concluded that chemoradiation was an option for good performance status elderly patients. However, the small numbers of elderly patients in these trials limit their generalizability.

There are also several phase II trials of chemoradiation in elderly patients. Westeel showed good tolerance of PAVE plus chemotherapy in all patients with limited disease and some patients with extensive disease. Median survival for the 25 patients with limited-stage disease was 70 weeks. Jeremic treated 75 patients with limited disease who were 70 years of age and older with carboplatin/etoposide and hyperfractionated radiotherapy (total dose of 45 Gy) and found a MS of 15 months and a five-year survival rate of 32% (99). One grade 4 toxicity (thrombocytopenia) but no treatment-associated death was observed, and the most common grade 3 side effects were leukopenia, esophagitis, and thrombocytopenia. Alternatively, Murray treated 55 limited-disease patients who were elderly, had poor performance status, or declined standard duration therapy, with an abbreviated course of one cycle of CAV and one cycle of carboplatin/etoposide with a lower dose of radiation (20–30 Gy). The MS was 54 weeks with a five-year survival rate of 18%. Although the regimen was well tolerated overall, there were three treatment-related deaths (100) . These studies suggest that chemoradiation may be effective and tolerable in some elderly patients, but further trials of chemotherapy alone in limited-disease small-cell lung cancer in the elderly are needed.

Chemotherapy in NSCLC

Chemotherapeutic regimens for advanced NSCLC are still usually based on platinum family compounds. Newer regimens in this category include combinations of cisplatin or carboplatin with paclitaxel, docetaxel, gemcitabine, or vinorelbine. Many of these regimens, therefore, carry the potential for significant toxicity in the elderly. Improved supportive care measures have had a major impact in improving feasibility and tolerability of such regimens for patients of all age groups. Development of modern antiemetics has markedly decreased both the incidence and severity of chemotherapy-induced nausea and vomiting (101). Weight loss and poor appetite remain matters of particular concern. However, Niiranen et al. (102) treated 89 patients over 70 years of age receiving chemotherapy for lung cancer with medroxyprogesterone acetate and reported a marked increase in appetite and weight gain and a decrease in chemotherapy-related side effects.

Chemoradiotherapy in NSCLC

Overall, patients with locally advanced NSCLC (medically inoperable Stage II/IIIA disease and unresectable Stage IIIA/B disease) benefit from combined modality treatment with chemoradiation (103–105). The benefit in elderly patients is more debatable. Several retrospective analyses of Radiation Therapy Oncology Group (RTOG) trials include retrospective information on subgroups of elderly patients. Movsas et al. reviewed 979 patients treated with radiation or combined chemoradiation and evaluated quality-adjusted survival. In the subgroup of patients over 70 years of age, the quality-adjusted survival was better when treated with radiotherapy alone (106). Werner-Wasik evaluated prognostic factors in 1999 patients from nine RTOG trials receiving radiation, 335 of whom also received chemotherapy. In univariate analysis, cisplatin-based chemoradiation was a good prognostic factor, but age over 70 years was a poor prognostic factor (MS: 7.6 months vs. 11.4 months, $P < 0.001$). Although it is unclear how many of the elderly patients enrolled received chemotherapy, further stratification showed that elderly patients with a Karnofsky performance status < 90 and pleural effusion did significantly worse than those with poor performance status and no effusion (107). Chemoradiotherapy was not beneficial in older patients randomized to radiotherapy alone versus combined modality therapy with cisplatin and vindesine and either standard or hyperfractionated radiotherapy in a phase III trial by Sause et al. This intergroup trial (including RTOG, ECOG, and SWOG) participation found better survival in the 490 patients in the overall population with chemotherapy plus standard radiation (radiation alone 11.4 months vs. chemotherapy with standard radiation 13.8 months vs. chemotherapy plus hyperfractionated radiation 12.3 months, $p = 0.03$). However, the subset of 66 patients who were 70 years of age and older had worse survival with chemoradiotherapy (MS with standard and hyperfractionated chemoradiation 10.9 months vs. radiation alone 13.1 months) (108).

Langer described more promising results for chemoradiation in the elderly in an analysis of another phase III trial, RTOG 9410. This trial randomized good-prognosis patients with unresectable NSCLC to three arms: (*i*) sequential radiotherapy and chemotherapy, (*ii*) concurrent chemoradiotherapy, or (*iii*) concurrent/hyperfractionated radiotherapy; cisplatin and vinblastine were used in arms *i* and *ii* and cisplatin and oral etoposide in arm *iii*. The 103 elderly patients in this trial had improved survival with concurrent chemoradiotherapy compared to hyperfractionated or sequential chemoradiotherapy (MS: 22.4 months vs. 16.4 months vs.10.8 months). Toxicity was greater in elderly patients in all three arms, with 75% of elderly patients versus 63% of younger patients having grade 4 or greater toxicity in the concurrent therapy arm. A 10% to 20% higher rate of severe neutropenia and 33% higher rate of severe esophagitis were also seen. Although the study is limited by the lack of a radiotherapy-only control, the survival benefit for good-prognosis elderly patients may outweigh the toxicity (109). These analyses suggest a role for chemoradiotherapy in good-prognosis elderly patients. However, this should be evaluated on a case-by-case basis.

Chemotherapy in Advanced NSCLC

Although chemotherapy may provide a two- to four-month MS advantage in advanced NSCLC, compared to best supportive care only, elderly patients are not always given the opportunity to achieve such benefit (110). Potosky's review of patients in the SEER database showed that the rates of administration of chemotherapy gradually decreased with age, from 58% in patients from 50 to 59 years to 16% in patients above 80 years (11). Concerns about tolerance of chemotherapy in the elderly cohort and increased comorbidity may effect such decisions. However, several randomized and nonrandomized trials of chemotherapy for advanced lung cancer in elderly patients have now been performed.

Single-agent chemotherapy regimens tested in elderly patients with advanced NSCLC include oral vinorelbine, gemcitabine, paclitaxel, and docetaxel. Colleoni et al. (111) and Gridelli et al. (112) examined the use of single-agent vinorelbine for the treatment of NSCLC. Response rates in the range of 15% to 25% with manageable myelosuppression were noted. In addition, Mattioli and Tripoli (113) noted an increase in quality of life and psychosocial functioning in 9 of 15 patients (median age: 70 years) treated for NSCLC with single-agent vinorelbine. A recent international expert panel review of advanced NSCLC treatment in the elderly (Gridelli et al.) evaluated phase II trials of several other single agents. Median survivals of 7.5 to 8.2 months in 108 patients treated with oral vinorelbine, 6.8 to 9.0 months in 163 patients treated in four studies of gemcitabine, 6.8 to 10.3 months in 116 patients treated in three studies of paclitaxel, and 5.0 months in 39 patients treated with docetaxel, were seen. Treatment was well tolerated with standard doses of gemcitabine. Efficacy was maintained, and toxicity improved with weekly low doses of the taxanes, paclitaxel and docetaxel, as compared to standard doses every three weeks (114).

The first large-scale, phase III trial of chemotherapy in elderly patients with NSCLC, the Elderly Lung Cancer Vinorelbine Study (ELVIS), showed benefit of single-agent chemotherapy over best supportive care. The ELVIS trial randomized 191 patients aged 70 years or older with Stage IIIB or IV NSCLC to either best supportive care or intravenous vinorelbine 30 mg/m^2 (days 1 and 8 every 21 days for up to six cycles). Enrollment did not reach the target of 350 patients, but a statistically significant improvement in overall survival and MS was seen with vinorelbine (MS: 28 weeks vs. 21 weeks, $p = 0.03$, one-year survival: 32% vs. 14%). Toxicity levels were acceptable, with only 10% of patients reporting grade 3 or 4 toxicity and less than 7% of patients stopping chemotherapy due to toxicity. Quality of life was measured using symptom review and functional assessment instruments. Patients in the vinorelbine arm had more chemotherapy-associated symptoms, including nausea, vomiting, neuropathy, and constipation, but fared better on lung cancer–related symptoms of cough, dyspnea pain, and fatigue, as well as measures of overall quality of life and function (115).

Because single-agent therapy was shown to be preferable to best supportive care in the elderly, numerous studies of combination therapy, primarily doublets both with and without platinum compounds, have been performed. Two phase III trials have compared the gemcitabine and vinorelbine doublet to single-agent therapy. Frasci et al. (116) published results of the Southern Italy Cooperative Oncology Group Trial, which randomized 120 patients aged 70 or older to vinorelbine or vinorelbine plus gemcitabine. Interim analysis showed significantly improved survival in the vinorelbine/gemcitabine combination arm (MS: 29 weeks vs. 18 weeks, $P = 0.01$). Deterioration of quality of life scores was delayed in the combination chemotherapy arm, although significantly higher toxicity rates were seen. The study showed an advantage for combination therapy, but has been criticized, as patients receiving single-agent vinorelbine only had survival rates comparable to patients historically receiving best supportive care. The results of this study conflict with those of the Multicenter Italian Lung Cancer in the Elderly Trial which randomized 698 patients aged 70 years or older with performance status of 0 to 2 and Stage IIIB or IV NSCLC to vinorelbine or gemcitabine or both vinorelbine and gemcitabine. Patients in all three arms had comparable MS and quality of life scores (MS: vinorelbine 36 weeks vs. vinorelbine/gemcitabine 30 weeks, $P = 0.93$; gemcitabine 28 weeks vs. vinorelbine/gemcitabine 30 weeks, $P = 0.65$). Quality of life questionnaires showed no significant differences in symptoms or function between the three arms.

However, toxicity was more severe in the combination chemotherapy arm. When compared to vinorelbine, the combination arm had a significantly increased incidence of thrombocytopenia. Compared to gemcitabine alone, combination chemotherapy had a statistically significant increase in anemia, neutropenia, nausea/ vomiting, mucositis, extravasation, cardiac toxicities, and constipation. The authors concluded that single-agent therapy was preferable to combination treatment (117).

Platinum-containing and non-platinum-containing doublets were found to confer a survival advantage compared to single-agent therapy in a phase III trial by Comella et al. (118). Two hundred and sixty-four patients with advanced NSCLC who were either over or below 70 years of age and had an ECOG performance status of 2 were randomized to gemcitabine/paclitaxel, gemcitabine/vinorelbine, gemcitabine alone, or vinorelbine alone. Toxicity was similar in all arms, but MS was improved in both doublet arms (MS: gemcitabine 5.1 months vs. paclitaxel 6.4 months vs. gemcitabine/paclitaxel 9.4 vs. gemcitabine/vinorelbine 9.7 months).

Platinum-based chemotherapy is considered the standard of care for most lung cancer patients. Information on the use of platinum-containing regimens in the elderly has been extracted from results of several large-scale phase III trials. Langer et al. compared the outcomes of 86 patients aged 70 years and older in ECOG 5592, in which 574 patients with advanced NSCLC were randomized to receive cisplatin with either etoposide or paclitaxel. Outcomes were not different among age groups (MS: 8.53 months in elderly patients vs. 9.05 months in younger patients; response rates: 21.5% vs. 23.3%; one-year survival: 38% vs. 28%). Quality of life scores were also similar. Toxicity, however, was greater in elderly patients, with significant increases in leukopenia and neuropsychiatric toxicity in older men and weight loss in older women (119). Langer et al. also reviewed the outcomes of elderly patients in ECOG 1592 randomized trial to cisplatin plus paclitaxel, cisplatin plus docetaxel, cisplatin plus gemcitabine, or carboplatin plus paclitaxel. Of the 1139 patients enrolled, 277 were 70 years of age or older, and there was no significant difference in MS (8.2 months vs. 8.3 months) or toxicity with increasing age. The results of two phase III SWOG trials were pooled by Kelly et al. (74) to assess treatment outcomes in the elderly. Of the 608 patients randomized to cisplatin versus cisplatin/vinorelbine in SWOG 9508, or cisplatin/vinorelbine versus paclitaxel/carboplatin in SWOG 9509, 117 were 70 years of age or older. The elderly patients had a nonsignificant decrease in MS (6.9 vs. 8.6 months, $P = 0.06$). No effect of age was found in multivariate analysis.

Novel agents, such as the epidermal growth factor receptor inhibitors, gefitinib and erlotinib, have shown benefit in some patients with advanced, treatment-refractory NSCLC. The targeted nature of these agents makes them potentially good choices for elderly patients because common hematologic and nonhematologic toxicities are decreased. Retrospective analysis of these agents from phase III trials has shown similar efficacy and tolerability between elderly and younger populations. Cappuzzo et al. showed a median response of 4.4 months to gefitinib in 40 previously treated elderly patients, with primarily mild dermatologic and gastrointestinal (diarrhea) toxicity (120).

Age would therefore not appear to be a contraindication to chemotherapy in either small-cell or NSCLC in appropriately selected patients. In fact, Albain et al. (121), using the 2531-patient SWOG advanced NSCLC database, identified age of at least 70 years as a positive predictive factor for survival. However, the choice of chemotherapeutic agents must be carefully considered in view of pre-existing comorbid conditions, and modern supportive care measures should be aggressively employed. Standard guidelines for lung cancer chemotherapy (such as re-evaluation for response after 2–3 cycles of chemotherapy) cannot be ignored, because increased toxicity can be expected if an extended course of treatment is undertaken. With appropriate diligence, increased survival due to chemotherapy with maintenance of good quality of life is possible for elderly patients with advanced lung cancer.

CONCLUSION

Lung cancer is the result of a life-long behavior (smoking) pattern that culminates in an increased risk of disease for the elderly. However, patients who develop this disease at a more advanced age may have a greater chance of having a localized and more treatable presentation. Accurate and timely detection and evaluation for therapy are therefore of particular importance in this age group. Improved techniques for both treatment and supportive care have increased the range of reasonable and tolerable therapies available to the aging population. These therapeutic options cannot be dismissed without careful evaluation of the stage of disease, comorbid disease, and individual desires for therapy. Assuming that the elderly as a group will not benefit from aggressive treatment for lung cancer would be a significant disservice to these patients.

REFERENCES

1. O'Rourke MA, Feussner JR, Feigl P, Laszlo J. Age trends of lung cancer stage at diagnosis. Implications for lung cancer screening in the elderly. JAMA 1987; 258(7):921–926.
2. Clinical characteristics, diagnosis and treatment of elderly patients with lung cancer at non-surgical institutions: a multicenter study. North-Eastern Italian Oncology Group. Neoplasms of the Elderly Committee. Tumori 1990; 76(5):429–433.
3. Kuo CW, Chen YM, Chao JY, Tsai CM, Perng RP. Non-small cell lung cancer in very young and very old patients. Chest 2000; 117(2):354–357.
4. Montella M, Gridelli C, Crispo A, et al. Has lung cancer in the elderly different characteristics at presentation? Oncol Rep 2002; 9(5):1093–1096.
5. Shibata A, Paganini-Hill A, Ross RK, Henderson BE. Dietary beta-carotene, cigarette smoking, and only lung cancer in men. Cancer Causes Control 1992; 3:207–214.
6. Goodman GE, Thornquist MD, Balmes J, et al. The Beta-Carotene and Retinol Efficacy Trial: incidence of lung cancer and cardiovascular disease mortality during 6-year follow-up after stopping beta-carotene and retinol supplements. J Natl Cancer Inst 2004; 96(23):1743–1750.
7. Hoffman D, Rivenson A, Chung FL, Wynden EL. Potential inhibitors of tobacco carcinogenesis. Ann NY Acad Sci 1993; 686:140–160.
8. Brooks DR, Palmer JR, Strom BL, Rosenberg L. Menthol cigarettes and risk of lung cancer. Am J Epidemiol 2003; 158:609–616.
9. Omenn GS, Goodman GE, Thornquist MD, et al. Risk factors for lung cancer and for intervention effects in CARET, the Beta-Carotene and Retinol Efficacy Trial. J Natl Cancer Inst 1996; 88(21):1550–1559.
10. DeMaria LC Jr, Cohen HJ. Characteristics of lung cancer in elderly patients. J Gerontol 1987; 42(5):540–545.
11. Tockman MS, Anthonisen NR, Wright EC, Donithan MG. Airways obstruction and the risk for lung cancer. Ann Intern Med 1987; 106(4):512–518.

12. Petty TL. Lung cancer and chronic obstructive pulmonary disease. Hematol Oncol Clin North Am 1997; 11(3):531–541.
13. Jack CI, Sheard JD, Lippitt B, Fromholtz A, Evans CC, Hind CR. Lung cancer in elderly patients: the role of induced sputum production to obtain a cytological diagnosis. Age Ageing 1993; 22(3):227–229.
14. Potosky AL, Saxman S, Wallace RB, Lynch CF. Population variations in the initial treatment of non-small-cell lung cancer. J Clin Oncol 2004; 22(16):3261–3268.
15. Shields TW. Surgical therapy for carcinoma of the lung. Clin Chest Med 1993; 14(1):121–147.
16. Smith TJ, Penberthy L, Desch CE, et al. Differences in initial treatment patterns and outcomes of lung cancer in the elderly. Lung Cancer 1995; 13(3):235–252.
17. O'Connell JB, Maggard MA, Ko CY. Cancer-directed surgery for localized disease: decreased use in the elderly. Ann Surg Oncol 2004; 11(11):962–969.
18. Jazieh AR, Kyasa MJ, Sethuraman G, Howington J. Disparities in surgical resection of early-stage non-small cell lung cancer. J Thorac Cardiovasc Surg 2002; 123(6):1173–1176.
19. Polednak AP. Disparities in surgical treatment of early-stage non-small-cell lung cancer. Yale J Biol Med 2001; 74(5):309–314.
20. Yellin A, Benfield JR. Surgery for bronchogenic carcinoma in the elderly. Am Rev Respir Dis 1985; 131(2):197.
21. Ginsberg RJ, Hill LD, Eagan RT, et al. Modern thirty-day operative mortality for surgical resections in lung cancer. J Thorac Cardiovasc Surg 1983; 86(5):654–658.
22. Whittle J, Steinberg EP, Anderson CF, Herbert R. Use of Medicare data to evaluate outcomes in elderly patients undergoing lung resection for lung cancer. Chest 1991; 100:729–734.
23. Sherman S, Guidot CE. The feasibility of thoracotomy for lung cancer in the elderly. JAMA 1987; 258(7):927–930.
24. Damhuis RA, Schutte PR. Resection rates and postoperative mortality in 7,899 patients with lung cancer. Eur Respir J 1996; 9(1):7–10.
25. Knott-Craig CJ, Howell CE, Parsons BD, Paulsen SM, Brown BR, Elkins RC. Improved results in the management of surgical candidates with lung cancer. Ann Thorac Surg 1997; 63(5):1405–1409.
26. Nanikawa S, Shimamoto A, Takao M, Yada I. Surgical treatment of lung cancer over 75 years old. Lung Cancer 1997; 18(suppl 1):115.
27. Breyer RH, Zippe C, Pharr WF, Jensik RJ, Kittle CF, Faber LP. Thoracotomy in patients over age seventy years. J Thorac Cardiovasc Surg 1981; 81:187–193.
28. Roxburgh JC, Thompson J, Goldstraw P. Hospital mortality and long-term survival after pulmonary resection in the elderly. Ann Thorac Surg 1991; 51(5):800–803.
29. Ishida T, Yokoyama H, Kaneko S, Sugio K, Sugimachi K. Long-term results of operations for non-small cell lung cancer in the elderly. Ann Thorac Surg 1990; 50:919–922.
30. Cangemi V, Volpino P, D'Andrea N, et al. Lung cancer surgery in elderly patients. Tumori 1996; 82:237–241.
31. Jie C, Wever AM, Huysmans HA, Franker HC, Weven-Hess J, Hermans J. Time trends and survival in patients presented for surgery with non-small-cell lung cancer 1969–1985. Eur J Cardio Thorac Surg 1990; 4:653–657.
32. Santambrogio L, Nosotti M, Bellavita N, Mezzetti M. Prospective study of surgical treatment of lung cancer in the elderly patient. J Corontol A Biol Sci Med Sci 1996; 51:M267–M269.
33. van Rens MT, de la Riviere AB, Elbers HR, van den Bosch JM. Prognostic assessment of 2,361 patients who underwent pulmonary resection for non-small cell lung cancer, stage I, II, and IIIA. Chest 2000; 117(2):374–379.
34. Shirakusa T, Tsutsui M, Iriki N, et al. Results of resection for bronchogenic carcinoma in patients over the age of 80. Thorax 1989; 44(3):189–191.

35. Pagni S, Federico JA, Ponn RB. Pulmonary resection for lung cancer in octogenarians. Ann Thorac Surg 1997; 63(3):785–789.
36. Shimamoto A, Yen G, Takao T, et al. Surgical treatment for primary lung cancer in octogenarians: the role of limited operations. Kyobu Geka 1998; 51(1):32–36.
37. Hurria A, Kris MG. Management of lung cancer in older adults. CA Cancer J Clin 2003; 53(6):325–341.
38. Fukuse T, Satoda N, Hijiya K, Fujinaga T. Importance of a comprehensive geriatric assessment in prediction of complications following thoracic surgery in elderly patients. Chest 2005; 127(3):886–891.
39. Francini A, Filosso PL, Podio F, et al. Quantitative perfusion lung scanning in the surgery of the lung cancer in the elderly. Lung Cancer 1997; 18(suppl 1):230.
40. Roviaro GC, Rebuffat C, Varoli F, et al. Major videothoracoscopic pulmonary resections. Endosc Surg Allied Technol 1993; 1(5–6):288–293.
41. Roviaro G, Varoli F, Rebuffat C, et al. Videothoracoscopic staging and treatment of lung cancer. Ann Thorac Surg 1995; 59(4):971–974.
42. Koren JP, Bocage JP, Geis WP, Caccavale RJ. Major thoracic surgery in octogenarians: the video-assisted thoracic surgery (VATS) approach. Surg Endosc 2003; 17(4): 632–635.
43. Hotta K, Matsuo K, Ueoka H, Kiura K, Tabata M, Tanimoto M. Role of adjuvant chemotherapy in patients with resected non-small-cell lung cancer: reappraisal with a meta-analysis of randomized controlled trials. J Clin Oncol 2004; 22(19):3860–3867.
44. Arriagada R, Bergman B, Dunant A, Le CT, Pignon JP, Vansteenkiste J. Cisplatin-based adjuvant chemotherapy in patients with completely resected non-small-cell lung cancer. N Engl J Med 2004; 350(4):351–360.
45. Kato H, Ichinose Y, Ohta M, et al. A randomized trial of adjuvant chemotherapy with Uracil-Tegafur for adenocarcinoma of the lung. N Engl J Med 2004; 350(17):1713–1721.
46. Vokes EE, Green MR. Clinical studies in non-small cell lung cancer: the CALGB experience. Cancer Invest 1998; 16(2):72–79.
47. Strauss GM, Herndon MA. Randomized clinical trial of adjuvant chemotherapy with paclitaxel and carboplatin following resection in Stage IB non-small cell lung cancer (NSCLC): Report of Cancer and Leukemia Group B (CALGB) Protocol 9633. J Clin Oncol 2004; 22(14S):7019.
48. Graham PH, Gebski VJ, Langlands AO. Radical radiotherapy for early nonsmall cell lung cancer. Int J Radiat Oncol Biol Phys 1995; 31(2):261–266.
49. Noordijk EM, vd Poest CE, Hermans J, Wever AM, Leer JW. Radiotherapy as an alternative to surgery in elderly patients with resectable lung cancer. Radiother Oncol 1988; 13(2):83–89.
50. Furuta M, Hayakawa K, Katano S, et al. Radiation therapy for stage I-II non-small cell lung cancer in patients aged 75 years and older. Jpn J Clin Oncol 1996; 26(2):95–98.
51. Gava A. Lung cancer radiation treatment in the elderly. Crit Rev Oncol Hematol 1999; 32(1):45–48.
52. Hayakawa K, Mitsuhashi N, Katano S, et al. High-dose radiation therapy for elderly patients with inoperable or unresectable non-small cell lung cancer. Lung Cancer 2001; 32(1):81–88.
53. Lonardi F, Pavanaro M, Coeli, M. Radiation Therapy (RT) of symptomatic advanced non small cell lung cancer (NSCLC) in the elderly [abstr]. Lung Cancer 1997; 18(suppl 1):130.
54. Atagi S, Furuse K, Kawahara M, et al. Phase II trail of daily low-dose carboplatin (CBDCA) and radiotherapy (RT) in elderly patients with unresectable locally advanced non-small cell lung cancer (NSCLC) [abstr]. Lung Cancer 1997; 18(suppl1);130.
55. Pignon T, Gregor A, Schaake KC, Roussel A, Van GM, Scalliet P. Age has no impact on acute and late toxicity of curative thoracic radiotherapy. Radiother Oncol 1998; 46(3):239–248.

56. Catell D, Steinfeld A, Donahue B. Lung cancer metastatic to brain in octogenarians. Lung Cancer 1997; 18(suppl 1):130.

57. Laaksonen R, Niiranen A, Iivanainen M, et al. Dementia-like, largely reversible syndrome after cranial irradiation and prolonged interferon treatment. Ann Clin Res 1988; 20(3):201–203.

58. Johnson BE, Patronas N, Hayes W, et al. Neurologic, computed cranial tomographic, and magnetic resonance imaging abnormalities in patients with small-cell lung cancer: further follow-up of 6- to 13-year survivors. J Clin Oncol 1990; 8(1):48–56.

59. Johnson BE, Becker B, Goff WB, et al. Neurologic, neuropsychologic, and computed cranial tomography scan abnormalities in 2- to 10-year survivors of small-cell lung cancer. J Clin Oncol 1985; 3(12):1659–1667.

60. Cull A, Gregor A, Hopwood P, et al. Neurological and cognitive impairment in long-term survivors of small cell lung cancer. Eur J Cancer 1994; 30A(8):1067–1074.

61. Gregor A, Cull A, Stephens RJ, et al. Prophylatic cranial irradiation is indicated following complete response to induction therapy in small cell lung cancer: results of a multi-centre co-ordinated trail. United Kingdom Co-ordinating Committee for Cancer Research (UKCCCR) and the European Organisation for Research and Treatment of Cancer (EORTC). Eur J Cancer 1997; 33(11):1717–1719.

62. Koga K, Kusumoto S, Watanabe K, Nishikawa K, Harada K, Ebihara H. Age factor relevant to the development of radiation pneumonitis in radiotherapy of lung cancer. Int J Radiat Oncol Biol Phys 1988; 14(2):367–371.

63. Numico G, Russi E, Merlano M. Best supportive care in non-small cell lung cancer: is there a role for radiotherapy and chemotherapy? Lung Cancer 2001; 32(3):213–226.

64. Albain KS, Crowley JJ, LeBlanc M, Livingston RB. Determinants of improved outcome in small-cell lung cancer: an analysis of the 2,580-patient Southwest Oncology Group data base. J Clin Oncol 1990; 8(9):1563–1574.

65. Osterlind K, Hansen HH, Hansen M, Dombernowsky P, Andersen PK. Long-term disease-free survival in small-cell carcinoma of the lung: a study of clinical determinants. J Clin Oncol 1986; 4(9):1307–1313.

66. Siu LL, Shepherd FA, Murray N, Feld R, Pater J, Zee B. Influence of age on the treatment of limited-stage small-cell lung cancer. J Clin Oncol 1996; 14(3):821–828.

67. Paccagnella A, Favaretto A. Treatment of small cell lung cancer (SCLC) in elderly patients (Meeting abstract). Proc ASCO 1996.

68. Yuen AR, Zou G, Turrisi AT, et al. Similar outcome of elderly patients in Intergroup Trial 0096: cisplatin, etoposide, and thoracic radiotherapy administered once or twice daily in limited stage small cell lung carcinoma. Cancer 2000; 89(9):1953–1960.

69. Ashley S, O'Brien M, Smith IE. Age is not an adverse predictive factor in the treatment of small cell lung cancer. Lung Cancer1997; 18(suppl 1):22–23.

70. Shepherd FA, Amdemichael E, Evans WK, et al. Treatment of small cell lung cancer in the elderly. J Am Geriatr Soc 1994; 42(1):64–70.

71. Nou E. Full chemotherapy in elderly patients with small cell bronchial carcinoma. Acta Oncol 1996; 34:399–406.

72. Oshita F, Kurata T, Kasai T, et al. Prospective evaluation of the feasibility of cisplatin-based chemotherapy for elderly lung cancer patients with normal organ functions. Jpn J Cancer Res 1995; 86(12):1198–1202.

73. Findlay MP, Griffin AM, Raghavan D, et al. Retrospective review of chemotherapy for small cell lung cancer in the elderly: does the end justify the means? Eur J Cancer 1991; 27(12):1597–1601.

74. Kelly P, O'Brien AA, Daly P, Clancy L. Small-cell lung cancer in elderly patients: the case for chemotherapy. Age Ageing 1991; 20(1):19–22.

75. Lind MJ, Margison JM, Cerny T, Thatcher N, Wilkinson PM. The effect of age on the pharmacokinetics of ifosfamide. Br J Clin Pharmacol 1990; 30(1):140–143.

76. Teramoto S, Fukuchi Y, Shu CY, Orimo H. Influences of cisplatin combination chemotherapy on oxygen radical generation by blood in elderly and adult patients with lung cancer. Chemotherapy 1995; 41(3):222–228.

77. Smit EF, Carney DN, Harford P, Sleijfer DT, Postmus PE. A phase II study of oral etoposide in elderly patients with small cell lung cancer. Thorax 1989; 44(8):631–633.

78. Carney DN, Grogan L, Smit EF, Harford P, Berendsen HH, Postmus PE. Single-agent oral etoposide for elderly small cell lung cancer patients. Semin Oncol 1990; 17(1 suppl 2):49–53.

79. Girling DJ. Comparison of oral etoposide and standard intravenous multidrug chemotherapy for small-cell lung cancer: a stopped multicentre randomised trial. Medical Research Council Lung Cancer Working Party. Lancet 1996; 348(9027):563–566.

80. Souhami RL, Spiro SG, Rudd RM, et al. Five-day oral etoposide treatment for advanced small-cell lung cancer: randomized comparison with intravenous chemotherapy. J Natl Cancer Inst 1997; 89(8):577–580.

81. Frasci G, Comella G, DelGaizo, et al. Carboplatin (CBDCA)-oral etoposide (VP-16) personalized dosing in elderly or poor performance status elderly NSCLC patients. Lung Cancer 1997; 18(suppl 1):38.

82. Berzinec P, Arpasova M, Kuzmova H. Carboplatin and etoposide in patients aged 75 years or older with small cell lung cancer. Lung Cancer 1997; 18(suppl 1):46.

83. Matsui K, Masuda N, Fukuoka M, et al. Phase II trial of carboplatin plus oral etoposide for elderly patients with small-cell lung cancer. Br J Cancer 1998; 77(11): 1961–1965.

84. Okamoto H, Watanabe K, Nishiwaki Y, et al. Phase II study of area under the plasma-concentration-versus-time curve-based carboplatin plus standard-dose intravenous etoposide in elderly patients with small-cell lung cancer. J Clin Oncol 1999; 17(11):3540–3545.

85. Samantas E, Skarlos DV, Pectasides D, et al. Combination chemotherapy with low doses of weekly carboplatin and oral etoposide in poor risk small cell lung cancer. Lung Cancer 1999; 23(2):159–168.

86. Shibata K, Nakatsumi Y, Kasahara K, Bando T, Fujimura M, Matsuda T. Analysis of thrombocytopenia due to carboplatin combined with etoposide in elderly patients with lung cancer. J Cancer Res Clin Oncol 1996; 122(7):437–442.

87. Evans WK, Radwi A, Tomiak E, et al. Oral etoposide and carboplatin. Effective therapy for elderly patients with small cell lung cancer. Am J Clin Oncol 1995; 18(2):149–155.

88. Raghavan D, Bishop JF, Stuart-Harris R, et al. Carboplatin-containing regimens for small cell lung cancer: implications for management in the elderly. Semin Oncol 1992; 19(1 suppl 2):12–16.

89. Carney DN. Carboplatin/etoposide combination chemotherapy in the treatment of poor prognosis patients with small cell lung cancer. Lung Cancer 1995; 12(suppl 3):S77–S83.

90. Westeel V, Murray N, Gelmon K, et al. New combination of the old drugs for elderly patients with small-cell lung cancer: a phase II study of the PAVE regimen. J Clin Oncol 1998; 16(5):1940–1947.

91. Neubauer M, Schwartz J, Caracandas J, et al. Results of a phase II study of weekly paclitaxel plus carboplatin in patients with extensive small-cell lung cancer with Eastern Cooperative Oncology Group Performance Status of 2, or age > or = 70 years. J Clin Oncol 2004; 22(10):1872–1877.

92. Grunberg SM, Crowley J, Hande KR, et al. Treatment of poor-prognosis extensive disease small-cell lung cancer with an all-oral regimen of etoposide and cyclophosphamide—a Southwest Oncology Group clinical and pharmacokinetic study. Cancer Chemother Pharmacol 1999; 44(6):461–468.

93. Stephens RJ, Girling DJ, Bleehen NM, Moghissi K, Yosef HM, Machin D. The role of post-operative radiotherapy in non-small-cell lung cancer: a multicentre randomised trial in patients with pathologically staged T1-2, N1-2, M0 disease. Medical Research Council Lung Cancer Working Party. Br J Cancer 1996; 74(4):632–639.

94. James LE, Gower NH, Rudd RM, et al. A randomised trial of low-dose/high-frequency chemotherapy as palliative treatment of poor-prognosis small-cell lung cancer: a Cancer Research Campaign trial. Br J Cancer 1996; 73(12):1563–1568.

95. Earl HM, Rudd RM, Spiro SG, et al. A randomised trial of planned versus as required chemotherapy in small cell lung cancer: a Cancer Research Campaign trial. Br J Cancer 1991; 64(3):566–572.

96. Ardizzoni A, Favaretto A, Boni L, et al. Platinum-etoposide chemotherapy in elderly patients with small-cell lung cancer: results of a randomized multicenter phase II study assessing attenuated-dose or full-dose with lenograstim prophylaxis—a Forza Operativa Nazionale Italiana Carcinoma Polmonare and Gruppo Studio Tumori Polmonari Veneto (FONICAP-GSTPV) study. J Clin Oncol 2005; 23(3):569–575.

97. Pignon JP, Arriagada R, Ihde DC, et al. A meta-analysis of thoracic radiotherapy for small-cell lung cancer. N Engl J Med 1992; 327(23):1618–1624.

98. Quon H, Shepherd FA, Payne DG, et al. The influence of age on the delivery, tolerance, and efficacy of thoracic irradiation in the combined modality treatment of limited stage small cell lung cancer. Int J Radiat Oncol Biol Phys 1999; 43(1):39–45.

99. Jeremic B, Shibamoto Y, Acimovic L, Milisavljevic S. Carboplatin, etoposide, and accelerated hyperfractionated radiotherapy for elderly patients with limited small cell lung carcinoma: a phase II study. Cancer 1998; 82(5):836–841.

100. Murray N, Grafton C, Shah A, et al. Abbreviated treatment for elderly, infirm, or non-compliant patients with limited-stage small-cell lung cancer. J Clin Oncol 1998; 16(10):3323–3328.

101. Grunberg SM, Hesketh PJ. Control of chemotherapy-induced emesis. N Engl J Med 1993; 329(24):1790–1796.

102. Niiranen A, Kajanti M, Tammilehto L, Mattson K. The clinical effect of medroxyprogesterone (MPA) in elderly patients with lung cancer. Am J Clin Oncol 1990; 13(2):113–116.

103. Chemotherapy in non-small cell lung cancer: a meta-analysis using updated data on individual patients from 52 randomised clinical trials. Non-small Cell Lung Cancer Collaborative Group. BMJ 1995; 311(7010):899–909.

104. Dillman RO, Seagren SL, Propert KJ, et al. A randomized trial of induction chemotherapy plus high-dose radiation versus radiation alone in stage III non-small-cell lung cancer. N Engl J Med 1990; 323(14):940–945.

105. Dillman RO, Herndon J, Seagren SL, Eaton WL Jr, Green MR. Improved survival in stage III non-small-cell lung cancer: seven-year follow-up of Cancer and Leukemia Group B (CALGB) 8433 trial. J Natl Cancer Inst 1996; 88(17):1210–1215.

106. Movsas B, Scott C, Sause W, et al. The benefit of treatment intensification is age and histology-dependent in patients with locally advanced non-small cell lung cancer (NSCLC): a quality-adjusted survival analysis of Radiation Therapy Oncology Group (RTOG) chemoradiation studies. Int J Radiat Oncol Biol Phys 1999; 45(5):1143–1149.

107. Werner-Wasik M, Scott C, Cox JD, et al. Recursive partitioning analysis of 1999 Radiation Therapy Oncology Group (RTOG) patients with locally-advanced non-small-cell lung cancer (LA-NSCLC): identification of five groups with different survival. Int J Radiat Oncol Biol Phys 2000; 48(5):1475–1482.

108. Sause W, Kolesar P, Taylor S IV, et al. Final results of phase III trial in regionally advanced unresectable non-small cell lung cancer: Radiation Therapy Oncology Group, Eastern Cooperative Oncology Group, and Southwest Oncology Group. Chest 2000; 117(2):358–364.

109. Langer CJ, Hsu C, Curran WJ, et al. Do elderly patients (pts) with locally advanced non-small cell lung cancer (NSCLC) benefit from combined modality therapy? A secondary analysis of RTOG 94-10. Int J Radiat Oncol Biol Phys 2001; 53(1 suppl 1):20–21.

110. Spira A, Ettinger DS. Multidisciplinary management of lung cancer. N Engl J Med 2004; 350(4):379–392.

111. Colleoni M, Gaion F, Nelli P, Colmellere GM, Manente P. Weekly variations in elderly patients with non-small-cell lung cancer. Tumori 1994; 80(6):448–452.

112. Gridelli C, Perrone F, Gallo C, et al. Vinorelbine is well tolerated and active in the treatment of elderly patients with advanced non-small cell lung cancer. A two-stage phase II study. Eur J Cancer 1997; 33(3):392–397.
113. Mattioli R, Tripoli NK. Corneal geometry reconstruction with the Keratron videokeratographer. Optom Vis Sci 1997; 74(11):881–894.
114. Gridelli C, Aapro M, Ardizzoni A, et al. Treatment of advanced non-small-cell lung cancer in the elderly: results of an international expert panel. J Clin Oncol 2005; 23(13):3125–3137.
115. Effects of vinorelbine on quality of life and survival of elderly patients with advanced non-small-cell lung cancer. The Elderly Lung Cancer Vinorelbine Italian Study Group. J Natl Cancer Inst 1999; 91(1):66–72.
116. Frasci G, Lorusso V, Panza N, et al. Gemcitabine plus vinorelbine versus vinorelbine alone in elderly patients with advanced non-small-cell lung cancer. J Clin Oncol 2000; 18(13):2529–2536.
117. Gridelli C, Perrone F, Gallo C, et al. Chemotherapy for elderly patients with advanced non-small-cell lung cancer: the Multicenter Italian Lung Cancer in the Elderly Study (MILES) phase III randomized trial. J Natl Cancer Inst 2003; 95(5):362–372.
118. Comella P, Frasci G, Carnicelli P, et al. Gemcitabine with either paclitaxel or vinorelbine vs paclitaxel or gemcitabine alone for elderly or unfit advanced non-small-cell lung cancer patients. Br J Cancer 2004; 91(3):489–497.
119. Langer CJ, Manola J, Bernardo P, et al. Cisplatin-based therapy for elderly patients with advanced non-small-cell lung cancer: implications of Eastern Cooperative Oncology Group 5592, a randomized trial. J Natl Cancer Inst 2002; 94(3):173–181.
120. Cappuzzo F, Bartolini S, Ceresoli GL, et al. Efficacy and tolerability of gefitinib in pretreated elderly patients with advanced non-small-cell lung cancer (NSCLC). Br J Cancer 2004; 90(1):82–86.
121. Albain KS, Crowley JJ, LeBlanc M, Livingston RB. Survival determinants in extensive-stage non-small-cell lung cancer: the Southwest Oncology Group experience. J Clin Oncol 1991; 9(9):1618–1626.

12

Prostate Cancer

Joseph S. Chan and Christopher W. Ryan
Oregon Health and Science University, Portland, Oregon, U.S.A.

Nicholas J. Vogelzang
Nevada Cancer Institute, Las Vegas, Nevada, U.S.A.

INTRODUCTION

Prostate cancer is the most common cancer in American men. Although prostate cancer does affect younger men, it is mostly a disease of the elderly, with a median age at diagnosis of 66 years (1). In 2005, the estimated number of new cases of prostate cancer is over 230,000—approximately one-third of all cancer cases in men (2). Prostate cancer is also the second leading cause of cancer death in men, with more than 30,000 deaths estimated for 2005. The cause of prostate cancer is unknown, although racial, genetic, and dietary factors have been implicated (1). Older age remains the greatest risk factor for development of prostate cancer. At autopsy, over two-thirds of men over 80 years of age have asymptomatic "latent" prostate cancer (3). The probability of developing prostate cancer increases from 1 in 39 during the ages of 40 to 59 to 1 in 7 during the ages of 60 to 79. While there are relatively few deaths from prostate cancer under the age of 60, it is the third leading cause of cancer death in men aged 60 to 79, and the second leading cause of cancer death in men aged 80 and over (2).

TUMOR BIOLOGY AND SCREENING

Prostate cancer is linked to several genetic loci, including the hereditary prostate cancer 1 (HPC1) gene. In a linkage analysis of 91 families, individuals linked to the HPC1 gene conferred an 88% lifetime probability of developing prostate cancer (4). There have been several other susceptibility loci identified with the three genetic mutations described. However, at present, the role of these genes is still unclear and only 5% to 10% of prostate cancer cases are associated with a strong family history of the disease (5). Variants in the androgen receptor and the vitamin D receptor have also been implicated in development of prostate cancer (6). Potential molecular markers that may determine prognostic significance are being investigated (7). These prognostic markers may become most important in the management of the elderly population with prostate cancer.

Clinicians must carefully consider the risks and benefits of prostate cancer screening and the therapeutic interventions that follow a diagnosis. Because the median time of death from a diagnosis of prostate cancer is 8 to 10 years, this risk/ benefit determination is especially pertinent in elderly patients. Sensitive prostate cancer screening is a recent phenomenon that began in the late 1980s with the introduction of prostate-specific antigen (PSA) testing, and improvements in transrectal ultrasonography and biopsy techniques. These advances, as well as greater public awareness of the disease, led to an explosive increase in prostate cancer diagnosis. Controversy still exists regarding screening recommendations.

Currently, the American Cancer Society recommends annual PSA blood test and digital rectal exam beginning at age 50 for all men with at least a 10-year life expectancy (8). Men at higher risk (African-American men or men with a strong family history of one or more first-degree relatives diagnosed at an early age) should be tested starting at age 45 (8). Individuals with multiple first-degree relatives affected at an early age or with an altered HPC1 gene may be candidates for annual screening, beginning at age 40 (9). Although there are no guidelines for when to stop PSA testing, the utility of screening men over 75 years of age is questionable (10).

The use of the PSA assay as a screening tool has been the center of much controversy. PSA is a serine protease of the kallikrein family, which is found only in prostatic tissue (11). The normal range that is in common use, regardless of age, is 0 to 4 ng/mL. Increases in prostatic volume, prostatic infarctions, ejaculation, and other nonspecific factors lead to an elevation of PSA level as men age, even in the absence of malignancy.

The low specificity of the PSA test can result in a high number of unnecessary biopsies. Age-specific ranges with higher levels of PSA accepted as "normal" for older patients have been proposed (Table 1) (12). PSA "density" (amount of PSA per unit volume of prostate gland, as determined by transrectal ultrasound) has also been proposed as a way to increase the value of the test. However, neither age-adjusted PSA measurements nor PSA density has increased the positive predictive value of PSA in older men. Both methods may miss up to 20% of significant prostate cancers. Currently, PSA testing has not been proven to increase overall survival. Many types of bias distort prediction for the value of PSA testing in overall survival. Length–time bias (the detection and treatment of early harmless cancer that would not become clinically relevant) is especially important in the elderly population. Treating these harmless tumors does not improve mortality and may significantly increase patient morbidity due to treatment side effects. The value of PSA testing

Table 1 PSA Age-Specific Reference Ranges

Age (years)	Serum PSA concentration (ng/mL)
40–49	0–2.5
50–59	0–3.5
60–69	0–4.5
70–79	0–6.5

Abbreviation: PSA, prostate-specific antigen.
Source: From Ref. 12.

in lowering prostate cancer mortality is currently being evaluated in large randomized controlled trials (13).

PSA has other roles besides that of a screening tool. PSA should drop to undetectable levels after radical prostatectomy for localized disease, and thus serves as a valuable tool for early detection of recurrence (14). Increasing PSA levels after treatment of metastatic disease is usually the earliest sign of relapse. Likewise, a decreasing PSA level during treatment of metastatic disease is frequently used for response assessment (15).

DIAGNOSIS AND STAGING

Prostate cancer usually causes few clinical symptoms in its early stages. As prostate cancer progresses locally, symptoms of urinary obstruction may occur, including hesitancy, weakness of stream, postvoid dribbling, incomplete voiding, and nocturia. However, many of these symptoms overlap with symptoms of benign prostatic hypertrophy. Most commonly, the disease is diagnosed after an elevated screening PSA and/or abnormal digital rectal exam. Pain from bony metastases occurs in late-stage disease and is now an uncommon initial presentation due to the prevalence of PSA screening. Anemia or pancytopenia may result from bone marrow replacement in advanced disease.

Staging of prostate cancer is described using the tumor, node, and metastases system (Table 2) (16). A typical staging workup includes measurement of PSA, digital rectal exam, and bone scan (if the PSA is $> 10 \, ng/mL$). Extracapsular or

Table 2 AJCC Prostate Cancer Staging

Stage I	
Found at time of TURP <5% of tissue resected Gleason 2–4	T1a G1
Stage II	
Found at time of TURP <5% of tissue resected Gleason 5–10	T1a G2–4
Found at time of TURP >5% of tissue resected	T1b
Tumor found at time of needle biopsy prompted by elevated PSA	T1c
Organ confined involving one-half of one lobe or less	T2a
Unilateral involving more than one-half of one lobe	T2b
Tumor involves both lobes	T2c
Stage III	
Extracapsular extension	T3a
Tumor invades seminal vesicle	T3b
Stage IV	
Invades bladder neck, external sphincter, rectum, levator muscles, or pelvic side-wall	T4
Metastatic disease pelvic nodes only	Any T N1
Metastatic disease to nonregional lymph nodes	Any T any N M1a
Metastatic disease to bone	Any T any N M1b
Metastatic disease to lung, liver, brain	Any T any N M1c

Abbreviations: AJCC, American Joint Committee on Cancer; TURP, transurethral resection of the prostate; PSA, prostate-specific antigen.
Source: From Ref. 16.

lymph node spread is difficult to assess clinically and may not be detected until the time of surgery. Computed tomography scan may be helpful for staging of patients with a high PSA and designing treatment portals for radiation therapy (17). Endorectal coil magnetic resonance imaging and transrectal ultrasound are accurate in determining extracapsular extension or seminal vesicle involvement to select patients for surgery (18,19).

The most common grading system in use is the Gleason system. A score of 2 to 10 is applied, based on the primary and secondary growth patterns of the tumor. The higher the grade, the more undifferentiated the tumor and the less discrete the glandular architecture. A higher grade is associated with a higher rate of local tumor spread and metastasis (20).

Further information on diagnosis and staging is included in the treatment section. Staging (Table 2) and method of diagnosis is often linked to the treatment of prostate cancer. This is especially true in the management of localized prostate cancer and treatment of the elderly patient.

TREATMENT

Localized Prostate Cancer

Stage 1 (T1aNoMoG1) prostate cancer is defined as a normal gland on rectal examination with less than 5% of tissue containing well-differentiated adenocarcinoma (Gleason sum <4). This stage of disease is usually diagnosed incidentally at the time of transurethral resection of the prostate (TURP). Stage T1a is often treated with observation alone, because disease progression is found to occur in only 2% of patients (21). Such conservative therapy has been challenged, because longer follow-up has shown disease progression in 16% of men followed for at least eight years after diagnosis (22). Lowe and Listrom found that the probability of disease progression increases with age and have recommended treatment for patients with a life expectancy of at least five years and with Gleason score ≥4 disease (23). Although stage T1a disease is unlikely to progress to clinical significance in the life span of many elderly men, annual PSA and rectal examinations remain necessary to monitor for disease progression.

Stage II prostate cancer consists of several entities, including moderate to high grade T1a, as well as T1b, T1c, and T2 tumors of any grade. T1b prostate cancer is defined as a normal gland on rectal examination with more than 5% of tissue containing adenocarcinoma. Again, this stage is found incidentally during TURP. Radical prostatectomy or radiation therapy are commonly offered, especially to men under 65 years of age, because median time to disease progression is four to five years and death from untreated cancer will occur in 50% of untreated patients within 10 to 15 years (24). Survival can improve to 70% to 90% at 10 to 15 years with treatment (25).

Stage T1c of prostate cancer was added to the tumor node metastasis staging system in 1992. It is defined as carcinoma found on needle biopsy solely from an elevated PSA level with no palpable tumor. These carcinomas have a tendency to be of higher grade and have higher tumor volumes than T1a tumors and clinically behave like T1b tumors. A 93% disease-free survival at eight years has been reported in T1c patients treated with radical prostatectomy (26). Deciding which elderly patients may benefit from definitive therapy should be based on pretreatment PSA levels and pathological findings at biopsy (27).

Stage T2a prostate cancer is defined as a palpable nodule localized to one lobe of the gland. Radical prostatectomy or radiotherapy have nearly the same efficacy, with a 50% to 60% survival at 10 years, although some evidence indicates a higher recurrence rate with radiotherapy (28). Interestingly, Alexander et al. noted that older patients with clinical stage T2a disease were found to have a higher pathological stage and grade at radical prostatectomy, possibly due to masking of prostatic induration by benign glandular hypertrophy (29). Stage T2b and T2c are defined as more extensive involvement of one lobe or involvement of both lobes of the prostate. These pathological stages can often be difficult to distinguish and, in clinical practice, the best prognostic indicators are probably the PSA level and Gleason score.

The management of clinically localized prostate cancer in the elderly is challenging. Without PSA substaging, nearly half of the patients thought to have organ-confined disease are found to have cancer spread beyond the prostate at the time of radical prostatectomy (30). With PSA-driven substaging, there is an increasing risk of nonorgan-confined disease with each incremental increase in the PSA above 4 ng/mL. For example, with PSA levels over 10 ng/mL, about 50% of patients have nonorgan-confined disease. The use of PSA testing, combined with clinical stage and Gleason score, can help predict the likelihood of lymph node spread, and thus stratify those patients who are more likely to achieve cure from radical prostatectomy (31). There are several nomograms published by Partin et al. and Kattan et al., which predict clinical stage and disease recurrence using PSA and Gleason score. These nomograms have been validated using data from an international contingent and are currently being used to identify patients at risk for failure after local therapy (32,33).

The efficacy of radical prostatectomy versus external beam radiotherapy in the management of localized prostate cancer has been a controversial topic for many years. The only randomized trial to date was small and not controlled for pretreatment PSA values, but indicated an advantage for radical prostatectomy (28). PSA or "biochemical" failure rates have been used to compare radiation and surgical outcomes in more recent series. Biochemical failure is defined as detectable levels of PSA (usually >0.2 ng/mL) after radical prostatectomy or a rising PSA on three consecutive occasions following a radiotherapy-induced nadir (usually <1.0 ng/mL). Although the PSA nadir is prognostic, there is no consensus for a specific level. When pretreatment PSA and Gleason score are used to stratify high-risk patients, some series suggest that radical prostatectomy offers improved biochemical relapse-free survival compared to radiation therapy (34). That position is controversial, because Lattanzi et al. estimate that a PSA of less than 8 ng/mL is the level at which the majority of patients can obtain long-term biochemical relapse-free control with radiation (35). A study of surgically staged cases of node-negative, localized prostate cancer revealed that although biochemical "cure" was not achieved with radiation therapy, cause-specific survival at 10 years still exceeded 80% (36). In 1997, an analysis of the surveillance epidemiology and end results (SEER) database implied a 10-year disease-specific survival advantage in age-matched cohorts for radical prostatectomy over both radiation therapy and conservative management. This effect was more significant in higher-grade tumors. However, comorbidities may be important in the selection of certain therapies and it is difficult to draw substantial conclusions about treatment modalities (37). Currently, young and healthy men are more likely to receive radical prostatectomy, while older men are more likely to receive radiation therapy. In summary, we believe that radiotherapy or surgery for prostate cancers are equivalent modalities when stratified by pretreatment PSA and Gleason scores.

Elderly men are often given the option of watchful waiting in the case of clinically localized disease. The Veterans Administration Cooperative Urological
Research Group was unable to show a survival benefit in patients with localized disease undergoing radical prostatectomy compared to observation alone; but this
study lacked statistical power (38). The study did conclude that localized prostate
cancer in patients older than 70 years with a low Gleason score (<7) is unlikely
to decrease that patient's life expectancy if no initial treatment is instituted. A nonrandomized observational study by Albertsen et al. suggested that observation alone
might be appropriate in older men who have low-volume, low-grade disease (39).
The study retrospectively examined men aged 65 to 75 years who were treated with
observation or hormonal therapy alone. Men with low-grade (Gleason 2–4) cancer
showed no reduction of life expectancy in comparison with the general population
whereas men with moderate-grade (Gleason 5–7) disease showed up to four- to
five-year reduction, and those with high-grade (Gleason 8–10) showed up to six-
to eight-year reduction. A follow-up analysis confirmed minimal risk of death from
prostate cancer at 20 years in patients with Gleason 2–4 tumors (six deaths per 1000
person-years) and high risk of death at 10 years in men with Gleason 8 to10 tumors
(121 deaths per 1000 person-years) (40). These studies suggest that conservative management is reasonable in elderly men with low-grade tumors, while definitive treatment should be considered for high-grade tumors. Management of men with
intermediate grade tumors remains debatable.

In 1993, the Prostate Patient Outcomes Research Team (PORT) published a
decision analysis for management of clinically localized prostate cancer that
accorded little benefit for curative intent therapy in elderly men (41). The group
modeled radiation therapy, radical prostatectomy, and watchful waiting, with the
benefit of treatment being a decrease in death or disability from metastatic disease.
They determined that there was less than a six-month improvement in quality-
adjusted survival for men between 70 and 75 years of age who received radiotherapy
or radical prostatectomy, and that in men older than 75 years, no benefits from
these therapies were seen in comparison to watchful waiting. Those favoring surgical or radiation treatment criticized the methodology of the PORT analysis, and a
repeat decision analysis with updated data suggested that aggressive therapy in men
with moderately or poorly differentiated cancers up to 75 years of age would be
beneficial (42,43).

In 2002, Holmberg et al. of the Scandinavian Prostate Cancer Group reported
the results of a randomized trial comparing radical prostatectomy with watchful
waiting in early stage prostate cancer (44). The results demonstrated an absolute
reduction of disease-specific mortality of approximately 7% and an absolute reduction of development of distant metastasis by 14%, eight years after radical prostatectomy. In addition, a 10-year follow-up of this trial published in 2005
demonstrated a significant benefit in prostate cancer–specific mortality and overall
survival in the radical prostatectomy group (45). However, an exploratory subgroup
analysis showed that this mortality benefit may be limited to patients younger
than 65. Importantly, this study was initiated in 1988 with 75% of patients diagnosed
with palpable disease and only 10% of patients diagnosed with elevated PSA. This is
certainly different from the patient population today which is mostly diagnosed by
an elevated PSA level. It is possible that in patients detected by early screening,
the risk of death from prostate cancer is lower, thus reducing the benefit of radical
prostatectomy. The Prostate Cancer Intervention Versus Observation Trial (PIVOT)
is a contemporary, prospective randomized trial comparing radical prostatectomy

with observation (46). PIVOT has completed accrual and, when mature, results from this trial will help better define the appropriate treatment of localized prostate cancer in the era of PSA-screening.

The decision between conservative versus definitive management of localized prostate cancer is not a trivial one, because side effects from treatment may have substantial negative effects on elderly patients. Poorer quality of life has been reported in men undergoing radical prostatectomy or radiation therapy, including significantly worse sexual, urinary, and bowel function (47). An analysis of radical prostatectomies performed on Medicare patients reported a 1.4% mortality rate for men aged 75 to 79 years and a 4.6% mortality rate in those aged over 79 years (48). Long-term complications from surgery may include impotence, incontinence, and urethral stricture. A survey of Medicare patients aged 65 years and older who had undergone radical prostatectomy reported that over 30% of men needed to use pads or clamps for wetness and 60% had absence of partial or full erections (49). The impairment of postoperative sexual function seems to be related to the age of the patient, with older patients faring worse (50). Although nerve-sparing radical prostatectomy has greatly decreased the incidence of postoperative impotence in recent years, these techniques have not been as beneficial in the older patient. Although overall potency rates after radical prostatectomy approach 75%, the rate for men over the age of 70 years is only 20% (51). Several types of treatment are available for postoperative or postradiation sexual dysfunction, including vacuum devices, oral or injection pharmacological therapy, and implantation of penile prosthesis (52).

Complications of radiotherapy may include acute toxicity, such as diarrhea, cystitis, and fatigue, and late toxicity, including proctitis, urinary incontinence, impotence, and urethral stricture (53). The incidence of urinary or rectosigmoid sequelae has been reported to be 3% for severe and 7% to 10% for moderate complications (54). Despite these risks, definitive radiation therapy is generally well tolerated in the elderly if comorbid conditions are absent.

Despite the potential complications of radical prostatectomy and radiation therapy, several studies indicate that quality of life may not be significantly reduced by therapy of curative intent. In addition, a study of a veteran population indicated that a majority of older patients were willing to accept both impotence and incontinence if there was a chance of at least 10% five-year survival advantage with treatment (55). A report in 2003 used a decision analytic Markov model, which demonstrated significantly improved life expectancy and quality-adjusted life expectancy in patients with poorly differentiated prostate cancer up to age 80 (56). An analysis of the Scandinavian Prostatic Group Trial indicated that overall quality of life may be similar in patients undergoing radical prostatectomy compared to watchful waiting (57). Although radical prostatectomy had an increased risk of erectile dysfunction and urinary leakage, it had a lower rate of urinary obstruction. The study also showed that patients in the watchful waiting group had more erectile dysfunction and urinary leakage than expected in the general population, indicating that tumor progression may be partly the cause for these side effects. Overall, subjective quality of life was similar in both groups. Open discussions need to be undertaken between the physician and patient regarding the risks and benefits of various treatment options. Other therapies such as brachytherapy and cryosurgery may prove to be well-tolerated alternatives for elderly patients, but further study is needed to determine the long-term outcome with these modalities (58).

Locally Invasive Disease

T3a, T3b, and T4 prostate cancer is defined as extension of tumor beyond the capsule of the gland and involving the seminal vesicles, pelvic side-wall, bladder, or rectum. The PSA is often above 20 ng/mL. Surgery, radiation therapy, and hormone therapy may be used singly, but most patients receive radiation therapy, which helps to control local symptoms, plus hormonal therapy prior to and during radiation to decrease the amount of tissue to be irradiated and increase symptom-free survival (59,60). Radiation Therapy Oncology Group (RTOG) Trial 85–31 evaluated the benefit of immediate hormonal therapy after radiation for locally advanced tumors and demonstrated improved survival at 10 years (49% vs. 39%) (61). A European Organization for Research and Treatment of Cancer (EORTC) trial also confirmed the benefit of immediate androgen suppression after radiation therapy and showed an improved five-year survival of 78% compared to 62%. Based on this data, radiation therapy plus hormonal therapy for one to three years is recommended for treatment of stage T3/T4 disease (62). The use of hormonal therapy alone is attractive for some elderly patients and may be a viable choice for men with significant comorbidities. In a randomized study comparing immediate versus delayed hormonal treatment in patients who did not receive local therapy, patients with delayed hormonal therapy had a higher frequency of pathological fracture, spinal cord compression, and ureteric obstruction (63). However, another study comparing immediate to delayed orchiectomy for elderly patients not undergoing curative treatment showed no significant improvement in quality of life or overall survival (64). Lastly, consideration of radical prostatectomy should not be ignored. A retrospective study of patients with clinical T3 disease reported a 73% 10-year local and recurrence-free survival after radical prostatectomy, but 78% of patients had received hormone therapy, radiotherapy, or both at some point after surgery. Also, the median PSA was low and many patients had pathological T2 disease and were overstaged (65).

Metastatic Disease

Late stage disease incorporates patients with positive pelvic nodes or distant metastasis. Previously, 25% to 30% of newly diagnosed prostate cancers in older men were metastatic at the time of diagnosis, but this figure has been greatly reduced due to early detection from PSA screening (66).

The management of node-positive disease is controversial. Most patients eventually die of their disease, whereas a minority survive long periods apparently free of further metastases. Five-year survival rates vary from 61% to 97%, partly as a function of the number and size of positive nodes (67). Some advocate aggressive therapy with radical prostatectomy or radiotherapy to control local, symptomatic spread of the disease. External beam radiation as a single modality treatment has shown mixed results, with some evidence suggesting a delay in disease progression, but no long-term survival benefit (68,69). A retrospective review of cases from patients in the M.D. Anderson Cancer Center Study seemed to demonstrate an improvement in disease progression in patients who receive local radiotherapy and androgen ablation compared to those who receive androgen ablation alone. There is some evidence that radical prostatectomy may show improved local control in comparison with expectant management. However, the possible benefit of surgical therapy in the node-positive patient is unlikely to overcome the risks and side effects, especially in elderly patients (67).

Early hormonal therapy has demonstrated value in the treatment of the node-positive patient. RTOG 85–31 included 173 patients with pathologically involved lymph nodes and demonstrated improved PSA control and lower incidence of distant metastases with radiation plus immediate androgen suppression, as well as an overall survival advantage on multivariate analysis (70). A small, randomized Eastern Cooperative Oncology Group study of immediate versus delayed androgen ablation in men found to have micrometastatic nodal disease at radical prostatectomy reported improved survival and reduced risk of recurrence with immediate hormone therapy (71). Another study by the EORTC reported that node-positive patients who did not receive local therapy suggested a benefit in early hormonal treatment (72). A retrospective review of cases from patients in the M.D. Anderson Cancer Center Study seemed to demonstrate an improvement in disease progression in patients who received local radiotherapy and androgen ablation compared with those who receive androgen ablation alone. At present, we recommend radiotherapy and early hormonal therapy for the treatment of node-positive disease.

Hormone ablation has been the mainstay of treatment for metastatic prostate cancer since Huggins and Hodges documented the palliative effects of castration in 1941 (73). Options for primary and androgen withdrawal include orchiectomy or injection of luteinizing hormone (LH)–releasing agonists. Orchiectomy remains the standard modality by which all other forms of hormonal therapy are measured. Although effective, this procedure can be psychologically detrimental and, like all forms of hormonal therapy, will cause decreased potency and hot flashes. Orchiectomy has the advantage of immediate hormonal control, relatively low cost, and elimination of issues of patient compliance. Despite these advantages, the majority of men choose a nonsurgical modality when given a choice between orchiectomy and other forms of therapy (74). The luteinizing hormone–releasing hormone (LHRH) agonists have become the most popular form of hormonal therapy, although these expensive agents have similar side effects and are less convenient than orchiectomy. The two analogues in common use in the United States are leuprolide and goserelin, which are administered via monthly injections, three- or four-monthly depot injections, or a 12-month implant (75). These agents have been shown to be as efficacious as orchiectomy. They rapidly bind to all LH receptors, causing an initial surge in LH production, followed by downregulation of LH production. The initial LH release and resultant rise in testosterone will cause a flare of disease activity when treatment is first begun. Because of this, patients with severe vertebral metastases or acute urethral obstruction should not be given LHRH agonists without the coadministration of an antiandrogen during the first few weeks of treatments (74).

Androgen blockade can also be accomplished by administration of antiandrogenic agents that competitively block binding of dihydrotestosterone to the androgen receptor. Examples include flutamide, biclutamide, and nilutamide. These drugs do not have the progestational side effects of the steroidal antiandrogens, cyproterone acetate and megesterol acetate, nor are they as effective as medical or surgical castration (76). The antiandrogens have hepatotoxic effects, and close monitoring of liver function may be a hardship for older patients. There has been intermittent enthusiasm for "total androgen blockade," using a combination of an antiandrogen with orchiectomy or LHRH agonists (77,78). The Southwest Oncology Group (SWOG) 8894 Study, the largest randomized study on total androgen blockade, did not show a significant benefit in overall survival (79). Other meta-analysis of total androgen blockade also do not confirm any meaningful benefit (80). The extra cost of daily oral treatment may be a drawback in older patients.

Nearly all patients with metastatic disease will eventually progress after initial hormone therapy, with a median time to PSA progression of 15 to 18 months and clinical progression of 24 to 36 months. Definitions of "androgen independent" or "hormone refractory" prostate cancer (HRPC) vary, but generally include patients with PSA progression on androgen deprivation and one or more other hormonal treatments. Second-line hormonal manipulations upon progression are commonly undertaken and can result in PSA declines, although the clinical significance of such maneuvers is not well defined. Withdrawal of antiandrogens for those patients progressing on total androgen blockade results in objective and/or PSA response in a minority of patients (81). The addition of an antiandrogen in those patients naïve to such agents can also result in response (82). Other second-line hormonal therapies include high-dose estrogen therapy or antiadrenal treatment with high-dose ketoconazole (83).

Once considered ineffective, cytotoxic chemotherapy now has an established role in the management of HRPC. Prior to the 1990s, no chemotherapeutic agent had shown significant clinical benefit in this patient population. Mitoxanrone, an anthracenedione with a favorable toxicity profile, received Food and Drug Administration approval for use in the management of hormone-refractory disease based on phase III evidence that it improved quality of life in men with symptomatic, advanced prostate cancer (84). Two randomized phase III trials compared mitoxantrone plus a glucocorticoid to a glucocorticoid alone in HRPC. Both trials showed an advantage for mitoxantrone in terms of pain control, improved quality of life, time to tumor progression, and decline in PSA (85,86). However, no overall survival advantage was demonstrated in these studies. Mitoxantrone remains a standard treatment option for symptomatic HRPC. Because of its favorable toxicity profile, it remains a reasonable choice for the treatment of symptomatic, elderly patients.

In 2004, two randomized studies demonstrated a survival advantage in HRPC with the use of docetaxel-based therapy. TAX 327 randomized hormone-refractory patients to treatment with docetaxel, either on a weekly or every three-week regimen plus daily prednisone, or to mitoxantrone plus prednisone (87). This study reported a median survival of 18.9 months with every three-week docetaxel/prednisone versus 16.5 months for patients receiving mitoxantrone/prednisone ($p = 0.009$). The docetaxel regimen also demonstrated better PSA response, pain control, and quality of life measurements. While patients on docetaxel had slightly more side effects, they were also more likely to complete treatment and had better quality of life scores. The patients were typical of prostate cancer patients with a median age of 68 and Karnofsky scores of 60 or higher. Subset analysis suggested an overall survival benefit in most groups, including patients older than 75 years (88). Another randomized study, SWOG 9916, reported a similar two-month survival benefit with a docetaxel plus estramustine regimen compared with mitoxantrone and prednisone (89).

Docetaxel-based therapy is now a standard treatment option for patients with hormone-refractory disease, improving both quality and quantity of life, regardless of patient age. Studies investigating the utility of docetaxel earlier in the course of the disease, including adjuvant studies for high-risk patients after local therapy, are being planned or are underway.

SUPPORTIVE CARE ISSUES

Skeletal complications are a significant cause of morbidity in men with advanced prostate cancer. Narcotic analgesics or nonsteroidal anti-inflammatory agents are vital tools in controlling cancer-related pain, but they must be administered with care, given their propensity to cause side effects in older patients. External beam radiation therapy is helpful in controlling individual sites of painful bony metastasis (90). Radiopharmaceuticals such as strontium-89 and samarium-153 are effective in managing multifocal bone pain (91,92). Radiopharmaceuticals can cause myelosuppression and integration with chemotherapy can be problematic. Spinal cord compression is a complication of bone metastasis for which the clinician should retain a high index of suspicion, and surgical or radiation therapy should not be delayed.

The bisphosphonate zoledronic acid decreases the incidence of skeletal complications including pathological fractures in hormone-refractory prostate cancer (93). Other less-potent bisphosphonates such as pamidronate have not demonstrated significant benefit in the management of the osteoblastic bone disease of prostate cancer (94). Potential complications of zoledronic acid therapy that should be considered in elderly patients include renal failure, especially in those with baseline dysfunction, and mandibular osteonecrosis in patients with poor dentition or those undergoing extensive dental work.

Osteoporosis is a frequent and under-diagnosed complication in men receiving androgen deprivation therapy. An increased risk of fracture has been reported in prostate cancer patients, which begins early after initiation of androgen deprivation. Approximately one-third of elderly men die within a year of sustaining a hip fracture, and fracture has been associated with poorer survival in prostate cancer patients (95). Hip fractures can cause a high degree of morbidity in the elderly patient and should be considered before initiation of therapy. Baseline and follow-up bone density screening should be performed for all men initiating androgen deprivation, and adequate calcium and vitamin D intake should be ensured. Institution of medical therapy with a bisphosphonate should be considered in osteoporotic patients as per published guidelines (96), including those patients with a T-score <2.5 and/or a history of osteoporotic fractures.

REFERENCES

1. Oesterling J, Fuks Z, Lee CT, Scher HI. Cancer of the prostate. In: DeVita VT Jr, Hellman S, Rosenberg SA, eds. Cancer Principles and Practice of Oncology. Philadelphia: Lippincott-Raven, 1997:1322–1386.
2. Jemal A, Murray T, Ward E, et al. Cancer statistics. CA Cancer J Clin 2005; 55:10–30.
3. Franks LM, Durh MB. Latency and progression in tumors: the natural history of prostate cancer. Proc Natl Acad Sci USA 1992; 89:3367–3371.
4. Smith JR, Freije D, Carpten JD, et al. Major susceptibility locus for prostate cancer on chromosome 1 suggested by a genome-wide search. Science 1996; 274:1371–1374.
5. Verhage BA, Kiemeney LA. Genetic susceptibility to prostate cancer: a review. Fam Cancer 2003; 2:57–67.
6. Ingles SA, Ross RK, Yu MC, et al. Association of prostate cancer risk with genetic polymorphisms in vitamin D receptor and androgen receptor. J Natl Cancer Inst 1997; 89:166–170.
7. Chin JL, Reiter RE. Molecular markers and prostate cancer prognosis. Clin Prostate Cancer 2004; 3(3):157–164.
8. Smith RA, Cokkinides V, Eyre HJ. American Cancer Society guidelines for the early detection of cancer, 2003. CA Cancer J Clin 2003; 53(1):27–43.
9. Gronberg H, Issacs SD, Smith JR, et al. Characteristics of prostate cancer in families potentially linked to the hereditary prostate cancer (HPC1) locus. JAMA 1997; 278: 1251–1255.

10. NCCN Clinical Practice Guidelines in Oncology, Prostate Cancer Early Detection, Jan 20, 2005.
11. Watt KWK, Lee PJ, M'Timkulu, et al. Human prostate-specific antigen: structural and functional similarity with serine protease. Proc Natl Acad Sci USA 1986; 83:3166–3170.
12. Oesterling JE, Jacobson SJ, Chute CG, et al. Serum prostate-specific antigen in a community-based population of healthy men. JAMA 1996; 80:83–98.
13. Wilson SS, Crawford ED. Screening for prostate cancer: current recommendations. Urol Clin N Am 2004; 31:219–226.
14. Stamey TA, Yang N, Hay AR, et al. Prostate-specific antigen as a serum marker for adenocarcinoma of the prostate. N Engl J Med 1987; 317:909–916.
15. Kelly WK, Scher HI, Mazumdar M, et al. Prostate specific antigen as a measure of disease outcome in hormone-refractory prostate cancer. J Clin Oncol 1999; 11:607–615.
16. Prostate. In: American Joint Committee on Cancer. AJCC Cancer Staging Manual. 6th ed. New York, NY: Springer, 2002:337–345.
17. Lee N, Newhouse JH, Olsson CA, et al. Which patients with newly diagnosed prostate cancer need a computed tomography scan of the abdomen and pelvis? An analysis based on 588 patients. Urology 1999; 54(3):490–494.
18. D'Amico AV, Schnall M, Whittington R, et al. Endorectal coil magnetic resonance imaging identifies locally advanced prostate cancer in select patients with clinically localized disease. Urology 1998; 51(3):449–454.
19. Garg S, Fortling B, Chadwick D, et al. Staging of prostate cancer using 3-dimensional transrectal ultrasound images: a pilot study. J Urol 1999; 162(4):1318–1321.
20. Gleason DF. Histologic grading of prostate cancer: a perspective. Hum Pathol 1992; 23:273–279.
21. Cantrell BB, DeKlerk DP, Eggleston JC, et al. Pathological of untreated stage A1 prostatic cancer: the influence of extent versus grade. J Urol 1981; 125:516–520.
22. Epstein JI, Paull G, Eggleston, et al. Prognosis of untreated stage A1 prostatic carcinoma: a study of 94 cases with extended follow up. J Urol 1986; 136:837–839.
23. Lowe BA, Listrom MB. Incidental carcinoma of the prostate: an analysis of the predictors of progression. J Urol 1988; 140:1340–1344.
24. Brockstein BE, Vogelzang NJ. Chemotherapy of genitourinary cancer. In: The Chemotherapy Source Book. Baltimore: Williams & Wilkins, 1996:1215–1251.
25. Elder JS, Gibbons RP, Correa RJ, et al. Efficacy of radical prostatectomy for stage A2 carcinoma of the prostate. Cancer 1985; 56:2151–2154.
26. Epstein JI, Walsh PC, Carmichael M, et al. Pathologic and clinical findings to predict tumor extent of nonpalpable (stage T1c) prostate cancer. JAMA 1994; 271:368–374.
27. Carter HB, Sauvageot J, Walsh PC, et al. Prospective evaluation of men with stage T1c adenocarcinoma of the prostate. J Urol 1997; 157:2206–2209.
28. Paulson DF, Lin GH, Hinshaw W, et al. Radical surgery versus radiotherapy for adenocarcinoma of the prostate. J Urol 1982; 128:502–504.
29. Alexander RB, Maguire MG, Epstein JI. Pathological stage is higher in older men with clinical stage B1 adenocarcinoma of the prostate. J Urol 1982; 128:502–504.
30. Garnick MB, Fair WR. Prostate cancer: emerging concepts. Part I. Ann Intern Med 1996; 125:119–125.
31. Partin AW, Kattan MW, Subong ENP, et al. Combination of PSA clinical stage and Gleason score to predict pathology in men with localized prostate cancer: a multiinstitutional update. JAMA 1997; 277(18):1445–1451.
32. Kattan MW, Wheeler TM, Scardino PT. A postoperative nomogram for disease recurrence following radical prostatectomy for prostate cancer. J Clin Oncol 1999; 17: 1499–1507.
33. Kattan MW, Zelefsky MJ, Kupelian PA, Scardino PT, Fuks Z, Leibel SA. Pretreatment nomogram for predicting the outcome of three-dimensional conformal radiotherapy in prostate cancer. J Clin Oncol 2000; 18(19):3252–3259.

34. Kupelian P, Katcher J, Levin H, et al. External beam radiotherapy versus radical prostatectomy for clinical stage T1–2 prostate cancer: therapeutic implications of stratification by pretreatment PSA levels and biopsy Gleason scores. Cancer J Sci Am 1997; 3:78–87.

35. Lattanzi JP, Hanlon AL, Hanks GE. Early stage prostate cancer treated with radiation therapy: stratifying an intermediate risk group. Int J Radiat Oncol Biol Phys 1997; 38:569–573.

36. Powell CR, Huisman TK, Riffenburgh RH, et al. Outcome for surgically staged localized prostate cancer treated with external beam radiation therapy. J Urol 1997; 157: 1754–1759.

37. Lu-Yao GL, Yao S. Population-based study of long-term survival in patients with clinically localized prostate cancer. Lancet 1997; 349(9056):906–910.

38. Graversen PH, Nielsen KT, Gasser TC, et al. Radical prostatectomy versus expectant primary treatment in stages I and II prostate cancer: a fifteen year follow-up. Urology 1990; 36:493–498.

39. Albertsen PC, Fryback DG, Storer BE, et al. Long-term survival among men with conservatively treated localized prostate cancer. JAMA 1995; 274:626–631.

40. Albertsen PC, Hanley JA, Fine J. 20-year outcome following conservative management of clinically localized prostate cancer. JAMA; 2005; 293:2095–2101.

41. Fleming C, Wasson JH, Albertsen PC, et al. A decision analysis of alternative treatment strategies for clinically localized prostate cancer. JAMA 1993; 269:2650–2658.

42. Beck JR, Kattan MW, Miles BJ. A critique of the decision analysis for clinically localized prostate cancer. J Urol 1994; 152:1894–1899.

43. Kattan MW, Cowen ME, Miles BJ, et al. Modeling the impact of comorbidity on the decision to treat localized prostate cancer. Med Decis Making 1996; 16:460.

44. Holmberg L, Bill-Axelson A, Helgesen, F. A randomized trial comparing radical prostatectomy with watchful waiting in early prostate cancer. N Engl J Med 2002; 347(11): 781–789.

45. Bill-Axelson A, Holmberg L, Ruutu M, et al. Radical prostatectomy versus watchful waiting in early prostate cancer. N Engl J Med 2005; 352(19):1977–1984.

46. Wilt TJ, Brawer MK. The prostate cancer intervention versus observation trial: a randomized trial comparing radical prostatectomy versus expectant management for the treatment of clinically localized prostate cancer. J Urol 1994; 152:1910–1914.

47. Litwin MS, Leake B, Hays RD, et al. Quality of life outcomes in men treated for localized prostate cancer. JAMA 1995; 273:129–135.

48. Lu-Yao GL, McLerran D, Wasson J, Wennberg JE. An assessment of radical prostatectomy. Time trends, geographic variation, and outcomes. The Prostate Patient Outcomes Research Team. JAMA 1993; 269:2633–2636.

49. Fowler FJ, Barry MJ, Lu-Yao G, et al. Patient-reported complications and follow-up treatment after radical prostatectomy. The national Medicare experience: 1988–1990. Urology 1993; 42:622–629.

50. Quinlan DM, Epstein JI, Carter BS, et al. Sexual function following radical prostatectomy: influence of preservation of neurovascular bundles. J Urol 1993; 145:998–1002.

51. Walsh PC. Retropubic prostatectomy for benign and malignant diseases. In: Marshall FF, ed. Operative Urology. Philadelphia: Saunders, 1991:264–289.

52. NIH Consensus Development Panel on Impotence. JAMA 1993; 270:93–90.

53. Dreicer R, Cooper CS, Williams RD. Management of prostate and bladder cancer in the elderly. Urol Clin North Am 1996; 23:87–97.

54. Perez CA, Hanks GE, Leibel SA. Localized carcinoma of the prostate (stages T1B, T1C, T2, and T3): a review of management with external beam radiation therapy. Cancer 1993; 72:3156–3173.

55. Mazur DJ, Merz JF. Older patients' willingness to trade off urologic adverse outcomes for a better chance of a five-year survival in the clinical setting of prostate cancer. J Am Geriatr Soc 1995; 43:979–984.

56. Alibhai SM, Naglie G, Nam R. Do older men benefit from curative therapy of localized prostate cancer? J Clin Oncol 2003; 21(17):3318–3327.
57. Steinbeck G, Helgesen F, Adolfsson J, et al. Quality of life after radical prostatectomy or watchful waiting. N Engl J Med 2002; 347(11):790–796.
58. Crook J, Lukka H, Klotz L, et al. Systemic overview of the evidence for brachytherapy in clinically localized prostate cancer. CMAJ 2001; 164(7):975–981.
59. Forman JD, Kumar R, Haas G, Montie J, Porter AT, Mesina CF. Neoadjuvant hormonal downsizing of localized carcinoma of the prostate: effects on the volume of normal tissue irradiation. Cancer Invest 1995; 13:8–15.
60. Pilepich MV, Krall JM, Al-Sarraf M, et al. Androgen deprivation with radiation therapy compared with radiation therapy alone for locally advanced prostate carcinoma: a randomized comparative trial of the Radiation Therapy Oncology Group. Urology 1995; 45:616–623.
61. Pilepich MV, Winter K, Lawton CA, et al. Androgen suppression adjuvant to definitive radiotherapy in prostate carcinoma—long-term results of phase III RTOG 85-31. Int J Radiat Oncol Biol Phys 2005; 61:1285–1290.
62. Bolla M, Collette L, Blank L, et al. Long-term results with immediate androgen suppression and external irradiation in patients with locally advanced prostate cancer (an EORTC study): a phase III randomized trial. Lancet 2002; 360:103–108.
63. Immediate versus deferred treatment for advanced prostatic cancer: initial results of the Medical Research Council Trial. The Medical Research Council Prostate Cancer Working Party Investigators Group. Br J Urol 1997; 79(2):235–246.
64. Studer UE, Dieter H, Silvia H, et al. Immediate versus deferred hormonal treatment for patients with prostate cancer who are not suitable for curative local treatment: results of the randomized trial SAKK 08/88. J Clin Oncol 2004; 22(20):4109–4118.
65. Ward JF, Slezak JM, Blute ML, et al. Radical prostatectomy for clinically advanced (cT3) prostate cancer since the advent of prostate-specific antigen testing: 15-year outcome. BJU Int 2005; 95:751–756.
66. Stephenson RA, Smart CR, Mineau GP, et al. The fall in incidence of prostate cancer: on the down side of a prostate specific antigen induced peak in incidence data from the Utah Cancer Registry. Cancer 1995; 77:1342–1348.
67. Steinberg GD, Epstein JI, Piantadosi S, et al. Management of stage D1 adenocarcinoma of the prostate: the Johns Hopkins experience 1974–1987. J Urol 1990; 122:1425–1432.
68. Smith JA, Haynes TH, Middleton RG. Impact of external irradiation on local symptoms and survival free of disease in patients with pelvic lymph node metastasis from adenocarcinoma of the prostate. J Urol 1984; 131:705–707.
69. Paulson DF, Clince WA, Koefoot RB, et al. Extended field radiation therapy versus delayed hormonal therapy in node positive prostatic adenocarcinoma. J Urol 1982; 172:935.
70. Lawton CA, Winter K, Grignon D, et al. Androgen suppression plus radiation versus radiation alone for patients with stage D_1/pathologic node-positive adenocarcinoma of the prostate: updated results based on National Prospective Randomized Trial Radiation Therapy Oncology Group 85-31. J Clin Oncol 2005; 23:800–807.
71. Messing EM, Manola J, Sarosdy M, et al. Immediate hormonal therapy compared with observation after radical prostatectomy and pelvic lymphadenectomy in men with node-positive prostate cancer. N Engl J Med 1999; 341(24):1781–1788.
72. Schroder FH, Kurth KH, Fossa SD, et al. Early versus delayed endocrine treatment of pN1-3 M0 prostate cancer without local treatment of the primary tumor: results of European Organization for the Research and Treatment of Cancer 30846-A phase III study. J Urol 2004; 172:923–927.
73. Huggins C, Hodges CV. Studies on prostatic cancer I: the effect of castration, estrogen and androgen injections on serum phosphatase in metastatic carcinoma of the prostate. Cancer Res 1941; 1:293–297.
74. Cassileth BR, Soloway MS, Vogelzang NJ, et al. Patient's choice of treatment in stage D prostate cancer. Urology 1989; 33(suppl 5):57–62.

75. Vogelzang NJ, Chodak G, Soloway MS, et al. Goserelin versus orchiectomy in the treatment of advanced prostate cancer: final results of a randomized trial. Urology 1995; 46:220–226.

76. Kolvenbag GJCM, Furr BJA. Bicalutamide development: from theory to therapy (review). Can J Sci Am 1997; 3:192–203.

77. Thrasher B, Crawford ED. Combined androgen blockade. In: Vogelzang NJ, Scardino PT, Shipley WU, et al, eds. Comprehensive Textbook of Genitourinary Oncology. Baltimore: Williams & Wilkins, 1995:875–884.

78. Prostate Cancer Trialist's Collaborative Group. Maximum androgen blockade in advanced prostate cancer: an overview of 22 randomized trials with 3283 deaths in 5710 patients. Lancet 1995; 346:265–269.

79. Eisenberger MA, Blumenstein BA, Crawford ED, et al. Bilateral orchiectomy with or without flutamide for metastatic prostate cancer. N Engl J Med 1998; 339(15): 1036–1042.

80. Samson DJ, Seidenfeld J, Schmitt B, et al. Systemic review and meta-analysis of monotherapy compared with combined androgen blockade for patients with advanced prostate carcinoma. Cancer 2002; 95(2):361–376.

81. Scher HI, Kelly WK. Flutamide withdrawal syndrome: its impact on clinical trials in hormone refractory prostate cancer. J Clin Oncol 1993; 11:1566–1572.

82. Labrie F, Dupont A, Giguere M, et al. Benefits of combination therapy with flutamide in patients relapsing after castration. Br J Urol 1988; 61(4):341.

83. Small EJ, Vogelzang NJ. Second line hormonal therapy for advanced prostate cancer: a shifting paradigm. J Clin Oncol 1997; 15(1):382–388.

84. Tannock IF, Osoba D, Stockler MR, et al. Chemotherapy with mitoxantrone plus prednisone or prednisone alone for symptomatic hormone-resistant prostate cancer: a Canadian randomized trial with palliative end points. J Clin Oncol 1996; 14:1756–1764.

85. Berry W, Dakhil S, Modiano M, et al. Phase III study of mitoxantrone plus low dose prednisone versus low dose prednisone alone in patients with asymptomatic hormone refractory prostate cancer. J Urol 2002; 168:2439–2443.

86. Kantoff PW, Halabi S, Conaway M, et al. Hydrocortisone with or without mitoxantrone in men with hormone-refractory prostate cancer: results of the Cancer and Leukemia Group B 9182 study. J Clin Oncol 1999; 17:2506–2513.

87. Tannock IF, de Wit R, Berry WR, et al. Docetaxel plus prednisone or mitoxantrone plus prednisone for advanced prostate cancer. N Eng J Med 2004; 351:1502–1512.

88. De Witt R, Eisenberger MA, Tannock IF. A multicenter phase III comparison of docetaxel + prednisone (P) and mitoxantrone (MTZ)+ P in patients with androgen-independent prostate cancer (AIPC): secondary analysis of survival in patient subgroups. The TAX 327 investigators. Proceedings of the European Society of Medical Oncology. Ann Oncol 2004; 15(suppl 3:iii12):abstr. number 44IN.

89. Petrylak DP, Tangen CM, Hussain MHA, et al. Docetaxel and estramustine compared with mitoxantrone and prednisone for advanced refractory prostate cancer. N Engl J Med 2004; 351:1513–1520.

90. Benson RC, Hasan JM, Jones AG, et al. External beam radiotherapy for palliation of pain from metastatic carcinoma of the prostate. J Urol 1981; 127:69–71.

91. Kobayashi K, Vokes EE, Vogelzang NJ, et al. A phase I study of suramin (NSC 34936) given by intermittent infusion without adaptive control in patients with advanced cancer. J Clin Oncol 1995; 13:2196–2207.

92. Porter AT, McEwan AJB, Powe JE, et al. Results of a randomized phase III trial to evaluate the efficacy of Strontium-89 adjuvant to local field external beam irradiation in the management of endocrine resistant prostate cancer. Int J Radiat Oncol Biol Phys 1993; 25:805–813.

93. Saad F, Gleason DM, Murray R, et al. A randomized placebo-controlled trial of zoledronic acid in patients with hormone refractory metastatic prostate carcinoma. J Natl Cancer Inst 2003; 94:1458.

94. Smith EJ, Smith MR, Seaman JJ, et al. Combined analysis of two multicenter, random-
     ized, placebo-controlled studies of pamidronate disodium for the palliation of bone pain
     in men with metastatic prostate cancer. J Clin Oncol 2003; 21(23):4277–4284.
95. Forsen L, Sogaard AJ, Meyer HE, Edna T, et al. Survival after hip fracture: short- and
     long-term excess mortality according to age and gender. Osteoporos Int 1999; 10:73–78.
96. Diamond TH, Higano CS, Smith MR, et al. Osteoperosis in men with prostate carci-
     noma receiving androgen-deprivation therapy. Cancer 2004; 100:892–899.

13

Colorectal Cancer in the Elderly

Peter C. Enzinger

Department of Medical Oncology, Dana-Farber Cancer Institute, Department of Medicine, Brigham and Women's Hospital, and Department of Medicine, Harvard Medical School, Boston, Massachusetts, U.S.A.

INTRODUCTION

Colorectal cancer accounts for approximately 10% of all new cancer cases and 10% of all cancer-related deaths in the United States (1). In fact, colorectal cancer causes more deaths than prostate cancer in men aged 60 to 79, and more deaths than breast cancer in women aged 80 years or older (1). Approximately 105,000 new cases of colon cancer and 40,000 new cases of rectal cancer are diagnosed in the United States every year (1). The probability of developing colorectal cancer increases from 0.06% in the first four decades of life to 3% to 4% in the sixth and seventh decades (1). The incidence of colorectal cancer increases from 18 cases per 100,000 persons under the age of 65, to 208 cases per 100,000 persons 65 to 74 years, to 348 cases per 100,000 persons aged 75 years or older (Fig. 1) (2). Similarly, the mortality rate increases from six cases per 100,000 persons under age 65, to 73 cases per 100,000 persons aged 65 to 74 years, to 164 cases per 100,000 persons aged 75 years or older (Fig. 2) (2). Although the five-year relative survival with this cancer is identical for persons under the age of 65 and for persons aged 65 to 74 years (66%), it declines to 60% for individuals aged 75 years or older (Fig. 3) (2). Thus, because of the increasing incidence and decreasing survival with advancing age, the great majority (83%) of the annual 57,000 colorectal cancer deaths will occur in men and women older than age 60 (1).

Most (2–7), but not all (8), studies have suggested that elderly patients present at the time of diagnosis with the same probabilities of having localized and advanced colon cancer as younger patients (Fig. 4) (2). In randomized studies, elderly patients are reported to have the same performance status and incidence of tumor-related symptoms as younger patients, but tend to have more disease-related weight loss (9). They also appear to have a greater incidence of right-sided (proximal) tumors (4,7,10–12) and higher rates of obstruction and perforation (5,10,13). This, in turn, results in a greater likelihood of acute presentations, leading to a higher perioperative mortality rate in this older age group (5,14,15). While some investigators have noted that overall survival is shorter in elderly patients, this difference is not significant if noncancer deaths are excluded (16). A population-based analysis, conducted by investigators at the National Institute on Aging, revealed that comorbid conditions,

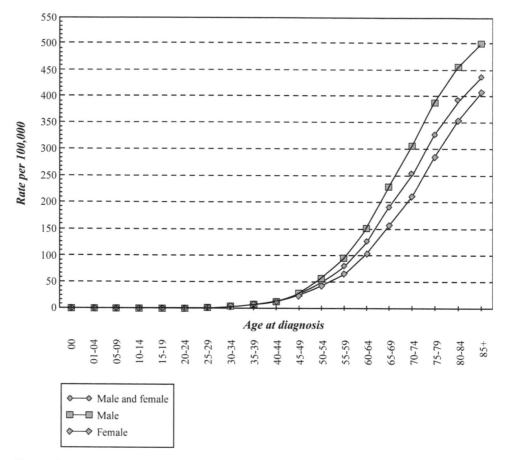

Figure 1 SEER incidence rates for colon and rectal cancer by sex for 1998–2002. *Abbreviation*: SEER, Surveillance Epidemiology and End Results. *Source*: From Ref. 2.

such as hypertension, heart disease, and chronic obstructive pulmonary disease, increased with age and were significant in predicting early mortality in older patients with colorectal cancer ($P = 0.0007$) (17).

Elderly patients with rectal cancer also tend to have similar symptoms at the time of presentation as do younger patients (13,18,19). In a retrospective study of 368 patients with rectal cancer, one group of investigators found almost the same distribution of early and advanced disease in older patients (>80 years) as in a younger cohort (5). Further, the distribution of cancers within the rectum (upper, middle, and lower) was nearly identical.

Risk Factors—Colorectal Cancer

As in younger individuals, most older persons have no clearly defined risk factors for the development of their colorectal cancer. Hereditary syndromes, such as familial adenomatosis polyposis (FAP) or hereditary nonpolyposis colorectal cancer (HNPCC), have less impact in this older age group, because the majority of cases (90% for FAP and 68–75% for HNPCC) are diagnosed before the age of 65 years (20,21). Many men are now being curatively treated with radiation for localized

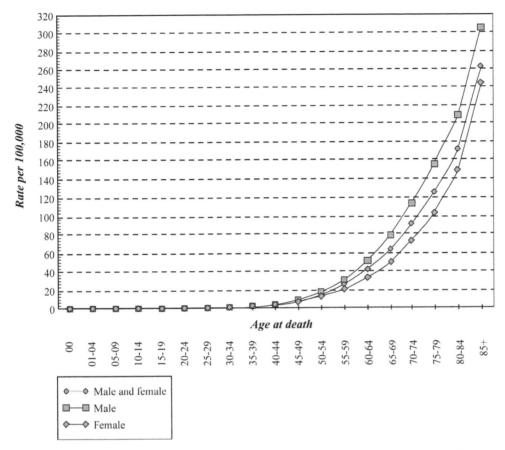

Figure 2 SEER mortality rates for colon and rectal cancer by sex for 1998–2002. *Abbreviation*: SEER, Surveillance Epidemiology and End Results. *Source*: From Ref. 2.

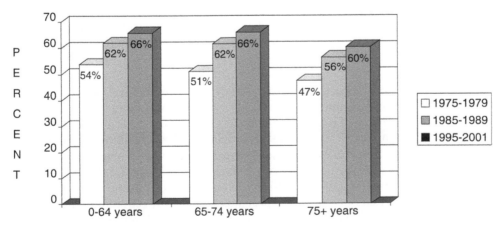

Figure 3 All-stage five-year survival by age group for colon and rectal cancer (SEER) nine registries for 1975–2001. *Abbreviation*: SEER, Surveillance Epidemiology and End Results.

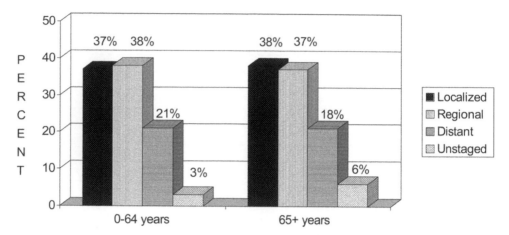

Figure 4   Stage distribution by age group for colon and rectal cancer (SEER) nine registries for 1988–2001. *Abbreviation*: SEER, Surveillance Epidemiology and End Results. *Source*: From Ref. 2.

prostate cancer. Long-term studies suggest that these men have a 70% increased risk of developing cancer in previously irradiated portions of the bowel (22). These men could potentially benefit from more frequent colorectal cancer screening than similarly aged individuals who have not been treated with radiation therapy.

Chemoprevention—Colorectal Cancer

Various dietary supplements and drugs have been proposed as chemopreventative agents for colorectal neoplasia. Of these, aspirin has been the most widely studied; the regular use of this drug appears to confer a significant risk reduction [relative risk (RR) 0.56–0.68] (23–25). Aspirin retards the development of the precursor lesions (i.e., aberrant crypt foci and microadenomas) of large bowel cancer, primarily through the inhibition of cyclooxygenase-2. Because many older persons now take aspirin to prevent coronary artery disease, and also because the impact of aspirin in the prevention of colorectal cancer appears to be cumulative over time (24,25), this drug likely has its greatest positive effect in elderly patients. A similar cumulative benefit (RR 0.25 with >15 years of intake) has been demonstrated with supplementation of folate, which is essential for orderly DNA methylation and synthesis (26). Here again, an intervention (i.e., change in diet) during midlife may have its greatest impact later in life.

In at least two prospective cohort studies, the use of postmenopausal estrogens has been shown to reduce the risk of colorectal cancer by approximately 30% (27,28). Possible mechanisms for this effect include the suppression of bile acid secretion, the alteration of DNA methylation, or the reduction of serum levels of mitogenic insulin-like growth factor I. Estrogen supplementation, however, has been associated with an increased risk for coronary heart disease, breast cancer, thromboembolic events, and early mortality in a large randomized study of postmenopausal women (29). Although the risk of colorectal cancer was significantly reduced in this trial, the results of this study have lead to the discontinuation of hormone replacement therapy in many older women, a change in practice that may increase the future incidence of colorectal cancer in this female cohort.

Most recently, it has been reported that statins, i.e., inhibitors of 3-hydroxy-3-methylglutaryl coenzyme A reductase–lipid-lowering agents, can significantly reduce the risk of colorectal cancer (30). As compared to individuals who did not use statins, individuals who used these agents for at least five years were able to reduce their RR of colorectal cancer by one half. Because statins are known to reduce the risk of cardiovascular events (31), further increased use of these agents, particularly in older patients, should reduce the risk of colorectal cancer in the future.

Screening—Colorectal Cancer

Approximately one in two persons will have an adenomatous polyp in their colon by the age of 70 (32). The risk of sporadic colorectal cancer can be reduced by 50% to 90% if adenomatous polyps are implicated by fecal occult blood testing (FOBT) or are visualized by barium enema, sigmoidoscopy, or colonoscopy and are then removed before they transform into a malignancy over a 5- to 10-year period (33–35).

Three randomized trials have demonstrated that routine FOBT can diminish colon cancer mortality by 15% to 20% during an 8- to 18-year follow-up period (36–38). Notably, in these trials, approximately one-third of patients were aged 65 years or older. The mortality benefit for this older group was slightly lower (10–16%) than for younger patients (19–23%) (36,37).

The benefits of screening sigmoidoscopy, double-contrast barium enema, and colonoscopy have, as yet, not been evaluated in randomized trials. Case–control studies, however, suggest that lower endoscopy and removal of polyps may decrease the incidence and mortality of colorectal carcinoma by 50% to 80% (33,34,39,40). Although colonoscopy appears to be particularly beneficial in older patients, who have a higher incidence of proximal neoplasms which are beyond the view of a flexible sigmoidoscopy (4,10,41), the risk of perforation from colonoscopy is higher than from sigmoidoscopy (odds ratio 1.8), and increases with advancing age (from 0.08% in persons aged 65 to 69 to 0.3% in persons aged 75 years or older) and the number of comorbidities (42). Therefore, screening decisions must be individualized for every elderly patient.

Based on these and other studies, a variety of screening strategies have been proposed for colorectal cancer (43–47). The American Cancer Society recommends that average-risk adults initiate screening at age 50. Options include (i) annual FOBT or fecal immunochemical test; (ii) flexible sigmoidoscopy every five years; (iii) annual FOBT or fecal immunochemical test plus flexible sigmoidoscopy every five years; (iv) colonoscopy every 10 years; or (v) double-contrast barium enema every five years (44,47). Similar recommendations have been made by the U.S. Preventive Services Task Force and the Multi-Society Task Force (45,46). The newest screening modality, computed tomographic colonography, i.e., "virtual colonoscopy," has not as yet been incorporated in these screening guidelines; questions remain about the sensitivity of this technology, particularly in comparison to the gold standard, colonoscopy (48).

In the United States, only a small percentage of persons at risk for colorectal neoplasia undergo routine screening (49). In response, Medicare now provides reimbursement for surveillance FOBT plus sigmoidoscopy or barium enema or colonoscopy for all beneficiaries. This has increased the prevalence of "screening within one year" for FOBT from 20% in persons under 65 years of age with health insurance (or 9% in persons without health insurance) to 26% in persons 65 years and older and the prevalence of "endoscopy within five years" from 37% in persons under 65 years of age with health insurance (or 19% in persons without health insurance) to 48% in persons aged 65 years or older (1). A similar effect was noted in a tele-phone survey conducted by the Centers for Disease Control and Prevention: men were asked if they had had undergone FOBT within the past year or a lower endo-scopy within the last five years (Fig. 5); the likelihood of having undergone either screening procedure increased from 40% in men aged 50 to 59, to 53% in men aged 60 to 69, and peaked (60%) in men aged 70 to 79, before decreasing again (52%) in men older than 80 years (50). Although these results represent an improvement in adherence to a colorectal screening program compared to previous years (49), these low percentages clearly remain unacceptable and will undoubtedly lead to a signifi-cant number of unnecessary deaths in the elderly during the next decade.

Because the risk of advanced neoplasia (51) and colorectal cancer (2) is highest in the oldest individuals, it seems doubtful that screening should be arbitrarily dis-continued after a certain age (52). In the United States, an individual who reaches the age of 80 has an average life expectancy of an additional 8.5 years; at age 85, average survival is 6.3 years (53). This estimate must be adjusted for the number and severity of chronic diseases affecting the individual, as well as his or her func-tional status. It may be reasonable to discontinue screening when life expectancy is shorter than the time a polyp progresses to a cancer, i.e., 5 to 10 years (54).

LOCALIZED COLORECTAL CANCER

Surgery—Localized Colon Cancer

Cancers of the colon are typically resected with a colectomy. Data on 20,862 patients undergoing surgery in 1997 for colon cancer from the Nationwide Inpatient Sample, a claims-based database, suggest that perioperative mortality increases gradually with advancing age until the age of 80 (0.8% in patients younger than 50 years of

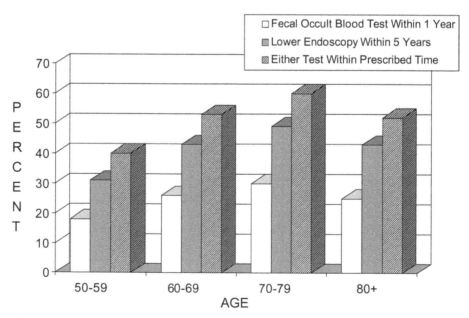

Figure 5 Proportion of men by age group, who are undergoing appropriate colorectal cancer screening. *Source*: From Ref. 50.

age, 1.3% for patients aged 51–65 years, and 2.9% for patients aged 66–80 years), after which a substantial increase in mortality is seen (6.9% for patients older than 80 years) (55). Earlier, age-related increases in 30-day mortality were documented in a cohort study of 15,390 patients who underwent resection of their colon cancer at Veteran's Administration Hospitals from 1990 to 2000 (7). In this study, 30-day mortality was 2.8% for patients less than 65 years of age and 5.6% for patients aged 65 years or older ($P < 0.0001$). Corresponding five-year cumulative survival was 57.6% and 46.6%, respectively ($P < 0.0001$).

Older patients in the Nationwide Inpatient Sample from 1997 had lower mortality rates at high-volume hospitals than at low-volume institutions: 3.1% versus 4.5% for patients older than 65 years ($P = 0.03$) (55). This effect was even more pronounced for patients older than 80 years, where 4.6% of patients died at high-volume centers compared to 7.3% at smaller institutions ($P = 0.04$). Therefore, it would be preferable that the oldest patients with colon cancer should undergo their resections at high-volume hospitals.

A tendency to perform less aggressive surgery in older patients may be evident from a recent analysis of 116,995 adults with localized colorectal cancer in the Surveillance, Epidemiology, and End Results (SEER) database (1988–2001). This retrospective study revealed that patients aged 71 years or older were half as likely to receive adequate lymph node evaluation (examination of at least 12 lymph nodes) as younger patients (56). Multiple studies have now demonstrated that inadequate lymph node evaluation correlates with inferior survival (57,58). These data would suggest that less aggressive surgical intervention predisposes elderly patients to a higher risk of recurrence and cancer-related death.

Increasingly, laparoscopic-assisted colectomies are being performed in the United States and elsewhere. Randomized studies indicate that patients undergoing this procedure have an outcome similar to that of patients undergoing an "open" colectomy, with slightly less postoperative pain and a one-day shorter hospital stay (59–61). This less invasive technique may be particularly beneficial in frail, elderly individuals. There is, however, continued concern that patients with more advanced disease may not undergo an adequate "cancer surgery" with this new technique. Small studies indicate that persons aged 75 years of or older tolerate laparoscopy-assisted colectomy as well as younger individuals (62).

Surgery—Localized Rectal Cancer

A radical resection with anastomosis or ostomy is the standard surgical procedure for cancer of the rectum. A Veteran's Administration study of 7243 patients who underwent surgery for their rectal cancer during the period of 1990 to 2000 revealed that 30-day mortality following resection for rectal cancer was 2.1% for patients younger than 65 years compared with 4.9% for patients aged 65 years or older ($P < 0.0001$) (7). Five-year survival was 59.9% versus 48.0%, respectively ($P < 0.0001$). French investigators reviewed the records of 92 surgical patients who were 80 years of age or older and matched these to records of 276 younger patients who underwent resection during the same time interval (5). The operative mortality was 8% in older patients and 4% in the younger patients ($P = NS$). Among elective surgeries, the operative mortality was nearly identical (3–4%). Although five-year overall survival was greater for younger patients, five-year cancer-specific survival was comparable for the two groups. This supports the conclusion that no arbitrary age limit should be set for rectal surgery in the elderly.

Adjuvant Therapy—Localized Colon Cancer

As a result of the publication of a National Institutes of Health consensus statement in 1990, 5-flurouracil (5-FU)–based adjuvant therapy has represented the standard of care for patients in the United States following the complete resection of colon cancer that has spread to regional lymph nodes (stage III disease). A benefit for post-operative chemotherapy has not been prospectively demonstrated in patients with fully resected, muscle-invasive, lymph node–negative (stage II) colon cancer (63). However, stage II cancers with high-risk features for recurrence (e.g., presentation with obstruction, perforation, or invasion into adjacent organs—stage IIb) are often treated by medical oncologists and are included in many randomized adjuvant trials.

Older patients receive adjuvant chemotherapy less often than their younger counterparts (Table 1) (10,64–66). A retrospective cohort study utilizing the SEER Medicare-linked database identified 6262 patients aged 65 years or older with resected stage III colon cancer from 1991 to 1996 (65). Overall, 55% of patients received adjuvant chemotherapy within three months of colon cancer resection. The likelihood of receiving treatment declined steeply with increasing age. Similar results were noted in an Italian study of 1014 patients with resected stage II or III colon cancer (69).

The reason for this age-related disparity in management is not entirely clear. In one study utilizing the California Cancer Registry, oncologists cited patient refusal, comorbid illness, or advanced age as the most common reasons for not providing chemotherapy to elderly patients with resected colon cancer (66). Financial considerations and logistical problems may also prevent some elderly from seeking care (70). Additionally, treatment for older patients is more frequently discontinued,

Table 1 Use of Chemotherapy for Colorectal Cancer by Age

	Age	Total number of patients	Percentage of patients treated	Hospitalizations for chemotherapy-related toxicity (%)
Stage III colon cancer (65)	65–69	1261	78	7
	70–74	1552	74	8
	75–79	1492	58	9
	80–84	1100	34	12
	85–89	604	11	13
Stage II/III rectal cancer (67)	65–69	367	60[a]	
	70–74	392	52[a]	
	75–79	301	36[a]	
	80–84	231	23[a]	
	85+	120	12[a]	
Stage IV colorectal cancer (68)	65–69	377	45	
	70–74	411	41	
	75–79	366	27	
	80–84	262	18	
	85+	214	5	

[a]Chemotherapy and radiation therapy.

suggesting a reluctance by physicians to treat older patients who have experienced some degree of side effects to chemotherapy (69).

A pooled analysis of 3351 patients, stratified by decade of life, from seven randomized trials evaluated the benefit of adjuvant chemotherapy in elderly persons with stage II or III colon cancer (71). In these trials, patients had been randomized to receive surgery alone or surgery followed by 5-FU–based chemotherapy. The primary conclusion of this pooled analysis was that elderly patients derive the same clinical benefit from postoperative chemotherapy as younger patients. Treatment-related toxicity was somewhat higher for older patients, yet such differences were only statistically significant for the likelihood of grade III or IV leukopenia (4% vs. 8%; $P = 0.05$).

Adjuvant chemotherapy also appeared to be slightly more toxic for elderly patients in a SEER- and Medicare-derived retrospective cohort study (65). Hospitalization for various chemotherapy-related toxicities increased steadily with advancing age (Table 1) (65). Similarly, prospective data from the Royal Marsden Hospital in London revealed slightly higher rates of grade III or IV toxicity in patients aged 70 years or older, reaching significance, however, only for stomatitis (11% vs. 19%; $P = 0.046$) (72).

Adjuvant chemotherapy for locally advanced colon cancer continues to evolve. A recent randomized trial, in which 35% of patients were 65 years of age or older, has suggested that disease-free survival can be enhanced if oxaliplatin, a third generation platinum analogue, is added to 5-FU and leucovorin (LV) (73). However, an overall survival advantage with this agent has, as yet, not been demonstrated in this trial. Although in subgroup analysis, the older patients had a slightly lower recurrence rate with the more aggressive triple chemotherapy regimen, the effect was less pronounced than in the younger patients and was not statistically significant. Toxicity specifically for these older patients has not been reported.

The oral 5-FU prodrug, capecitabine, has recently demonstrated an efficacy similar to that of monthly intravenous 5-FU and LV (Mayo Clinic Regimen) in the adjuvant setting (74). A subgroup analysis in 391 patients aged 70 years or older suggests that capecitabine causes less severe overall toxicity than the 5-FU or LV combination (75). Additionally, the incidence of severe adverse events for patients aged 65 years or older who received capecitabine in this study was nearly identical to younger patients. Therefore, postoperative treatment with this agent may be another option for older patients with resected high-risk colon cancer.

In conclusion, it appears that postoperative chemotherapy in stage III colon cancer is as beneficial in elderly patients as it is in younger individuals. A slight increase in toxicity should not prevent the clinician from treating these older patients, although increased vigilance during chemotherapy is warranted.

Adjuvant Therapy—Localized Rectal Cancer

Chemoradiation after surgery reduces the local recurrence rate and increases disease-free survival in patients with deeply invasive (T3-4) or lymph node–positive rectal cancer (76,77). Although there are few data to suggest that elderly patients respond any differently to chemoradiotherapy than younger patients, they are less frequently referred to oncologists for this treatment (Table 1) (78). Analyses of linked SEER and Medicare databases identified patients aged 65 years or older with stage II or III rectal cancer who underwent surgical resection between 1992 and 1996 (67,79). In this group of patients, 57% received postoperative radiation therapy and 42%

received postoperative chemotherapy and radiation. Increasing age corresponded inversely with the percentage of patients who received adjuvant therapy (Table 1). Overall, chemoradiation therapy was associated with a 17% reduced risk of death among all cases (RR 0.83), with a 29% reduced risk of death in stage III patients (RR 0.71), but no statistically significant improvement in stage II cases, similar to the results reported in younger patients.

Based on California Cancer Registry data, it is likely that the decreased use of adjuvant therapy for rectal cancer with increasing age is attributable to comorbid illnesses, patient refusal, problems with transportation, and suboptimal family support (66). Additionally, radiation therapy is more toxic in older patients (80); older patients appear to be at an increased risk for radiation enteritis (81), probably because of pre-existing conditions, such as hypertension, vascular disease, diabetes, and prior abdominal surgery.

Postoperative Surveillance—Localized Colorectal Cancer

There is general agreement that all patients with resected colorectal cancer should undergo regular surveillance screening with colonoscopy and carcinoembryonic antigen carcinoembryonic antigen testing (82). Analysis of 52,283 Medicare beneficiaries treated for locoregional colorectal cancer between 1986 and 1996 suggests that younger patients are more likely to undergo periodic surveillance endoscopies and that the median time to first follow-up endoscopy is significantly shorter ($P < 0.0001$) for patients at younger ages (83).

ADVANCED COLORECTAL CANCER

Surgery—Advanced Colorectal Cancer

Removal of the primary cancer is indicated in patients who have an (impending) obstruction, uncontrollable bleeding, or oligometastatic disease that may potentially be cured with aggressive therapy (84). In spite of these restrictive criteria, a recent pattern of care study, utilizing data from the SEER Program, revealed that the majority of patients aged 65 years or older with stage IV colorectal cancer undergo resection of their primary tumor (85). Overall, 72% of patients underwent this primary cancer–directed surgery. The percentage of patients undergoing surgery declined gradually from 76% in patients who were 65 to 69 years old, to 70% in patients who were 80 to 84 years old, and then dropped to 62% in patients who were 85 years of age or older.

In this pattern of care study, the 30-day mortality was 10% for all patients (85). However, higher perioperative mortality rates for elderly patients with advanced colorectal cancer have been reported elsewhere; in patients 70 to 79 years of age, the mortality may be as high as 21%, and in octogenarians, it may reach 38% (86,87). Overall, improvements in surgical techniques and postoperative care have led to a decrease in operative mortality, particularly in older patients, at many hospitals over the past two decades (88), so that current operative survival figures for elderly patients now approach those reported for younger patients a decade ago (89).

Elderly patients with oligometastatic disease or isolated recurrences of their colorectal cancer may be candidates for a "curative-intent" resection. In a series from the Memorial Sloan-Kettering Cancer Center, 128 patients aged 70 years of age or older underwent liver resection for metastatic colorectal cancer between 1985 and 1994

(90). While these patients experienced a 4% perioperative mortality rate and a 42% complication rate, their median survival was 40 months, and five-year survival rate was 35%. These older patients had an outcome similar to that to 449 patients less than 70 years of age who underwent comparable liver resections during the same time period. Additionally, studies have shown that appropriately selected elderly patients can tolerate resection of colorectal metastases to the lungs with an outcome similar to that seen in younger patients, with acceptable morbidity and mortality (91,92).

Chemotherapy—Advanced Colorectal Cancer

Palliative chemotherapy remains the mainstay of treatment for patients with unresectable or metastatic colorectal cancer. Although multiple studies have demonstrated a similar benefit for older as well as for younger patients, SEER data document that the usage of chemotherapy in patients with advanced colorectal cancer falls with increasing age (Table 1) (68).

5-Fluorouracil

Until the early 1990s, the only active treatment for advanced colorectal cancer was the use of 5-FU, a thymidylate synthase inhibitor. Multiple studies have now demonstrated that this agent, given as a bolus with LV or as an infusion with or without LV, is effective and well tolerated in the elderly population, with similar response rates and overall survival compared to younger cohorts (9,72,93–97).

Folprecht et al. carried out a pooled analysis of 22 randomized European trials in which patients received palliative 5-FU–based therapy (9). They identified 629 patients aged 70 years or older and compared them to 3196 patients younger than 70 years. Outcome for these elderly patients did not differ significantly from the younger patients: response and survival was 23.9% and 10.8 months for the older patients and 21.1% and 11.3 months for the younger patients ($P=0.14$ and 0.31, respectively).

A second pooled analysis of 1748 patients with advanced colorectal cancer treated with 5-FU–based therapy was conducted by the North Central Cancer Treatment Group (NCCTG) (93). Patients were divided into quartiles by age: less than 56 years, 56 to 65 years, 66 to 70 years, and greater than 70 years. No significant differences in response rate ($P=0.90$), time to tumor progression ($P=0.25$), or overall survival ($P=0.42$), were seen among these groups.

Clinicians at the Royal Marsden Hospital in London collected prospective data on 658 patients younger than 70 years of age and 186 patients older than 70 who received palliative 5-FU–based therapy between 1990 and 1997 (72). They found no difference in dose-intensity, response rate, or median failure-free survival time. Although the one-year survival was nearly identical between the two groups (44% and 48%, respectively), the median overall survival was shorter for the older patients (9.6 months vs. 11.5 months; $P=0.04$), likely owing to competing comorbidities.

Age-related differences in 5-FU–related toxicity have been observed in some (93,98–100), but not all (70,94,96), studies. In the NCCTG pooled analysis, patients aged 65 years or older had higher overall severe toxicity than their younger counterparts (53% vs. 46%; $P=0.01$) (93). Statistically significant differences in severe diarrhea and stomatitis were noted (Table 2). A second study noted higher rates of nonhematologic toxicity and hand–foot syndrome in older patients (99). By contrast, in the Royal Marsden study, rates of overall and severe toxicity were nearly identical

Table 2 Severe Toxicity to 5-Fluorouracil–Based Therapy by Age in a Pooled Analysis of 1748 Patients with Advanced Colorectal Cancer Treated by the NCCTG (93)

Severe toxicity (NCI CTC grade ≥ 3)	Age			P-value[a]
	<66 Years (%)	66–70 years (%)	>70 years (%)	
Any	46	53	53	0.01
Diarrhea	16	23	21	0.01
Leukopenia	14	18	17	0.23
Nausea/vomiting	9	9	9	0.95
Stomatitis	13	18	17	0.03
Infection	2	5	4	0.02

[a]The P-value compares the rate of toxicity for the three age groups using a χ^2-test with two degrees of freedom.
Abbreviations: NCI, National Cancer Institute; CTC, Common Toxicity Criteria; NCCTG, North Central Cancer Treatment Group.
Source: From Ref. 93.

for younger and older patients in all categories (72). Furthermore, there were no statistical differences in average length of inpatient stay between the two groups.

Capecitabine

The oral 5-FU prodrug, capecitabine, has demonstrated an efficacy similar to that of intravenous 5-FU plus LV in advanced colorectal cancer (101). In one study of 51 patients older than 70 years with metastatic colorectal cancer, the overall response rate was 24%, and the overall survival time was 11 months (102). Severe treatment-related toxicity was noted in only 12% of patients. These results are similar to those seen in younger individuals treated with capecitabine (101), or in persons older than 70 years treated with 5-FU (9). Preliminary results from another study of 99 patients older than 65 years with advanced colorectal cancer treated with capecitabine confirm these findings (103).

Irinotecan

Irinotecan, a topoisomerase I inhibitor, is another active drug in the treatment of metastatic colorectal cancer. It is converted by the liver into two active metabolites, SN-38 and SN-38 glucuronide; plasma levels of these metabolites are thought to be predictive of toxicity. Pharmacokinetic studies have revealed no significant differences in the plasma levels of these irinotecan metabolites in older and younger patients (104). A multi-institutional phase II study found similar grade III or IV toxicity in 85 patients who were 65 years or older and in 90 patients younger than 65 years receiving a weekly schedule of this agent (105). Irinotecan may also be given as a single dose every three weeks—in which case, the dose is generally lowered by 15% for patients aged 70 years or older (106). In a trial comparing the weekly and the triweekly dosing regimens of this drug as second-line therapy for metastatic disease, more than one-third of 291 patients were at least 70 years of age (107). Age did not affect survival or time to progression. Patients aged 70 years or older, however, were at increased risk of grade III/IV neutropenia and grade III/IV diarrhea compared to patients younger than 70 years of age. In another trial, 72 patients aged 70 years or older with advanced colorectal cancer received irinotecan every three weeks (108). No significant differences in outcome were noted for these patients compared to

267 patients younger than 70 years. Although elderly patients had a higher incidence of neutropenia than younger patients ($P = 0.0228$), no significant differences in overall toxicity were found ($P = 0.218$).

Oxaliplatin

Oxaliplatin is a third generation platinum analogue, which induces platinum–DNA adducts, inhibiting the replication of DNA (109). Although it has limited activity as a single agent in colorectal cancer, oxaliplatin has notable synergy with 5-FU and LV (110). This combination, known as "FOLFOX," has demonstrated superior efficacy in advanced colorectal cancer, and is currently the most commonly employed regimen in the United States and Europe for this indication (111,112). Univariate analysis of one pivotal trial has suggested that age, as a continuous variable, is not a significant prognostic factor for patients treated with the FOLFOX regimen ($P = 0.739$) (111). In fact, patients older than 65 years had a response rate identical to that of younger patients. Similar results were noted in a Swiss observational study, where 33 patients older than 70 years compared favorably to 104 younger patients (113). Additional studies have reported that various FOLFOX combinations are active and well tolerated in older individuals (114–118).

Bevacizumab

The humanized monoclonal antibody, bevacizumab, binds to the vascular epidermal growth factor. It can reduce the vascularity of tumors, leading to hypoxia and necrosis (119,120), and also appears to lower interstitial fluid pressure in cancer nodules, promoting diffusion of other chemotherapeutic agents into these tumors (121). Two pivotal studies in patients with advanced colorectal cancer have established that this agent significantly enhances the efficacy of 5-FU–based therapy with either irinotecan (122) or oxaliplatin (123). Treatment effect in these studies appeared to be consistent for patients of all age groups, including patients as old as 85. A third study in advanced colorectal cancer, specifically geared to older persons ($\geq$65 years), or those individuals of poor performance status, compared bolus 5-FU and LV alone or the same regimen in combination with bevacizumab (124). Enhanced response and survival was again noted in those patients (mean age, 71 years) receiving this monoclonal antibody.

Although older persons, as well as younger individuals, generally appear to tolerate bevacizumab, a higher incidence of arterial thrombotic events (myocardial infarction, stroke, or peripheral arterial thrombotic event) in patients older than 64 years has been documented (125). In multivariate analysis, older persons had a 2.24-fold greater risk (7.1%) of developing an arterial thrombotic event compared to younger individuals. In elderly patients who had previously experienced an arterial thrombotic event, this risk increased to 17.9%, as compared to 2.2% for older individuals receiving standard chemotherapy alone. Therefore, bevacizumab should be avoided in elderly patients with a history of atherosclerosis-related disease.

Cetuximab

Cetuximab is a chimerized monoclonal antibody to the epidermal growth factor receptor (126). Blockade of this receptor in colorectal cancer cells induces apoptosis and cell death. In individuals with extensively treated metastatic colorectal cancer, this agent can induce significant tumor regressions in 11% of patients; in combination with irinotecan, this rate of response increases to 23% (127). The most common severe toxicities to this agent include dyspnea, asthenia, acneiform rash, and hypersensitivity reaction (127). Specific data concerning efficacy and toxicity for this agent in elderly patients are not yet available.

Combination Chemotherapy

Various trials have evaluated combination chemotherapy in elderly patients with metastatic colorectal cancer. These have included combinations of irinotecan and bolus 5-FU/LV (128,129), irinotecan and infusional 5-FU/LV (115,130), irinotecan and capecitabine (131), oxaliplatin and infusional 5-FU (FOLFOX) (115,116,118,132), oxaliplatin and capecitabine (CAPOX) (133,134), and irinotecan and oxaliplatin (IROX) (135). These trials uniformly revealed that response to chemotherapy, median survival times, and degree of toxicity in these elderly patients appear to be similar to what is observed in younger patients (115,116,118,128–135).

CLINICAL TRIALS

Whereas 70% to 75% of colorectal cancers are diagnosed in patients older than 65 years of age, only 40% to 48% of patients enrolled in NCI-sponsored or cooperative group trials are drawn from this age group (136–140). The most recent data (2000–2002) from NCI-sponsored cooperative group trials suggest that this under-representation of elderly patients with colorectal cancer has not improved in the past several years (compared with 1996–1998) (140). During the 2000–2002 time period, only 2% of colorectal cancer patients aged 65 to 74 years and 0.5% of colorectal cancer patients aged 75 years or older enrolled in NCI-sponsored trials. This is substantially less than the 4% enrollment recorded for patients aged 30 to 64 years.

A possible explanation for these discrepancies may be related to financial constraints (141). However, a similarly low rate of enrollment for older patients has been documented in Canada, where the national health care program provides reimbursement for all health care costs (142). More plausible explanations for the lack of participation of elderly patients in clinical trials may include lack of social and home care support, physician reluctance to offer research protocols to older individuals, difficulties with access to clinics and hospitals, potential noncoverage of investigational treatments by Medicare, patient refusal, increasing concomitant medication usage and comorbidities with advancing age, and availability of fewer trials specifically aimed at elderly patients (139,141).

CONCLUSION

Although colorectal cancer is primarily a disease of the elderly, the treatments for this condition have generally been designed for and evaluated in younger patients. Nonetheless, treatment of the elderly is generally well tolerated. Many operative procedures once thought too dangerous for young patients can now be performed safely in otherwise healthy octogenarians. Likewise, radiation therapy is well tolerated in older individuals, perhaps with slight increases in bone marrow suppression and small bowel toxicity. Most chemotherapeutic agents cause slightly increased toxicity in elderly patients. The therapeutic benefit for adjuvant treatment for colorectal cancers appears to be age-independent. For the more advanced cancers, however, survival benefits for older individuals are marginal, and the value of such treatment in elderly or infirm patients must be balanced with potential toxicities, which may diminish quality of life. At present, too few elderly patients are enrolled in clinical trials. Prospective studies involving older patients should evaluate the efficacy, toxicity, and quality of life in this important and rapidly expanding age group.

REFERENCES

1. Jemal A, Murray T, Ward E, et al. Cancer statistics, 2005. CA Cancer J Clin 2005; 55(1):10–30.
2. Ries L, Eisner M, Kosary C, et al. SEER cancer statistics review, 1975–2002. http:// seer.cancer.gov/csr/1975_2002/. Bethesda, MD: National Cancer Institute, 2005.
3. Yancik R, Ries L. Cancer in older persons. Cancer 1994; 74:1995–2003.
4. Zhang B, Fattah A, Nakama H. Characteristics and survival rate of elderly patients with colorectal cancer detected by immunochemical occult blood screening. Hepatogastroenterology 2000; 47(32):414–418.
5. Barrier A, Ferro L, Houry S, Lacaine F, Huguier M. Rectal cancer surgery in patients more than 80 years of age. Am J Surg 2003; 185(1):54–57.
6. Demetriades H, Kanellos I, Vasiliadis K, et al. Age-associated prognosis following curative resection for colorectal cancer. Tech Coloproctol 2004; 8(suppl 1):S144–S146.
7. Rabeneck L, Davila JA, Thompson M, El-Serag HB. Outcomes in elderly patients following surgery for colorectal cancer in the Veterans Affairs health care system. Aliment Pharmacol Ther 2004; 20(10):1115–1124.
8. Jessup J, McGinnis L, Steele G, Menck H, Winchester D. The National Cancer Data Base. Report on colon cancer. Cancer 1996; 78(4):918–926.
9. Folprecht G, Cunningham D, Ross P, et al. Efficacy of 5-fluorouracil-based chemotherapy in elderly patients with metastatic colorectal cancer: a pooled analysis of clinical trials. Ann Oncol 2004; 15(9):1330–1338.
10. Coburn M, Pricolo V, Soderberg C. Factors affecting prognosis and management of carcinoma of the colon and rectum in patients more than eighty years of age. J Am Coll Surg 1994; 179(1):65–69.
11. Arai T, Takubo K, Sawabe M, Esaki Y. Pathologic characteristics of colorectal cancer in the elderly: a retrospective study of 947 surgical cases. J Clin Gastroenterol 2000; 31(1):67–72.
12. Koketsu S, Watanabe T, Tada T, Kanazawa T, Ueda E, Nagawa H. Sporadic colorectal cancer in elderly people. Hepatogastroenterology 2003; 50(54):1749–1752.
13. Paksoy M, Ipek T, Colak T, Cebeci H. Influence of age on prognosis and management of patients with colorectal carcinoma. Eur J Surg 1999; 165(1):55–59.
14. Mulcahy H, Patchett S, Daly L, O'Donoghue D. Prognosis of elderly patients with large bowel cancer. Br J Surg 1994; 81(5):736–738.
15. Damhuis R, Wereldsma J, Wiggers T. The influence of age on resection rates and postoperative mortality in 6,457 patients with colorectal cancer. Int J Colorectal Dis 1996; 11(1):45–48.
16. Adloff M, Ollier J, Schloegel M, Arnaud J, Serrat M. Colorectal cancer in patients over the age of 80 years. Ann Chir 1993; 47(6):492–496.
17. Yancik R, Wesley M, Ries L, et al. Comorbidity and age as predictors of risk for early mortality of male and female colon carcinoma patients. Cancer 1998; 82(11):2123–2134.
18. Irvin T. Prognosis of colorectal cancer in the elderly. Br J Cancer 1988; 75(5): 419–421.
19. Curless R, French J, Williams G, James O. Comparison of gastrointestinal symptoms in colorectal carcinoma patients and community controls with respect to age. Gut 1994; 35(9):1267–1270.
20. Burt R. Hereditary aspects of the polyposis syndromes. Hematol Oncol Ann 1994; 2:163–170.

21. Burke W, Petersen G, Lynch P, et al. Recommendations for follow-up care of individuals with an inherited predisposition to cancer. I. Hereditary nonpolyposis colon cancer. Cancer Genetics Studies Consortium. JAMA 1997; 277(11):915–919.

22. Baxter NN, Tepper JE, Durham SB, Rothenberger DA, Virnig BA. Increased risk of rectal cancer after prostate radiation: a population-based study. Gastroenterology 2005; 128(4):819–824.

23. Thun M, Namboodiri M, Heath C. Aspirin use and reduced risk of fatal colon cancer. N Engl J Med 1991; 325(23):1593–1596.

24. Giovannucci E, Rimm E, Stampfer M, Colditz G, Asherio A, Willett W. Aspirin use and the risk for colorectal cancer and adenoma in male health professionals. Ann Intern Med 1994; 121(4):241–246.

25. Giovannucci E, Egan K, Hunter D, et al. Aspirin and the risk of colorectal cancer in women. N Engl J Med 1995; 333(10):609–614.

26. Giovannucci E, Stampfer M, Colditz G, et al. Multivitamin use, folate, and colon cancer in women in the Nurses' Health Study. Ann Intern Med 1998; 129(7):517–524.

27. Calle E, Miracle-McMahill H, Thun M, Heath C. Estrogen replacement therapy and the risk of fatal colon cancer in a prospective cohort of postmenopausal women. J Natl Cancer Inst 1995; 87(7):517–523.

28. Grodstein F, Martinez E, Platz E, et al. Postmenopausal hormone use and risk for colorectal cancer and adenoma. Ann Intern Med 1998; 128(9):705–712.

29. Rossouw J, Anderson G, Prentice R, et al. Risks and benefits of estrogen plus progestin in healthy postmenopausal women: principal results from the Women's Health Initiative randomized controlled trial. JAMA 2002; 288(3):321–333.

30. Poynter JN, Gruber SB, Higgins PD, et al. Statins and the risk of colorectal cancer. N Engl J Med 2005; 352(21):2184–2192.

31. Cannon CP, Braunwald E, McCabe CH, et al. Intensive versus moderate lipid lowering with statins after acute coronary syndromes. N Engl J Med 2004; 350(15):1495–1504 (Epub 2004 Mar 8).

32. Williams A, Balasooriya B, Day D. Polyps and cancer of the large bowel: a necropsy study in Liverpool. Gut 1982; 23(10):835–842.

33. Muller A, Sonnenberg A. Prevention of colorectal cancer by flexible endoscopy and polypectomy. A case-control study of 32,702 veterans. Ann Intern Med 1995; 123(12): 904–910.

34. Winawer S, Zauber A, Ho M, et al. Prevention of colorectal cancer by colonoscopic polypectomy. N Engl J Med 1993; 329(27):1977–1981.

35. Fearon E, Vogelstein B. A genetic model for colorectal tumorigenesis. Cell 1990; 61(5): 759–767.

36. Kronborg O, Fenger C, Olsen J, Jorgensen O, Sondergaard O. Randomized study of screening for colorectal cancer with faecal-occult-blood test. Lancet 1996; 348(9040): 1467–1471.

37. Hardcastle J, Chamberlain J, Robinson M, et al. Randomised controlled trial of faecal-occult-blood screening for colorectal cancer. Lancet 1996; 348(9040):1472–1477.

38. Mandel J, Church T, Bond J, et al. The effect of fecal occult-blood screening on the incidence of colorectal cancer. N Engl J Med 2000; 343(22):1603–1607.

39. Selby J, Friedman G, Quesenberry C, Weiss N. A case-control study of screening sigmoidoscopy and mortality from colorectal cancer. N Engl J Med 1992; 326(10): 653–657.

40. Newcomb P, Norfleet R, Storer B, Surawicz T, Marcus P. Screening sigmoidoscopy and colorectal cancer mortality. J Natl Cancer Inst 1992; 84(20):1572–1575.

41. Arora A, Singh P. Colonoscopy in patients 80 years of age and older is safe, with high success rate and diagnostic yield. Gastrointest Endosc 2004; 60(3):408–413.

42. Gatto N, Frucht H, Sundararajan V, Jacobson J, Grann V, Neugut A. Risk of perforation after colonoscopy and sigmoidoscopy: a population-based study. J Natl Cancer Inst 2003; 95(3):230–236.

43. Levin B, Barthel J, David D, et al. NCCN colorectal cancer screening practice guidelines. Oncology 1999; 13(5A):152–179.
44. Smith RA, von Eschenbach AC, Wender R, et al. American Cancer Society guidelines for the early detection of cancer: update of early detection guidelines for prostate, colorectal, and endometrial cancers. Also: update 2001–testing for early lung cancer detection. CA Cancer J Clin 2001; 51(1):38–75; quiz 7–80.
45. Force UPST. Screening for colorectal cancer: recommendation and rationale. Ann Intern Med 2002; 137(2):129–131.
46. Winawer S, Fletcher R, Rex D, et al. Colorectal cancer screening and surveillance: clinical guidelines and rationale—update based on new evidence. Gastroenterology 2003; 124(2):544–560.
47. Levin B, Brooks D, Smith RA, Stone A. Emerging technologies in screening for colorectal cancer: CT colonography, immunochemical fecal occult blood tests, and stool screening using molecular markers. CA Cancer J Clin 2003; 53(1):44–55.
48. Mulhall BP, Veerappan GR, Jackson JL. Meta-analysis: computed tomographic colonography. Ann Intern Med 2005; 142(8):635–650.
49. Vernon S. Participation in colorectal cancer screening: a review. J Natl Cancer Inst 1997; 89(19):1406–1422.
50. Sirovich B, Schwartz L, Woloshin S. Screening men for prostate and colorectal cancer in the United States. Does practice reflect evidence? JAMA 2003; 289(11):1415–1420.
51. Stevens T, Burke CA. Colonoscopy screening in the elderly—when to stop? Am J Gastroenterol 2003; 98(8):1881–1885.
52. Clark AJ, Stockton D, Elder A, Wilson RG, Dunlop MG. Assessment of outcomes after colorectal cancer resection in the elderly as a rationale for screening and early detection. Br J Surg 2004; 91(10):1345–1351.
53. Vital Statistics. http://www.census.gov/prod/2001pubs/statab/sec02.pdf. 2001. (Accessed May 8, 2003).
54. Bond JH. Polyp guideline: diagnosis, treatment, and surveillance for patients with colorectal polyps. Practice Parameters Committee of the American College of Gastroenterology. Am J Gastroenterol 2000; 95(11):3053–3063.
55. Dimick JB, Cowan JA Jr, Upchurch GR Jr, Colletti LM. Hospital volume and surgical outcomes for elderly patients with colorectal cancer in the United States. J Surg Res 2003; 114(1):50–56.
56. Baxter NN, Virnig DJ, Rothenberger DA, Morris AM, Jessurun J, Virnig BA. Lymph node evaluation in colorectal cancer patients: a population-based study. J Natl Cancer Inst 2005; 97(3):219–225.
57. Swanson RS, Compton CC, Stewart AK, Bland KI. The prognosis of T3N0 colon cancer is dependent on the number of lymph nodes examined. Ann Surg Oncol 2003; 10(1):65–71.
58. Le Voyer TE, Sigurdson ER, Hanlon AL, et al. Colon cancer survival is associated with increasing number of lymph nodes analyzed: a secondary survey of Intergroup Trial INT-0089. J Clin Oncol 2003; 21(15):2912–2919.
59. Weeks JC, Nelson H, Gelber S, Sargent D, Schroeder G. Short-term quality-of-life outcomes following laparoscopic-assisted colectomy vs open colectomy for colon cancer: a randomized trial. JAMA 2002; 287(3):321–328.
60. Leung KL, Kwok SP, Lam SC, et al. Laparoscopic resection of rectosigmoid carcinoma: prospective randomised trial. Lancet 2004; 363(9416):1187–1192.
61. A comparison of laparoscopically assisted and open colectomy for colon cancer. N Engl J Med 2004; 350(20):2050–2059.
62. Sklow B, Read T, Birnbaum E, Fry R, Fleshman J. Age and type of procedure influence the choice of patients for laparoscopic colectomy. Surg Endosc 2003; 17(6):923–929 (Epub 2003 Mar 7).
63. Moertel C, Fleming T, Macdonald J, et al. Intergroup study of fluorouracil plus levamisole as adjuvant therapy for stage II/Dukes' B2 colon cancer. J Clin Oncol 1995; 13(12):2936–2943.

64. Sundarajan V, Grann V, Jacobson J, Ahsan H, Neugut A. Variations in the use of adjuvant chemotherapy for node-positive colon cancer in the elderly: a population-based study. Cancer J 2001; 7(3):213–218.

65. Schrag D, Cramer L, Bach P, Begg C. Age and adjuvant chemotherapy use after surgery for stage III colon cancer. J Natl Cancer Inst 2001; 93(11):850–857.

66. Ayanian JZ, Zaslavsky AM, Fuchs CS, et al. Use of adjuvant chemotherapy and radiation therapy for colorectal cancer in a population-based cohort. J Clin Oncol 2003; 21(7):1293–1300.

67. Schrag D, Gelfand S, Bach P, Guillem J, Minsky B, Begg C. Who gets adjuvant treatment for stage II and III rectal cancer? Insight from the Surveillance, Epidemiology, and End Results–Medicare. J Clin Oncol 2001; 19(17):3712–3718.

68. Sundararajan V, Grann V, Neugut A. Population based variation in the use of chemotherapy for colorectal cancer in the elderly. Proc Am Soc Clin Oncol 1999; 18:A1598.

69. Ashele C, Guglielmi A, Tixi L, et al. Adjuvant treatment of colorectal cancer in the elderly. Cancer Control 1995; 2(2 suppl 1):36–38.

70. Mandelblatt J, Yabroff K, Kerner J. Equitable access to cancer services: a review of barriers to quality care. Cancer 1999; 86:2378–2390.

71. Sargent D, Goldberg R, Jacobson J, et al. A pooled analysis of adjuvant chemotherapy for resected colon cancer in elderly patients. N Engl J Med 2001; 345(15):1091–1097.

72. Popescu R, Norman A, Ross P, Parikh B, Cunningham D. Adjuvant or palliative chemotherapy for colorectal cancer in patients 70 years or older. J Clin Oncol 1999; 17(8):2412–2418.

73. Andre T, Boni C, Mounedji-Boudiaf L, et al. Oxaliplatin, fluorouracil, and leucovorin as adjuvant treatment for colon cancer. N Engl J Med 2004; 350(23):2343–2351.

74. Twelves C, Wong A, Nowacki MP, et al. Capecitabine as adjuvant treatment for stage III colon cancer. N Engl J Med 2005; 352(26):2696–2704.

75. Diaz-Rubio E, Burris H, Douillard J, et al. Safety of capecitabine (X) compared to fluorouracil/leucovorin (5-FU/LV) for the adjuvant treatment of elderly colon cancer patients (pts). J Clin Oncol 2004; 22(14S):3737.

76. Gastrointestinal-Tumor-Study-Group. Prolongation of the disease-free interval in surgically treated rectal carcinoma. N Engl J Med 1985; 312(23):1465–1472.

77. NIH Consensus Conference. Adjuvant therapy for patients with colon and rectal cancer. JAMA 1990; 264:1444–1450.

78. Newcomb P, Carbone P. Cancer treatment and age: patient perspectives. J Natl Cancer Inst 1993; 85:1580–1584.

79. Neugut A, Fleischauer A, Sundarajan V, et al. Use of adjuvant chemotherapy and radiation therapy for rectal cancer among the elderly: a population-based study. J Clin Oncol 2002; 20(11):2643–2650.

80. Ooi B, Tjandra J, Green M. Morbidities of adjuvant chemotherapy and radiotherapy for resectable rectal cancer: an overview. Dis Colon Rectum 1999; 42:403–418.

81. Farniok K, Levitt S. The role of radiation therapy in the treatment of colorectal cancer. Implications for the older patient. Cancer 1994; 74(7 suppl):2154–2159.

82. Benson A, Desch C, Flynn P, et al. 2000 update of American Society of Clinical Oncology colorectal cancer surveillance guidelines. J Clin Oncol 2000; 18(20):3586–3588.

83. Knopf K, Warren J, Feuer E, Brown M. Bowel surveillance patterns after a diagnosis of colorectal cancer in Medicare beneficiaries. Gastrointest Endosc 2001; 54(5):563–571.

84. Engstrom P, Benson A, Choti M, et al. Colon cancer: clinical practice guidelines in oncology. J Nat Comp Cancer Network 2003; 1(1):40–63.

85. Temple LK, Hsieh L, Wong WD, Saltz L, Schrag D. Use of surgery among elderly patients with stage IV colorectal cancer. J Clin Oncol 2004; 22(17):3475–3484.

86. Lewis A, Khoury G. Resection for colorectal cancer in the very old: are the risks too high? Br Med J (Clin Res Ed) 1988; 296(6620):459–461.

87. Whittle J, Steinberg E, Anderson G, Herbert R. Results of colectomy in elderly patients with colon cancer, based on Medicare claims data. Am J Surg 1992; 163(6):572–576.

88. Arveux I, Boutron M, El Mrini T, et al. Colon cancer in the elderly: evidence for major improvements in health care and survival. Br J Cancer 1997; 76(7):963–967.
89. Catena F, Pasqualini E, Tonini V, Avanzolini A, Campione O. Emergency surgery for patients with colorectal cancer over 90 years of age. Hepatogastroenterology 2002; 49(48):1538–1539.
90. Fong Y, Blumgart L, Fortner J, Brennan M. Pancreatic or liver resection for malignancy is safe and effective for the elderly. Ann Surg 1995; 222(4):426–434.
91. Girard P, Ducreux M, Baldeyrou P, et al. Surgery for lung metastases from colorectal cancer: analysis of prognostic factors. J Clin Oncol 1996; 14(7):2047–2053.
92. Okumura S, Kondo H, Tsuboi M, et al. Pulmonary resection for metastatic colorectal cancer: experiences with 159 patients. J Thorac Cardiovasc Surg 1996; 112(4):867–874.
93. D'Andre S, Sargent DJ, Cha SS, et al. 5-Fluorouracil-based chemotherapy for advanced colorectal cancer in elderly patients: a North Central Cancer Treatment Group study. Clin Colorectal Cancer 2005; 4(5):325–331.
94. Chiara S, Nobile M, Vincenti M, et al. Advanced colorectal cancer in the elderly: results of consecutive trials with 5-fluorouracil-based chemotherapy. Cancer Chemother Pharmacol 1998; 42(4):336–340.
95. Weinerman B, Rayner H, Venne A, Fietz C, Ghesquire F. Increased incidence and severity of stomatitis (S) in women treated with 5-fluorouracil (F) and leucovorin (L). Proc Am Soc Clin Oncol 1998; 17:A1176.
96. Magne N, Francois E, Broisin L, et al. Palliative 5-fluorouracil-based chemotherapy for advanced colorectal cancer in the elderly: results of a 10-year experience. Am J Clin Oncol 2002; 25(2):126–130.
97. Daniele B, Rosati G, Tambaro R, et al. First-line chemotherapy with fluorouracil and folinic acid for advanced colorectal cancer in elderly patients: a phase II study. J Clin Gastroenterol 2003; 36(3):228–233.
98. Stein B, Petrelli N, Douglass H, Driscoll D, Arcangeli G, Meropol N. Age and sex are independant predictors of 5-fluorouracil toxicity. Analysis of a large scale phase III trial. Cancer 1995; 75(1):11–17.
99. Meta-Analysis Group in Cancer. Efficacy of intravenous continuous infusion of fluorouracil compared with bolus administration in advanced colorectal cancer. J Clin Oncol 1998; 16(1):301–308.
100. Zalcberg J, Kerr D, Seymour L, Palmer M. Haematological and non-haematological toxicity after 5-fluorouracil and leucovorin in patients with advanced colorectal cancer is significantly associated with gender, increasing age and cycle number. Tomudex International Study Group. Eur J Cancer 1998; 34(12):1871–1875.
101. Van Cutsem E, Hoff PM, Harper P, et al. Oral capecitabine verses intravenous 5-fluorouracil and leucovorin: integrated efficacy data and novel analyses from two large, randomised, phase III trials. Br J Cancer 2004; 90(6):1190–1197.
102. Feliu J, Escudero P, Llosa F, et al. Capecitabine as first-line treatment for patients older than 70 years with metastatic colorectal cancer: an Oncopaz Cooperative Group study. J Clin Oncol 2005; 23(13):3104–3111.
103. Jonker D, Vincent M, Kerr I, et al. Dose reduced first-line capecitabine monotherapy in older and less fit patients with advanced colorectal cancer (ACRC)[abstr.]. Proc Gastrointestinal Symp 2004; 1:212.
104. Schaaf L, Ichhpurani N, Elfring G, Wolf M, Rothenberg M, Von Hoff D. Influence of age on the pharmacokinetics of irinotecan (CPT-11) and its metabolites, SN-38 and SN-38 glucuronide (SN-38G), in patients with previously treated colorectal cancer. Proc Am Soc Clin Oncol 1997; 16:A708.
105. Pazdur R, Zinner R, Rothenberg M, et al. Age as a risk factor in irinotecan (CPT-11) treatment of 5-FU refractory colorectal cancer. Proc Am Soc Clin Oncol 1997;16:A921.
106. Cunningham D, Pyrhoenen S, James R, et al. Randomized trial of irinotecan plus supportive care versus supportive care alone after fluorouracil failure for patients with metastatic colorectal cancer. Lancet 1998; 352:1413–1418.

107. Fuchs C, Moore M, Harker G, Villa L, Rinaldi D, Hecht J. Phase III comparison of two irinotecan dosing regimens in second-line therapy of metastatic colorectal cancer. J Clin Oncol 2003; 21(5):807–814.
108. Chau I, Norman AR, Cunningham D, et al. Elderly patients with fluoropyrimidine and thymidylate synthase inhibitor-resistant advanced colorectal cancer derive similar benefit without excessive toxicity when treated with irinotecan monotherapy. Br J Cancer 2004; 91(8):1453–1458.
109. Raymond E, Faivre S, Woynarowski JM, Chaney SG. Oxaliplatin: mechanism of action and antineoplastic activity. Semin Oncol 1998; 25(2 suppl 5):4–12.
110. Rothenberg ML, Oza AM, Bigelow RH, et al. Superiority of oxaliplatin and fluorouracil-leucovorin compared with either therapy alone in patients with progressive colorectal cancer after irinotecan and fluorouracil-leucovorin: interim results of a phase III trial. J Clin Oncol 2003; 21(11):2059–2069.
111. de Gramont A, Figer A, Seymour M, et al. Leucovorin and fluorouracil with or without oxaliplatin as first-line treatment in advanced colorectal cancer. J Clin Oncol 2000; 18(16):2938–2947.
112. Goldberg RM, Sargent DJ, Morton RF, et al. A randomized controlled trial of fluorouracil plus leucovorin, irinotecan, and oxaliplatin combinations in patients with previously untreated metastatic colorectal cancer. J Clin Oncol 2004; 22(1):23–30.
113. Exquis B, Aapro M, Kohler S. Oxaliplatin (with 5FU and leucovorin) in patients above age 70 ("elderly") suffering from metastatic colorectal cancer: an observational study. J Clin Oncol 2004; 22(14S):8042.
114. Aparicio T, Desrame J, Lecomte T, et al. Oxaliplatin- or irinotecan-based chemotherapy for metastatic colorectal cancer in the elderly. Br J Cancer 2003; 89(8):1439–1444.
115. Nardi M, Mare M, Zavettieri M, et al. Folfiri (CPT11/LV5FU2) and FOLFOX4 (oxaliplatin/LV5FU2): two safety regimens in elderly fit patients with metastatic colorectal cancer (MCRC). J Clin Oncol 2004; 22(14S):3711.
116. Mattioli R, Massacesi C, Recchia F, et al. High activity and reduced neurotoxicity of bi-fractionated oxaliplatin plus 5-fluorouracil/leucovorin for elderly patients with advanced colorectal cancer. Ann Oncol 2005; 16(7):1147–1151 (Epub 2005 Apr 22).
117. Figer A, Perez N, Carola E, et al. 5-Fluorouracil, folinic acid and oxaliplatin (FOLFOX) in very old patients with metastatic colorectal cancer. Proc Am Soc Clin Oncol 2004; 23:263; A3571.
118. Gruenberger T, Schuell B, Kornek GV, Scheithauer W. Elderly patients do benefit from oxaliplatin based neoadjuvant chemotherapy in resectable colorectal cancer liver metastases. J Clin Oncol 2005; 23(16S):271s.
119. Jain RK. Normalizing tumor vasculature with anti-angiogenic therapy: a new paradigm for combination therapy. Nat Med 2001; 7(9):987–989.
120. Willett CG, Boucher Y, di Tomaso E, et al. Direct evidence that the VEGF-specific antibody bevacizumab has antivascular effects in human rectal cancer. Nat Med 2004; 10(2):145–147 (Epub 2004 Jan 25).
121. Wildiers H, Guetens G, De Boeck G, et al. Effect of antivascular endothelial growth factor treatment on the intratumoral uptake of CPT-11. Br J Cancer 2003; 88(12):1979–1986.
122. Hurwitz H, Fehrenbacher L, Novotny W, et al. Bevacizumab plus irinotecan, fluorouracil, and leucovorin for metastatic colorectal cancer. N Engl J Med 2004; 350(23):2335–2342.
123. Giantonio B, Catalano P, Meropol NJ, et al. High-dose bevacizumab improves survival when combined with FOLFOX4 in previously treated advanced colorectal cancer: Results from the Eastern Cooperative Oncology Group (ECOG) study E3200. J Clin Oncol ASCO Annu Meet Proc 2005; 23(16S):1s.
124. Kabbinavar FF, Schulz J, McCleod M, et al. Addition of bevacizumab to bolus fluorouracil and leucovorin in first-line metastatic colorectal cancer: results of a randomized phase II trial. J Clin Oncol 2005; 23(16):3697–3705 (Epub 2005 Feb 28).

125. Skillings JR, Johnson D, Miller K, et al. Arterial thromboembolic events (ATEs) in a pooled analysis of 5 randomized, controlled trials (RCTs) of bevacizumab (BV) with chemotherapy. J Clin Oncol 2005; 23(16S):196s.

126. Mendelsohn J. Targeting the epidermal growth factor receptor for cancer therapy. J Clin Oncol 2002; 20(18 suppl):1S–13S.

127. Cunningham D, Humblet Y, Siena S, et al. Cetuximab monotherapy and cetuximab plus irinotecan in irinotecan-refractory metastatic colorectal cancer. N Engl J Med 2004; 351(4):337–345.

128. Saltz L, Cox J, Blanke C, et al. Irinotecan plus fluorouracil and leucovorin for metastatic colorectal cancer. N Engl J Med 2000; 343(13):905–914.

129. Knight R, Miller L, Elfring G, Pirotta N, Locker P, Saltz L. Evaluation of age, gender, performance status (PS), and organ dysfunction as predictors of toxicity with first-line irinotecan (C), fluorouracil (F), leucovorin (L) therapy of metastatic colorectal cancer (MCRC). Proc Am Soc Clin Oncol 2001; 20:A534.

130. Sastre J, Marcuello E, Masutti B, et al. Irinotecan in combination with fluorouracil in a 48-hour continuous infusion as first-line chemotherapy for elderly patients with metastatic colorectal cancer: a Spanish Cooperative Group for the Treatment of Digestive Tumors study. J Clin Oncol 2005; 23(15):3545–3551.

131. Bollina R, Beretta G, Toniolo D, et al. Capecitabine (C) and irinotecan (I)(CAPIRI): A good combination in elderly patients (pts) with advanced colorectal cancer (ACRC) as first line chemotherapy (CT). Preliminary results of a phase II trial. Proc Am Soc Clin Oncol 2003; 22:A1332.

132. Berretta M, Buonadonna A, Rupolo M, et al. Comparison between elderly and non-elderly patients (PTS), of efficacy and tolerabilitiy of FOLFOX2 schedule in advanced colorectal cancer (COL). Proc Am Soc Clin Oncol 2001; 20:A2195.

133. Carreca I, Comella P, Maiorino L, et al. Oral capecitabine plus oxaliplatin (XELOX regimen) in elderly patients with advanced colorectal carcinoma (ACC). Southern Italy Cooperative Oncology Group (SICOG 0108) phase II study. Proc Am Soc Clin Oncol 2003; 22:A2939.

134. Twelves C, Butts C, Cassidy J, et al. XELOX (capecitabine plus oxaliplatin), a safe and active first-line regimen for elderly patients with metastatic colorectal cancer (MCRC): post-hoc analysis of a large phase II study. J Clin Oncol 2004; 22(14S).

135. Bollina R, Toniolo D, Belloni P, Cozzi C, Clerici M. Oxaliplatin (LOHP) and irinotecan (CPT-11)-OXIRI: phase I/II study in 5-FU (F) refractory advanced colorectal cancer (ACRC) elderly patients (pts), a second line treatment. Proc Am Soc Clin Oncol 2001; 20:A1625.

136. Trimble E, Carter C, Cain D, Freidlin B, Ungerleider R, Friedman M. Representation of older patients in cancer treatment trials. Cancer 1994; 74:2208–2214.

137. Yancik R. Cancer burden in the aged: an epidemiologic and demographic overview. Cancer 1997; 80:1273–1283.

138. Hutchins L, Unger J, Crowley J, Coltman C, Albain K. Underrepresentation of patients 65 years of age or older in cancer-treatment trials. N Engl J Med 1999; 341(27):2061–2067.

139. Talarico L, Chen G, Pazdur R. Enrollment of elderly patients in clinical trials for cancer drug registration: a 7-year experience by the US Food and Drug Administration. J Clin Oncol 2004; 22(22):4626–4631.

140. Murthy VH, Krumholz HM, Gross CP. Participation in cancer clinical trials: race-, sex-, and age-based disparities. JAMA 2004; 291(22):2720–2726.

141. Klabunde C, Springer B, Butler B, White M, Atkins J. Factors influencing enrollment in clinical trials for cancer treatment. South Med J 1999; 92(12):1189–1193.

142. Yee K, JL P, Pho L, Zee B, Siu L. Enrollment of older patients in cancer treatment trials in Canada: why is age a barrier? J Clin Oncol 2003; 21(8):1618–1623.

14

Ovarian Cancer

Nicholas C. Lambrou and Meredith P. Crisp
*Division of Gynecologic Oncology, Department of Obstetrics and Gynecology,
University of Miami School of Medicine, Miami, Florida, U.S.A.*

Robert E. Bristow
*Department of Gynecology and Obstetrics, The Kelly Gynecologic Oncology Service,
The Johns Hopkins Medical Institutions, Baltimore, Maryland, U.S.A.*

INTRODUCTION

The incidence of ovarian carcinoma increases with advancing age, with a peak incidence during the seventh decade of life and continues to elevate until 80 years of age. Despite the high prevalence of ovarian cancer in the elderly, the management of these patients is often less aggressive than that of their younger counterparts with the result being that many elderly cancer patients undergo inadequate treatment. Although some data suggest that age is a negative prognostic factor, there is no evidence that age alone should preclude one from standard therapy. In fact, the majority of elderly patients will be able to tolerate the standard of care for ovarian cancer including initial surgical cytoreduction followed by platinum and taxane chemotherapy. Because functional status does not show a reliable correlation with either tumor stage or comorbidity, each patient's comorbidities should be assessed independently. For those elderly patients with significant medical comorbidity, the extent of surgery and the aggressiveness of chemotherapy should be tailored to the individual's extent of disease, symptoms, overall health, and life goals. In addition, enhanced cooperation between geriatricians and oncologists may help in the pretreatment assessment of elderly patients and improve treatment guidelines in this population.

Ovarian Cancer Statistics

In 2004, there were an estimated 25,580 new cases of ovarian cancer with 16,090 estimated deaths annually (1). Dramatic improvements in healthcare and a decrease in mortality have resulted in an increased life expectancy among people living in developed countries. In western countries, a woman's life expectancy was 81.1 years in 1991 and is anticipated to reach 90.4 years by 2020 (2,3). As a result, the incidence of cancer-bearing patients aged 70 or older may also be expected to increase (4–6). The incidence of ovarian cancer increases with advancing age with a peak incidence during the seventh decade of life and continues to elevate until 80 years of age. Thirty to forty percent of malignant ovarian neoplasms occur after the age of 65 (7,8). Despite the high prevalence of ovarian cancer in the elderly, the management of these patients is often less aggressive than that of their younger counterparts, with the result being that many elderly cancer patients undergo inadequate treatment (9–13).

Patterns of Care Among Ovarian Cancer Patients

In one of the earliest published reports examining patterns of care among elderly patients with ovarian cancer, Ries (12) analyzed data for over 22,000 women diagnosed between 1973 and 1987 within the Surveillance, Epidemiology, and End Results (SEER) program. When stratified by stage, age was a significant determinant of survival. Five-year survival for women less than 45 years of age was 45% compared to only 8% for those 85 years of age and over. Over 40% of women aged 85 years or older did not receive definitive treatment for their disease. In addition, when treatment was given, younger women received multimodality therapy more often than their older counterparts who received more single modality treatments such as surgery alone or chemotherapy or hormonal therapy alone. More recent SEER data, depicted in Table 1, reveals continued differences in survival between patients 65 years of age or older and those younger than 65 (1).

Further evidence that older women received less aggressive therapy and had poorer survival rates was published in 1994. Hightower et al. (13) analyzed data by the American College of Surgeons Cancer Commission to investigate differences in patterns of care among the elderly. In this study, the survival and care of patients who were 80 years of age or older was compared to that of those less than 80 years of age. Of 12,316 patients diagnosed between 1983 and 1988, 1115 were 80 years or older. Survival was significantly lower among patients over the age of 80. Most elderly ovarian cancer patients were cared for by nononcologists such as general surgeons (31%) and obstetricians/gynecologists (29%). Older patients had fewer total abdominal hysterectomies, bilateral salpingo-oophorectomies, and omentectomies than their younger counterparts. Optimal tumor-debulking rates were significantly lower for women 80 years or older. Adjuvant chemotherapy was also less likely to be given to older patients than to younger patients (42% vs. 69%, $P < 0.0001$).

It has recently been reported that although 60% of ovarian cancers arise in women 65 years of age or older, only 20% to 40% of patients who are enrolled

Table 1 Five-Year Survival for Ovarian Cancer (1995–2000)

Disease location	Age < 65 yr	Age > 65 yr
All stages combined	55.7	28.8
Localized	93.2	93.8
Regional	74.8	59.1
Distant	37.1	19.6
Unstaged	41.9	13.2

Data from nine SEER areas. Rates based on population-based registries from follow-up of patients into 2001 from Connecticut, Utah, New Mexico, Hawaii, Iowa, Atlanta, Seattle-Puget Sound, Detroit, and San Francisco-Oakland.
Abbreviation: SEER, Surveillance Epidemiology and End Results.
Source: From Ref. 1.

in phase II and III trials are over this age range, and a majority are less than 70 years of age (14,15). Markman et al. (16) reported on "The Memorial Sloan-Kettering Cancer Center experience" of clinical trial enrollment for women with ovarian cancer after primary surgical therapy. Forty-six percent of the younger patients were entered into an intensive initial chemotherapy trial compared to only 17% of older patients. The reported reason for lower enrollment in the older population was an excessive prevalence of comorbid conditions such as heart disease. In addition, there was a fourfold higher rate of referrals to this institution for both initial treatment and salvage therapy among younger women when compared to their older counterparts. This observation suggests that older patients are less likely to be referred for secondary experimental programs.

Recent reports have demonstrated that older women with ovarian cancer are less likely to receive standard recommended treatment (17) and are less likely to be seen by a gynecologic oncologist during the diagnosis or treatment (18). Carney et al. (18) performed a statewide population-based study in Utah between 1992 and 1998. Of the 848 cases of epithelial ovarian cancer identified, fewer than 25% of women aged 70 or older were seen by a gynecologic oncologist, compared to 55% of women who were 40 to 59 years of age and 42.6% of patients 60 to 69 years of age. Furthermore, this study noted a significantly increased survival for patients with advanced disease who were treated by a gynecologic oncologist (median survival time: 26 months) when compared to those treated by a nongynecologic oncologist (median survival time: 15 months).

SCREENING

Ovarian cancer metastatic to the pelvis or abdomen is diagnosed in approximately 90% of patients, and survival rates are less than 30% for patients with advanced disease. In contrast, the fraction of patients with Stage I ovarian cancer at diagnosis have a 90% five-year survival (19). For this reason, screening strategies are desired to detect ovarian cancer at an early stage. Several strategies to screen for early detection of ovarian cancer have been proposed, including ultrasound, serum cancer antigen (CA)-125, combination of ultrasound and serum CA-125, and proteomic analysis of serum.

DePriest et al. investigated 3220 postmenopausal women (mean age: 60 years) who were asymptomatic at the time of ultrasound examination (20). In this study, an ovarian volume greater than 10 cm^3 or papillary projections in the lumen of a cystic tumor were considered abnormal. Repeat ultrasounds were performed on patients with an abnormal initial scan. If abnormalities were still noted on the repeat scan, the morphology index of the tumor (including volume, structure of septae, and structure of cyst wall), serum CA-125, and exploratory surgery were undertaken. If no abnormalities were noted on initial scan, patients were followed up with a repeat scan in one year. A persistent abnormality was noted in 44 (1.4%) patients who then underwent laparotomy. Of these patients, one was diagnosed with Stage IIIB and two with Stage IA upon pathology examination of specimens. Of note, no abnormal serum CA-125 levels or pelvic examinations were noted on patients with ovarian cancer in this study (20). Other studies have evaluated the use of various morphology index-scoring systems in an attempt to improve the sensitivity and specificity of the ovarian cancer–screening ultrasound. Sassone et al. achieved 100% sensitivity and 83% specificity when using wall structure, septations, thickness of the cyst wall, and echogenicity to differentiate between malignant and benign ovarian masses (21). In a multi-institutional study, DePriest et al. used a morphology index including ovarian volume, structure of septae, and structure of cyst wall. This study noted 89% sensitivity and 46% positive predictive value for determination of ovarian neoplasms (22).

CA-125 is a glycoprotein expressed in normal tissues originally derived from coelomic epithelia such as peritoneum, pleura, pericardium, fallopian tubes, and endometrium. CA-125, a nonspecific biomarker for ovarian cancer, has not proven to be an effective screening tool for the general population. However, it is useful during the evaluation of a patient with a pelvic mass and for monitoring treatment effect (23). Elevated serum CA-125 is also associated with several nonmalignant conditions such as uterine fibroids, endometriosis, pregnancy, pelvic inflammatory disease, and tubo-ovarian abscess (24–26) as well as other nongynecologic conditions such as cirrhosis, diverticulitis, and renal failure. In addition, other primary malignancies with intra-abdominal metastases such as pancreatic, breast, colon, and uterine cancer may be associated with an elevated CA-125. Despite the possibility of false-positive results, CA-125 above 65 U/mL has been shown to have a sensitivity of 97% and specificity of 78% in patients with a pelvic mass, who are postmenopausal (27).

A new technology known as proteomic profiling uses an analysis of cellular protein alterations in serum and may show promise in differentiating malignant versus ovarian lesions, with potential for identifying early stage ovarian cancer (28,29). However, at present, this technology is of uncertain clinical value.

DIAGNOSIS AND STAGING

Approximately 75% of patients with epithelial ovarian cancer are diagnosed when their disease has spread throughout the peritoneal cavity. Most commonly, patients will present with abdominal discomfort or pain. This is generally followed closely by abdominal distention due to the presence of intra-abdominal masses and/or malignant ascites. Gastrointestinal symptoms are nonspecific but include nausea, early satiety, constipation, or obstipation, and less frequently, urinary symptoms (30). If disease has progressed to involve the lungs as exemplified by the presence of pulmonary metastases or by malignant pleural effusions, the patient may present with complaints of shortness of breath and lethargy. Patients with early-stage ovarian cancer tend to have symptoms of mass effect (67%) rather than constitutional symptoms (9%). Mass-effect symptoms include constipation, urinary frequency, pelvic pressure, and palpable mass. Unfortunately, these symptoms are reported by only two-thirds of patients with early ovarian cancer (31).

The five-year survival of patients with epithelial ovarian cancer correlates directly with tumor stage. The Federation Internationale de Gynecologie et d'obstetrique staging system, revised in 1985, is presented in Table 2. With the exception of Stage IV disease, which can be diagnosed by a cytologically positive pleural fluid, computed tomography–guided biopsy of intraparenchymal liver lesions, or other pathologic evidence of distant spread, the stage of disease is only accurately determined by an exploratory surgical assessment (i.e., laparotomy or laparoscopy). Laparotomy should be performed through a vertical midline incision to allow access to the upper abdomen. Peritoneal lavage or aspiration of ascites is performed to obtain specimens for cytologic analysis. Suspicious areas throughout the abdomen and pelvis should be biopsied, including adhesions, with separate specimens sent from the pelvis, right and left paracolic gutters, and the undersurfaces of the right

Table 2 Carcinoma of the Ovary

Stage	I	Growth limited to the ovaries
	IA	Growth limited to one ovary; no ascites containing malignant cells. No tumor on the external surface; capsule intact
	IB	Growth limited to both ovaries; no ascites containing malignant cells. No tumor on the external surface; capsule intact
	IC	Tumor classified as either Stage IA or IB but with tumor on the surface of one or both ovaries, with ruptured capsule(s), with ascites containing malignant cells or with positive peritoneal washings
Stage	II	Growth involving one or both ovaries, with pelvic extension
	IIA	Extension and/or metastases to the uterus and/or tubes
	IIB	Extension to other pelvic tissues
	IIC	Tumor classified as either Stage IIA or IIB but with tumor on the surface of one or both ovaries, with capsule(s) ruptured, or with ascites containing malignant cells or with positive peritoneal washings
Stage	III	Tumor involving one or both ovaries with peritoneal implants outside the pelvis and/or positive retroperitoneal or inguinal nodes. Superficial liver metastasis equals Stage III. Tumor is limited to the true pelvis but with histologically proven malignant extension to small bowel or omentum
	IIIA	Tumor grossly limited to the true pelvis with negative nodes but with histologically confirmed microscopic seeding of abdominal peritoneal surfaces
	IIIB	Tumor of one or both ovaries with histologically confirmed implants of abdominal peritoneal surfaces, none exceeding 2 cm in diameter; nodes are negative
	IIIC	Abdominal implants greater than 2 cm in diameter and/or positive retroperitoneal or inguinal nodes
Stage	IV	Growth involving one or both ovaries, with distant metastases. If pleural effusion is present, there must be positive cytological findings to allot a case to Stage IV. Parenchymal liver metastasis equals Stage IV

and left hemidiaphragms. All intestinal surfaces should be evaluated, and an omentectomy with random peritoneal biopsies should be performed. Pelvic and aortic lymph-node sampling is also required. When a thorough and methodical staging is performed, a significant number of patients initially felt to have localized disease will be upstaged. In a report by Young et al. (32), 31% of women thought to have Stage I or II ovarian cancer at initial surgery were upstaged at repeat surgical staging. Of these patients, 77% were upstaged to Stage III. In a report by McGowan et al. (33), gynecologic oncologists performed adequate surgical staging in 97% of cases, compared to 52% of cases performed by an obstetrician/gynecologist and just 32% of cases attended to by general surgeons. In this report, of the 291 women evaluated, 46% had been inadequately staged for their disease.

TREATMENT

Surgical Cytoreduction

In addition to the prognostic importance of accurate staging, surgical cytoreduction (or debulking) has proven to be an integral component in the management of epithelial ovarian cancer. The volume of residual disease following cytoreductive surgery is inversely related to survival (34–37). Current criteria for optimal cytoreduction imply residual tumor nodules no greater than 1 cm in diameter. Patients who have been optimally cytoreduced have approximately a 22-month median survival advantage when compared to patients with suboptimal cytoreduction (residual disease >1 cm in maximum diameter). Hoskins et al. analyzed Gynecologic Oncology Group (GOG) data and noted a significant improvement in survival in patients who had 1 to 2 cm residual disease as compared to those having greater than 2 cm residual disease (38). In addition to the survival benefits of cytoreductive surgery, recent reports also confirm that aggressive primary cytoreductive operations are associated with minimal morbidity and mortality when performed by experienced surgeons (39). Most of the studies supporting the survival benefit of cytoreductive surgery have included both Stage III and Stage IV patients. Four recent retrospective reports have examined cytoreductive surgery in patients with Stage IV disease separately and have consistently demonstrated a statistically significant improvement in survival when left with small-volume residual disease (40–42).

Surgery for Ovarian Cancer in the Elderly

Although several studies have reported that elderly patients undergo proportionally fewer and less aggressive surgeries for primary treatment of ovarian cancer than their younger counterparts (43–45), relatively little data exist on the influence of age alone on surgical outcomes. Several large trials have shown that healthy elderly patients can tolerate most oncologic treatments as well as younger patients (14,46), despite the widely held belief that elderly patients may not tolerate radical surgical intervention. One should also consider that the elderly patients in these studies may have been selected on the basis of performance status, age, and the absence of serious medical illnesses and may not be representative of the elderly population at large. In a recent series by Cloven et al. (43), 16 of 18 patients with ovarian cancer over 80 years of age underwent primary debulking surgery. Twenty-five percent were optimally cytoreduced, and 38% of patients experienced major postoperative morbidity. Seventy-five percent of patients spent time in the intensive care unit; however, the majority of patients were discharged home and received postoperative chemotherapy. Most patients in this group had one or more preexisting medical illnesses and an advanced American Society of Anesthesiologists score.

In contrast, a retrospective study by Wright et al. reviewed a total of 175 patients, 129 younger and 46 older than 70 years, who underwent exploratory laparotomy during 1996–2002 for a pelvic mass (47). They report that cytoreduction (defined as 1 cm for the largest tumor diameter) was achieved in 81% and 82% of patients 70 and older versus those younger than 70 years of age, respectively. Additionally, similar hospital stay, distribution of stage, postoperative complications, and survival were noted in the two groups (47).

Giannice et al. (45) conclude in their retrospective review that age alone should not preclude lymphadenectomy in elderly patients. This study reviewed surgical cases of patients aged 70 and older with endometrial and ovarian cancer from 1986 to 1996. In this study, 85% of ovarian cancer patients with indicated lymphadenectomy did not receive this procedure, age being cited as the only documented reason for omission of this procedure. In the patients with endometrial and ovarian cancer who did undergo lymphadenectomy, no significant difference in intraoperative complications, blood loss or transfusion, required reintervention, time interval with ileus, or hospital stay in the postoperative period was noted when compared with matched controls who did not get lymphadenectomy. Authors also reported similar comorbid conditions such as cardiovascular disease, hypertension, diabetes mellitus, and obesity in both groups (45).

In another recent report by Bruchim et al. (44), patients with epithelial ovarian cancer were retrospectively reviewed and stratified according to age less than or greater than or equal to 70. The group of elderly patients had fewer primary debulking surgeries and was more likely to receive neoadjuvant chemotherapy. However, age did not appear to be a limiting factor in achieving optimal debulking in those patients who did undergo surgery. In this study, nearly 92% of the younger patients entered a first-line chemotherapy regimen compared to 65% of the older patients. Of note, hematologic toxicity was more severe among the elderly patients who did receive chemotherapy.

A study noted that as age increases, patients were less likely to receive chemotherapy. Sundararajan et al. reviewed SEER data from 1992 to 1996, with attention to 1775 women who were 65 years of age or older. Although 80% of patients underwent some cancer-related surgery and 83% received some chemotherapy, increased age was associated with lesser chance of receiving chemotherapy. Of note, only 43% of women 85 years or older were treated with chemotherapy. Additionally, those patients with two or more comorbidities or those of Hispanic descent who were 75 years of age or older were less likely to receive chemotherapy than those 65 to 74 years of age (48).

Chemotherapy

Surgery alone is rarely curative for patients with ovarian cancer. Chemotherapeutic agents from a wide variety of different classes have shown activity against ovarian cancer. With the establishment of platinum-based therapy and introduction of the taxanes, the past two decades have shown dramatic improvements in chemotherapy-response rates and progression-free survival. Paclitaxel was reported to have significant activity in the treatment of advanced ovarian carcinoma in 1989 (49). After a series of phase I and phase II trials establishing the activity of paclitaxel, two prospective randomized trials comparing cisplatin plus paclitaxel versus cisplatin plus cyclophosphamide demonstrated the superiority of the paclitaxel-containing regimen (50,51). Later prospective randomized trials comparing paclitaxel–carboplatin versus paclitaxel–cisplatin have demonstrated decreased toxicity with the carboplatin regimen with no difference in efficacy (52,53). With these results, paclitaxel plus carboplatin is now considered the first-line treatment for most patients with advanced ovarian cancer.

Chemotherapy for Ovarian Cancer in the Elderly

Cooperative trials have shown that healthy elderly people can tolerate most chemotherapy regimens as well as their younger counterparts. However, this observation may not necessarily apply to the subset of elderly patients with significant medical comorbidity. A recent review by Ceccaroni et al. (6) suggests that the use of a multidimensional geriatric evaluation may be useful in evaluating elderly patients for chemotherapy. Similarly, Monfardini et al. (54) have published the Multidimensional Assessment of Cancer in the Elderly Comprehensive Geriatric Assessment scale in elderly cancer patients and have proposed its use in clinical trials. Repetto et al. (55) recently published a review describing a clinical approach to the geriatric oncology patient. Table 3 summarizes the variety of some current methods used to assess the effects of aging.

It is evident that many parameters may be used to assess elderly patients and that the majority of these are nonspecific. Cooperation between geriatricians and oncologists is a potential strategy to improve the pretreatment assessment.

In elderly patients, several pharmacodynamic changes may shift the balance of cytotoxic treatments in favor of increased toxicity and decreased efficacy.

Table 3 Assessment of Aging

Laboratory assessment	
Serum creatinine	Nonspecific
Serum osmolarity	Nonspecific
Circulating levels of cytokines (IL-6, TNF)	Nonsensitive to early aging
Cystine/acid-soluble thiol ratio	Nonspecific
D-dimer levels	Nonspecific
Serum growth hormones	Experimental
Physical assessment	
Stature	Nonspecific; may be influenced by cancer and malnutrition
Hand-grasp	May predict development of functional disability
Lower extremities strength	Experimental
Raising from chair	Useful to establish difficulties in movement; no relationship to functional dependence or life expectancy
CGA	
Functional status	
ADL and IADL	Relationship to life expectancy and tolerance of chemotherapy
Comorbidity	
Number of comorbid conditions	Relationship to life expectancy and tolerance of chemotherapy
Mental status	
Folstein minimental status	Relationship to life expectancy and dependence
Emotional conditions	
GDS	Relationship to survival; may indicate motivation to receive treatment
Nutritional status	
MNA	Reversible condition; possible relationship to survival
Polypharmacy	Risk of drug interactions
Geriatric syndromes (delerium, dementia, depression, falls, incontinence, spontaneous bone fractures, neglect and abuse, failure to thrive)	Relationship to survival, functional dependence

Abbreviations: ADL, activities of daily living; CGA, comprehensive geriatric assessment; GDS, geriatric depression scale; IADL, instrumental activities of daily living; IL-6, interleukin 6; MNA, mininutritional assessment; TNF, tumor necrosis factor.
Source: From Ref. 55.

Molecular changes associated with age, which may lead to a higher prevalence of drug resistance include a reduction in tumor growth rate and a resistance to apoptosis (6,56–58). Theoretically, a reduction in lean body mass and increase in body fat may occur with age, which can influence drug distribution. However, currently no significant correlation has been found between age and drug clearance, dose, or toxicity (6). Several studies have demonstrated that despite an age-related decrease in patient's creatinine clearance of many drugs, total clearance does not change, and this observation may be due to an increase in hepatic clearance (6,59,60). Myelotoxicity is the most commonly encountered chemotherapy-related toxicity and may occur more frequently in the elderly. An Eastern Cooperative Oncology Group review showed that commonly used chemotherapeutic agents (for nine disease sites) were significantly more myelotoxic in patients aged 70 years or older than in those less than 70 (61). However, the increased toxicity appeared to be mostly limited to methotrexate and 1-(2-chloroethyl)-3-(4-methylcyclohexyl)-1-nitrosourea. In the Mayo clinic experience of women with ovarian cancer enrolled in phase III trials (46), progressively larger dose reductions were required for treatment continuation with advancing age; however, chemotherapy was generally well tolerated across all age groups.

In a recent review of advanced ovarian cancer in the elderly by Chiara et al. (62), no significant difference in toxicity was evident in patients 65 years of age or older treated with cisplatin-based chemotherapy when compared with younger patients. Nevertheless, interruption of chemotherapy due to toxicity was more frequent among the elderly. Thyss et al. (63) demonstrated that cisplatin could be safely administered (at doses ranging from 60 to $100 \, mg/m^2$) without excessive toxicity in patients older than 80 years with normal renal function. In a recent Italian trial, carboplatin ($230 \, mg/m^2$ intravenously every 28 days) along with mitoxantrone was well tolerated when administered to 82 ovarian cancer patients who were older than 70 years. Similar data in the setting of second-line treatment have also shown no difference in toxicity comparing patients 65 years and older versus younger counterparts (64).

The largest study evaluating chemotherapy tolerance in elderly oncology patients with gynecologic malignancies is based on the experience of women treated between 1990 and 2000 in four Italian centers (2). Of 148 patients reviewed, the median age was 73 years (range: 70–84) and 37% were more than 75 years of age. Nearly 70% of the patients were treated for ovarian cancer. One or more coexisting medical illnesses were present in nearly 80% of the patients. Of the patients subjected to a first-line chemotherapy, 96 (64.9%) received platinum-based treatment with no taxane (Group 1), 42 (28.4%) received combined platinum–paclitaxel regimens (Group 2), and 10 (6.8%) received taxane-based treatment with no platinum (Group 3). Table 4 summarizes the toxicity data stratified according to the type of first-line chemotherapy administered (2). No significant differences were observed in performance status before, during, or at the completion of first-line chemotherapy. Of the 103 ovarian cancer patients, 74 (71.9%) received combination chemotherapy and 38 (36.9%) received first-line treatment with platinum and taxanes. There were 38.2% grade 3 to 4 hematologic toxicities reported, and 6.8% of the patients discontinued treatment because of the toxicity. No significant association was seen between the number of comorbidities and toxicities. This study confirms previous reports that indicate that elderly patients with adequate renal and hepatic function tolerate standard chemotherapy regimens with equivalent toxicity profiles and no significant difference in treatment delays or discontinuations (46,64–66).

Table 4 Grade 3 to 4 Toxicity in Elderly Women Observed During a First-Line Regimen by Chemotherapy Group

Characteristic	Total	Group 1, platinum-based	Group 2, combination	Group 3, taxane only
Number of patients (%)	148 (100)	96 (64.9)	42 (28.4)	10 (6.8)
Hematological	66 (44.6)	44 (45.8)	20 (47.6)	2 (20)
Gastrointestinal	1 (0.7)	1 (1.0)	–	–
Acoustic	2 (1.4)	1 (1.0)	1 (2.4)	–
Cardiac	–	–	–	–
Renal	–	–	–	–
Neurological	–	–	–	–
Total	69 (46.6)	46 (47.9)	21 (50)	2 (20)
Discontinuation	6 (4)	6 (6.2)	–	–
Dose reduction	23 (15.5)	18 (18.8)	5 (11.9)	–
Treatment delay	25 (16.9)	20 (20.8)	4 (9.5)	1 (10)

Source: From Ref. 2.

AGE AS A PROGNOSTIC FACTOR

Marchetti et al. report that despite aggressive cytoreduction and chemotherapy for patients older than 65 years of age, median survival differed significantly (22.0 months vs. 36.7 months) from younger patients. This study notes that only 79% of elderly patients underwent optimal surgery (largest tumor diameter <2 cm), compared with 97% of younger patients. Also, more elderly patients received dose-reduced chemotherapy during the first three cycles (67). Although this research is limited by its small sample size, retrospective analysis, and differences in surgery and chemotherapy, it does suggest that age may be a poor prognostic indicator for ovarian cancer.

In a 1993 publication by Thigpen et al., 2123 patients enrolled in six GOG trials were reviewed to determine prognostic factors for ovarian cancer. One of the poor prognostic indicators noted was age over 69 years. After accounting for residual disease, drug therapy including dose, and stage of disease, prognosis was still less favorable for this group. Additionally, this study indicated that elderly patients tolerated aggressive therapy as well as their younger counterparts did (68). Although these studies present interesting data, it is still unknown why age may be a poor prognostic indicator of disease in ovarian cancer.

FOLLOW-UP

Advanced-stage ovarian cancer maintains a high risk of recurrence (50–60%) even after achieving a complete clinical remission to primary therapy. At our institutions, patients who have completed therapy return every three months for two years, then every six months for two years thereafter if they are without evidence of disease. During follow-up, patients undergo a physical examination, including pelvic and rectovaginal examination. Additionally, serum CA-125 is obtained. If recurrence is suspected based on examination, CA-125 level, or reported symptoms, then further radiographic imaging is obtained.

SUPPORTIVE CARE ISSUES

In view of the high mortality among elderly patients with advanced disease, end-of-life care is often required for these patients. Intra-abdominal structures, namely the intestine, are often involved in progressive ovarian cancer and may lead to intestinal obstruction. If the obstruction is partial, it can often be managed conservatively. Ultimately, however as disease progresses, women often undergo surgery for relief of bowel obstruction. In some situations, this may require a permanent colostomy, gastrostomy, or other surgical interventions. In a report by Rubin et al. at Memorial Sloan-Kettering Cancer Center, 54 procedures for intestinal obstruction were reviewed. In 43 of the 54 operations, surgical correction of the obstruction was possible. Seventy-nine percent of the postoperative patients were able to leave the hospital tolerating low-residue or regular diet. Additionally, the group undergoing procedures to correct obstruction were noted to have a survival of 6.8 months (69). For those patients with inoperable obstruction, octreotide has been shown to decrease emesis, limiting pain and discomfort at the time of death (70).

Pain management is a critical component in the management of advanced ovarian cancer and is often one of the few areas in which we, as care-providers, are able to help our patients. In a recent study, moderate to severe pain was noted in 50% of communicative patients in the few days prior to their death (71). Various pain medications can be utilized, but in patients with emesis or bowel obstruction, transdermal or oral transmucosal pain medications may be required when oral medications are no longer tolerated (72). Careful attention to the patient's symptoms is integral to achieving adequate pain relief, and consultation with pain specialists is often indicated.

Psychosocial well-being is an important aspect to be addressed throughout diagnosis and treatment, but is probably never more important than during end-of-life discussions. A study performed by Roberts et al. reported patient preferences and attitude obtained through a questionnaire filled in by benign gynecology patients and patients at various stages of gynecologic cancer. Patients desired their physician to display compassion (64%) and "straight talk" (96%). Fear of pain (63%), developing total dependence (46%), and losing control (48%) were major results of their cancer diagnosis. Through the same questionnaire, patients reported that continued hope was facilitated through their religious devotion. The authors concluded that physicians should provide education to patients so that their fears can be alleviated, their power can be maintained throughout their medical experience, and they can make educated decisions about care (73).

Depression is a psychological concern for many cancer patients and can influence one's quality of life. Patients may report helplessness, hopelessness, guilt, or worthlessness. Additionally, weight loss, disturbed sleep patterns, anorexia, and decreased activity may be signs of depression in patients. Treatment may include counseling or pharmacotherapy (72,74). Physicians dealing with oncology patients must be attentive to their patients' treatment preferences and establish advanced directives early in their care. "Do not resuscitate" orders and interventions such as intravenous fluids, nutritional support, and antibiotics are topics that may be discussed when appropriate (75). When a patient is deemed to have less than six months of life and no further treatment is intended, hospice care may be instituted. Hospice allows for palliative care while allowing as comfortable a death as possible and providing family members with education on the bereavement process (75).

SUMMARY

Treatment of ovarian cancer among elderly patients should be individualized. Limited data is available to indicate that age is a negative prognostic indicator. Additionally, the majority of elderly patients will be able to tolerate the standard of care for ovarian cancer including initial surgical cytoreduction followed by platinum and taxane chemotherapy. Because functional status does not show a reliable correlation with either tumor stage or comorbidity, each patient's comorbidities should be assessed independently. For those elderly patients with significant medical comorbidity, the extent of surgery and the aggressiveness of chemotherapy should be tailored to the individual's extent of disease, symptoms, overall health, and life goals. There are few clinical trials specifically designed for older patients, and the number of elderly patients referred to existing trials is limited. A concerted effort should be made to enter older persons into treatment protocols. In addition, enhanced cooperation between geriatricians and gynecologic oncologists may help in the pretreatment assessment of elderly patients and improve treatment guidelines in this population. When end-of-life care is indicated, a consortium of health care providers may help to provide palliative care.

REFERENCES

1. Ries LAG, Eisner MP, Kosary CL, et al., eds. SEER Cancer Statistics Review, 1975–2001. Bethesda, MD: National Cancer Institute, 2004. http://seer.cancer.gov/csr/1975_2001/.
2. Ceccaroni M, D'Agostino G, Ferrandina G, Gadducci A, et al. Gynecologic malignancies in elderly patients: Is age 70 a limit to standard-dose chemotherapy? An Italian retrospective toxicity multicentric study. Gynecol Oncol 2002; 85(3):445–450.
3. Lesur A, Riso M. Evaluation of elderly patients for fitness to receive treatment. Onc Prac 1998; 2:9–11.
4. Aapro MS. Geriatric oncology still has a long way to go. Onc Prac 1998; 2:2.
5. Boyle P. Trends in cancer mortality in Europe. Eur J Cancer 1992; 28(1):7–8.
6. Ceccaroni M, De Iaco P, Scambia G, Bovicelli L. Chemotherapy in elderly gynecologic cancer patients aged over 70 years: facts and controversies. Women's Oncol 2002; Rev 2: 385–394.
7. Pecorelli S, Odicino F, Maisonneuve P, et al. Carcinoma of the ovary. Annual report on the results of treatment of gynecological cancer. J Epidemiol Biostat 1998; 3:75–102.
8. Berek JS. Epithelial ovarian cancer. In: Berek JS, Hacker NF, eds. Practical Gynecologic Oncology. 3rd. Lippincott: Williams & Wilkins, 2002:457.
9. Fentiman IS. Denying surgery to elderly people with cancer. Onc Prac 1998; 2:12.
10. Fentiman IS, Tirelli U, Monfardini S, et al. Cancer in the elderly: Why so badly treated? Lancet 1990; 335:1020–1022.
11. Berkman B, Rohan B, Sampson S. Myths and biases related to cancer in the elderly. Cancer 1994; 74(suppl 7):2004–2008.
12. Ries LA. Ovarian cancer. Survival and treatment differences by age. Cancer 1993; 71(suppl 7):524–529.
13. Hightower RD, Nguyen HN, Averette HE, Hoskins W, Harrison T, Steren A. National survey of ovarian carcinoma. IV: Patterns of care and related survival for older patients. Cancer 1994; 73(2):377–383.
14. Aapro M, Extermann M, Repetto L. Evaluation of the elderly with cancer. Ann Oncol 2000; 11(suppl 3):223–229.
15. Monfardini S, Sorio R, Boes GH, Kaye S, Serraino D. Entry and evaluation of elderly patients in European Organization for Research and Treatment of Cancer (EORTC) new drug development studies. Cancer 1995; 76:333–338.

16. Markman M, Lewis JL Jr, Saigo P, et al. Epithelial ovarian cancer in the elderly. The Memorial Sloan Kettering Cancer Center experience. Cancer 1993; 71(suppl 2):634–637.

17. Munoz KA, Harlan LC, Trimble EL. Patterns of care for women with ovarian caner in the United States. J Clin Oncol 1997; 15(11):3408–3415.

18. Carney ME, Lancaster JM, Ford C, Tsodikov A, Wiggins CL. A population-based study of patterns of care for ovarian cancer: who is seen by a gynecologic oncologist and who is not? Gynecol Oncol 2002; 84(1):36–42.

19. Jacobs I, Menon U. Progress and challenges in screening for early detection of ovarian cancer. Mol Cell Proteom 2004; 3(4):355–366.

20. DePriest PD, vanNagell JR, Gallion HH, et al. Ovarian cancer screening in asymptomatic postmenopausal women. Gynecol Oncol 1993; 51(2):205–209.

21. Sassone AM, Timor-Tritsch IE, Artner A, Westhoff C, Warren WB. Transvaginal sonographic characterization of ovarian disease: evaluation of a new scoring system to predict ovarian malignany. Obstet Gynecol 1991; 78(1):70–76.

22. DePriest PD, Varner E, Powell J, et al. The efficacy of a sonographic morphology index in identifying ovarian cancer: a multi-institutional investigation. Gynecol Oncol 1994; 55(2):174–178.

23. Olt GJ, Berchuck A, Bast RC. Gynecologic tumor markers. Sem Surg Onc 1990; 6(6): 305–313.

24. Marci CI, Vasilev SA. Highly elevated CA125 and tubo-ovarian abscess mimicking ovarian carcinoma. Gynecol Obstet Invest 1994; 37:143–144.

25. Halila H, Stenman U, Seppala M. Ovarian cancer antigen CA-125 levels in pelvic inflammatory disease and pregnancy. Cancer 1986; 57(2):1327–1329.

26. Vasilev SA, Schlaerth JB, Campeau J, Morrow CP. Serum CA 125 levels in preoperative evaluation of pelvic masses. Obstet Gynecol 1988; 71:751–756.

27. Malkasian GD Jr, Knapp RC, Lavin PT, et al. Preoperative evaluation of serum CA 125 levels in premenopausal and postmenopausal patients with pelvic masses: discrimination of benign from malignant disease. Am J Obstet Gynecol 1988; 159(2):341–346.

28. Zhang Z, Bast RC, Yu Y, et al. Three biomarkers identified from serum proteomic analysis for the detection of early stage ovarian cancer. Cancer Res 2004; 64(16):5882–5890.

29. Petricoin EF III, Ardekani AM, Hitt BA, et al. Use of proteomic patterns in serum to identify ovarian cancer. Lancet 2202; 359(9603):572–577.

30. Ozols RF, Rubin SC, Thomas GM, Robboy SJ. Epithelial ovarian cancer. In: Hoskins WJ, Perez CA, Young RC, eds. Principles and Practice of Gynecologic Oncology. 3rd. Lippincott: Williams & Wilkins, 2000:981.

31. Attanucci CA, Ball HG, Zweizig SL, et al. Differences in symptoms between patients with benign and malignant ovarian neoplasms. Am J Obstet Gynecol 2004; 190(5): 1435–1437.

32. Young RC, Decker DG, Wharton JT, et al. Staging laparotomy in early ovarian cancer. JAMA 1983; 250(22):3072–3076.

33. McGowan L, Lesher LP, Norris HJ, Barnett M. Misstaging of ovarian cancer. Obstet Gynecol 1985; 65(4):568.

34. Delgado G, Oram DH, Petrilli ES. Stage III epithelial ovarian cancer: the role of maximal surgical reduction. Gynecol Oncol 1984; 18(3):293–298.

35. Vogl S, Pagano M, Kaplan B, Greenwald E, Arseneau J, Bennett B. Cisplatin based combination chemotherapy for advanced ovarian cancer: high overall response rate with curative potential only in women with small tumor burdens. Cancer 1983; 51(11): 2024–2030.

36. Redman JR, Petrini GR, Saigon PE, Geller NL, Hakes TB. Prognostic factors in advanced ovarian carcinoma. J Clin Oncol 1986; 4(4):515–523.

37. Louie K, Ozols R, Myers E, et al. Long term results of cisplatin-containing combination chemotherapy regimen for the treatment of advanced ovarian carcinoma. J Clin Oncol 1986; 4(11):1579–1585.

38. Hoskins WJ, McGuire WP, Brady MF, et al. The effect of diameter of largest residual disease on survival after primary cytoreductive surgery in patients with suboptimal residual epithelial ovarian carincoma. Am J Obstet Gynecol 1994; 170(4):974–979.

39. Venesmaa P, Ylikorkala O. Morbidity and mortality associated with primary and repeat operations for ovarian cancer. Obstet Gynecol 1992; 79:168.

40. Bristow RE, Montz FJ, Lagasse LD, Leuchter RS, Karlan BY. Survival impact of surgical cytoreduction in Stage IV epithelial ovarian cancer. Gynecol Oncol 1999; 72(3): 278–287.

41. Curtin JP, Malik R, Venkatraman ES, Barakat RR, Hoskins WJ. Stage IV ovarian cancer: impact of surgical debulking. Gynecol Oncol 1997; 64(1):9–12.

42. Liu PC, Benjamin I, Morgan MA, King SA, Mikuta JJ, Rubin SC. Effect of surgical debulking on survival in Stage IV ovarian cancer. Gynecol Oncol 1997; 64(1):4–8.

43. Cloven NG, Manetta A, Berman ML, Kohler MF, DiSaia PJ. Management of ovarian cancer in patients older than 80 years of age. Gynecol Oncol 1999; 73(1):137–139.

44. Bruchim I, Altaras M, Fishman A. Age contrasts in clinical characteristics and pattern of care in patients with epithelial ovarian cancer. Gynecol Oncol 2002; 86(3): 274–278.

45. Giannice R, Tommaso S, Gerrandina G, et al. Systematic pelvic and aortic lymphadenectomy in elderly gynecologic oncology patients. Cancer 2001; 92(10):2562–2568.

46. Edmonson JH, Su J, Krook JE. Treatment of ovarian cancer in elderly women. Mayo Clinic North Central Cancer Treatment Group studies. Cancer 1993; 71(2):615–617.

47. Wright J, Herzog T, Powell M. Morbidity of cytoreductive surgery in the elderly. Am J Obstet Gynecol 2004; 190(5):1398–1400.

48. Sundararajan V, Hershman D, Grann V, et al. Variations in the use of chemotherapy for elderly patients with advanced ovarian cancer: a population-based study. J Clin Oncol 2002; 20(1):173–178.

49. McGuire WP, Ozols RF. Chemotherapy of advanced ovarian cancer. Semin Oncol 1998; 25(3):340.

50. McGuire WP, Hoskins WJ, Brady MF, et al. Cyclophosphamide and cisplatin compared with paclitaxel and cisplatin in patients with stage III and stage IV ovarian cancer. N Engl J Med 1996; 334(1):1–6.

51. Stuart G, Bertelson K, Mangioni C, et al. Updated analysis shows a highly significant improved overall survival (OS) for cisplatin-paclitaxel as first line treatment of advanced ovarian cancer; mature results of the EORTC-GCCG, NOCOVA, NCTC, CT and Scottish intergroup trial. Proc Am Soc Clin Oncol 1998; 17:361.

52. du Bois A, Lueck HJ, Meier W, et al. Cisplatin/paclitaxel vs. carboplatin/paclitaxel in ovarian cancer: update of an Arbeitsgermeinschaft Gynaekologische Onkologie (AGO) Study Group Trial. Proc Am Soc Clin Oncol 1990; 18:356.

53. Ozols RF, Bundy BN, Fowler J, et al. Randomized phase II trial of cisplatin/paclitaxel versus carboplatin/paclitaxel in optimal Stage III epithelial ovarian cancer: a Gynecologic Oncology Group trial (GOG 158). Proc Am Soc Clin Oncol 1999; 18:1373.

54. Monfardini S, Ferrucci L, Fratino L, et al. Validation of a multidimensional evaluation scale for use in elderly cancer patients. Cancer 1996; 77(2):395–401.

55. Repetto L, Venturino A, Fratino L, et al. Geriatric oncology: a clinical approach to the older patient with cancer. Eur J Cancer 2003; 39(7):870–880.

56. Baker SD, Grochow LB. Pharmacology of cancer chemotherapy in the older person. Clin Geriatr Med 1997; 13:169–184.

57. Ershler WB, Longo D. Aging and cancer: issues of basic and clinical science. J Natl Cancer Inst 1997; 89(20):1489–1497.

58. Campisi J. Aging and cancer: the double-edged sword of proliferative senescence. J Am Geriatr Soc 1997; 45(4):482–488.

59. Balducci L, Extermann M. Cancer chemotherapy in the older patient: what the medical oncologist needs to know. Cancer 1997; 80(7):1317–1322.

60. Burkowski JM, Duerr M, Donehower RC, et al. Relation between age and clearance rate of nine investigational anticancer drugs from phase I pharmacokinetic data. Cancer Chemother Pharmacol 1994; 33:493–496.

61. Begg CB, Elson PJ, Carbone PP. A study of excess hematology toxicity in elderly patients treated on cancer chemotherapy protocols. In: Yancik K, Yates JW, eds. Cancer in the Elderly. An Approach to Early Detection and Treatment. New York: Springer-Verlag, 1989:149–163.

62. Chiara S, Lionetto R, Vincenti M, Bruzzone M, et al. Advanced ovarian cancer in the elderly: results of consecutive trials with cisplatin-based chemotherapy. Crit Rev Oncol Hematol 2001; 37(1):27–34.

63. Thyss A, Saudes L, Otto J, et al. Renal tolerance of cisplatin in patients more than 80 years old. J Clin Oncol 1994; 12(10):2121–2125.

64. Gronlund B, Hogdall C, Hansen HH, Endgelholm SA. Performance status rather than age is the key prognostic factor in second-line treatment of elderly patients with epithelial ovarian carcinoma. Cancer 2002; 94(7):1961–1967.

65. Gershenson DM, Mitchell MF, Atkinson N, et al. Age contrasts in patients with advanced epithelial ovarian cancer. The M.D. Anderson Cancer Center experience. Cancer 1993; 71(suppl 2):638–643.

66. Bicher A, Sarosy G, Kohn E, et al. Age does not influence taxol dose intensity in recurrent carcinoma of the ovary. Cancer 1993; 71(suppl 2):594–600.

67. Marchetti DL, Lele SB, Priore RL, et al. Treatment of advanced ovarian carcinoma in the elderly. Gynecol Oncol 1993; 49(1):36–91.

68. Thigpen T, Brady MF, Omura GA, et al. Age as a prognostic factor for ovarian carcinoma. The Gynecologic Oncology Group Experience. Cancer 1993; 71(suppl 2):606–614.

69. Rubin SC, Hoskins WJ, Benjamin I, et al. Palliative surgery for intestinal obstruction in advanced ovarian cancer. Gynecol Oncol 1989; 34(1):16–19.

70. Mangili G, Franchi M, Mariani A, et al. Octreotide in the management of bowel obstruction in terminal ovarian cancer. Gynecol Oncol 1996; 61(3):345–348.

71. The SUPPORT principal investigators. A controlled trial to improve care for seriously ill hospitalized patients. The study to understand prognoses and preferences for outcomes and risks of treatments (SUPPORT). JAMA 1995; 274(20):1591–1598.

72. Abrahm JL. Care without chemotherapy: the role of the palliative care team. Cancer J 2002; 8(5):357–363.

73. Roberts JA, Brown D, Elkins T, et al. Factors influencing views of patients with gynecologic cancer about end-of-life decisions. Am J Obstet Gynecol 1997; 176(1 Pt 1):166–172.

74. Block SD. Assessing and managing depression in the terminally ill patient. Ann Intern Med 2000; 132(3):209–218.

75. Matulonis UA. End of life issues in older patients. Sem in Oncol 2004; 31(2):274–281.

15

Cervical, Endometrial, and Vulvar Cancer

David H. Moore
*Department of Obstetrics and Gynecologic, Indiana University School of Medicine,
Indianapolis, Indiana, U.S.A.*

INTRODUCTION

During the 20th century, the number of persons under 65 years of age living in the United States tripled; however, the number of persons over 65 years of age increased by a factor of 11 (1). The older population is expected to double by the year 2030. The percentage of women 65 years of age and older has also increased from 13.1% in 1980 to 14.6% in 1990 (2). The incidence of most cancers increases with age. Approximately 50% of all cancers—and 60% of cancer deaths—occur in people over 65 years of age (3). Cancer is the leading cause of mortality in women between the ages of 35 and 75 years. As the population continues to age, and the number of older cancer patients continues to increase, it is essential that the medical community not only study cancer biology and clinical care relevant to the aged, but also appreciate the unique concerns and quality of life expectations of the elderly. For these patients, it is unfortunate that much of what we know about the diagnosis, treatment, and prognosis of specific cancers is derived from studies conducted in younger patient populations (4).

Cancers arising in the female reproductive organs are some of the more common malignancies in women. Gynecologic cancers comprise approximately 12% of all new cancer diagnoses and 10% of all cancer deaths among women in the United States (5). It is the intent of this chapter to discuss the epidemiology, presenting symptoms, diagnostic and staging procedures, and treatment of cancers of the cervix, endometrium, and vulva. Furthermore, the differences in cancer biology and/or clinical management between younger and older patients will be highlighted.

CERVICAL CANCER

Worldwide, cervical cancer is third only to breast and colorectal cancer in the incidence and mortality of cancers in women (6). In industrialized countries, cervical cancer is less common because of the implementation of cytological screening programs based on the Papanicolaou (Pap) smear. Cervical cancer is still the third most common gynecologic cancer in the United States with approximately 10,370 new cases (1.6% of all cancers in women) and 3710 deaths each year (5). Approximately

85% to 90% of invasive cervical cancers are squamous cell carcinomas and 10% to 15% are adenocarcinomas.

Epidemiology

The influence of sexual behaviors has long been recognized as important to the development of cervical carcinoma. First intercourse at an early age, multiple sexual partners, and high parity are all important risk factors (7,8). Weaker associations have been suggested for cigarette smoking and the use of oral contraceptives. Carcinogens present in cigarette smoke are concentrated in cervical mucus (9) and may interfere with the local immunity (10). Several studies have clearly linked exposure to cigarette smoke to an increased risk for developing cervical cancer (11,12). Among women with only one lifetime sexual partner, past and current high-risk sexual behaviors by the male partner have a substantial role in the development of cervical carcinogenesis (13). Conversely, male circumcision is associated with a reduced risk of cervical cancer in their current sexual partners (14). These factors suggest that a sexually transmitted agent may be responsible, and the agent that has long been implicated is the family of human papillomaviruses (HPV) (15,16). Over 80 subtypes of HPV have been identified, each with a predilection to infect specific tissue sites. The types most prevalent in squamous cell carcinoma of the cervix are HPV 16 and HPV 18, and these are rarely isolated in women who have not had sexual intercourse (17–19). The oncogenic potential of HPV is, in part, a result of integration of viral DNA into the host cell and expression of viral transforming proteins such as E6 and E7. E6 binds to and enhances the degradation of the p53 gene product, which is important in cell cycle regulation, and the E7 protein binds to and functionally inactivates the gene product of the retinoblastoma tumor-suppressor gene. It is interesting that p53 mutations are present in a very few patients with cervical carcinoma without associated HPV (20). Only a minority of women who harbor HPV develop cervical neoplasia, suggesting that other factors such as nutritional or immunological status may also be important.

Screening

Since the advent of Pap, screening the incidence of cervical cancer has steadily declined. Many women are diagnosed and treated with preinvasive disease (cervical intraepithelial neoplasia). Pap smear screening is thus a means of primary prevention. An abnormal Pap test prompts further evaluation (colposcopy and biopsy), which in turn leads to a determination of continued but closer clinical follow-up versus treatment, depending upon biopsy results. Most cases of preinvasive cervical neoplasia may be treated with office or outpatient surgical procedures such as cryotherapy, laser, loop electrosurgical excision procedure, or cone biopsy. Selected patients may also be treated with hysterectomy. There is some controversy concerning the ideal frequency of cytological screening, but the American College of Obstetrics and Gynecology and the American Cancer Society currently recommend that annual screening commence approximately three years after the onset of vaginal intercourse, or no later than 21 years of age (21). After initiation, cervical screening should be performed annually with conventional cervical cytology smears, or every two years using liquid-based cytology. At or after the age of 30, women who have had three consecutive, technically satisfactory normal cytology results may be screened every two to three years (unless they have a history of "in utero" diethylstilbestrol exposure, are

HIV positive, or are immunocompromised). Mathematical modeling predicts that, in comparison to annual screening, the excess risk of cervical cancer with less frequent screening intervals is approximately three cases per 100,000 women (22). Despite the proven efficacy of cytological screening, many women remain unscreened. Fifty percent of the women with newly diagnosed invasive cervical cancer have never had a Pap smear, and another 10% have not had a Pap smear in five years (23). Categories of women who tend to be underscreened include those who are postmenopausal, uninsured, of an ethnic minority, rural, and elderly. In the United States, about 25% of the cervical cancer cases and 41% of the deaths occur in women who are 65 years of age or older. In addition, approximately one-half of women older than 60 years have not had a Pap smear in three years, even though many have seen a physician for other medical needs.

Diagnosis and Clinical Evaluation

Patients with cervical cancer may present with complaints of pain, vaginal bleeding or discharge, or postcoital spotting (Fig. 1). Patients diagnosed through cytological screening programs are often asymptomatic and usually have earlier-stage disease. The diagnosis is confirmed through tissue biopsy. Cervical cancer spreads primarily by means of local infiltration into surrounding tissues. Lateral extension may result in renal failure from ureteral obstruction. Invasion into the bladder or rectum may also occur. Cervical cancers may also metastasize via lymphatic dissemination to regional lymph nodes, and uncommonly by vascular dissemination to distant

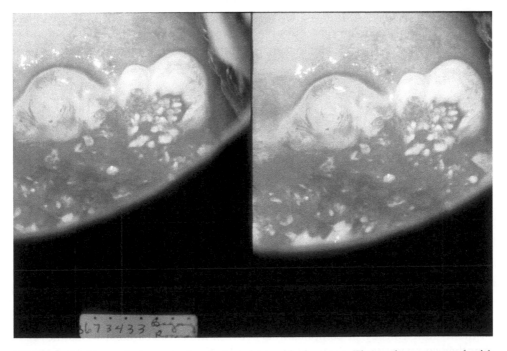

Figure 1 Colposcopic images of early invasive cervical cancer. The patient presented with complaints of post-coital spotting of three months duration. Pap smear = HSIL (high-grade squamous intraepithelial lesion). Biopsy of the lesion seen on colposcopic examination = invasive (4 mm) squamous cell carcinoma.

Table 1 FIGO Staging Classification for Cervical Cancer

Stage 0	Carcinoma in situ, intraepithelial carcinoma
Stage IA1	Tumor confined to the cervix, identified only microscopically, measured invasion of stroma ≤3 mm in depth and ≤7 mm in width
Stage IA2	Tumor confined to the cervix, identified only microscopically, measured invasion of stroma >3 and ≤5 mm in depth and ≤7 mm in width
Stage IB1	Tumor confined to the cervix, preclinical lesions greater than IA or clinical lesions ≤4 cm in diameter
Stage IB2	Tumor confined to the cervix, clinical lesions >4 cm in diameter
Stage IIA	Tumor extends beyond the cervix, involves the vagina but not the lower one-third, no obvious parametrial involvement
Stage IIB	Tumor extends beyond the cervix, obvious parametrial involvement but does not extend to the pelvic sidewall
Stage IIIA	Tumor extends beyond the cervix, involves the lower one-third of the vagina
Stage IIIB	Tumor extends beyond the cervix with extension to the pelvic wall and/or hydronephrosis or nonfunctioning kidney
Stage IVA	Spread of the tumor to adjacent organs (bladder, rectum)
Stage IVB	Spread of the tumor to organs beyond the pelvis

Abbreviation: FIGO, International Federation of Gynecology and Oncology.

organs (24). The International Federation of Gynecology and Oncology (FIGO) staging system for cervical carcinoma is detailed in Table 1.

Only the results of palpation, inspection, colposcopy, endocervical curettage, hysteroscopy, cystoscopy, proctoscopy or barium enema, intravenous pyelography, and chest X ray can be used to assign stage. Bladder or rectal involvement should be confirmed by biopsy. Although the results of imaging studies such as lymphangiography, computed tomography, and magnetic resonance imaging, and the findings of operative procedures, including laparoscopy or open lymphadenectomy are of prognostic value and may influence treatment planning, they may not be used to assign FIGO stage.

Treatment—Early-Stage Disease

Approximately 50% of women with cervical cancer present with tumors clinically confined to the cervix. Patients with stage IA1 (microinvasive) cervical cancers may be treated with nonradical hysterectomy, or cone biopsy if preservation of fertility is desired. For patients with stage IA2–IIA disease, radical hysterectomy or radiation therapy are appropriate treatment options. Comparative studies suggest that either therapy is equally effective in the treatment of early-stage cervical cancer. Morley and Seski compared 208 women treated with radical hysterectomy versus 193 women treated with pelvic radiation therapy at the University of Michigan between 1945 through 1975. The corrected five-year survival rates for surgical versus radiation treatment were 91% versus 87%, respectively. Prior to the early 1960s, women were placed in a modified alternating series, and thereafter entered into a randomized alternating series. During these two time-periods, there were no differences in therapeutic efficacy or complications between the two treatment modalities (25). Another comparative analysis was reported by Volterrani et al. from the National Cancer Institute of Milan in 1983. Among the 250 women treated for stage IB cervical cancer, 127 received radiation therapy and 123 underwent surgery. The five-year disease-free survival rate was 91% in the radiation therapy group versus 89% in the surgical group. However, only 37 women in the surgical group actually underwent radical hysterectomy whereas the other 86 underwent lymph node dissection. Furthermore, all patients received postoperative brachytherapy (26). Two prospective randomized trials of surgery versus radiotherapy have been reported. With follow-up ranging from 1 to 3.5 years, Roddick and Greenelaw reported disease-free survival rates of 42% (21/50) with surgery versus 60% (30/50) for radiation therapy. Unfortunately, this study included patients with stage III–IV disease (27). Landoni et al. randomized 343 evaluable patients with stage IB–IIA cervical carcinoma to radical hysterectomy versus radiation therapy. Postoperative radiation therapy was prescribed for patients with positive or close surgical margins, microscopic infiltration of tumor into the parametrium, or positive lymph nodes. With a median follow-up of 87 months, the disease-free and overall survival rates were identical in the two treatment groups (28).

There are substantial selection biases affecting the choice of treatment. Most published studies reveal that surgical series tend to consist primarily of younger, thinner, healthier patients of ten times with smaller tumors. In contrast, patients selected for radiation therapy tend to be older and have more coexisting medical problems. One of the perceived advantages of surgery for younger patients is diminished vaginal fibrosis and atrophy and therefore better sexual function, along with the potential for preserved ovarian function. Radiation therapy has the distinct advantages of outpatient treatment, better physical performance "during" therapy, and fewer severe short-term complications. Unfortunately, no prospective study has been conducted with appropriate measurements of psychosexual or other quality of life parameters. To choose therapy based solely on age is without scientific merit.

Patients who undergo radical hysterectomy and prove to have positive lymph nodes are at a high risk for recurrence. Postoperative pelvic radiation therapy is administered to these patients. To determine whether adjuvant chemotherapy might prove beneficial, Tattersall et al. randomized patients with positive pelvic lymph nodes to pelvic radiation therapy versus chemotherapy consisting of cisplatin plus vinblastine plus bleomycin. There was no difference in disease-free or overall survival in the two groups, nor was there any difference in the pattern of recurrence (29). Killackey et al. conducted a nonrandomized comparative study of radiation therapy alone versus sequential chemotherapy followed by radiation therapy. Chemotherapy consisted of cisplatin plus bleomycin, with or without ifosfamide/mesna. With a mean follow-up of 37 months, there was a 14% recurrence rate in the radiation alone group versus no recurrences in the chemotherapy plus radiation group (30). Peters et al. reported results from a trial conducted by the Southwest Oncology Group and the Gynecologic Oncology Group (GOG) to determine if concurrent radiation therapy and cisplatin plus 5-fluorouracil (5-FU) chemotherapy is superior to radiation therapy alone, in patients with positive surgical margins, positive parametrial disease, or pelvic lymph node metastasis. The three-year survival rate was significantly improved for women who received radiation plus concomitant chemotherapy (87%) versus radiation therapy alone (77%) (31).

Tumor size is a significant risk factor for recurrence and is reflected in the FIGO staging classification. Radical hysterectomy as primary treatment for stage IB2 "bulky" cervical cancer is feasible; however, many of these patients will prove to have clinicopathological risk factors that will lead to the administration of postoperative radiation therapy. In the series reported by Landoni et al., 80% of surgically treated patients with tumors larger than 4 cm in diameter required postoperative pelvic radiation therapy (28). Given the relatively high risk for treatment-related complications when radical surgery and radiation therapy are combined, the decision to routinely operate on women who are likely to require subsequent radiation treatments must be questioned. The knowledge that pelvic recurrences are more common among patients with larger tumors, who are treated with primary radiation therapy, prompted the study of hysterectomy following radiation therapy as a means of improving local control and cure rates. In a retrospective analysis of patients with bulky cervical tumors, treated with either radiation therapy followed by extrafascial hysterectomy or radiation therapy alone, Durrance et al. reported a lower pelvic recurrence rate for the surgical group (32). Gallion et al. found not only a lower pelvic recurrence rate, but also an overall improved survival, for patients treated with radiation therapy followed by hysterectomy (33). In 1991, the GOG completed a prospective, randomized trial of radiation therapy with or without hysterectomy for patients with stage IB2 cervical tumors. Although hysterectomy appeared to reduce the rate of local recurrence, there was no improvement in overall survival (34). Subsequently, the GOG conducted a trial of weekly cisplatin plus radiation therapy versus radiation therapy alone in patients with bulky stage IB2 cervical cancer. Hysterectomy was performed three to six weeks after the conclusion of radiation-based treatment. The rates of progression-free and overall survival were significantly higher in the group receiving concurrent cisplatin (35). Unfortunately, the GOG initiated a randomized trial of radical hysterectomy (with postoperative radiation therapy for specified risk factors) versus radiation therapy plus concurrent cisplatin chemotherapy, which was closed for lack of accrual. In the absence of data from unbiased, prospective comparative trials, either surgery or radiation therapy with concurrent chemotherapy may be considered appropriate treatments for bulky stage I disease.

Treatment—Locally Advanced Disease

Many years ago, primary radiation therapy surpassed surgery as the preferred treatment for locally advanced cervical cancer. Not only was local control better, but radiation therapy also allowed for the preservation of bowel and rectal function. Chemotherapy has been increasingly used in combination with radiation for the treatment of many cancers in an attempt to improve outcome. The mechanisms of drug–radiation interactions are poorly understood compared to the identified benefits. Plausible mechanisms of interaction leading to enhanced clinical effect may include: modification of the slope of the dose–response curves; inhibition of sublethal damage repair; inhibition of recovery from potentially lethal damage; alterations in cellular kinetics; decreases in tumor bulk leading to improved blood supply, tissue oxygenation, and increased radiosensitivity (36). The GOG conducted a trial of hydroxyurea versus placebo concomitant to radiation therapy in patients with stage IIIB–IV cervical cancer. There were several problems with the conduct of this study. Pretreatment evaluation of the aortic lymph nodes was not required. Among the 190 women entered in this study, only 104 were evaluable for toxicity and only 97 were evaluable for survival. The incidence of leukopenia in the hydroxyurea-treated group was significant. Complete tumor regression was reported for 68% in the hydroxyurea group versus 49% in the placebo group. The estimated median survival was also improved with hydroxyurea as compared to placebo (19.5 months vs. 10.7 months) (37). Subsequently, the GOG conducted a randomized trial of misonidazole versus hydroxyurea in combination with radiation therapy in patients with stage IIB–IVA cervical cancer. An eligibility requirement for this trial was negative aortic lymph nodes based on pretreatment surgical staging. Among 296 evaluable patients, the median progression-free interval was 42.9 months for the hydroxyurea group versus 40.4 months for the misonidazole group. The initial report of this trial did not detect a survival difference between the two arms although the pelvic failure rate was higher in the misonidazole group (23.6%) versus the hydroxyurea group (18.0%), and the overall recurrence rate was higher in the misonidazole group versus the hydroxyurea group (43.9% vs. 36.7%, respectively) (38). In a subsequent report from this trial after extended follow-up, there was both a progression-free and survival advantage in the hydroxyurea arm (39). The Radiation Therapy Oncology Group (RTOG) reported their results from a trial of radiation therapy with or without misonidazole and found that misonidazole plus radiation was no better than radiation therapy alone (40).

Cisplatin is widely regarded as one of the most active cytotoxic agents in the treatment of cervical cancer and has been frequently studied either alone or in combination with other cytotoxic drugs (usually 5-FU) as a "radiation sensitizer." Whitney et al. published their results from a trial of cisplatin plus 5-FU plus radiation versus hydroxyurea plus radiation therapy, for the treatment of locally advanced cervical carcinoma. All patients underwent pretreatment surgical staging and had stage IIB–IVA cervical cancer with negative common iliac and aortic lymph nodes. Disease progression occurred in 43% of the patients randomized to cisplatin plus 5-FU versus 53% of the patients randomized to hydroxyurea. Progression-free survival was significantly better in the cisplatin plus 5-FU arm ($P = 0.033$). The three-year survival rate for women who received cisplatin plus 5-FU versus hydroxyurea was 67% versus 57%, respectively (41). Another trial confirmed the superiority of cisplatin plus 5-FU chemoradiation for the treatment of locally advanced cervical cancer. Morris et al. reported results from an RTOG trial of pelvic radiation therapy and concurrent cisplatin plus 5-FU chemotherapy versus pelvic plus aortic radiation therapy. Estimated cumulative five-year survival rates for patients treated with chemotherapy versus radiation therapy alone were 73% versus 58%, respectively. A significant difference in disease-free survival was also seen in favor of the chemotherapy arm. The addition of chemotherapy to radiation therapy was effective in reducing both the frequency of local recurrences and distant metastasis (42). Two other GOG trials demonstrated improved results with radiation therapy and concurrent chemotherapy. Rose et al. reported a three-arm trial of pelvic radiation therapy plus concurrent chemotherapy: cisplatin alone versus hydroxyurea alone versus cisplatin plus hydroxyurea plus 5-FU. All patients had stage IIB–IVA cervical cancer with surgically confirmed negative common iliac and aortic lymph nodes. Patients randomized to either of the cisplatin-containing arms had significant improvements in progression-free and overall survival over patients who received hydroxyurea. Because treatment with cisplatin alone was equally effective and less toxic than treatment with the three-drug combination, the authors recommended weekly cisplatin as the standard drug for chemoradiation therapy of cervical cancer (43). Keys et al. showed that the rates of progression-free and overall survival were significantly higher with the addition of weekly cisplatin to pelvic radiation therapy (35). Not only did these randomized controlled studies identify a significant survival advantage from the addition of chemotherapy to radiation therapy, but also the degree of benefit attained through concurrent chemotherapy was remarkably similar across the four trials. These important results changed the standard of care for the treatment of patients with locally advanced cervical cancer to chemoradiation therapy and formed the basis for a 1999 National Cancer Institute Clinical Announcement.

Treatment—Recurrent/Metastatic Disease

The prognosis is extremely poor for patients with recurrent or metastatic cervical cancer that cannot be surgically resected for treatment with radiation therapy with a curative intent. Systemic chemotherapy is a therapeutic option for these patients, although no trial to date has compared chemotherapy to the best supportive care in this setting. For almost 25 years cisplatin has been regarded as the most active single-agent for the treatment of cervical carcinoma (44). Phase III studies have not confirmed an advantage with either higher doses or alternative infusion schedules of cisplatin (45,46). A number of phase III trials have investigated the use of other active drugs in combination with cisplatin. Omura et al. showed a higher objective response rate and progression-free survival with cisplatin plus ifosfamide; however, there was no improvement in overall survival, and toxicity with combination therapy was significantly increased (47). Another phase III trial demonstrated no advantage with the addition of bleomycin to the cisplatin plus ifosfamide combination (48). More recently, the GOG compared single-agent cisplatin to a combination of cisplatin plus paclitaxel, with quality of life assessments included among outcomes measures. The combination of cisplatin plus paclitaxel yielded a higher objective response rate, longer progression-free survival, and greater toxicity—without an apparent decrement in patient reported quality of life (49). Long et al. presented results of a prospective randomized trial comparing cisplatin versus cisplatin plus topotecan, which for the first time, demonstrated an improvement in overall survival with the combination regimen (50). Although improvements in response rates and in the rates of progression-free and overall survival have been attained with cisplatin-containing combinations, women with advanced/recurrent cervical carcinoma ultimately do poorly, and median survival remains less than one year. Whenever available, these patients should seek participation in prospective trials in the hope of identifying a more active and more effective therapy.

Cervical Cancer in the Elderly Patient

Elderly women with cervical cancer have a worse prognosis. In her review of 17,119 cases of cervical cancer in the Surveillance, Epidemiology, and End Results (SEER) database, Kosary reported that the five-year relative survival rates steadily decreased as age increased: under 30 years old (88%); 30 to 39 years (81%); 40 to 49 years (71%); 50 to 59 years (63%); 60 to 69 years (58%); and 70 years and older (46%) (51). The poor prognosis associated with advancing age was independent of disease extent at diagnosis. At all FIGO stages (except stage IA), elderly women did worse (51). In a review of GOG data, it was noted that increasing age was associated with a poorer performance status and more advanced-stage disease (52).

It is unclear whether these age-based differences in survival reflect differences in cervical cancer biology, clinical presentation (FIGO stage), or treatment efficacy. Baay et al. reported no difference between younger and older cervical cancer patients with respect to the prevalence of HPV types (53). Similarly, Gostout et al. found that tumors from older patients with cervical cancer were extremely similar to those from younger patients with respect to HPV types, (infrequent) occurrence of p53 mutations, and human leukocyte antigen types (54). In contrast, Saito et al. from Japan found that the presence of HPV DNA was higher in the younger versus older patients (84% vs. 50%, respectively). The prevalence of HPV types differed between younger and older patients, but the overexpression of p53 did not (55).

Thus, differences in tumor biology between younger and older patients—if they exist—would not appear to reflect differences in HPV prevalence or p53 function. There are data to suggest that elderly women with cervical cancer may not receive appropriate treatment. In a review of the National Cancer Institute's SEER database, Trimble et al. found that 9% of women diagnosed with invasive cervical cancer received no therapy for their disease. Lack of therapy was associated with a later stage of disease at diagnosis, older age, and unmarried status. More than 16% of women over 65 years of age with stage IIB–IV cervical cancer received no treatment (56). Wright et al. reviewed a large hospital-based tumor registry and identified 1582 patients treated for cervical cancer. Comparing younger (<70 years of age) versus older (≥70 years of age) patients, they found that elderly patients who presented with a more advanced-stage disease were more likely to have a nonsquamous histology, and were less likely to undergo surgical treatment (54% vs. 16%, respectively). Elderly women were nine times more likely to receive no treatment (57).

In a series of patients undergoing radical hysterectomy for the treatment of cervical cancer, Choi et al. found no differences in mean operating time, mean blood loss, perioperative transfusion, frequency of intraoperative injuries, duration of hospital stay, and postoperative complications between younger (ages 41–50 years) and older (ages ≥65 years) women (58). Others have also shown that selected elderly patients with cervical cancer can undergo radical pelvic surgery without appreciable increases in operative time, blood loss and transfusion rates, postoperative stay, and postoperative or long-term complications (59). Even if surgical therapy is inappropriate due to the extent of disease or coexisting medical conditions, radiation therapy can still be administered. Age should not be considered a deterrent to receiving appropriate cancer treatment. There is one report of a 104-year-old woman with stage IIIB cervical cancer, who received radiation therapy and is without any evidence of recurrence five years later (age 109 years) (60).

More information is needed regarding the epidemiology of cervical cancer in the older versus younger patients. Given the worse prognosis associated with aging, it is important that elderly women be given the opportunity to participate in cervical cancer screening programs. Several reports suggest that Pap smear screening of the elderly is cost effective (61,62). Finally, the eligibility criteria for clinical trials participation should not inappropriately exclude elderly women.

ENDOMETRIAL CANCER

In the United States, cancer of the uterine corpus is the fourth most common cancer in women (6% of all cancers in women) and the most common gynecologic malignancy. There are an estimated 40,880 new cases and 7310 deaths from uterine cancer each year (5). Sarcomas account for 3% to 5% and adenocarcinomas arising from the uterine endometrium account for 95% to 97% of uterine cancers. The focus of this section will be endometrial cancer.

Epidemiology

Obesity, diabetes mellitus, and hypertension are widely recognized risk factors for the development of endometrial cancer (63). The development of endometrial cancer in obese women is believed to be mediated by enhanced production of endogenous estrogen via the peripheral conversion of adrenal steroids (androstenedione) by the aromatase found in adipocytes (64). The level of risk is proportional to the degree of obesity, and is increased 10-fold for women who are more than 50 pounds (23 kg) overweight (65). Estrogen is a common theme for endometrial cancer; hence, prolonged use of unopposed estrogens, history of nulliparity or infertility, chronic anovulation, early age at menarche or late age at menopause are accepted risk factors. Conversely, pregnancy or the use of hormonal contraception decreases the risk for developing endometrial cancer (66). The use of postmenopausal estrogen therapy increases endometrial cancer risk; however, women who use estrogen in combination with a progestin are actually at a lower risk of developing endometrial carcinoma as compared to those who never used hormone replacement therapy (67). Tamoxifen is a selective estrogen receptor modulator commonly used to reduce the risk for recurrence in estrogen receptor–positive breast cancer. The effect of tamoxifen on the endometrium is that of a weak estrogen; consequently, the risk of developing endometrial cancer with tamoxifen therapy is two to three times higher than that of age-matched populations (68,69). Inheritable genetic factors contribute to a small percentage of cases. Endometrial cancer is the most common extracolonic malignancy to arise in women with Lynch II (hereditary nonpolyposis colorectal cancer) syndrome. Most germline mutations have been detected in three DNA mismatch repair genes: human Mut-S Homolog 2 (MSH2), human Mut-L Homolog 1 (MLH1), and MSH6. The cumulative lifetime risk of developing endometrial cancer for women who are germline mutation carriers is approximately 25% to 40%. Also, these patients tend to develop endometrial cancer at a younger age (mean age of 47 years vs. 62 years for sporadic cases) (70,71).

Endometrial cancer is a disease associated with aging. Three-fourths of endometrial cancers occur in postmenopausal women, and the incidence increases from approximately 12 cases per 100,000 women at the age of 40 to 84 cases per 100,000 women at the age of 60 (72). There is emerging evidence that endometrial cancer arises in two distinct scenarios. Type I cancers are associated with the classic risk factors discussed above, and appear to arise from a background atypical hyperplasia. These cancers tend to be well differentiated, are the typical endometrioid histological type, and occur in relatively younger women. Common molecular alterations in Type I endometrial cancers include mutations or deletions of the Phosphatase and Tensin Homolog (PTEN) tumor suppressor gene and microsatellite instability (73,74). In contrast, Type II cancers tend to arise from an atrophic endometrium in the absence of estrogen influence and are usually found in older women. These cancers are typically poorly differentiated and may display a more clinically aggressive histological subtype such as adenosquamous, serous, or clear cell carcinoma. Molecular alterations associated with Type II endometrial cancers include mutations in the p53 tumor suppressor gene and either increased expression or amplification of the human epidermal growth factor receptor 2/neuroblastoma (HER-2/neu) proto-oncogene (75,76). Thus, molecular mechanisms for the derivation of endometrial cancers found in younger versus older patients may be different.

Screening

There is no screening test for endometrial cancer. Pap smears are abnormal in only 30% to 50% of women known to have endometrial cancer. Various cytological and histological sampling methods have been devised and studied, but eventually discarded as a potential screening test for asymptomatic women, because of high cost or low sensitivity. Ultrasonography is widely available and may be performed with minimal patient discomfort. The functional basis of ultrasound evaluation is to assess endometrial thickness and complexity. As a screening test, however, it is costly and cannot be recommended. The ineffectiveness of biopsy and ultrasound screening for endometrial cancer is best illustrated in studies of women receiving tamoxifen for breast cancer chemoprevention or treatment. These women are already being seen on a regular basis by the medical community and are at increased risk for developing endometrial cancer. The estimated annual risk of endometrial cancer in tamoxifen-treated patients is approximately 2 per 1000 women (77). Despite concerns raised in earlier case series, these women do not have a worse prognosis compared to other patients with endometrial cancer. Because of subepithelial stromal hypertrophy induced by tamoxifen, the mean endometrial thickness as measured by ultrasound among tamoxifen users (10 mm) is markedly greater than the endometrial thickness among control patients (4 mm) (78). Even though a thickness greater than the 5 mm threshold prompts most clinicians to proceed with biopsy, almost all patients taking tamoxifen will prove not to have significant endometrial pathology in the absence of bleeding (79,80).

Diagnosis and Clinical Evaluation

Despite the unavailability of a cost-effective screening test, over 90% of patients with endometrial cancer will present with disease clinically confined to the uterus. Furthermore, in the vast majority of cases, patients present with abnormal bleeding. Approximately 25% of cases occur in premenopausal women, from whom abnormal menstruation—often of longstanding duration—is a frequent complaint. Oral contraceptive pills and progestin therapy are contraindicated in the patient with undiagnosed vaginal bleeding. Although the presence of malignant disease is usually excluded, postmenopausal patients who present with bleeding should be evaluated for the possibility of endometrial cancer. The diagnosis may be suggested by ultrasonography, but it is established with office endometrial biopsy, or dilation and curettage in the operating suite. Hysteroscopy may be useful to assist with tissue collection and can also be performed as an office procedure. Endometrial cancer spreads by local infiltration, lymphatic dissemination, and transperitoneal seeding. Rarely, hematogenous dissemination may also occur. Because over 95% of women with endometrial cancer undergo primary surgical therapy, and clinical staging is inaccurate, the FIGO staging classification for endometrial cancer is based on surgical–pathological findings (Table 2).

Surgical Treatment

For the 90% of women with cancer clinically confined to the uterus, optimal surgical management consists of total abdominal hysterectomy (TAH), bilateral salpingo-oophorectomy (BSO), pelvic washings for cytological evaluation, pelvic and aortic lymph node biopsies, and abdominal exploration. This operation accomplishes removal of the primary tumor, assessment of prognostic factors, and tissue sampling from areas at risk for metastatic disease. Such an operative approach facilitates rational postoperative treatment planning. Most gynecological surgeons are not trained in lymph node dissection procedures. In experienced hands, pelvic and aortic lymphadenectomy do not significantly contribute to increased postoperative morbidity (81–83). A prospective study reported by the GOG provides important information on the relationship between tumor grade, depth of myometrial invasion, and lymph node metastasis for stage I endometrial cancer (84). Given the low risk (<3%) of lymph node metastasis for stage I grade 1 endometrial adenocarcinoma, it is questionable whether lymph node dissection is necessary in all of these patients.

Table 2 FIGO Staging Classification for Uterine Cancer

Stage IA	Tumor limited to the endometrium
Stage IB	Invasion to less than one-half the myometrium
Stage IC	Invasion to more than one-half the myometrium
Stage IIA	Endocervical glandular involvement only
Stage IIB	Cervical stromal invasion
Stage IIIA	Tumor invades the serosa and/or adnexae, and/or positive peritoneal cytology
Stage IIIB	Vaginal metastasis
Stage IIIC	Metastasis to the pelvic and/or aortic lymph nodes
Stage IVA	Tumor invasion of the bladder or rectum
Stage IVB	Distant metastasis including intra-abdominal and/or inguinal lymph nodes

Note: Cases of carcinoma of the corpus should be graded according to the degree of histologic differentiation as follows: Grade 1 = 5% or less of a nonsquamous or nonmorular solid-growth pattern. Grade 2 = 6% to 50% of a nonsquamous or nonmorular solid-growth pattern. Grade 3 = more than 50% of a nonsquamous or nonmorular solid-growth pattern.
Abbreviation: FIGO, International Federation of Gynecology and Oncology.

Furthermore, the risk of aortic lymph node metastasis was negligible if pelvic lymph nodes were negative. In this series, almost 50% of positive lymph nodes were not detected by intraoperative inspection or palpation, and thus these cursory procedures are insufficient for patients at significant risk for nodal disease (84). Sood et al. conducted a retrospective study of preoperative cancer antigen (CA)-125 levels from 210 women undergoing surgical treatment for endometrial cancer. Elevated CA-125 levels (>35 U/mL) correlated with higher stage, higher grade, increased depth of myometrial invasion, positive cytology, lymph node metastasis, and reduced survival. Conversely, they suggested that patients with well-differentiated tumors and preoperative CA-125 <20 U/mL be considered for vaginal hysterectomy, because of a less than 3% risk of missing extrauterine disease (85). Patients with grade 2 to 3 endometrial cancer should undergo pelvic and aortic lymph node biopsy. Cragun et al. conducted a retrospective study of 509 patients who underwent surgical staging for endometrial cancer at their institution. Although the number of lymph nodes removed was not predictive of survival among patients with grade 1 to 2 cancers, among patients with poorly differentiated (grade 3) cancers, those having more than 11 pelvic nodes removed had improved overall survival compared with patients with 11 or fewer nodes removed (86). Other investigators have suggested a possible therapeutic benefit of lymphadenectomy beyond the premise of surgical staging, to both determine the need for and direct postoperative therapy. Bristow et al. reported their results for 41 women with stage IIIC endometrial cancer and grossly positive pelvic ($N=41$) and aortic ($N = 20$) lymph nodes. Patients with completely resected nodal disease had a significantly longer disease-specific survival as compared to patients with residual nodal disease (87).

For the morbidly obese patient with endometrial cancer, abdominal surgery can be a formidable exercise for the surgeon, and the risk for wound infection, separation, or dehiscence, and other postoperative complications can be high. For many of these women who have well-differentiated cancers, lower risk for lymph node metastasis, and a better overall prognosis, vaginal hysterectomy may be preferable. Although vaginal hysterectomy should not be considered the standard operative procedure for endometrial cancer, for selected patients it appears to yield long-term survival rates comparable to those with abdominal surgery (88–90). A newer approach to the surgical management of endometrial cancer is laparoscopy. Total laparoscopic hysterectomy or laparoscopic-assisted vaginal hysterectomy with BSO allows for resection of the primary tumor, and when combined with laparoscopic pelvic and aortic lymph node biopsy, offers the same prospects for accurate surgical staging as abdominal surgery but with lower treatment-related morbidity. Both retrospective and prospective cohort studies suggest that laparoscopic procedures are comparable to abdominal hysterectomy with respect to frequency of recurrence and survival (91,92). Tozzi et al. conducted a multivariate analysis to identify risk factors for postoperative complications among 122 patients undergoing laparoscopic ($N = 63$) or abdominal ($N = 59$) procedures for endometrial cancer. They found that age more than 65 years, weight more than 80 kg, Quetelet index more than 30, and the presence of comorbid medical conditions were predictive of postoperative complications. Furthermore, in these high-risk patients, a laparoscopic-vaginal approach significantly reduced the rate of complications (93). Thus, elderly women with endometrial cancer and coexisting medical problems should not be considered ineligible for laparoscopic surgery, and in fact, this technique may reduce their risk for postoperative complications.

Postoperative Treatment

Based on surgical–pathological staging, patients may be grouped into three risk categories for recurrence (Table 3).

Patients at low risk (<5%) for recurrence do not benefit from postoperative treatment (Fig. 2). The role of postoperative radiation therapy for patients at intermediate risk for recurrence has been addressed in three randomized controlled trials. Over 20 years ago, Aalders et al. at the Norwegian Radium Hospital conducted a randomized trial of vaginal brachytherapy and hysterectomy versus with/without postoperative pelvic radiation therapy. Although patients who received postoperative pelvic radiation therapy had a lower risk of pelvic recurrence, and a potential survival benefit was realized in the subset of patients with stage ICG3 disease, there was no overall improvement in survival with the addition of postoperative radiation

Table 3 Endometrial Cancer: Risk Factors for Recurrence

Low risk
Stage IA
Stage IB (and absence of capillary lymphatic space invasion)
Grade 1–2
Intermediate risk
Stage IA (grade 3)
Stage IB (presence of capillary lymphatic space invasion)
Stage IC (any tumor grade)
Positive peritoneal cytology
Occult cervical involvement (stage II)
High risk
Stage IIIA (except positive peritoneal cytology only)
Stage IIIB
Stage IIIC
Stage IVA
Stage IVB

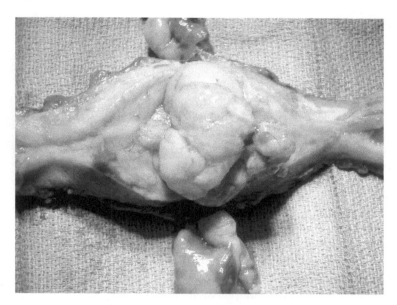

Figure 2 Hysterectomy specimen opened to reveal a polypoid tumor filling much of the endometrial cavity. Microscopic examination revealed grade 2 endometrial cancer with 3 mm invasion (total myometrial thickness 14 mm), no capillary-lymphatic space involvement, no metastasis to adnexal structures, pelvic or aortic lymph nodes.

therapy (94). A second study was conducted in the Netherlands and involved 715 women with endometrial cancer, who underwent TAH/BSO, lymph node palpation, and biopsy of suspicious lymph nodes. Surgical staging was otherwise not required. The study included patients with papillary serous, clear cell, and adenosquamous cell histological types. Patients were randomized to receive postoperative pelvic radiation therapy versus no further treatment (control group). Although postoperative radiation therapy reduced the rate of local recurrence, survival was not improved. Patients less than 60 years of age had a 4% risk of recurrence versus a 10% risk in older patients. Older patients also had a threefold higher risk of cancer-related death (95). In a subsequent analysis, for patients who had had a recurrence and had received treatment, the investigators found that survival was significantly better in the patient group who had not received postoperative radiation therapy. Treatment for vaginal recurrence yielded an 89% complete response rate and 65% five-year survival rate among patients in the control group (96). A third study of adjuvant pelvic radiation therapy was conducted by the GOG. After surgical staging, which included pelvic and aortic lymph node biopsies, there were 392 eligible patients randomized to receive pelvic radiation therapy versus no further treatment. Consistent with the two European studies, pelvic radiation therapy reduced the incidence of local recurrence without an improvement in overall survival. There was a subgroup of "high intermediate risk" patients, which accounted for approximately two-thirds of all cancer-related deaths. This subgroup included patients over 70 years of age with one risk factor (i.e., grade 2–3, lymphovascular invasion, or outer-third myometrial invasion), patients over 50 years of age with two risk factors, or patients of any age with three risk factors. In this high intermediate risk group of patients, pelvic radiation therapy both reduced the incidence of recurrence and increased recurrence-free survival (97). Thus, all three randomized controlled trials have demonstrated that pelvic radiation therapy reduces the incidence of local recurrence among intermediate-risk patients without an apparent improvement in survival. Each trial suggested an improvement in survival with radiation therapy for elderly patients or those with grade 3 tumors and/or deep myometrial invasion; however, differences were not significant due to insufficient study power.

High-risk patients should receive postoperative therapy. When endometrial cancer has metastasized to the aortic lymph nodes, a combination of pelvic plus aortic ("extended-field") radiation therapy is effective (98,99). When pelvic lymph nodes are positive but aortic lymph nodes are negative, some investigators have achieved excellent therapeutic results with pelvic radiation therapy alone (100). Patients with small-volume residual stage IVB endometrial cancer confined to the abdominal cavity may be salvaged with whole abdominal radiation therapy (101,102). The GOG conducted a phase II trial of whole abdominal radiation therapy for patients with stage III–IV endometrial cancer with tumor debulking to < 2 cm residual. Three-year recurrence-free survival rate was 29% for endometrioid and 27% for high-risk (papillary serous, clear cell) histological types. All long-term survivors were patients with no gross residual disease (103). Patients with stage IIIA disease on the basis of positive pelvic cytology alone have a good prognosis without adjuvant therapy, and should not be considered for these more aggressive radiation therapy programs (104). There has been a recent paradigm shift from radiation therapy alone to the use of adjuvant chemotherapy in high-risk patients. The GOG presented results from a phase III randomized study of whole abdominal radiation therapy versus cisplatin plus doxorubicin chemotherapy in high-risk endometrial cancer. With median follow-up of 52 months, there were significant improvements in both progression-free survival and overall survival in favor of adjuvant chemotherapy. Recurrences were frequent and occurred predominantly in the abdomen and pelvis in both arms (105). In an effort to further improve long-term survival in these high-risk patients, investigators have administered both radiation therapy and chemotherapy as postoperative treatment. The RTOG conducted a phase II study of pelvic radiation therapy combined with cisplatin chemotherapy (days 1 and 28) followed by four cycles of cisplatin plus paclitaxel chemotherapy. At two years, the pelvic and distant recurrence rates were 2% and 17%, respectively. Disease-free survival was 83% and overall survival was 90%. Severe acute toxicity was primarily hematologic. Grade 3 to 4 chronic toxicity was experienced by 18% of patients including four patients with small bowel complications (106).

Advanced/Recurrent Disease

A small subset of patients with recurrent endometrial cancer in the central pelvis after receiving both surgery and radiation therapy, may be salvaged with pelvic exenteration. The majority of patients with advanced/recurrent disease will not be cured. Selected patients with well-differentiated tumors expressing estrogen and progesterone receptors will respond well to progestin therapy (107,108). For other patients— and those who fail progestin therapy—cytotoxic chemotherapy is available as a palliative treatment. Drugs with significant single-agent activity in the treatment of endometrial cancer, include doxorubicin (109), cisplatin (110), ifosfamide (111), topotecan (112), and paclitaxel (113). Subsequent trials have demonstrated a significantly greater response rate and improved progression-free survival with combination therapy versus single-agent therapy. The GOG showed that the addition of cyclophosphamide to doxorubicin increased the response rate at a cost of greater toxicity and without any appreciable improvement in survival (114). The addition of cisplatin to doxorubicin resulted in a significantly higher response rate and progression-free survival, but also resulted in greater toxicity with no improvement in overall survival (115). Circadian timed administration of cisplatin plus doxorubicin does not have any clinical advantage over conventional drug administration schedules (116). Carboplatin plus paclitaxel is another effective combination against endometrial cancer (117). Furthermore, this treatment may be administered on an outpatient basis and may be a reasonable alternative to cisplatin plus paclitaxel in elderly patients due to less anticipated nausea and vomiting, neurotoxicity, and nephrotoxicity. However, substitution of carboplatin for cisplatin will result in greater myelosuppression, and should be used with caution in patients who have previously received radiation therapy. The most active systemic chemotherapy as demonstrated in a large multi-institution trial is the three-drug combination of cisplatin plus doxorubicin plus paclitaxel. The objective response rate was 57% (22% complete responses) and both progression-free survival and overall survival were significantly improved over cisplatin plus doxorubicin. Neurotoxicity was greater, and growth factors must be administered for hematopoietic support (118).

Endometrial Cancer in the Elderly Patient

There are considerable data that suggest elderly women with endometrial cancer have worse outcomes. Morrow et al. from the GOG reviewed the relationship between surgical–pathological risk factors and outcomes for patients with stages I–II endometrial cancer, who underwent hysterectomy with/without postoperative radiation therapy. The relative risk for recurrence was 1.8 times greater for patients more than 75 years of age and 1.4 times greater for patients 65 to 75 years of age (119). In an analysis of 41,120 cases from the SEER database, Kosary noted a steady decrease in the five-year survival rate with increasing age: less than 40 years (93%); 40 to 49 years (92%); 50 to 59 years (91%); 60 to 69 years (85%); and 70 years and older (71%). Within each FIGO stage, the five-year survival rate also declines with increasing age (51). Aziz et al. evaluated the effects of age and race on prognosis of 279 patients with endometrial cancer. In general, endometrial cancers in older patients were of higher clinical stage, higher grade, and deeper myometrial invasion. Overall, younger patients had a median survival of 200 months versus 90 months for older patients. Age was a very important prognostic factor in endometrial cancer in both races, although the effect of age appeared to be more pronounced in older black patients (120).

There is emerging evidence that elderly women with endometrial cancer do worse because they have worse cancers. As previously discussed, there are two types of endometrial cancer. Type I endometrial cancers usually occur in women who are younger and have classic risk factors (e.g., obesity, diabetes mellitus, nulliparity, infertility, and exogenous estrogen therapy). Type I cancers are grade 1 or 2, infrequently have deep myometrial invasion or lymph node metastasis, and have a good prognosis. On the other hand, type II endometrial cancers typically do not have estrogen-related features, are poorly differentiated, are often of high-risk histology (papillary serous, clear cell, or adenosquamous), frequently have deep myometrial invasion or lymph node metastasis, and are associated with a worse prognosis (121). Hoffman et al. studied histological specimens from 35 women aged 75 to 92 years with endometrial cancer. Only 23% of specimens were stage I, grade 1. The majority of tumors were deeply invasive or metastatic (stage IC–IV). Only 57% were "endometrioid" types and 43% were nonendometrioid types including papillary serous, clear cell, squamous, or undifferentiated (122). The proportion of type II cancers among elderly women with endometrial cancer is high.

Aside from tumor biology considerations, another reason that the elderly women with endometrial cancer may do worse is because of the presence of coexisting medical conditions precluding operative treatment. For these medically inoperable patients, radiation therapy alone can be curative (123,124). However, the effectiveness of primary radiation therapy for endometrial cancer in elderly (vs. younger) women is offset by the tendency of these patients to die of their underlying medical conditions (125). There are unfortunately few studies addressing treatment administered to younger versus older patients with endometrial cancer. Truong et al. conducted a population-based analysis in a cohort of 401 patients with endometrial cancer referred to the British Columbia Cancer Agency (Vancouver Island Centre) from 1989 to 1996. The age distribution of patients was: less than 65 (37%), 65 to 74 (38%), and above 75 (25%) years. In stage IC disease, the use of postoperative radiation therapy declined with increasing age. Although surgical therapy for endometrial cancer was not influenced by age or the presence of comorbid conditions, reduced use of postoperative radiation therapy resulted in a higher pelvic/vaginal relapse rate in elderly patients. In a multivariate analysis, age at diagnosis, performance status, stage and grade of tumor, presence of lymphovascular invasion, and surgery and radiation therapy use—but not Charlson comorbidity score—were significant predictors of overall survival. The authors concluded that chronologic age alone should not preclude patients from receiving optimal local therapy (126).

VULVAR CANCER

Invasive cancers of the vulva constitute approximately 5% of all gynecologic cancers. It is the fourth most common gynecologic cancer in the United States, with approximately 3870 new cases and 870 deaths from vulvar cancer each year (5). Although malignant melanomas, carcinomas of the Bartholin gland, various sarcomas, and a number of other cutaneous tumors may arise on the vulva, squamous cell carcinomas account for over 90% of invasive vulvar carcinomas. Unless otherwise specified, "vulvar cancer" implies a squamous cell carcinoma. Most of what is known about vulvar cancer is derived from studies of squamous cell carcinomas, which will be the focus of this section.

Epidemiology

Vulvar cancer has traditionally been considered a disease of the elderly. Most cases occur during the sixth decade of life, although approximately 15% of vulvar cancers occur in women less than 40 years of age (127,128). It has been reported in very young women (129) and during pregnancy (130). The epidemiology of vulvar cancer is not well understood. Hypertension, diabetes mellitus, and obesity are associated with vulvar carcinoma (131); however, more recent studies have not confirmed the etiologic significance of these diagnoses (132).

Neoplasias of the lower genital tract have several risk factors in common. An important risk factor for the development of vulvar neoplasia is a history of neoplasia elsewhere in the lower genital tract. Chronic vulvar dermatoses such as lichen sclerosis and squamous cell hyperplasia are often found simultaneously with squamous cell carcinoma and have been suggested as precursor lesions of vulvar cancer (Fig. 3). A longitudinal study of 350 patients with lichen sclerosis showed that only 3% developed invasive vulvar cancer (133). A link between cigarette smoking and vulvar carcinoma has been confirmed by two case–control studies (132,134).

There is a strong association between HPV infection and vulvar neoplasia. HPV DNA has been isolated from both invasive and "carcinoma in situ" lesions (135,136). HPV DNA can be identified in approximately 70% to 80% of intraepithelial lesions, but is seen in only 10% to 50% of invasive lesions. Brinton et al. conducted a case–control analysis and identified women with a history of genital condylomata, those with a previous abnormal Pap smear, and those who smoked as having an increased risk for developing vulvar cancer. Those who both smoked and had a history of genital warts had a 35-fold increase in risk when compared with women without these factors (132).

Recent observations have suggested that squamous cell carcinoma of the vulva may have two different etiologies (137,138). Trimble et al. described two histologic subtypes—with basaloid or warty features—that are associated with HPV, versus keratinizing squamous carcinomas, which usually are not associated with HPV. The so-called basaloid or warty carcinomas are associated with risk factors typical of cervical carcinoma, including: early age at first intercourse; a number of sexual partners during lifetime; prior abnormal Pap smears; smoking; and lower socioeconomic status. These risk factors are often absent in keratinizing squamous carcinomas (139). Flowers et al. have found mutations in the p53 tumor suppressor gene to be frequent in HPV-negative vulvar carcinomas versus those associated with HPV (140). Thus, a final common pathway in the development of vulvar carcinoma appears to be inactivation of the p53 tumor suppressor gene, either by genetic mutation (in HPV-negative tumors) or through functional inactivation of p53 gene products through the expression of HPV E6 viral oncoproteins. There presently does not seem to be any prognostic difference between HPV-positive and HPV-negative vulvar carcinomas (141,142).

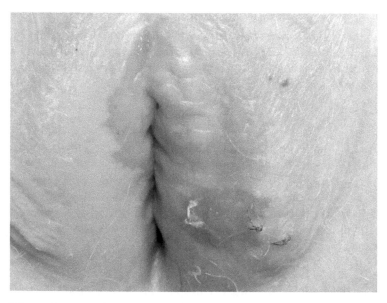

Figure 3 Early invasive squamous cell carcinoma of the vulva (biopsy site marked with suture material) arising from a generalized background of lichen sclerosis.

Screening

There is no effective screening procedure for vulvar cancer aside from a meticulous inspection of the external genitalia at the time of the annual gynecological examination. The vast majority of women who present with vulvar neoplasia have symptoms of vulvar burning or pruritis, pain, bleeding, or a mass (Fig. 4). The initial step in the management of vulvar cancer may be easily accomplished with an office punch biopsy under local analgesia. Other vulvar lesions such as large condylomata accuminata or verrucous carcinomas, Paget's disease, or extensive vulvar intraepithelial neoplasia-III (carcinoma in situ) may mimic an invasive squamous cell carcinoma and a histological confirmation will prevent the delay of appropriate treatment.

Diagnosis and Clinical Evaluation

Vulvar cancers metastasize by three routes: local growth and infiltration; embolization to groin lymph nodes; and vascular dissemination to distant sites (rare). Treatment planning in all patients should include pelvic examination with careful palpation of the groin lymph nodes. For large tumors encroaching on the urethra or bladder, a cystourethroscopy with biopsy may provide useful information. Lower gastrointestinal (GI) endoscopy or barium enema may be useful for the evaluation of tumors extending to the anus or infiltrating the rectovaginal septum. In 1988, the FIGO staging classification for vulvar cancer was changed and based on surgical-pathological findings (Table 4).

There were several reasons for this change: practically all patients with vulvar carcinoma undergo operative treatment, including biopsy of the inguinal-femoral lymph nodes, as part of primary therapy; the presence of cancer metastatic to the

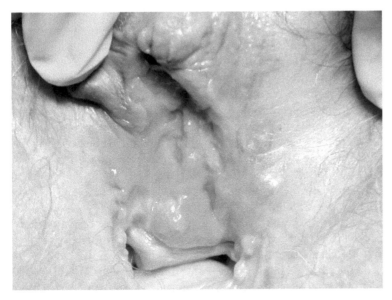

Figure 4 The patient is a 53-year-old who had undergone previous laser and excisional procedures for VIN (vulva intraepithelial neoplasia). She had missed follow-up appointments for almost two years when she presented with complaints of vulva pain and dysuria. Biopsy of the lesion infiltrating the vestibule, external urethral meatus and clitoris revealed squamous cell carcinoma.

Table 4 FIGO Staging Classification for Carcinoma of the Vulva

Stage 0	Carcinoma in situ, intraepithelial carcinoma
Stage I	Tumor confined to the vulva and/or perineum, ≤2 cm in greatest diameter
Stage II	Tumor confined to the vulva and/or perineum, >2 cm in greatest diameter
Stage III	Tumor of any size with adjacent spread to the lower urethra and/or the vagina, or the anus, and/or unilateral regional lymph node metastasis
Stage IVA	Tumor invades the upper urethra, bladder mucosa, rectal mucosa, or pelvic bone, and/or bilateral regional lymph node metastasis
Stage IVB	Any distant metastasis including pelvic lymph nodes

Abbreviation: FIGO, International Federation of Gynecology and Oncology.

groin lymph nodes is the single most important prognostic factor for recurrence and survival; the accuracy of clinical evaluation of the groin lymph nodes is poor.

Treatment

Radical deep resection of the entire vulva, with dissection of the groin lymph nodes, became standard therapy for vulvar cancer in the mid-20th century. Surgical refinements by Taussig (143) and Way (144) greatly improved survival, particularly when tumors could be removed entirely and the lymph nodes proved to be uninvolved. The disadvantages of these procedures include a high risk for postoperative complications, including wound breakdown, infection, groin lymphocyst formation, and lower extremity lymphedema. Furthermore, these procedures can lead to permanent disfigurement with negative effects on body image and sexual function. More recently, surgeons have attempted a more individualized approach to the resection of vulvar carcinomas. DiSaia et al. were the first to describe a successful and more conservative resection in patients with stage I vulvar cancer (145). Subsequent reports have applied this same technique to patients with larger primary tumors (146,147). Various terms have been used to describe this surgery, including "radical wide excision," "radical hemivulvectomy," or "partial radical vulvectomy." Combined with the removal of groin lymph nodes through separate incisions instead of through an en bloc excision of intervening vulva and perineum (148), the morbidity of vulvar surgery has been greatly reduced without compromising efficacy. For tumors that do not encroach upon midline structures, removal of the ipsilateral groin lymph nodes is sufficient. When the ipsilateral lymph nodes are negative, the likelihood for metastasis to the contralateral groin is exceedingly small (146,149,150).

Radiation therapy has an established role in the treatment of vulvar cancer, usually in the postoperative setting. The GOG conducted a randomized controlled trial of pelvic lymph node dissection versus groin irradiation in patients with metastasis to the inguinal–femoral lymph nodes, confirming the superiority of radiation therapy over a more extensive surgical dissection (151). Attempts to replace groin lymph node dissection with elective groin irradiation have been unsuccessful (152). Primary radiation therapy has been used as an alternative to ultraradical surgery (e.g., pelvic exenteration) for patients with locally advanced vulvar carcinomas, and it has also been investigated as an alternative to surgery for patients with smaller tumors (153,154). The GOG conducted a large, prospective phase II trial of preoperative chemotherapy (cisplatin plus 5-FU) and radiation therapy in patients with locally advanced tumors that were deemed unresectable by standard radical vulvectomy. A complete clinical tumor response was noted in 33 of the 71 (47%) patients. Only 2 of the 71 patients (3%) still had unresectable disease after chemoradiation, and for only three patients it was not possible to preserve urinary and/or GI integrity (155).

Predictors of survival in vulvar cancer include the presence and the number of involved groin lymph nodes, FIGO stage, and age. Five-year survival rates range from stage I, 80%; stage II, 70%; stage III, 65%; to stage IV, 24% (51).

Vulvar Cancer in the Elderly Patient

Elderly women with vulvar cancer appear to have a worse prognosis (156). Five-year survival rates decline from 87% for women less than 40 years of age to 66% for women over the age of 70 years (51). Whether these age-based differences in survival reflect differences in tumor biology, clinical presentation (FIGO stage), or treatment selection is unknown. In a multivariate regression analysis of patients treated for squamous cell carcinoma of the vulva, a poorer survival rate was associated with smoking, parity (patients who had more than three children), body mass index more than 27, and age (older than 73 years) (157). Hyde et al. assessed the impact of various clinical and pathological variables on outcome in a series of elderly ($\geq$80 years of age) women with vulvar carcinoma. Standard therapy was administered to 57 of the 75 (76%) patients. When all variables were assessed in the subgroup that received standard treatment, only performance status and extracapsular lymph node involvement were found to be independent prognostic factors for survival. Thus, performance status should be considered when individualizing treatment for vulvar carcinoma in elderly patients (158). In a review of 62 women with squamous cell carcinoma of the vulva, Heatley noted that older women were more likely to have clinical features associated with poor clinical outcome including: high grade tumors; large tumors; and higher FIGO stage (159).

Consistent with what has been reported for other cancers, there is evidence that elderly women with vulvar cancer are more likely to receive inadequate therapy. In a review of the Geneva Tumor Registry, Vlastos et al. identified 230 women treated for vulvar carcinoma between 1979 and 1999. Treatments were compared for women 80 years and older versus younger patients. The majority of cancers in older women were diagnosed at more advanced stages. Furthermore, elderly women were more likely to have either inadequate therapy or no treatment. Less aggressive therapy in these women correlated with poorer outcome (160). The mainstay of vulvar cancer treatment is surgery, and age per se is not a contraindication to surgical treatment. There is one case report of radical vulvectomy successfully performed in a 101-year-old patient (161). Even if surgery is contraindicated due to severe medical comorbidities, patients with vulvar cancer may still receive radiation therapy, most often with a curative intent. Elderly patients with vulvar carcinoma should not go untreated. Ulutin et al. reported results for a more limited surgery followed with radiation therapy. Median age of patients was 67 years. With median follow-up of 35 months, the local recurrence rate was 18%, the five-year survival rate was 60%, and disease-specific survival rate was 69%. There were no delays in completing planned treatment or treatment-related deaths. The authors concluded that this approach could be offered as an alternative to radical surgery with less morbidity (162).

Elderly women with vulvar cancer are often faced with problems of long-term disability and disfigurement from radical surgery and/or radiation therapy. Although surgical treatment over the past 30 years has become more conservative, vulvar surgery still affects body image, sexual function, and psychosocial well-being. Unfortunately, very few studies have adequately addressed these problems. It will become increasingly important that we not only develop better treatments for vulvar carcinoma, but also understand the impact of those treatments on the quantity and quality of life of elderly patients.

CONCLUSIONS

The risk for developing gynecological cancer increases with age. Elderly patients with cancers of the cervix, endometrium, or vulva appear to have a poorer prognosis. Assuming that age is an independent prognostic factor for survival, is it because elderly patients are "just old" that they present with more advanced-stage disease, have more biologically aggressive tumors, or receive substandard therapy? If elderly patients receive less than optimal therapy, is it because of medical conditions that complicate the delivery of standard therapy, physician or family biases, or unique patient expectations and needs? Are there genetic and biological differences between gynecological cancers arising in older and younger patients and, if so, can therapies be developed to exploit these differences? It will be difficult to design and study better treatments for elderly patients with cancer when they are frequently underrepresented, if not excluded from clinical trial participation (163–165). As the population ages, it is imperative that we better understand and care for the elderly cancer patient.

REFERENCES

1. U.S. Census Bureau, Office of Statistics. Statistical brief: sixty-five plus in the United States. Washington, D.C., 1997.
2. U.S. Bureau of the Census. Current Population Reports, series P-25, No. 1045.
3. Yancik R. Frame of reference: old age as the context for the prevention and treatment of cancer. In: Yancik R, ed. Perspectives on Prevention and Treatment of Cancer in the Elderly. New York: Raven Press, 1983:5–17.
4. Silliman RA, Balducci L, Goodwin JS, et al. Breast cancer in old age: what we know, don't know, and do. J Natl Cancer Inst 1993; 85:190–199.
5. American Cancer Society, Inc. 2005 surveillance research: www.cancer.org.
6. Pisani P, Parkin DM, Bray F, Ferlay J. Estimates of the worldwide mortality from 25 cancers in 1990. Int J Cancer 1999; 83:18–29.
7. Brinton LA, Hamman RF, Huggins GR, et al. Sexual and reproductive risk factors for invasive squamous cell cervical cancer. J Natl Cancer Inst 1987; 79:23–30.
8. La Vecchia C, Franceschi S, Decarli A, et al. Sexual factors, venereal diseases, and the risk of intraepithelial and invasive cervical neoplasia. Cancer 1986; 58:935–941.
9. Hellberg D, Nilsson S, Haley NJ, et al. Smoking and cervical intraepithelial neoplasia: nicotine and cotinine in serum and cervical mucus in smokers and nonsmokers. Am J Obstet Gynecol 1988; 158:910–913.
10. Barton SE, Maddox PH, Jenkins D, et al. Effect of cigarette smoking on cervical epithelial immunity: a mechanism for neoplastic change? Lancet 1988; 2:652–654.
11. Slattery ML, Robison LM, Schuman KL, et al. Cigarette smoking and exposure to passive smoke are risk factors for cervical cancer. JAMA 1989; 261:1593–1598.

12. Sood AK. Cigarette smoking and cervical cancer: meta-analysis and critical review of recent studies. FAX 1991; 6:31–36.
13. Agarwal SS, Sehgal A, Sardana S, Kumar A, Luthra UK. Role of male behavior in cervical carcinogenesis among women with one lifetime sexual partner. Cancer 1993; 72: 1666–1669.
14. Castellsague X, Bosch FX, Munoz N, et al. Male circumcision, penile human papillomavirus infection, and cervical cancer in female partners. N Engl J Med 2002; 346: 1105–1112.
15. Schiffman MH. Recent progress in defining the epidemiology of human papillomavirus infection and cervical neoplasia. J Natl Cancer Inst 1992; 84:394–398.
16. Hines JF, Jenson AB, Barnes WA. Human papillomaviruses: their clinical significance in the management of cervical carcinoma. Oncology 1995; 9:279–285.
17. Das BC, Gopalkrishna V, Das DK, et al. Human papillomavirus DNA sequences in adenocarcinoma of the uterine cervix in Indian women. Cancer 1993; 72:147–153.
18. Koutsky LA, Holmes KK, Critchlow CW, et al. A cohort study of the risk of cervical intraepithelial neoplasia grade 2 or 3 in relation to papillomavirus infection. N Engl J Med 1992; 327:1272–1278.
19. Rylander E, Ruusuvaara L, Almstromer MW, et al. The absence of vaginal human papillomavirus 16 DNA in women who have not experienced sexual intercourse. Obstet Gynecol 1994; 83:735–737.
20. Paquette RL, Lee YY, Wilczynski SP, et al. Mutations of p53 and human papillomavirus infection in cervical carcinoma. Cancer 1993; 72:1272–1280.
21. Saslow D, Runowicz CD, Solomon D, et al. American Cancer Society guideline for the early detection of cervical neoplasia and cancer. CA Cancer J Clin 2002; 52:342–362.
22. Sawaya GF, McConnell KJ, Kulasingam SL, et al. Risk of cervical cancer associated with extending the interval between cervical-cancer screenings. N Engl J Med 2003; 349:1501–1509.
23. Parkin DM, Pisani P, Ferlay J. Global cancer statistics. CA Cancer J Clin 1999; 49: 33–64.
24. Moore DH. Anatomy, natural history, and patterns of spread of invasive cervical cancer. In: Rubin SC, Hoskins WJ, eds. Cervical Cancer and Preinvasive Neoplasia. Philadelphia: Lippincott-Raven, 1996:161–170.
25. Morley GW, Seski JC. Radical pelvic surgery versus radiation therapy for stage I carcinoma of the cervix (exclusive of microinvasion). Am J Obstet Gynecol 1976; 126: 785–798.
26. Volterrani F, Feltre L, Sigurta D, Di Giuseppe M, Luciani L. Radiotherapy versus surgery in the treatment of cervix stage Ib cancer. Int J Radiat Oncol Biol Phys 1983; 9:1781–1784.
27. Roddick JW, Greenelaw RH. Treatment of cervical cancer: a randomized study of operation and radiation. Am J Obstet Gynecol 1971; 109:754–764.
28. Landoni F, Maneo A, Colombo A, et al. Randomised study of radical surgery versus radiotherapy for stage Ib-IIa cervical cancer. Lancet 1997; 350:535–540.
29. Tattersall MHN, Ramirez C, Coppleson M. A randomized trial of adjuvant chemotherapy after radical hysterectomy in stage Ib-IIa cervical cancer patients with pelvic lymph node metastases. Gynecol Oncol 1992; 46:176–181.
30. Killackey MA, Boardman L, Carroll DS. Adjuvant chemotherapy and radiation in patients with poor prognostic stage Ib/IIa cervical cancer. Gynecol Oncol 1993; 49: 377–379.
31. Peters WA, Liu PY, Barrett RJ, et al. Concurrent chemotherapy and pelvic radiation therapy compared with pelvic radiation therapy alone as adjuvant therapy after radical surgery in high-risk early-stage cancer of the cervix. J Clin Oncol 2000; 18:1606.
32. Durrance FY, Fletcher GH, Rutledge FN. Analysis of central recurrent disease in stages I and II squamous cell carcinomas of the cervix on intact uterus. Am J Roentgenol 1969; 106:831–838.

33. Gallion HH, Van Nagell JR Jr, Donaldson ES, et al. Combined radiation therapy and extrafascial hysterectomy in the treatment of stage IB barrel-shaped cervical cancer. Cancer 1985; 56:262–265.

34. Keys HM, Bundy BN, Stehman FB, et al. Radiation therapy with and without extrafascial hysterectomy for bulky stage IB cervical carcinoma: a randomized trial of the Gynecologic Oncology Group. Gynecol Oncol 2003; 89:343–353.

35. Keys HM, Bundy BN, Stehman FB, et al. Cisplatin, radiation, and adjuvant hysterectomy compared with radiation and adjuvant hysterectomy for bulky stage IB cervical carcinoma. N Engl J Med 1999; 340:1154–1161.

36. Fu KK. Biological basis for the interaction of chemotherapeutic agents and radiation therapy. Cancer 1985; 55:2123–2130.

37. Hreshchyshyn MM, Aron BS, Boronow RC, Franklin EW, Shingleton HM, Blessing JA. Hydroxyurea or placebo combined with radiation to treat stages IIIB and IV cervical cancer confined to the pelvis. Int J Radiat Oncol Biol Phys 1979; 5:317–322.

38. Stehman FB, Bundy BN, Keys H, Currie JL, Mortel R, Creasman WT. A randomized trial of hydroxyurea versus misonidazole adjunct to radiation therapy in carcinoma of the cervix: A preliminary report of a Gynecologic Oncology Group study. Am J Obstet Gynecol 1988; 159:87–94.

39. Stehman FB, Bundy BN, Thomas G, et al. Hydroxyurea versus misonidazole with radiation in cervical carcinoma: long-term follow-up of a Gynecologic Oncology Group trial. J Clin Oncol 1993; 11:1523–1528.

40. Leibel S, Bauer M, Wasserman T, et al. Radiotherapy with or without misonidazole for patients with stage IIIB or stage IVA squamous cell carcinoma of the uterine cervix: preliminary report of a Radiation Therapy Oncology Group randomized trial. Int J Radiat Oncol Biol Phys 1987; 13:541–549.

41. Whitney CW, Sause W, Bundy BN, et al. A randomized comparison of fluorouracil plus cisplatin versus hydroxyurea as an adjunct to radiation therapy in stages IIB-IVA carcinoma of the cervix with negative para-aortic lymph nodes: a Gynecologic Oncology Group and Southwest Oncology Group study. J Clin Oncol 1999; 17:1339–1348.

42. Morris M, Eifel PJ, Lu J, et al. Pelvic radiation with concurrent chemotherapy versus pelvic and para-aortic radiation for high-risk cervical cancer: a randomized Radiation Therapy Oncology Group clinical trial. N Engl J Med 1999; 340:1137–1143.

43. Rose PG, Bundy BN, Watkins EB, et al. Concurrent cisplatin based radiotherapy and chemotherapy for locally-advanced cervical cancer. N Engl J Med 1999; 340:1144–1153.

44. Thigpen JT, Singleton H, Homesley H, Lagasse L, Blessing J. cis-Platinum in treatment of advanced or recurrent squamous cell carcinoma of the cervix: a phase II trial of the Gynecologic Oncology Group. Cancer 1981; 48:899–903.

45. Bonomi P, Blessing JA, Stehman FB, DiSaia PJ, Walton L, Major FJ. Randomized trial of three cisplatin dose schedules in squamous-cell carcinoma of the cervix: a Gynecologic Oncology Group study. J Clin Oncol 1985; 3:1079–1085.

46. Thigpen JT, Blessing JA, DiSaia PJ, Fowler WC, Hatch KD. A randomized comparison of rapid versus prolonged (24 hr) infusion of cisplatin in therapy of squamous cell carcinoma of the uterine cervix: a Gynecologic Oncology Group study. Gynecol Oncol 1989; 32:198–202.

47. Omura GA, Blessing JA, Vaccarello L, et al. A randomized trial of cisplatin versus cisplatin plus mitolactol versus cisplatin plus ifosfamide in advanced squamous carcinoma of the cervix: a Gynecologic Oncology Group study. J Clin Oncol 1997; 15:165–171.

48. Bloss JD, Blessing JA, Behrens BC, et al. Randomized trial of cisplatin and ifosfamide with or without bleomycin in squamous carcinoma of the cervix: a Gynecologic Oncology Group study. J Clin Oncol 2002; 20:1832–1837.

49. Moore DH, Blessing JA, McQuellon RP, et al. Phase III study of cisplatin with or without paclitaxel in stage IVB, recurrent, or persistent squamous cell carcinoma of the cervix: a Gynecologic Oncology Group trial. J Clin Oncol 2004; 22:3113–3119.

50. Long HJ, Bundy BN, Grendys EC, et al. Randomized phase III trial of cisplatin vs. cisplatin plus topotecan vs. MVAC in stage IVB, recurrent or persistent carcinoma of the uterine cervix: a Gynecologic Oncology Group study [abstr.]. Gynecol Oncol 2004; 92:397.

51. Kosary CL. FIGO stage, histology, histologic grade, age and race as prognostic factors in determining survival for cancers of the female gynecological system: an analysis of 1973–87 SEER cases of cancers of the endometrium, cervix, ovary, vulva, and vagina. Semin Surg Oncol 1994; 10:31–46.

52. Stehman FB, Bundy BN, DiSaia PJ, et al. Carcinoma of the cervix treated with radiation therapy: a multi-variate analysis of prognostic variables in the Gynecologic Oncology Group. Cancer 1991; 67:2776–2785.

53. Baay MF, Tjalma WA, Weyler J, et al. Prevalence of human papillomavirus in elderly women with cervical cancer. Gynecol Obstet Invest 2001; 52:248–251.

54. Gostout BS, Podratz KC, McGovern RM, Persing DH. Cervical cancer in older women: a molecular analysis of human papillomavirus types, HLA types, and p53 mutations. Am J Obstet Gynecol 1998; 179:56–61.

55. Saito J, Hoshiai H, Noda K. Type of human papillomavirus and expression of p53 in elderly women with cervical cancer. Gynecol Obstet Invest 2000; 49:190–193.

56. Trimble EL, Harlan LC, Clegg LX. Untreated cervical cancer in the United States. Gynecol Oncol 2005; 96:271–277.

57. Wright JD, Gibb RK, Geevarghese S, et al. Cervical carcinoma in the elderly: an analysis of patterns of care and outcome. Cancer 2005; 103:85–91.

58. Choi YS, Kim YH, Kang S, et al. Feasibility of radical surgery in the management of elderly patients with uterine cervical cancer in Korea. Gynecol Obstet Invest 2005; 59:165–170.

59. Levrant SG, Fruchter RG, Maiman M. Radical hysterectomy for cervical cancer: morbidity and survival in relation to weight and age. Gynecol Oncol 1992; 45:317–322.

60. Sakurai H, Niibe H, Suzuki M, Nakano T. A 104-year-old woman with advanced cervical carcinoma of the uterus. Gynecol Oncol 2004; 92:713–715.

61. Mandelblatt J, Gopaul I, Wistreich M. Gynecological care of elderly women: another look at Papanicolaou smear testing. JAMA 1986; 256:367–371.

62. Mandelblatt J, Fahs MC. The cost-effectiveness of cervical cancer screening for low-income elderly women. JAMA 1988; 259:2409–2413.

63. Wharton JT, Mikuta JJ, Mettlin C, et al. Risk factors and current management in carcinoma of the endometrium. Surg Gynecol Obstet 1986; 162:515–520.

64. Judd HL, Shamonki IM, Frumar AM, Lagasse LD. Origin of serum estradiol in postmenopausal women. Obstet Gynecol 1982; 59:680–686.

65. Dubeau L. Etiology and detection of gynecologic cancer. In: Morrow CP, Curtin JP, Townsend DE, eds. Synopsis of Gynecologic Oncology. 4th ed. New York: Churchill Livingstone, 1993:1–22.

66. The Cancer and Steroid Hormone Study of the Centers for Disease Control and the National Institute of Child Health and Human Development. Combination oral contraceptive use and the risk of endometrial cancer. JAMA 1987; 257:796–800.

67. Million Women Study Collaborators. Endometrial cancer and hormone-replacement therapy in the Million Women Study. Lancet 2005; 365:1543–1551.

68. Sismondi P, Biglia N, Volpi E, et al. Tamoxifen and endometrial cancer. Ann NY Acad Sci 1994; 734:310–321.

69. Fisher B, Costantino JP, Redmond CT, et al. Endometrial cancer in tamoxifen-treated breast cancer patients: findings from the National Surgical Adjuvant Breast and Bowel Project (NSABP) B-14. J Natl Cancer Inst 1994; 86:527–537.

70. Vasen HF, Stormorken A, Menko FH, et al. MSH2 mutation carriers are at higher risk of cancer than MLH1 mutation carriers: a study of hereditary nonpolyposis colorectal cancer families. J Clin Oncol 2001; 19:4074–4080.

71. Watson P, Vasen HF, Mecklin J, et al. The risk of endometrial cancer in hereditary nonpolyposis colorectal cancer. Am J Med 1994; 96:516–520.

72. Kosary CL, Reis LAG, Miller BA, et al., eds. SEER Cancer Statistics Review, 1973–1992: Tables and Graphs. Bethesda, MD: National Cancer Institute (NIH Publication #95–2789), 1995:171–181.

73. Risinger JI, Hayes AK, Berchuck A, Barrett JC. PTEN/MMAC1 mutations in endometrial cancers. Cancer Res 1997; 57:4736.

74. Kong D, Suzuki A, Zou TT, et al. PTEN1 is frequently mutated in primary endometrial carcinomas. Nat Genet 1997; 17:143.

75. Kohler MF, Carney P, Dodge R, et al. p53 overexpression in advanced-stage endometrial adenocarcinoma. Am J Obstet Gynecol 1996; 175:1246–1252.

76. Khalifa MA, Mannel RS, Haraway SD, et al. Expression of EGFR, HER-2/*neu*, p53, and PCNA in endometrioid, serous papillary, and clear cell endometrial adenocarcinomas. Gynecol Oncol 1994; 53:84–92.

77. Barakat RR. The effect of tamoxifen on the endometrium. Oncology 1995; 9:129–139.

78. Lahti E, Blanco G, Kauppila A, Apaja-Sarkkinen M, Taskinen PJ, Laatikainen T. Endometrial changes in postmenopausal breast cancer patients receiving tamoxifen. Obstet Gynecol 1993; 81:660–664.

79. Bertelli G, Venturini M, Del Mastro L, et al. Tamoxifen and the endometrium: findings of pelvic ultrasound examination and endometrial biopsy in asymptomatic breast cancer patients. Breast Cancer Res Treat 1998; 47:41–46.

80. Love CD, Muir BB, Scrimgeour JB, Leonard RC, Dillon P, Dixon JM. Investigation of endometrial abnormalities in asymptomatic women treated with tamoxifen and an evaluation of the role of endometrial screening. J Clin Oncol 1999; 17:2050–2054.

81. Homesley HD, Kadar N, Barrett RJ, Lentz SS. Selective pelvic and periaortic lymphadenectomy does not increase morbidity in surgical staging of endometrial carcinoma. Am J Obstet Gynecol 1992; 167:1225–1230.

82. Larson DM, Johnson K, Olson KA. Pelvic and para-aortic lymphadenectomy for surgical staging of endometrial cancer: morbidity and mortality. Obstet Gynecol 1992; 79:993–1001.

83. Moore DH, Fowler WC, Walton LA, Droegemueller W. Morbidity of lymph node sampling in cancers of the uterine corpus and cervix. Obstet Gynecol 1984; 74:180–184.

84. Boronow RC, Morrow CP, Creasman WT, et al. Surgical staging in endometrial cancer: clinical-pathologic findings of a prospective study. Obstet Gynecol 1984; 63:825–832.

85. Sood AK, Buller RE, Burger RA, Dawson JD, Sorosky JI, Berman M. Value of preoperative CA 125 level in the management of uterine cancer and prediction of clinical outcome. Obstet Gynecol 1997; 90:441–447.

86. Cragun JM, Havrilesky LJ, Calingaert B, et al. Retrospective analysis of selective lymphadenectomy in apparent early-stage endometrial cancer. J Clin Oncol 2005; 23: 3668–3675.

87. Bristow Re, Zahurak ML, Alexander CJ, Zellars RC, Montz FJ. FIGO stage IIIC endometrial carcinoma: resection of macroscopic nodal disease and other determinants of survival. Int J Gynecol Cancer 2003; 13:64–672.

88. Peters WA, Andersen WA, Thornton WN, Morley GW. The selective use of vaginal hysterectomy in the management of adenocarcinoma of the endometrium. Am J Obstet Gynecol 1983; 146:285–291.

89. Massi G, Savino L, Susini T. Vaginal hysterectomy versus abdominal hysterectomy for the treatment of stage I endometrial adenocarcinoma. Am J Obstet Gynecol 1996; 174: 1320–1326.

90. Lelle RJ, Morley GW, Peters WA. The role of vaginal hysterectomy in the treatment of endometrial carcinoma. Int J Gynecol Cancer 1994; 4:342–347.

91. Obermair A, Manolitsas TP, Leung Y, Hammond IG, McCartney AJ. Total laparoscopic hysterectomy versus total abdominal hysterectomy for obese women with endometrial cancer. Int J Gynecol Cancer 2005; 15:319–324.

92. Tozzi R, Malur S, Koehler C, Schneider A. Laparoscopy versus laparotomy in endometrial cancer: first analysis of survival of a randomized prospective study. J Minim Invasive Gynecol 2005; 12:130–136.

93. Tozzi R, Malur S, Koehler C, Schneider A. Analysis of morbidity in patients with endometrial cancer: is there a commitment to offer laparoscopy? Gynecol Oncol 2005; 97:4–9.

94. Aalders J, Abeler V, Kolstad P, Onsrud M. Postoperative external irradiation and prognostic parameters in stage I endometrial carcinoma. Clinical and histopathologic study of 540 patients. Obstet Gynecol 1980; 56:419–426.

95. Creutzberg CL, van Putten WLJ, Koper PCM, et al. Surgery and postoperative radiotherapy versus surgery alone for patients with stage 1 endometrial carcinoma: multicentre randomised trial. Lancet 2000; 355:1404–1411.

96. Creutzberg CL, van Putten WLJ, Koper PC, et al. Survival after relapse in patients with endometrial cancer: results from a randomized trial. Gynecol Oncol 2003; 89:201–209.

97. Keys HM, Roberts JA, Brunetto VL, et al. A phase III trial of surgery with or without adjunctive external pelvic radiation therapy in intermediate risk endometrial adenocarcinoma: a Gynecologic Oncology Group study. Gynecol Oncol 2004; 744–751.

98. Potish RA, Twiggs LB, Adcock LL, et al. Paraaortic lymph node radiotherapy in cancer of the uterine corpus. Obstet Gynecol 1985; 65:251–256.

99. Rose PG, Cha SD, Tak WK, et al. Radiation therapy for surgically proven para-aortic node metastasis in endometrial carcinoma. Int J Radiat Oncol Biol Phys 1992; 24:229–233.

100. Nelson G, Randall M, Sutton G, Moore D, Hurteau J, Look K. FIGO stage IIIC endometrial carcinoma with metastases confined to pelvic lymph nodes: analysis of treatment outcomes, prognostic variables, and failure patterns following adjuvant radiation therapy. Gynecol Oncol 1999; 75:211–214.

101. Greer BE, Hamberger AD. Treatment of intraperitoneal metastatic adenocarcinoma of the endometrium by the whole-abdomen moving-strip technique and pelvic boost irradiation. Gynecol Oncol 1983; 16:356–373.

102. Loeffler JS, Rosen EM, Niloff JM, et al. Whole abdominal irradiation for tumors of the uterine corpus. Cancer 1988; 61:1332–1335.

103. Sutton G, Axelrod JH, Bundy BN, et al. Whole abdominal radiotherapy in the adjuvant treatment of patients with stage III and IV endometrial cancer: a Gynecologic Oncology Group study. Gynecol Oncol 2005; 97:755–763.

104. Slomovitz BM, Ramondetta LM, Lee CM, et al. Heterogeneity of stage IIIA endometrial carcinomas: implications for adjuvant therapy. Int J Gynecol Cancer 2005; 15:510–516.

105. Randall ME, Brunetto G, Muss H, et al. Whole abdominal radiotherapy versus combination doxorubicin-cisplatin chemotherapy in advanced endometrial carcinoma: a randomized phase III trial of the Gynecologic Oncology Group [abstr.]. Proc ASCO 2003; 22:2.

106. Greven K, Winter K, Underhill K, Fontenesci J, Cooper J, Burke T. Preliminary analysis of RTOG 9708: adjuvant postoperative radiotherapy combined with cisplatin/paclitaxel chemotherapy after surgery for patients with high-risk endometrial cancer. Int J Radiat Oncol Biol Phys 2004; 59:168–173.

107. Ingram SS, Rosenman J, Heath R, Morgan TM, Moore D, Varia M. The predictive value of progesterone receptor levels in endometrial cancer. Int J Radiat Oncol Biol Phys 1989; 17:21–27.

108. Lentz SS, Brady MF, Major FJ, et al. High-dose megestrol acetate in advanced or recurrent endometrial cancer: a Gynecologic Oncology Group study. J Clin Oncol 1996; 14:357–361.

109. Thigpen JT, Buchsbaum HJ, Mangan C, Blessing JA. Phase II trial of adriamycin in the treatment of advanced or recurrent endometrial carcinoma: a Gynecologic Oncology Group study. Cancer Treat Rep 1979; 63:21–27.

110. Thigpen JT, Blessing JA, Homesley H, et al. Phase II trial of cisplatin as first-line chemotherapy in patients with advanced or recurrent endometrial carcinoma: a Gynecologic Oncology Group study. Gynecol Oncol 1989; 33:68–70.

111. Sutton GP, Blessing JA, DeMars LR, Moore D, Burke TW, Grendys EC. A phase II Gynecologic Oncology Group trial of ifosfamide and mesna in advanced or recurrent adenocarcinoma of the endometrium. Gynecol Oncol 1996; 63:25–27.

112. Wadler S, Levy DE, Lincoln ST, Soori GS, Schink JC, Goldberg G. Topotecan is an active agent in the first-line treatment of metastatic or recurrent endometrial carcinoma: Eastern Cooperative Oncology Group study E3E93. J Clin Oncol 2003; 21:2110–2114.

113. Lissoni A, Zanetta G, Losa G, et al. Phase II study of paclitaxel as salvage treatment in advanced endometrial cancer. Ann Oncol 1996; 7:861–863.

114. Thigpen JT, Blessing JA, DiSaia PJ, Yordan E, Carson LF, Evers C. A randomized comparison of doxorubicin alone versus doxorubicin plus cyclophosphamide in the management of advanced or recurrent endometrial carcinoma: a Gynecologic Oncology Group study. J Clin Oncol 1994; 12:1408–1414.

115. Thigpen JT, Brady MF, Homesley HD, Malfetano J, DuBeshter B, Burger RA, Liao S. Phase III trial of doxorubicin with or without cisplatin in advanced endometrial carcinoma: a Gynecologic Oncology Group study. J Clin Oncol 2004; 22:3902–3908.

116. Gallion HH, Brunetto VL, Cibull M, et al. Randomized phase III trial of standard timed doxorubicin plus cisplatin versus circadian timed doxorubicin plus cisplatin in stage III and IV or recurrent endometrial carcinoma: a Gynecologic Oncology Group study. J Clin Oncol 2003; 21:3808–3813.

117. Hoskins PJ, Swenerton KD, Pike JA, et al. Paclitaxel and carboplatin, alone or with irradiation, in advanced or recurrent endometrial cancer: a phase II study. J Clin Oncol 2001; 19:4048–4053.

118. Fleming GF, Brunetto VL, Cella D, et al. Phase III trial of doxorubicin plus cisplatin with or without paclitaxel plus filgrastim in advanced endometrial carcinoma: a Gynecologic Oncology Group study. J Clin Oncol 2004; 22:2159–2166.

119. Morrow CP, Bundy BN, Kurman RJ, et al. Relationship between surgical-pathological risk factors and outcome in clinical stage I and II carcinoma of the endometrium: a Gynecologic Oncology Group study. Gynecol Oncol 1991; 40:55–65.

120. Aziz H, Hussain F, Edelman S, et al. Age and race as prognostic factors in endometrial carcinoma. Am J Clin Oncol 1996; 19:595–600.

121. Bokhman JV. Two pathogenetic types of endometrial carcinoma. Gynecol Oncol 1983; 15:10–17.

122. Hoffman K, Nekhlyudov L, Deligdisch L. Endometrial carcinoma in elderly women. Gynecol Oncol 1995; 58:198–201.

123. Kupelian PA, Eifel PJ, Tornos C, et al. Treatment of endometrial carcinoma with radiation therapy alone. Int J Radiat Oncol Biol Phys 1993; 27:817–824.

124. Rose PG, Baker S, Kern M, et al. Primary radiation therapy for endometrial carcinoma: a case controlled study. Int J Radiat Oncol Biol Phys 1993; 27:585–590.

125. Chao CKS, Grigsby PW, Perez CA, et al. Medically inoperable stage I endometrial carcinoma: a few dilemmas in radiotherapeutic management. Int J Radiat Oncol Biol Phys 1996; 34:27–31.

126. Truong PT, Kader HA, Lacy B, et al. The effects of age and comorbidity on treatment and outcomes in women with endometrial cancer. Am J Clin Oncol 2005; 28:157–164.

127. Zaino RJ. Carcinoma of the vulva, urethra, and Bartholin's glands. In: Wilkinson EJ, ed. Pathology of the Vulva and Vagina. New York: Churchill Livingstone, 1987: 119–153.

128. Henson D, Tarone R. An epidemiologic study of cancer of the cervix, vagina, and vulva based on the Third National Cancer Survey in the United States. Am J Obstet Gynecol 1977; 129:525–532.

129. Nilsson T, Malmstrom H, Simonsen E, Trope C. Case report: a 16-year-old girl with invasive carcinoma in the vulva. Acta Obstet Gynecol Scand 1990; 69:551–552.

130. Moore DH, Fowler WC, Currie JL, Walton LA. Case report: squamous cell carcinoma of the vulva in pregnancy. Gynecol Oncol 1991; 41:74–77.

131. Franklin EW, Rutledge FD. Epidemiology of epidermoid carcinoma of the vulva. Obstet Gynecol 1972; 39:165.

132. Brinton LA, Nasca PC, Mallin K, et al. Case-control study of cancer of the vulva. Obstet Gynecol 1990; 75:859.

133. Thomas RHM, Ridley CM, McGibbon DH, Black MM. Lichen sclerosus et atrophicus and autoimmunity: a study of 350 women. Br J Dermatol 1988; 118:41–46.

134. Mabuchi K, Bross DS, Kessler II. Epidemiology of cancer of the vulva: a case control study. Cancer 1985; 55:1843–1848.

135. Ansink AC, Krul MRL, DeWeger RA, et al. Human papillomavirus, lichen sclerosus, and squamous cell carcinoma of the vulva: detection and prognostic significance. Gynecol Oncol 1994; 52:180.

136. Downey GO, Okagaki T, Ostrow RS, et al. Condylomatous carcinoma of the vulva with special reference to human papillomavirus DNA. Obstet Gynecol 1988; 72:68.

137. Hording U, Junge J, Daugaard S, et al. Vulvar squamous cell carcinoma and papillomaviruses: indications for two different etiologies. Gynecol Oncol 1994; 52:241–246.

138. Trimble CL, Hildesheim A, Brinton LA, et al. Heterogeneous etiology of squamous carcinoma of the vulva. Obstet Gynecol 1996; 87:59–64.

139. Trimble CL, Hildesheim A, Brinton LA, Shah KV, Kurman RJ. Heterogeneous etiology of squamous carcinoma of the vulva. Obstet Gynecol 1996; 87:59.

140. Flowers LC, Wistuba II, Scurry J, Muller CY, et al. Genetic changes during multistage pathogenesis of human papillomavirus positive and negative vulvar carcinomas. J Soc Gynecol Invest 1999; 6:213.

141. Nuovo GJ, Delvenne P, MacConnell P, et al. Correlation of histology and detection of human papillomavirus DNA in vulvar cancers. Gynecol Oncol 1991; 43:275–280.

142. Kurman RJ, Toki T, Schiffman MH. Basaloid and warty carcinoma of the vulva. Am J Surg Pathol 1993; 17:133–145.

143. Taussig FJ. An analysis of 155 cases of vulvar carcinoma. Am J Obstet Gynecol 1949; 40:764–769.

144. Way S. The anatomy of the lymphatic drainage of the vulva and its influence on the radical operation for carcinoma. Ann R Coll Surg Engl 1948; 3:187–209.

145. DiSaia PJ, Creasman WT, Rich WM. An alternative approach to early cancer of the vulva. Am J Obstet Gynecol 1979; 133:825–832.

146. Burke TJ, Levenback C, Coleman RL, et al. Surgical therapy of T1 and T2 vulvar carcinoma: further experience with radical wide excision and selective inguinal lymphadenectomy. Gynecol Oncol 1994; 57:515–520.

147. Berman ML, Soper JT, Creasman WT, et al. Conservative surgical management of superficially invasive stage I vulvar carcinoma. Gynecol Oncol 1989; 35:352–357.

148. Hacker NF, Leuchter RS, Berek JS, et al. Radical vulvectomy and bilateral inguinal lymphadenectomy through separate groin incisions. Obstet Gynecol 1981; 58:574–579.

149. Hacker NF. Current treatment of small vulvar cancers. Oncology 1990; 4:21–25.

150. Stehman FB, Bundy BN, Dvoretsky PM, Creasman WT. Early stage I carcinoma of the vulva treated with ipsilateral superficial inguinal lymphadenectomy and modified radical hemivulvectomy: a prospective study of the Gynecologic Oncology Group. Obstet Gynecol 1992; 79:490–497.

151. Homesley HD, Bundy BN, Sedlis A, Adcock L. Radiation therapy versus pelvic node resection for carcinoma of the vulva with positive groin nodes. Obstet Gynecol 1986; 68:733–740.

152. Stehman FB, Bundy BN, Thomas G, et al. Groin dissection versus groin irradiation in carcinoma of the vulva. Int J Radiat Oncol Biol Phys 1992; 24:389–396.

153. Boronow RC, Hickman BT, Reagan MT, Smith A, Steadham RE. Combined therapy as an alternative to exenteration for locally advanced vulvovaginal cancer: II. Results,

complications, and dosimetric and surgical considerations. Am J Clin Oncol 1987; 10:171.

154. Perez CA, Grigsby PW, Galakatos A, et al. Radiation therapy in management of carcinoma of the vulva with emphasis on conservative therapy. Cancer 1993; 71: 3707–3716.

155. Moore DH, Thomas GM, Montana GS, Bundy BN, Gallup DG, Olt G. Preoperative chemoradiation for advanced vulvar cancer: a phase II study of the Gynecologic Oncology Group. Int J Radiat Oncol Biol Phys 1998; 42:1317–1323.

156. Rosen C, Malmstrom H. Invasive cancer of the vulva. Gynecol Oncol 1997; 65:213–217.

157. Kouvaris JR, Kouloulias VE, Loghis CD, Balafouta EJ, Miliadou AC, Vlahos LJ. Minor prognostic factors in squamous cell vulvar carcinoma. Eur J Gynaecol Oncol 2001; 22:305–308.

158. Hyde SE, Ansink AC, Burger MP, Schilthuis MS, van der Velden J. The impact of performance status on survival in patients of 80 years and older with vulvar cancer. Gynecol Oncol 2002; 84:388–393.

159. Heatley MK. Prognostic factors associated with vulval carcinoma in women aged above and below 65 years. J Obstet Gynaecol 2003; 23:664–665.

160. Vlastos AT, Usel M, Beffa V, et al. Treatment patterns of vulvar cancer in the elderly. Surg Oncol 2004; 13:187–191.

161. Olejek A, Kozak-Darmas I, Ziolkowski A, Rembielak-Stawecka B. Surgical treatment of vulvar cancer in 101-year old patient—a case report. Ginekol Pol 2002; 73:908–912.

162. Ulutin HC, Pak Y, Dede M. Can radiotherapy be a treatment option for elderly women with invasive vulvar carcinoma without radical surgery? Eur J Gynaecol Oncol 2002; 23:426–428.

163. Townsley C, Pond GR, Peloza B, et al. Analysis of treatment practices for elderly cancer patients in Ontario, Canada. J Clin Oncol 2005; 23:3802–3810.

164. Lewis JH, Kilgore ML, Goldman DP, et al. Participation of patients 65 years of age or older in cancer clinical trials. J Clin Oncol 2003; 21:1383–1389.

165. Yee KWL, Pater JL, Pho L, Zee B, Siu LL. Enrollment of older patients in cancer treatment trials in Canada: why is age a barrier? J Clin Oncol 2003; 21:1618–1623.

16

Genitourinary Cancer

George K. Philips
Hematology/Oncology Unit, University of Vermont College of Medicine and
Fletcher Allen Health Care, Burlington, Vermont, U.S.A.

INTRODUCTION

The most common genitourinary cancers (excluding the gynecologic malignancies discussed in other chapters) are prostate, urothelial, renal, and testicular cancers, in decreasing order of frequency of occurrence as well as deaths. This group of cancers is also known as "urologic cancers." Prostate and testicular cancers (of which the vast majority are germ cell tumors) are restricted to men. Germ cell tumors (testicular typically in men) do rarely develop in women, however, and are typically of ovarian origin, but may be extragonadal in either sex. The common genitourinary cancers described above are most frequently found in older populations with the exception of testicular cancer, which typically occurs in young men. Prostate cancer is discussed elsewhere in this textbook; hence this chapter will be devoted mainly to urothelial and renal cancers with a brief account of pertinent issues in testicular tumors.

With the exception of testicular cancer, genitourinary cancers including prostate cancer have historically lagged in benefiting from a collaborative multidisciplinary approach to research, training, and patient care that has brought many advances and successes in the areas of breast, colorectal, and lung cancer in areas spanning screening, predictive risk modeling, management of early and late stage disease, and tumor biology. However, beginning in the 1990s, acceleration in the field of urologic oncology (also termed genitourinary oncology) has resulted from increased public and physician awareness of this group of cancers, rising funding levels from governmental and private sources, interdisciplinary collaboration among medical specialties, and international attention. The field has benefited from (a) strong organized voices of advocacy for testicular cancer (e.g., Lance Armstrong Foundation, www.laf.org), prostate cancer (e.g., USTOO, www.ustoo.org), and kidney cancer (National Kidney Cancer Association, www.nkca.org), (b) personal testimonials of important public figures including celebrities and politicians as well as (c) public awareness programs of the U.S. government, such as the U.S. postal stamp in support of prostate cancer (1). Strong leadership from the National Cancer Institute, broad and burgeoning interest from an increasing number of medical and radiation oncologists in addition to urologists (who in recent years have formed the Society of Urologic Oncology as well as initiated the development of postresidency fellowship training in urologic oncology), as well as developmental therapeutics within the pharmaceutical industry, are together advancing the science and practice of urologic oncology.

At the same time, similar progress in the field of geriatric oncology has led to some convergence in interest, particularly with respect to prostate cancer. However, the other genitourinary cancers have not experienced a similar focused interest in the elderly, who are therefore approached in a manner similar to younger and fitter patients, using some combination of best medical judgment and generalization from other better studied older cancer populations. However, selected age-specific information for the genitourinary cancers is available, albeit embedded in the general literature on these cancers and specific treatment modalities. The current review summarizes available general and age-specific information that will help support a rational multidisciplinary approach to older patients with these cancers.

TESTICULAR CANCER

Epidemiology and Demographics of Germ Cell Tumors

Testicular cancer is typically a cancer that occurs in young men. This includes the common varieties of germ cell tumors (seminomatous and nonseminomatous), which are uncommonly found in men above the age of 60 and rarely above the age of 70 years. This age predilection also applies to gonadal (usually ovarian) germ cell tumors in women as well as extragonadal (i.e., nontesticular) germ cell tumors, which often arise from midline structures such as the retroperitoneum and mediastinum.

Spermatocytic Seminoma

Spermatocytic seminoma is an uncommon histologic variant of testicular seminoma occurring in older men, and has an indolent course and tends to be localized to the testes (Stage I) at diagnosis, and therefore carries a particularly good prognosis following initial therapy. Ultrasound or computed tomography (CT) scanning typically shows speckled calcification within the tumor mass (2). In a series of 771 testicular seminoma patients diagnosed over a period of two decades at a single institution, 13 (1.7%) had spermatocytic histology (3). The median age was 62 years but included a few significantly younger adults. All patients had Stage I disease and not one of the five patients treated with postorchiectomy abdominal radiation or the seven who participated in a surveillance program, relapsed after a median follow-up of 8.5 years. Despite the small numbers of patients so studied with spermatocytic seminoma, a policy of surveillance following inguinal orchiectomy may be reasonably preferred with the expectation of a cure proportion approaching 100%. The rare relapse can easily be salvaged with radiation or chemotherapy with a very high probability of cure.

Treatment of Testicular Germ Cell Tumors in Older Patients

The treatment of the common testicular germ cell tumors in the elderly population has not been prospectively compared to experiences of toxicity and efficacy in younger patients. Clinical experience suggests that inguinal orchiectomy as well as pelvic and para-aortic radiation should be just as feasible and effective as in younger patients with early stage disease. For advanced or recurrent germ cell tumors, standard chemotherapy options (cisplatin, and etoposide with or without bleomycin) should be offered on the basis of prognostic classification into good risk or poor risk categories (4) and the presence of pulmonary comorbidities that would compound the risks associated with bleomycin-induced pulmonary toxicity. Based on general principles, myelosuppression can be expected to be greater in an elderly population but not prohibitively so for a highly curative chemotherapy regimen (see Chapter 5).

Survivorship Issues in Older Men

The long-term mortality after curative treatment of testicular germ cell tumors with orchiectomy and prophylactic irradiation or chemotherapy in young adults, appears to increase with time. A variety of secondary malignancies have been described in long-term survivors. Over a four-decade period of follow up of 477 men treated with curative orchiectomy and prophylactic abdominal or mediastinal irradiation for testicular seminoma, the standardized mortality ratio (SMR) was elevated nearly twofold for overall actuarial survival as well as cardiac and cancer-specific causes (5). The difference in SMR became evident mainly after 15 years of follow-up. The 10-, 20-, 30-, and 40-year actuarial survivals were 93%, 79%, 59%, and 26%, respectively, and the median age for cardiac death was 62 years (range 35–87 years) and for cancer death, 59 years (range 22–78 years). Seven secondary testicular cancers occurred between 2.3 and 12.1 years. In a second large study, cardiovascular events and deaths were found to be increased in radiation- as well as chemotherapy-treated testicular cancer patients by 10 years (6). Therefore, long-term monitoring of health status of older survivors of testicular cancer curatively treated in young adulthood, especially those who received irradiation or chemotherapy, appears to be prudent.

Among long-term survivors of unilateral testicular cancer who have undergone unilateral orchiectomy and additional treatments such as chemotherapy, the risk of hypogonadism was elevated 3.8-fold and related to the intensity of treatment (7). Hence, the syndrome of androgen deficiency in older males needs to be suspected, tested for with a serum testosterone level, and managed accordingly with androgen supplementation. Complications of hypogonadism may include anemia, muscle atrophy, sexual dysfunction, and bone mineral loss with attendant risk of osteoporotic fractures (8).

Other Testicular Cancers of Older Men

The testicular malignancies that are typically seen in older men are rare but far less easily cured. These include metastases from a variety of solid tumors as well as hematologic malignancies. However, the dominant primary tumor of the testes in older men is non-Hodgkin's lymphoma (NHL). The finding of testicular NHL, usually after orchiectomy for a testicular mass presumed to be a germ cell tumor, should always lead to a complete standard staging workup for lymphoma including bone marrow biopsy. The Sheffield Lymphoma Group reported on 30 patients seen over three decades, with a median age of 74 years (range 38–87) with 63% being over 70 years of age and all patients having had orchiectomy as the initial procedure (9). The International Extranodal Lymphoma Study Group retrospectively examined the clinical features and outcome of 373 primary testicular diffuse, large B-cell lymphomas (10). Most presentations were of early Stage I or II disease diagnosed at a median age of 66 years (19–91). Median overall survival was 4.8 years without a clear plateau to suggest a cured fraction. However, favorable prognostic factors included low international prognostic index score, absence of B-symptoms, use of anthracyclines, and prophylactic

Table 1 Approach to Testicular Cancer in the Elderly

Testicular germ cell tumors are rare in an older age group with the exception of spermatocytic
  seminoma, which carries an excellent prognosis for cure with surveillance for Stage I disease
Testicular NHL is found more often in the elderly and has a poor prognosis even in early
  stages. Multimodality treatment is recommended
Survivors of testicular cancers have a higher rate of cardiac events and increased cardiac
  mortality decades after initial curative treatment and require long-term follow-up for
  cardiovascular and cancer events as well as hypogonadism
The general approach to treatment of germ cell tumors in the elderly should follow the same
  principles as in younger patients with curative intent

Abbreviation: NHL, non-Hodgkin's lymphoma.

scrotal radiotherapy. Fifty-two percent of patients had relapsed by 7.6 years, most
commonly at extranodal sites (140/195 relapses) with a persistent risk of recurrence
in the contralateral testis in patients not given scrotal radiotherapy. In summary, stage
for stage, primary testicular NHL appears to carry a poorer long-term prognosis and
a reduced chance of cure relative to nodal and other extranodal sites of NHL. A multimodal treatment approach is strongly recommended.

Key issues regarding testicular cancer in the elderly are summarized in Table 1.

UROTHELIAL CARCINOMA (BLADDER CANCER)

Epidemiology

Urothelial carcinoma includes epithelial cancers of the urinary tract comprising the
renal pelvis, ureters, bladder, and urethra. Bladder cancer is a disease of older persons and is the second most common genitourinary cancer in the United States after
prostate cancer. The American Cancer Society estimated that in 2005, there would be
63,210 new diagnoses of bladder cancer (excluding the smaller numbers arising from
the remaining urothelial tract) and 13,180 deaths in the United States (11). This
represents approximately 4.5% of all cancers and cancer deaths. Compared to
women, men develop bladder cancer three times as often (47,010 vs. 16,200 projected
for 2005) and die twice as often from bladder cancer (8970 vs. 4210 in 2005). Based
on the U.S. National Cancer Institute's Surveillance Epidemiology and End Results
(SEER) program, the majority of cases of bladder cancer occur in the sixth to eighth
decades of life, with only about 17% of cases occurring before 55 years of age and
11% above the age of 85 (12). The median ages at diagnosis and death were 73
and 78 years, respectively, across all races and genders.

Tumor Biology, Histology, and Etiology

About 90% of bladder and other urothelial tract cancers arising from the epithelial
lining of the urinary tract are histologically classified as "transitional cell" carcinomas. The remainder is comprised of squamous, adenocarcinoma, and small cell
carcinoma histologies (13). Occasionally mixed histologies of various carcinomas
albeit usually with a dominant "transitional cell" histology are seen. It is now
suggested that the term "transitional cell" be replaced by "urothelial" carcinoma.
Nonepithelial tumors of the urinary tract such as lymphomas, sarcomas, and pheo-
chromocytomas, as well as metastases to the bladder are quite rare.

Cigarette smoking is the strongest etiologic risk factor for the development of urothelial carcinoma, causing field cancerization of the uroepithelium with a latency period of about two decades. Cigarette smoking accounts for one-third to half of all bladder cancers, but workers in the dye, rubber, leather, paint, and metalworking occupations may have elevated risks (14). Chronic inflammation induced by the use of chronic indwelling urinary catheters by patients with spinal cord injury is associated with the development of squamous cell carcinoma of the bladder, perhaps in up to 10% of patients after 10 years (15). Bilharzial bladder cancer, which is associated with infestation with *Schistosoma hematobium*, is common in endemic zones of the Middle East, Africa, Asia, and South America, but is most prevalent in Egypt where about 60% of all bladder cancers are of squamous histology. Bilharzial squamous cell carcinoma of the bladder occurs in the seventh decade of life (compared to the fifth decade of life in the uncommon nonbilharzial squamous carcinoma in Western countries), and tends to present at a more advanced stage (16). Fluid intake, regardless of type of beverage, appeared to protect (relative risk of 0.49) against the development of bladder cancer in the prospective Health Professionals Follow-Up study (17). Elimination of smoking and, possibly, reduction of arsenic in the water supply, appear to reverse the risk of bladder cancer over decades (18). In the absence of a prospective randomized trial with any of a variety of urine tests available for early detection, there is no widely available and universally recommended screening test or policy for the early detection of bladder cancer in healthy individuals. Voided urine NMP22 is a Food and Drug Administration (FDA)–approved test for screening for recurrent bladder cancer after transurethral resection, which complements cystoscopy moderately well and is economically viable (19–21). A new point-of-care proteomic assay for urinary NMP22 showed a sensitivity of 56% and specificity of 86% compared to 16% and 99%, respectively for urine cytology (22). In the absence of a proven test for mass screening, a low threshold of suspicion of the presence of bladder cancer in the event of unexplained gross or microscopic hematuria is a prudent recommendation in older individuals. In this situation, further evaluation would include urine cytology or referral to a urologist for cystoscopy.

Diagnosis and Staging

Over 90% of urothelial tract carcinomas occur in the bladder with most of the remainder arising from the renal pelvis and less than 2% from the ureter or proximal two-thirds of the urethra. Ureteral and renal pelvic origins are denoted as "upper tract" disease. Less than 10% of urothelial carcinomas present with metastatic disease, while of the remainder, about two-thirds present with low-risk superficial disease and one-third with muscle-invasive disease. However, approximately one-third of patients with superficial disease will progress to muscle-invasive disease, and a substantial proportion of the latter (~30–60%) will have recurrence with metastatic disease. The most common diagnostic procedures employed in the initial evaluation of bladder cancer are urine cytology, cystoscopy, and/or retrograde ureteroscopy, CT scan of the abdomen and pelvis, and intravenous pyelogram to rule out "upper tract" disease. Once anatomical localization is accomplished by direct visualization or imaging studies, pathologic confirmation is obtained by transurethral biopsy or complete resection of a cystoscopically accessible tumor. For renal masses representing invasive renal pelvic urothelial carcinomas, pathologic diagnosis is obtained by urine cytology or percutaneous CT-guided biopsy, and can usually be readily distinguished from primary renal cell carcinomas. All these procedures can be expected to be well tolerated in elderly patients; however, if renal function is compromised on the basis of age, comorbidity, and urinary outflow tract obstruction by tumor, the use of intravenous contrast should be reconsidered in the diagnostic evaluation.

Imaging studies [chest X ray, CT, or magnetic resonance imaging (MRI) scan of abdomen and pelvis, and bone scan] and the pathologic findings of the initial tumor support staging of urothelial carcinomas. Positron emission tomography does not have an established role in the evaluation of bladder cancer (23). The newer tumor node metastase (TNM) staging for urothelial carcinoma has replaced the older Jewett system (24), although both recognize the prognostic importance and therapeutic relevance of depth of invasion of the primary tumor, as well as nodal and distant metastatic involvement. There is no known association between patient age at presentation and stage of disease at presentation. Upper tract lesions tend to have a more advanced stage and grade at presentation (25). The 1997 TNM staging (26) definitions for bladder cancer are summarized below along with the five-year overall survival by stage grouping.

Primary tumor (T)

 TX Primary tumor cannot be assessed
 TO No evidence of primary tumor
 Ta Noninvasive papillary carcinoma
 Tis Carcinoma in situ: "flat tumor"
 T1 Tumor invades subepithelial connective tissue
 T2 Tumor invades muscle
   T2a Tumor invades superficial muscle (inner half)
   T2b Tumor invades deep muscle (outer half)
 T3 Tumor invades perivesical tissue
   T3a Microscopically
   T3b Macroscopically (extravesical mass)
T4 Tumor invades any of the following: prostate, uterus, vagina, pelvic wall, abdominal wall
 T4a Tumor invades prostate, uterus, vagina
 T4b Tumor invades pelvic wall, abdominal wall

Regional lymph nodes (N)[a]

 NX Regional lymph nodes cannot be assessed
 N0 No regional lymph node metastasis
 N1 Metastasis in a single lymph node, 2 cm or less in greatest dimension
 N2 Metastasis in a single lymph node, more than 2 cm but not more than 5 cm in greatest dimension; or multiple lymph nodes, none more than 5 cm in greatest dimension
 N3 Metastasis in a lymph node more than 5 cm in greatest dimension

Distant metastasis (M)

 MX distant metastasis cannot be assessed
 M0 No distant metastasis
 M1 Distant metastasis

Stage grouping				Approximate five-year survival %	
0a	Ta	N0	M0	(Stage 0)	> 90
0is	Tis	N0	M0		
I	T1	N0	M0	(Stage I)	> 80
II	T2	N0	M0	(Stage II)	40–70
	T3a	N0	M0		
III	T3b	N0	M0	(Stage III)	10–30
	T4a	N0	M0		

(Continued)

(Continued)

Stage grouping				Approximate five-year survival %	
IV	T4b	N0	M0	(Stage IV)	< 10
	Any	T N1	M0		
	Any	T N2	M0		
	Any	T N3	M0		
	Any	T N	M1		

[a]Regional lymph nodes are those within the true pelvis; all others are distant lymph nodes.

Management of Urothelial Carcinoma

The initial care of a patient with urothelial carcinoma is often undertaken by a urologist and if only superficial disease is discovered, then transurethral resection and periodic surveillance with cystoscopies with repeated resections as necessary is continued. However, patients with muscle-invasive and more advanced urothelial carcinomas are best served by a multidisciplinary team consisting additionally of a radiation and medical oncologist because of evolving multidisciplinary standards of care and broadening treatment options. In these more advanced stages, treatment options tend to be more complex and multimodal, toxicities have the potential to interact with age, and attention to age-associated comorbidities is necessary to establish a management plan with an optimal risk–benefit ratio that is also respectful of patient preferences. However, in general, older age by itself does not indicate a poor prognosis, for the disease or a substantially lower likelihood of benefiting from standard interventions. The management of bladder cancer is the paradigm for management of cancers arising from other parts of the urothelial tract and is broadly divided into treatment approaches to superficial, muscle-invasive, and advanced (metastatic) disease.

Superficial Bladder Cancer

Superficial disease (Ta, Tis, and T1) carries a good prognosis, although two-thirds of patients will experience a recurrence (usually superficial) and up to one-third of patients will progress to muscle-invasive disease over the long term (27). Standard initial therapy is to achieve maximal transurethral resection of bladder tumor performed under general anesthesia, with the goal of eradicating the tumor, which is feasible in most elderly patients. Serious complications are rare but may include severe or prolonged hematuria and bladder perforation. Unfortunately, the natural history of superficial bladder cancer despite effective intervention is characterized by recurrence, the prognostic factors for which include high tumor grade (G3 vs. G1 or G2), depth (T1 vs. Ta), pattern of recurrences (frequency), and in some studies, over-expression of p53 or the epidermal growth factor receptor (EGFR) (28–32). The goal of intravesical therapy in high-risk superficial disease is either treatment of residual disease (e.g., Tis) to eliminate it, or adjuvant therapy to reduce the future development of recurrent or progressive disease and the need for cystectomy.

Muscle-Invasive Bladder Cancer

Radical Cystectomy

In the United States, radical cystectomy has traditionally been the preferred approach for definitive treatment of muscle-invasive bladder cancer, although radiation therapy is not infrequently employed in Europe and elsewhere (33). Radical cystectomy is a major abdominal operative procedure performed under general anesthesia with a perioperative mortality averaging about 2% to 3% and significant perioperative morbidity, prolonged time to recovery, and learning to cope with the urinary diversion procedure. However, the operation may not be as frequently performed in the elderly especially in non–tertiary health care settings because of a concern for surgical mortality and morbidity. At centers of excellence in the developing world, postoperative mortality is significant at about 5% (of 41) for patients above 70 years of age and 8.6% (of 197) for younger patients (34). In an important pattern of care study using a Medicare database for patients above 65 years of age, cystectomy was shown to confer a substantial survival benefit (35). Yet, cystectomy rates in Stage II and III disease declined from about 60% (of 1991 patients) in a "big metro" area to 23% in "metro" areas to 2% in rural areas. Furthermore, the second most common treatment strategy in this older population was no treatment at all, including no chemotherapy or radiation. Cystectomy was performed more often (24–31%) in men between the ages of 65 and 74 years compared to those 75 to 79 years (13%) and patients 85 or older (5%), and was strikingly associated inversely with the presence of comorbidity. In 404 patients aged 70 years or older (median 74 years) undergoing radical cystectomy at the University of Southern California by experienced urologists between 1971 and 1996, the postoperative mortality rate was 3% (11/762) among patients aged 70 to 79 years and 0% (0/52) in those aged 80 plus. Although overall survival was slightly less among these elderly patients compared to an under-70 cohort, presumably from other comorbidities, bladder cancer recurrence rates were the same suggesting a similar efficacy for the operation in elderly patients. However, early postoperative complications were more common in the elderly (32% vs. 25%). In an updated analysis at the same institution, elderly patients were more likely to have extravesical disease, less likely to receive adjuvant chemotherapy, and not surprisingly experienced a higher risk of disease recurrence; however, rates of nodal involvement and p53 mutation were similar across age groups (36). In a contemporary health department community-based survey of 8228 operated patients in England, in-hospital mortality (in the context of an average length of stay of 19 days) following a radical cystectomy rose from 1.6% among patients younger than 60 years, to 3.6% among patients in their 60s, to 6.3% in patients in their 70s and 10.3% for those at least 80 years old, along with longer hospital stays (37). In a number of case series of radical cystectomy since the 1970s, performed by a single surgeon or at a single institution with fewer than 100 elderly patients studied per series, perioperative mortality ranged from 0% to 6% and perioperative morbidity ranged as high as 60% (38–46). Perioperative morbidity and mortality tended to be somewhat higher in these series than in younger patients. Typical complications (which frequently prolonged hospitalization) included urine leak, intestinal anastomotic leak, acute renal failure, cardiovascular or thromboembolic events, and infections. Comorbidities at baseline were frequent and hospitalization frequently exceeded one week. Nevertheless, these authors felt that radical cystectomy was a viable and valuable treatment option that should, with judicious patient selection, be offered to elderly patients including those in their 80s. Therefore, age alone should not represent a barrier to patients otherwise suitable for radical cystectomy. The experience of the center as well as the surgeon may play a role in maintaining optimal outcomes for radical cystectomy in the elderly, particularly for in-hospital mortality, length of stay, and cost of the procedure (47). The fact that authors of surgical series advocate radical cystectomy in the elderly, while this practice is avoided in a community-based study (48), indirectly suggests a possible impact of the practice environment on outcomes following radical cystectomy.

Neoadjuvant and adjuvant chemotherapy have been used more frequently in recent years owing to emerging data from randomized clinical trials indicating a modest but real overall survival advantage (33,49–51). The chemotherapy regimens used are generally those found to be effective in the metastatic setting, such as the combination of methotrexate, vinblastine, doxorubicin (Adriamycin®) and cisplatin (MVAC), cyclophosphamide, mitoxantrone, and vinblastine, or cisplatin plus gemcitabine (GC). These regimens are given for three to four cycles and are generally associated with less morbidity and mortality (0–1%) than when given in the metastatic setting (33,50). In the two large randomized trials of neoadjuvant chemotherapy, the greatest number of enrollees were in their 60s, with a significant proportion in their 70s and a small number in their 80s (33,50). Furthermore, despite the generally appreciated higher risk of chemotherapy-induced toxicity in the elderly, this did not interfere with the ability of patients to undergo planned radical cystectomy in the neoadjuvant chemotherapy arms of the trials except in the rare event of death (33,50). Therefore, age alone is not a barrier to a patient receiving neoadjuvant or adjuvant chemotherapy in conjunction with a radical cystectomy or radiation therapy.

Radiation Therapy

Radical radiation therapy is less widely accepted for curative treatment of muscle-invasive bladder cancer in the United States, although bladder cancer is highly sensitive to radiation therapy and lends itself to organ preservation strategies (52). Radical radiation with or without neoadjuvant or concurrent chemotherapy is a valid and feasible treatment strategy for organ preservation in patients who are averse to urinary diversion procedures and motivated by quality of life considerations (53,54). There has been no definitive randomized controlled trial comparing radical cystectomy to initial radiation therapy in establishing equivalence for cancer control, survival, or quality of life. In the absence of such evidence, radiation has been frequently reserved for frail or older patients, or those with significant comorbidities (55,56). Radiation therapy–based treatment strategies generally yield a complete response rate of 50% to 70% as well as bladder preservation in 50% to 80% of the survivors, an overall five-year survival of about 40% to 50%, with about 30% to 40% of patients alive with an intact bladder at five years. Deaths are more often due to development of distant metastases and competing causes and not from local recurrence in the intact bladder, which can be effectively salvaged by cystectomy.

The outcome of radiation-based (including chemoradiation for bladder preservation) treatment is dependent on case selection, use of radiosensitizing chemotherapy, and tumor-related prognostic factors. Selective bladder preservation is typically undertaken at tertiary care centers with strong multimodality teams (53,57). Patients in radiation-based series may be understaged compared to surgical series because of less sensitive detection of extravesical and nodal involvement by imaging compared to pathologic examination, leading to a case selection bias favoring surgical series. On the other hand, unlike older radiation series (54), modern bladder preservation series are more likely to exclude patients with bulky local disease or substantial extravesical spread, hydronephrosis from ureteral obstruction, and those without a maximal or visibly complete transurethral resection of tumor, which would favor long-term outcome in a radiation-based series. In a randomized trial, the concurrent use of single-agent cisplatin chemotherapy has been shown to improve complete response rates and enhance local control (i.e., reduce pelvic failure) without affecting distant metastatic spread (58). Although more complex combination chemotherapy regimens using cisplatin, methotrexate, vinblastine, fluorouracil, and paclitaxel have been employed with acceptable toxicity prior to or concurrent with radiation in selective bladder preservation programs, the added value of these more complex regimens to local and distant cancer control has not been established in randomized controlled trials (57,59–61). Hyperfractionated radiation, which may improve local control over once-daily fractionation schedules, has also been used with acceptable tolerability in multicenter studies (57,60). The common toxicities associated with radiation therapy are irritative bladder and bowel symptoms, skin reactions, erectile dysfunction, and fatigue. Rarely a cystectomy or partial bowel resection is required for late but severe mucosal damage causing bleeding from a friable surface or bladder contracture (54,62). Cost, complexity, and intensity of long-term monitoring for recurrence are higher with a bladder preservation approach than with radical cystectomy, particularly because salvage cystectomy may be required for recurrence even up to 10 years following chemoradiation (53,63). The increasing use of an orthotopic neobladder instead of a diverting ileostomy reduces the attractiveness of a bladder-sparing approach with respect to preserving the native bladder to enhance quality of life. Furthermore, the use of neoadjuvant full-dose systemic combination chemotherapy as part of a bladder preservation protocol is occasionally associated with significant toxicity, including a few deaths from neutropenic sepsis (4%), and coronary and venous thromboembolic events and Grade 3 or 4 toxicity in half the patients in one multi-institutional trial cooperative group trial (60). Therefore, although age is not a contraindication to a bladder preservation approach, patient and regimen selection is critical to successful implementation of a bladder preservation protocol. In this context, it is important to note that adjuvant (i.e., following chemoradiation) chemotherapy is now being introduced in more recent bladder preservation protocols, and preliminary evidence suggests that it is feasible although moderately toxic especially with respect to myelosuppression (60).

Prognostic factors for outcome after radiation or chemoradiation for muscle-invasive bladder cancer include tumor stage (62,64–66), Her-2 and epidermal growth factor receptor (EGFR) expression (67), completeness of transurethral resection of tumor (54), performance status (62), and achievement of complete remission (68). Older patients have a poorer overall survival in major part from competing causes of death, as well as poorer tolerance of therapy and possibly more aggressive tumor biology leading to a greater risk of recurrence (64,65,68).

Results of radiation therapy in elderly or frail ("unfit") patients have been variable. In 36 radical radiotherapy–treated patients between 71 and 89 years of age with an Eastern Cooperative Oncology Group (ECOG) performance status of 0 or 1, the median survival was two years, toxicity was low, and a trend to better survival with an accelerated compared to conventional dose schedule was noted (69). Among 89 patients deemed too old or frail for conventional radiation, a split-course schedule was used to treat T1–T4 bladder cancer with 10 to 12 fractions of a mean dose of 45 Gray over a mean of 48 days (70). Complete remission was achieved in 31% of patients; acute mild radiation reaction reactions occurred in 60% of patients but only 8% experienced Grade 2 to 3 toxicity. In 94 patients with a median age of 78 years given split-course radiation with a two-week break to a total dose of about 60 Gray in six weeks, median survival was only 13.9 months and half the patients were hospitalized for acute gastrointestinal or urogenital toxicity (71). Higher T-stage, poorer tolerance of therapy (defined as hospitalization for toxicity), and a better performance status influenced survival. In a retrospective review of 45 patients with a median age of 75 years (72–87), with a Charlson comorbidity index (which accounts for age) score of more than 2, external beam radiation with continuous daily fractionation (~190 cgy/day) was given with curative intent to a total dose of 60 Gray to the bladder and regional nodes (72). Modest toxicity without any hospitalization was observed and a median survival of 21.5 months was achieved. In summary, conventional and alternate schedules of external radiation with curative or palliative intent are feasible in elderly or frail patients, with achievement of clinically meaningful outcomes with respect to tumor control; however, survival, and sometimes tolerance, is poor in this cohort at least in part owing to adverse case selection bias.

Chemoradiation alone or as part of a bladder preservation strategy is certainly feasible in older patients in the seventh and eighth and even ninth decades of life, and such patients have been included in these protocols and can be expected to achieve similar benefits as younger patients when matched for performance status and tumor stage (33,54,58,61,73). Although somewhat lower tolerance to both radiation and chemotherapy is likely compared with younger patients, age alone does not constitute adequate reason to determine feasibility of treatment; rather performance status, frailty, comorbidities, patient preferences and goals, and tumor characteristics (tumor stage, ureteral obstruction, etc.) should bear on the choice between radiation alone, a bladder preservation approach, or a radical cystectomy. Indeed, as a purely palliative procedure, radiation alone is highly effective at rapidly controlling gross hematuria from a bladder tumor (74,75).

Muscle-invasive bladder cancer is a potentially curable disease state for which several treatment options are available even for the elderly population. However, judicious application of an optimal treatment requires multidisciplinary collaboration to capture all the available options, especially for the very old or frail patient. "Upper tract" muscle-invasive disease arising from the renal pelvis or ureter is treated using the same general principles as for bladder cancer but typically nephroureterectomy is the standard curative approach.

Metastatic (Advanced) Urothelial Carcinoma

Advanced urothelial carcinoma is incurable with a median survival despite therapy ranging from 12 to 18 months and fewer than 15% of treated patients alive at five years (76–78). While about a third of patients present with de novo metastatic disease, the majority experience distant recurrences occurring several years after definitive therapy for muscle-invasive disease. These patients are frequently elderly with significant comorbidities, occasionally have a history of hydronephrosis or ureteral obstruction by bladder tumor, and some have had urinary tract manipulations or instrumentation for urinary diversion procedures or have undergone prior nephroureterectomy for "upper tract" primary tumors. Consequently, up to a third of patients at presentation may have renal dysfunction defined as an abnormal serum creatinine or a creatinine clearance below 50 mL/min.

Age and Prognostic Factors

Neither age nor renal function have been shown to impact survival of patients with metastatic urothelial carcinoma treated with MVAC at a single institution (79). However, Karnofsky performance status and the presence of visceral metastases (to liver, lung, or bone as opposed to nodal metastases) were identified as powerful independent prognostic factors for both response and overall survival (79). These findings have been duplicated in clinical trial series of patients treated with cisplatin and gemcitabine (78), cisplatin and docetaxel (80), carboplatin and gemcitabine (80), or the combination of cisplatin, paclitaxel, and gemcitabine (81). These prognostic factors play a powerful role through case selection bias in defining the tumor response and survival outcomes observed in Phase II trials. A drift in performance status criteria and case selection over the decades has tended to favor improved outcomes in modern series. Compared to older trials that allowed patients with an ECOG performance status (ECOG PS) of 3 to be entered (82,83), some modern trials are dominated by patients with an ECOG PS of 0 to 1 (84). Bajorin has suggested that a predictive model based on the distribution of two prognostic factors—performance status and visceral metastases—in a clinical trial cohort of advanced urothelial cancer patients treated with chemotherapy, can assist in the interpretation of Phase II trial results and establish whether the new regimen warrants testing in a Phase III randomized trial (85). Such a process could improve the process of rational selection of promising new treatment regimens and through such efficiencies, potentially hasten improvements in the standard of care, given the limited number of patients with advanced urothelial cancer who are available to participate in clinical trials. Although age has no independent prognostic value, age-based selection into clinical trials may occur indirectly. For example, trials incorporating the nephrotoxic agent, cisplatin, have typically required "adequate" renal function usually defined by a calculated creatinine clearance exceeding 40 to 60 mL/min, criteria which are less likely to be met at older ages (83,86,87). Only rarely has an explicit upper age limit been placed on clinical trial entry, e.g., 80 years (86). Age-associated comorbidities can compound the toxicity experiences of such patients treated with chemotherapy. A small but significant number of patients treated with combination chemotherapy for metastatic bladder cancer can develop deep venous thrombosis and pulmonary embolism (88), as well as cerebrovascular ischemic events.

Standard Chemotherapy Regimens

The standard current chemotherapy regimens for advanced urothelial carcinoma have been determined through carefully conducted randomized clinical trials over the past two decades. The addition of cisplatin to methotrexate plus vinblastine conferred a survival benefit (89). Carboplatin has shown inferior results to cisplatin for response and survival in otherwise similar combination regimens (90,91). Until recently, the standard combination chemotherapy regimen was MVAC, based on its superiority for survival compared to single-agent cisplatin (77,83); the combination of cisplatin, cyclophosphamide, and doxorubicin (86); as well as docetaxel plus cisplatin (92). The cisplatin–gemcitabine combination has in recent years become an accepted practice following a randomized controlled trial that demonstrated less toxicity including myelosuppression, hospitalizations, supportive care needs, and toxic deaths (1% vs. 3%) for this regimen, but with similar survival (13.8 months vs. 14.8 months) and response proportions (49% vs. 46%) compared to MVAC (87). However, a critical analysis of the noninferiority design of this trial calls for caution in assumptions of equivalence of the two regimens for prolonging survival in advanced urothelial carcinoma (93). Dose-escalated MVAC did not show superiority over standard-dose MVAC for survival but patients in the high-dose arm of the trial that used colony-stimulating factor support, experienced less hematologic toxicity (94). The additional survival benefits for triple-agent chemotherapy regimens (81,84,95) await testing in randomized controlled trials that are ongoing. The benefits of addition of any of the new classes of molecularly and mechanism-targeted agents to a standard chemotherapy regimen remains unknown.

Treatment Regimens for Elderly, "Unfit," or Renally Impaired Patients

Because advanced urothelial cancer patients are frequently elderly or have renal dysfunction, trials of chemotherapy regimens specifically directed at this population have been conducted. Because of the known nephrotoxicity of cisplatin, these regimens have often included carboplatin dosed to an area-under-the-curve of 4.5 to 6, or other agents without a substantial urinary excretion profile, such as the taxanes or gemcitabine either in combination with carboplatin or as "non-platinum doublets." It should be remembered that non–cisplatin containing chemotherapy regimens have never been shown to confer a survival benefit, and that the accumulated evidence to date suggests that response and survival are potentially worse with carboplatin- (89–91) and taxane-containing (92,96,97) regimens. Therefore, such regimens should be employed in a palliative context with expectations of an objective response in the 30% to 60% range. Clearly, regimens employing a combination of carboplatin and gemcitabine (98–100), carboplatin and paclitaxel (101–106), gemcitabine plus either paclitaxel or docetaxel (107–112), or an anthracycline (113,114) have either been shown to be feasible or are potentially so in older patients or those with moderate degrees of renal dysfunction. The major toxicity of most of these regimens is myelosuppression however, and older patients are particularly susceptible to this and related complications. Platinum plus gemcitabine-based regimens are notable for significant thrombocytopenia; however, platelet transfusions are generally unnecessary (87). In an exploratory analysis of a large cohort of patients with advanced urothelial carcinoma treated with cisplatin and non–cisplatin containing regimens, there was a significantly higher risk of Grade 3 or 4 neutropenia (55% vs. 37%), as well as nephrotoxicity (28% vs. 10%) among patients more than 70 years old versus those younger, but survival for the two age cohorts was similar (80). Other toxicities of concern, particularly in the elderly, would be cisplatin-induced ototoxicity and cisplatin- or paclitaxel-induced neuropathy, which could interact adversely with preexisting medical conditions, frailty, and disabilities.

In summary, suitable single-agent or combination chemotherapy regimes are available for the treatment of advanced urothelial carcinoma in older or renally impaired patients. These regimens probably do not confer a survival benefit and are associated with an increased risk of toxicity in the elderly; hence judicious selection of a chemotherapy regimen appropriate to individual age, comorbidities, and patient preferences is necessary to match the goals of an individualized palliative care plan. Neutropenia and its complications may be ameliorated by the use of granulocyte colony-stimulating factor (115). The successful incorporation of less toxic molecularly targeted agents into treatment programs may facilitate achievement of an improved therapeutic ratio. Such efforts are ongoing and are based on the rich molecular targets widely present in urothelial carcinoma such as the EGFR that could potentially be exploited therapeutically (116–118).

Key issues in the management of urothelial carcinoma in the elderly are summarized in Table 2.

KIDNEY CANCER

Presentation

Renal cell carcinoma, even until the late 1990s, has invited a nihilistic view of its relentlessly downward course in the metastatic setting, although at the same time, surprising observers with its unusual behavior such as spontaneous regression,

Table 2 Approach to Urothelial Cancer in the Elderly

Urothelial carcinomas frequently occur in the elderly; however, age is not an independent
prognostic factor for cancer control at any stage
Radical cystectomy for muscle-invasive disease is associated with a small increase in
perioperative morbidity and mortality in older patients, but nevertheless is an effective and
feasible curative procedure in many patients
Multidisciplinary collaboration is necessary to facilitate perioperative chemotherapy, bladder
preservation chemoradiation approaches, or radical radiation alone for muscle-invasive
disease
Survival in metastatic urothelial carcinoma is governed by the presence of visceral metastases
and performance status and not by age
Chemotherapy for advanced urothelial carcinoma is associated with a greater risk of
nephrotoxicity and myelosuppression in the elderly; however, suitable non-nephrotoxic
regimens have been designed for these populations

prolonged periods of disease stability in occasional patients, resistance to chemotherapy but sensitivity to immunologic intervention (119). With the widespread use of abdominal imaging and the frequent finding of incidental renal masses, the classic presentation with the triad of flank pain, gross hematuria, and a palpable abdominal mass occurs less than 20% of the time although this probably remains more common in the developing world where up to half the patients may still present in this manner (120). Therefore, in modern health care settings, the key evaluative issues surround the radiographic evaluation of renal cysts or masses for possible malignancy, which have been extensively reviewed (121–123). Other common presenting symptoms of the "Internist's tumor" include a number of paraneoplastic syndromes such as weight loss, fever, anemia, hypertension, hypercalcemia, erythrocytosis (polycythemia secondary to erythropoietin overproduction), and nonmetastatic elevation in liver function tests also known as Stauffer's syndrome (124–126). The approach to the management of renal cell carcinoma should ideally be undertaken by a team, in particular a urologist and medical oncologist, that has a special understanding of the natural history of this peculiar cancer as well as experience with the unconventional interventions that are known to be effective for the management of this disease especially in the metastatic setting (Table 3).

Epidemiology and Etiology

In the United States, renal cell carcinoma was estimated to be diagnosed in 22,080 men (with 7870 deaths) and 13,630 women (with 4610 deaths). Its global burden is expected to be similarly low relative to other common cancers (breast, colorectal, and lung), which are roughly 10 times as frequent. Nevertheless, the incidence of kidney cancer has been rising steadily in the United States for inexplicable reasons. Between 1975 and 1995, the incidence of renal cell carcinoma increased by 2.3% yearly among white men, 3.1% among white women, 3.9% among black men, and 4.3% among black women (127). The annual incidence is marginally higher in African-Americans than Caucasians, but nearly twice as common in men as it is in women. Because of a simultaneous fall in renal pelvis carcinoma (which is subsumed under the "kidney cancer" site in the SEER categorization) and the overall rise in renal cell carcinoma mortality, this epidemiologic trend cannot be explained solely by more frequent detection of early tumors secondary to the widespread use of abdominal imaging studies (127). The reasons for the steady and continued rise in

Table 3 Approach to Kidney Cancer in the Elderly

The prognosis of kidney cancer at all stages appears to be independent of age and all interventions should be assumed to have similar benefits in older patients. A nihilistic approach to the disease is not warranted at any age

Radical nephrectomy with curative intent is easily performed without excessive perioperative mortality in older patients. A laparoscopic procedure may be especially advantageous to the older patient

Elderly patients are candidates for a variety of systemic therapies for metastatic disease. However, the use of high dose interleukin 2 regimens may be restricted by its toxicities, which can be prohibitive in the presence of organ dysfunction or comorbidities prevalent in the elderly

Management considerations for advanced disease in older patients should include observation, interferon alpha, cytoreductive nephrectomy, resection of a solitary metastasis, zoledronic acid for bony metastasis, and participation in clinical trials

Fascinating information regarding the genetics and biology of clear cell carcinoma is emerging, for which promising molecularly targeted agents are being tested in ongoing clinical trials

---

renal cell carcinoma remain unknown. The population burden of renal cancer is too low to justify mass screening. In an asymptomatic older cohort of patients in an aneurysm mass screening study who underwent abdominal ultrasonography, in 6678 subjects (U.S. veterans aged 50–79 years) simple renal cysts were found in 9.4% and solid lesions in 0.33% (128). The mean age for the 15 pathologically confirmed renal cell carcinoma patients was 69 (61–81) with a mean tumor diameter of 5.8 cm; 13 had clear cell histology and three died of recurrence within two years. These tumor characteristics are not substantially different from an unscreened population and the low detection rate does not support the use of a screening strategy. Furthermore, the rate of previously unsuspected kidney cancer detected only at autopsy is less than 1% (129).

Although the approximate median age at diagnosis (across gender and ethnicity) is 65 years and the median age at death is 71 years in the National Cancer Institute's SEER database for 1998–2002, it should be noted that 26% of cases are diagnosed between the ages of 65 and 74 years, 20% between 75 and 84, and 6% at age 85 and older (130).

The major risk factors for the development of renal cell carcinoma are the presence of a somatic mutation for the von Hippel Lindau (VHL) gene on chromosome 3 (100-fold relative risk) as well as chronic dialysis (32-fold relative risk) (125). Other risk factors such as smoking, obesity (131), family history, and hypertension have far more modest associations (1.5-fold–3-fold relative risk), but may contribute a larger number of cases in the population because of the widespread prevalence of these exposure factors. Whether reversal of population obesity and smoking trends will be associated with a decline in the disease is unclear.

Histology, Biology, and Genetic Syndromes

The four main histologic types of renal cell carcinoma are clear cell (75%), papillary (15%), chromophobe (5%), and oncocytoma (3–5%). Occasionally, urothelial (transitional cell) carcinoma of the renal pelvis may mimic a renal mass through direct extension into the renal parenchyma. However, rarer noncarcinoma histologies such as lymphoma or plasmacytoma, solid tumor metastasis, and soft tissue sarcoma, some of which require a different approach than a radical nephrectomy, also lie in the differential diagnosis of a renal mass.

Clear cell carcinoma is characterized by its origin in proximal tubular cells, loss of the VHL tumor suppressor gene, and deregulation of the hypoxia inducible factor (HIF)-mediated gene transcription leading to overexpression of vascular endothelial growth factor and an array of other growth factors that represent potential targets for intervention (132). Clear cell and Type I and Type II papillary cell carcinomas are associated with classic genetic syndromes with characteristic phenotypic expression (positive family history with multiple bilateral renal tumors) by disrupting the VHL, c-met, and Birt Hogg Dube tumor suppressor genes, respectively, which have been the subject of an excellent recent review (133).

Diagnosis, Staging, and Prognostic Factors

The pathologic diagnosis of localized renal cell carcinoma in the United States is frequently made at radical nephrectomy because of concerns that in less than 1% of cases, a diagnostic needle biopsy or fine needle aspirate will lead to tumor seeding of the needle track. As a consequence, however, pathologic findings will rarely reveal a relatively benign lesion such as oncocytoma or a lymphoma, for which nephrectomy may not have been justifiable as the optimal treatment. While paraaortic lymph node sampling or dissection at the time of radical nephrectomy can provide prognostic information, it has no therapeutic value and so is not consistently performed. The conventional initial evaluation for diagnosis and staging includes urinalysis, urine cytology, abdomen and pelvis CT scan, chest X ray, hemagram, renal and liver function tests, measurement of calcium and lactate dehydrogenase (LDH). Bone and brain scans are indicated for symptoms. CT scans of the chest are more sensitive for detection of pulmonary metastases, a common metastatic site, and are frequently obtained these days instead of a chest X ray.

The grading of renal cell carcinoma is based on the Fuhrman nuclear grade, which is a powerful independent predictor of recurrence and survival after nephrectomy (134). The staging of renal cell carcinoma shown below was last revised in 2002 by the American Joint Commission on Cancer and carries prognostic value as shown in the adjacent stage-specific survival figures.

Primary tumor (T)
   TX: Primary tumor cannot be assessed
   T0: No evidence of primary tumor
   T1: Tumor 7 cm or less, limited to kidney
   T2: Tumor greater than 7 cm, limited to kidney
   T3: Tumor extends into major veins/adrenal/perinephric tissue; not beyond Gerota's
        fascia
      T3a: Tumor invades adrenal/perinephric fat
      T3b: Tumor extends into renal vein(s) or vena cava below diaphragm
      T3c: Tumor extends into van cava above diaphragm
   T4: Tumor invades beyond Gerota's fascia

Regional lymph nodes (N)
   NX: Regional nodes cannot be assessed
   N0: No regional lymph node metastasis

(Continued)

(*Continued*)

N1: Metastasis in a single regional lymph node
N2: Metastasis in more than one regional lymph node
Distant metastasis (M)
  MX: Distant metastasis cannot be assessed
  M0: No distant metastasis
  M1: Distant metastasis

Stage grouping				Five-year survival%
Stage I	T1	N0	M0	80
Stage II	T2	N0	M0	60
Stage III	T1-2	N0	M0	40
	T3	N0-1	M0	
Stage IV	T4	N0-1	M0	10–20
	Any T	N2	M0	
	Any T	Any N	M1	

The prognosis of resected renal cell carcinoma is primarily determined by grade and stage. Additionally, histologic features such as sarcomatoid differentiation, inferior performance status (135), or patient symptoms (136) and possibly serum markers of inflammation, but not age, carry a higher risk of recurrence. Gene expression signatures that predict recurrence and metastases are emerging (137). Independent prognostic factors for advanced disease were derived by Memorial Sloan Kettering Cancer Center (MSKCC) from a data set of 670 untreated patients aged 18 to 82 years (median 58 years) entered on clinical trials of immunotherapy, chemotherapy, and hormones at that institution between 1975 and 1995 (138). Independent prognostic variables (risk factors) conferring a poor survival outcome were found to be high LDH, low hemoglobin, higher corrected serum calcium, lower Karnofsky performance status, and prior nephrectomy; however age was not examined in the preliminary univariate analysis in developing the final model. Three risk groups with 0 (25% of patients), 1 or 2 (53% of patients), and 3 to 5 (22% of patients) of these risk factors were identified with discriminating median survivals of 19.9, 10.3, and 3.9 months and one-year survivals of 71%, 42%, and 12%, respectively (138,139). The Cleveland Clinic validated the MSKCC prognostic model in 353 previously untreated patients and additionally found prior radiotherapy and the presence of lung, liver, or retroperitoneal nodal metastases, but not age (which was analyzed in the model) to confer a poor prognosis. In 425 patients with metastatic disease in prospective European trials, age ($<$ 50 years vs. $\geq$50 years) was not a significant prognostic factor in univariate analysis (140). Instead, a multivariate analysis showed neutrophil count $\geq$6500, LDH $\geq$220 U/L, C reactive protein $\geq$11 mg/L, time from diagnosis to metastatic disease $\geq$3 years, number of metastatic sites $\geq$3, and presence of bone metastases to be independently predictive of poor survival outcome.

Management

Nephrectomy
Open radical nephrectomy is the standard curative approach for localized renal cell carcinoma even when renal vein or inferior vena cava invasion has occurred. In a

small study comparing 27 patients aged less than 70 years with 10 older patients, no significant difference in presentation, receipt of curative intent nephrectomy (23/27 vs. 7/10, respectively), or survival could be detected (141). However, among 735 patients presenting to the Rotterdam Comprehensive Cancer Center, patients aged 70 years and above had a significantly lower resection rate than younger patients (63% vs. 82%, $P < 0.001$); however, the postoperative mortality of 3.8% was not age related (142).

Nephron-sparing surgery (partial nephrectomy) may be an option in patients with kidney cancer developing in a solitary kidney, both kidneys, or other clinical situations in which preservation of renal function is important (143), a situation that is more likely to be present in older patients with comorbidities such as longstanding hypertension and diabetes. Nephron-sparing surgery achieves the same results as the open procedure in comparison cohorts that have been followed for many years for cancer-specific survival, even among patients with tumors up to 7 cm in diameter (144). A higher incidence of local recurrence but a lower risk of renal insufficiency at 10 years is observed with the nephron-sparing procedure (145). Laparoscopic radical nephrectomy has increasingly become a routine practice at specialized centers with surgeons experienced in the technique, with ongoing diffusion into community practice. This is an acceptable procedure satisfying the principles of cancer surgery for Stage T1 to T3a tumors (143,146). Although no randomized comparisons have been performed, single institution experiences have strongly suggested significant reduction in postoperative pain, blood loss, and hospital stay, which are likely to be of value to the older patient as well as those patients for whom further systemic therapy is planned after cytoreductive nephrectomy for advanced renal cell carcinoma (147). Following laparascopic nephrectomy in 93 patients (63 with localized renal cell carcinoma), older patients (>65 years) appear to have the same perioperative experiences as younger ones with respect to operative time (approximately four hours), blood loss (<200 mL), and postoperative complications, but have a statistically significant, marginally longer hospital stay (5.7 days vs. 5 days) (148). Other options such as CT-guided or laparoscopic cryoablation and radiofrequency ablation are being performed in increasing numbers for smaller tumors at selected centers, and have not entered common clinical practice.

Two randomized controlled trials have shown a survival benefit for performing a cytoreductive nephrectomy preceding interferon immunotherapy for advanced renal cell carcinoma compared to interferon alone (149,150). Although objective tumor responses in metastatic sites were rare, a significant three- to six-month additional survival benefit was accrued depending on baseline performance status. Only one postoperative death was noted in 98 nephrectomies (149). The primary tumor tends to be larger in patients with metastatic disease than in those with localized disease. Nevertheless, experienced surgeons using the laparoscopic technique, have been able to perform comparably successful nephrectomies with respect to postoperative pain control, blood loss (~300 mL), hospital stay (~1.7 days), and operative time (~3.1 hours), but with possibly more complications than when localized renal cancer is curatively resected (151). Intuitively, a laparoscopic cytoreductive nephrectomy should be an attractive consideration in elderly patients with metastatic renal cell carcinoma. However, additional data on perioperative morbidity in such patients who are burdened with metastatic disease and tend to have larger tumors is needed, especially if patients who are unfit for the open procedure are accepted to undergo a laparoscopy.

Adjuvant Therapy

Adjuvant therapy following curative intent resection for locally advanced or high-risk renal cell carcinoma has been investigated with negative results. Several randomized trials, some of which were flawed by design or on account of low power, have shown no benefit for adjuvant therapy for either progression-free or overall survival with the use of high dose interleukin-2 (IL-2), alpha interferon, or fluorouracil chemotherapy (135,152,153). Adjuvant radiation to the nephrectomy bed to reduce local recurrence is controversial and not standard practice. Therefore, the standard practice after successful radical nephrectomy is surveillance for recurrence.

Management of Advanced Renal Cell Carcinoma

Renal cell carcinoma is unusual in terms of its sensitivity to immunologic therapy and relative resistance to chemotherapy. The FDA approved high dose IL-2 (aldesleukin) for the treatment of metastatic renal cell carcinoma in 1992, based on the observation of durable complete remission lasting several years in a small proportion of patients so treated (154). Interferon alpha has been shown to confer a survival benefit in two randomized controlled trials. The larger trial conducted by the British Medical Research Council randomized 335 patients to medroxyprogesterone acetate or a three-month course of interferon alpha at 10 million units three times a week subcutaneously, and detected a 12% absolute survival benefit at one year and a prolongation in median survival from 6 to 8.5 months (155). A second randomized trial in 160 patients showed a seven-month median survival advantage for interferon plus vinblastine versus vinblastine alone, each regimen administered for a year (156). Two other negative trials were underpowered to detect a true difference of this magnitude. Because of these positive results for interferon therapy as well as the beneficial impact on survival for cytoreductive nephrectomy preceding interferon, MSKCC investigators determined outcomes for a cohort of 463 patients entered on MSKCC interferon-based clinical trials, 55% of who had undergone prior nephrectomy, in order to define a comparator standard for clinical trials. The median age was 59 (range 20–81), median survival was 13 months with 30% alive at two years and 10% alive at five years, and median progression-free survival was 4.7 months. Although age was not examined, independent prognostic factors for inferior survival were lower hemoglobin, higher LDH, higher corrected serum calcium, lower performance status, and shorter interval from diagnosis to interferon treatment. These risk factors allowed separation into low (0 risk factors), intermediate (1–2 risk factors), and high (3–5 risk factors) risk groups with median survivals of 30, 14, and 5 months, respectively (157). Age per se should not to be a major consideration in determining qualification of appropriate patients to receive interferon therapy. However, toxicity of interferon can be significant and may interact adversely with other age dependent factors including reduced cognitive capacity, and frailty, as well as other independent conditions such as depressed mood or poor performance status resulting from cancer cachexia. In an adjuvant trial of interferon (in which disease-related symptoms are few), 16 of 140 (11.4%) patients experienced Grade 4 toxicity, including neutropenia, myalgia, fatigue, depression, and neurologic toxicity (135). In this study, which included participation by patients aged 70 to 79 years, approximately one-third of patients discontinued interferon for Grade 3 or 4 toxicities, most commonly for flu-like symptoms, fatigue, or myalgias. Toxic deaths are rare but suicides from depression have been reported. Drug-induced hypothyroidism may complicate fatigue. Therefore interferon therapy should be closely monitored, particularly in the elderly patient, so that dose reductions and treatment interruptions can be undertaken in a timely fashion to maintain quality of life.

IL-2 or aldesleukin may be given in a high-dose, intravenous short-term schedule in the hospital with intent to achieve a durable (>5 years) complete remission viewed as a cure in 5% to 10% of patients so treated, or as an outpatient low-dose subcutaneous regimen with intent to achieve a response only without expectation of a survival benefit. In an adjuvant trial of high-dose IL-2 in 69 patients, the age range of participants was 25 to 64 years (151). Although conducted at experienced centers and in a nonmetastatic setting (in which disease-related symptoms will be few), toxicities were severe and included Grade 3 or 4 hypotension (52%), gastrointestinal symptoms (27%), electrolyte changes (27%), constitutional symptoms (18%), renal failure (15%), hepatic toxicities (15%), cardiac arrhythmias (9%), and central nervous system toxicities (9%). Other common toxicities include edema, weight gain, and hypoxia. Not infrequently, patients require monitoring in an intensive care unit until recovery. Toxicities are of similar nature but are less frequent and of a lower grade (especially hypotension) in low-dose IL-2 regimens used for the treatment of metastatic disease (158,159). Even in the metastatic disease setting, patients treated with IL-2 tend to be of younger age (e.g., median age 48) and excellent ECOG performance status of 0 to 1 (159). Clearly the nature and degree of toxicities of IL-2 are prohibitive for many older patients with or without known age-associated comorbidities. Patient selection is important and achieved in part by rigorous pretreatment cardiac, pulmonary, and other organ function screening. Clinical experience is essential in achieving zero treatment-related mortality as opposed to the 3% to 4% mortality in the years immediately following introduction of this therapy (160,161).

Various combinations of immunotherapy, chemotherapy, and other biologic agents for the treatment of advanced renal cell carcinoma have been attempted, generally with additive toxicities but without added benefit. The most promising avenues of current research involve exploiting the HIF and vascular endothelial growth factor pathways (162) as well as other tyrosine kinase and growth factor signaling pathways (163) that appear to be critical to the pathogenesis and phenotype of the common, clear cell carcinoma histologic subtype. These new classes of agents have shown beneficial effects on progression-free survival and tumor response, and appear to have a unique side-effect profile consisting of skin reactions, diarrhea, proteinuria, and hypertension which at first glance, do not appear to preclude their use in elderly patients.

Resection of a solitary metastasis may result in prolonged survival and potential cure in a small number of patients, especially those with metachronous presentations, a longer disease-free interval since nephrectomy, and fewer metastases that are amenable to complete resection (164–166). Administration of zoledronic acid to patients with bony metastases significantly delays or prevents skeletal-related complications of malignancy (pathological fracture, bone pain, spinal cord compression, need for surgery, or radiation to bone) and may even delay tumor progression at skeletal sites (167). Care should be taken to monitor renal function during zoledronic acid administration, especially in the elderly or in those who have had a prior nephrectomy and consequently have compromised renal function and reserve.

Choice of Therapy in Older Patients with Advanced Renal Cell Carcinoma

It is important that treatment be individualized for older patients by a team of physicians who are experienced in the management of renal cell carcinoma. Observation until disease progression is a valid option in patients who are asymptomatic and are experiencing a not uncommon prolonged period of disease stability, or even very occasionally, spontaneous tumor regression. Few older patients will be eligible for high-dose IL-2 because of comorbidities that can be worsened by drug toxicity leading to intolerance or life-threatening complications. Participation in clinical trials, particularly of active new agents with acceptable toxicity, should be routinely considered for a disease with few currently available, effective treatments. It should be recognized that age by itself is not recognized as a prognostic or predictive factor for response or survival; hence, given the short median survival of patients with advanced renal cell carcinoma, even elderly patients stand to benefit from effective treatments that are otherwise appropriate for that individual.

REFERENCES

1. Woloshin S, Schwartz LM. The U.S. Postal Service and cancer screening—stamps of approval? N Engl J Med 1999; 340(11):884–887.
2. Raghavan D, Skinner E. Genitourinary cancer in the elderly. Semin Oncol 2004; 31(2): 249–263.
3. Chung PW, Bayley AJ, Sweet J, et al. Spermatocytic seminoma: a review. Eur Urol 2004; 45(4):495–498.
4. International Germ Cell Consensus Classification: a prognostic factor-based staging system for metastatic germ cell cancers. International Germ Cell Cancer Collaborative Group. J Clin Oncol 1997; 15(2):594–603.
5. Zagars GK, Ballo MT, Lee AK, Strom SS. Mortality after cure of testicular seminoma. J Clin Oncol 2004; 22(4):640–647.
6. Huddart RA, Norman A, Shahidi M, et al. Cardiovascular disease as a long-term complication of treatment for testicular cancer. J Clin Oncol 2003; 21(8):1513–1523.
7. Nord C, Bjoro T, Ellingsen D, et al. Gonadal hormones in long-term survivors 10 years after treatment for unilateral testicular cancer. Eur Urol 2003; 44(3):322–328.
8. Shahinian VB, Kuo YF, Freeman JL, Goodwin JS. Risk of fracture after androgen deprivation for prostate cancer. N Engl J Med 2005; 352(2):154–164.
9. Darby S, Hancock BW. Localised non-Hodgkin lymphoma of the testis: the Sheffield Lymphoma Group experience. Int J Oncol 2005; 26(4):1093–1099.
10. Zucca E, Conconi A, Mughal TI, et al. Patterns of outcome and prognostic factors in primary large-cell lymphoma of the testis in a survey by the International Extranodal Lymphoma Study Group. J Clin Oncol 2003; 21(1):20–27.
11. www.cancer.org accessed May 9th, 2005.
12. http://seer.cancer.gov/csr accessed May 9th, 2005.
13. Manunta A, Vincendeau S, Kiriakou G, Lobel B, Guille F. Non-transitional cell bladder carcinomas. BJU Int 2005; 95(4):497–502.
14. Silverman DT, Hartge P, Morrison AS, Devesa SS. Epidemiology of bladder cancer. Hematol Oncol Clin North Am 1992; 6(1):1–30.
15. Navon JD, Soliman H, Khonsari F, Ahlering T. Screening cystoscopy and survival of spinal cord injured patients with squamous cell cancer of the bladder. J Urol 1997; 157(6):2109–2111.
16. Shokeir AA. Squamous cell carcinoma of the bladder: pathology, diagnosis and treatment. BJU Int 2004; 93(2):216–220.
17. Michaud DS, Spiegelman D, Clinton SK, et al. Fluid intake and the risk of bladder cancer in men. N Engl J Med 1999; 340(18):1390–1397.
18. Yang CY, Chiu HF, Chang CC, Ho SC, Wu TN. Bladder cancer mortality reduction after installation of a tap-water supply system in an arsenious-endemic area in south-western Taiwan. Environ Res 2005; 98(1):127–132.

19. Soloway MS, Briggman V, Carpinito GA, et al. Use of a new tumor marker, urinary NMP22, in the detection of occult or rapidly recurring transitional cell carcinoma of the urinary tract following surgical treatment. J Urol 1996; 156(2 Pt 1):363–367.

20. Lachaine J, Valiquette L, Crott R. Economic evaluation of NMP22 in the management of bladder cancer. Can J Urol 2000; 7(2):974–980.

21. Zaher A, Sheridan T. Tumor markers in the detection of recurrent transitional cell carcinoma of the bladder: a brief review. Acta Cytol 2001; 45(4):575–581.

22. Grossman HB, Messing E, Soloway M, et al. Detection of bladder cancer using a point-of-care proteomic assay. JAMA 2005; 293(7):810–816.

23. Schoder H, Larson SM. Positron emission tomography for prostate, bladder, and renal cancer. Semin Nucl Med 2004; 34(4):274–292.

24. Jewett HJ. The historical development of the staging of bladder tumors: personal reminiscences. Urol Surv 1977; 27(2):37–40.

25. Stewart GD, Bariol SV, Grigor KM, Tolley DA, McNeill SA. A comparison of the pathology of transitional cell carcinoma of the bladder and upper urinary tract. BJU Int 2005; 95(6):791–793.

26. AJCC Cancer Staging Manual. American Joint Committee on Cancer, editor. 5th ed. Lippincott-Raven, 1997:241–246.

27. Amling CL. Diagnosis and management of superficial bladder cancer. Curr Probl Cancer 2001; 25(4):219–278.

28. Millan-Rodriguez F, Chechile-Toniolo G, Salvador-Bayarri J, Palou J, Vicente-Rodriguez J. Multivariate analysis of the prognostic factors of primary superficial bladder cancer. J Urol 2000; 163(1):73–78.

29. Kondo T, Onitsuka S, Ryoji O, et al. Analysis of prognostic factors related to primary superficial bladder cancer tumor recurrence in prophylactic intravesical epirubicin therapy. Int J Urol 1999; 6(4):178–183.

30. Tetu B, Fradet Y, Allard P, Veilleux C, Roberge N, Bernard P. Prevalence and clinical significance of HER/2neu, p53 and Rb expression in primary superficial bladder cancer. J Urol 1996; 155(5):1784–1788.

31. Serth J, Kuczyk MA, Bokemeyer C, et al. p53 immunohistochemistry as an independent prognostic factor for superficial transitional cell carcinoma of the bladder. Br J Cancer 1995; 71(1):201–205.

32. Lipponen P, Eskelinen M. Expression of epidermal growth factor receptor in bladder cancer as related to established prognostic factors, oncoprotein (c-erbB-2, p53) expression and long-term prognosis. Br J Cancer 1994; 69(6):1120–1125.

33. Neoadjuvant cisplatin, methotrexate, and vinblastine chemotherapy for muscle-invasive bladder cancer: a randomised controlled trial. International collaboration of trialists. Lancet 1999; 354(9178):533–540.

34. Gupta NP, Goel R, Hemal AK, et al. Radical cystectomy in septuagenarian patients with bladder cancer. Int Urol Nephrol 2004; 36(3):353–358.

35. Schrag D, Mitra N, Xu F, et al. Cystectomy for muscle-invasive bladder cancer: patterns and outcomes of care in the Medicare population. Urology 2005; 65(6): 1118–1125.

36. Clark PE, Stein JP, Groshen SG, et al. Radical cystectomy in the elderly. Cancer 2005; 104(1):36–43.

37. Nuttall MC, van der MJ, McIntosh G, Gillatt D, Emberton M. Changes in patient characteristics and outcomes for radical cystectomy in England. BJU Int 2005; 95(4):513–516.

38. Chang SS, Alberts G, Cookson MS, Smith JA Jr. Radical cystectomy is safe in elderly patients at high risk. J Urol 2001; 166(3):938–941.

39. Kursh ED, Rabin R, Persky L. Is cystectomy a safe procedure in elderly patients with carcinoma of the bladder? J Urol 1977; 118(1 Pt 1):40–42.

40. Lance RS, Dinney CP, Swanson D, et al. Radical cystectomy for invasive bladder cancer in the octogenarian. Oncol Rep 2001; 8(4):723–726.

41. Leibovitch I, Avigad I, Ben Chaim J, Nativ O, Goldwasser B. Is it justified to avoid radical cystoprostatectomy in elderly patients with invasive transitional cell carcinoma of the bladder? Cancer 1993; 71(10):3098–3101.

42. Soulie M, Straub M, Game X, et al. A multicenter study of the morbidity of radical cystectomy in select elderly patients with bladder cancer. J Urol 2002; 167(3): 1325–1328.

43. Stroumbakis N, Herr HW, Cookson MS, Fair WR. Radical cystectomy in the octogenarian. J Urol 1997; 158(6):2113–2117.

44. Wood DP Jr, Montie JE, Maatman TJ, Beck GJ. Radical cystectomy for carcinoma of the bladder in the elderly patient. J Urol 1987; 138(1):46–48.

45. Zingg EJ, Bornet B, Bishop MC. Urinary diversion in the elderly patient. Eur Urol 1980; 6(6):347–351.

46. Zebic N, Weinknecht S, Kroepfl D. Radical cystectomy in patients aged $> /= 75$ years: an updated review of patients treated with curative and palliative intent. BJU Int 2005; 95(9):1211–1214.

47. Konety BR, Dhawan V, Allareddy V, Joslyn SA. Impact of hospital and surgeon volume on in-hospital mortality from radical cystectomy: data from the health care utilization project. J Urol 2005; 173(5):1695–1700.

48. Schrag D, Mitra N, Xu F, et al. Cystectomy for muscle-invasive bladder cancer: patterns and outcomes of care in the Medicare population. Urology 2005; 65(6): 1118–1125.

49. Neoadjuvant chemotherapy in invasive bladder cancer: a systematic review and meta-analysis. Lancet 2003; 361(9373):1927–1934.

50. Grossman HB, Natale RB, Tangen CM, et al. Neoadjuvant chemotherapy plus cystectomy compared with cystectomy alone for locally advanced bladder cancer. N Engl J Med 2003; 349(9):859–866.

51. Vale CL. Neoadjuvant chemotherapy in invasive bladder cancer: Update of a Systematic Review and Meta-Analysis of Individual Patient Data Advanced Bladder Cancer (ABC) Meta-analysis Collaboration. Eur Urol 2005; 48:202–205.

52. Gospodarowicz M. Radiotherapy and organ preservation in bladder cancer: are we ignoring the evidence? J Clin Oncol 2002; 20(14):3048–3050.

53. Kim HL, Steinberg GD. The current status of bladder preservation in the treatment of muscle invasive bladder cancer. J Urol 2000; 164(3 Pt 1):627–632.

54. Rodel C, Grabenbauer GG, Kuhn R, et al. Combined-modality treatment and selective organ preservation in invasive bladder cancer: long-term results. J Clin Oncol 2002; 20(14):3061–3071.

55. Konety BR, Joslyn SA. Factors influencing aggressive therapy for bladder cancer: an analysis of data from the SEER program. J Urol 2003; 170(5):1765–1771.

56. Chahal R, Sundaram SK, Iddenden R, Forman DF, Weston PM, Harrison SC. A study of the morbidity, mortality and long-term survival following radical cystectomy and radical radiotherapy in the treatment of invasive bladder cancer in Yorkshire. Eur Urol 2003; 43(3):246–257.

57. Shipley WU, Zietman AL, Kaufman DS, Coen JJ, Sandler HM. Selective bladder preservation by trimodality therapy for patients with muscularis propria-invasive bladder cancer and who are cystectomy candidates—the Massachusetts General Hospital and Radiation Therapy Oncology Group experiences. Semin Radiat Oncol 2005; 15(1):36–41.

58. Coppin CM, Gospodarowicz MK, James K, et al. Improved local control of invasive bladder cancer by concurrent cisplatin and preoperative or definitive radiation. The National Cancer Institute of Canada Clinical Trials Group. J Clin Oncol 1996; 14(11):2901–2907.

59. Kaufman DS, Shipley WU, Griffin PP, Heney NM, Althausen AF, Efird JT. Selective bladder preservation by combination treatment of invasive bladder cancer. N Engl J Med 1993; 329(19):1377–1382.

60. Shipley WU, Kaufman DS, Tester WJ, Pilepich MV, Sandler HM. Overview of bladder cancer trials in the Radiation Therapy Oncology Group. Cancer 2003; 97(8 suppl): 2115–2119.

61. Shipley WU, Winter KA, Kaufman DS, et al. Phase III trial of neoadjuvant chemotherapy in patients with invasive bladder cancer treated with selective bladder preservation by combined radiation therapy and chemotherapy: initial results of Radiation Therapy Oncology Group 89–03. J Clin Oncol 1998; 16(11):3576–3583.

62. Fokdal L, Hoyer M, von der MH. Treatment outcome and prognostic variables for local control and survival in patients receiving radical radiotherapy for urinary bladder cancer. Acta Oncol 2004; 43(8):749–757.

63. Cooke PW, Dunn JA, Latief T, Bathers S, James ND, Wallace DM. Long-term risk of salvage cystectomy after radiotherapy for muscle-invasive bladder cancer. Eur Urol 2000; 38(3):279–286.

64. Fossa SD, Waehre H, Aass N, Jacobsen AB, Olsen DR, Ous S. Bladder cancer definitive radiation therapy of muscle-invasive bladder cancer. A retrospective analysis of 317 patients. Cancer 1993; 72(10):3036–3043.

65. Moonen L, vd Voet H, de Nijs R, Hart AA, Horenblas S, Bartelink H. Muscle-invasive bladder cancer treated with external beam radiotherapy: pretreatment prognostic factors and the predictive value of cystoscopic re-evaluation during treatment. Radiother Oncol 1998; 49(2):149–155.

66. Gospodarowicz MK, Hawkins NV, Rawlings GA, et al. Radical radiotherapy for muscle invasive transitional cell carcinoma of the bladder: failure analysis. J Urol 1989; 142(6):1448–1453.

67. Chakravarti A, Winter K, Wu CL, et al. Expression of the epidermal growth factor receptor and Her-2 are predictors of favorable outcome and reduced complete response rates, respectively, in patients with muscle-invading bladder cancers treated by concurrent radiation and cisplatin-based chemotherapy: a report from the Radiation Therapy Oncology Group. Int J Radiat Oncol Biol Phys 2005; 62(2):309–317.

68. Pollack A, Zagars GK, Swanson DA. Muscle-invasive bladder cancer treated with external beam radiotherapy: prognostic factors. Int J Radiat Oncol Biol Phys 1994; 30(2):267–277.

69. Agranovich A, Czaykowski P, Hui D, Pickles T, Kwan W. Radiotherapy for muscle-invasive urinary bladder cancer in elderly patients. Can J Urol 2003; 10(6):2056–2061.

70. Vrouvas J, Dodwell D, Ash D, Probst H. Split course radiotherapy for bladder cancer in elderly unfit patients. Clin Oncol (R Coll Radiol) 1995; 7(3):193–195.

71. Sengelov L, Klintorp S, Havsteen H, Kamby C, Hansen SL, von der MH. Treatment outcome following radiotherapy in elderly patients with bladder cancer. Radiother Oncol 1997; 44(1):53–58.

72. Santacaterina A, Settineri N, De Renzis C, et al. Muscle-invasive bladder cancer in elderly-unfit patients with concomitant illness: can a curative radiation therapy be delivered? Tumori 2002; 88(5):390–394.

73. Raghavan D, Grundy R, Greenaway TM, et al. Pre-emptive (neo-adjuvant) chemotherapy prior to radical radiotherapy for fit septuagenarians with bladder cancer: age itself is not a contra-indication. Br J Urol 1988; 62(2):154–159.

74. Widmark A, Flodgren P, Damber JE, Hellsten S, Cavallin-Stahl E. A systematic overview of radiation therapy effects in urinary bladder cancer. Acta Oncol 2003; 42(5/6):567–581.

75. McLaren DB, Morrey D, Mason MD. Hypofractionated radiotherapy for muscle invasive bladder cancer in the elderly. Radiother Oncol 1997; 43(2):171–174.

76. Hussain SA, James ND. The systemic treatment of advanced and metastatic bladder cancer. Lancet Oncol 2003; 4(8):489–497.

77. Saxman SB, Propert KJ, Einhorn LH, et al. Long-term follow-up of a phase III intergroup study of cisplatin alone or in combination with methotrexate, vinblastine, and

doxorubicin in patients with metastatic urothelial carcinoma: a cooperative group study. J Clin Oncol 1997; 15(7):2564–2569.

78. Stadler WM, Hayden A, von der MH, et al. Long-term survival in phase II trials of gemcitabine plus cisplatin for advanced transitional cell cancer. Urol Oncol 2002; 7(4):153–157.

79. Bajorin DF, Dodd PM, Mazumdar M, et al. Long-term survival in metastatic transitional-cell carcinoma and prognostic factors predicting outcome of therapy. J Clin Oncol 1999; 17(10):3173–3181.

80. Bamias A, Efstathiou E, Moulopoulos LA, et al. The outcome of elderly patients with advanced urothelial carcinoma after platinum-based combination chemotherapy. Ann Oncol 2005; 16(2):307–313.

81. Bellmunt J, Albanell J, Paz-Ares L, et al. Pretreatment prognostic factors for survival in patients with advanced urothelial tumors treated in a phase I/II trial with paclitaxel, cisplatin, and gemcitabine. Cancer 2002; 95(4):751–757.

82. Hillcoat BL, Raghavan D, Matthews J, et al. A randomized trial of cisplatin versus cisplatin plus methotrexate in advanced cancer of the urothelial tract. J Clin Oncol 1989; 7(6):706–709.

83. Loehrer PJ Sr, Einhorn LH, Elson PJ, et al. A randomized comparison of cisplatin alone or in combination with methotrexate, vinblastine, and doxorubicin in patients with metastatic urothelial carcinoma: a cooperative group study. J Clin Oncol 1992; 10(7):1066–1073.

84. Hussain M, Vaishampayan U, Du W, Redman B, Smith DC. Combination paclitaxel, carboplatin, and gemcitabine is an active treatment for advanced urothelial cancer. J Clin Oncol 2001; 19(9):2527–2533.

85. Bajorin D. The phase III candidate: can we improve the science of selection? J Clin Oncol 2004; 22(2):211–213.

86. Logothetis CJ, Dexeus FH, Finn L, et al. A prospective randomized trial comparing MVAC and CISCA chemotherapy for patients with metastatic urothelial tumors. J Clin Oncol 1990; 8(6):1050–1055.

87. von der MH, Hansen SW, Roberts JT, et al. Gemcitabine and cisplatin versus methotrexate, vinblastine, doxorubicin, and cisplatin in advanced or metastatic bladder cancer: results of a large, randomized, multinational, multicenter, phase III study. J Clin Oncol 2000; 18(17):3068–3077.

88. Tannock I, Gospodarowicz M, Connolly J, Jewett M. M-VAC (methotrexate, vinblastine, doxorubicin and cisplatin) chemotherapy for transitional cell carcinoma: the Princess Margaret Hospital experience. J Urol 1989; 142(2 Pt 1):289–292.

89. Mead GM, Russell M, Clark P, et al. A randomized trial comparing methotrexate and vinblastine (MV) with cisplatin, methotrexate and vinblastine (CMV) in advanced transitional cell carcinoma: results and a report on prognostic factors in a Medical Research Council study. MRC Advanced Bladder Cancer Working Party. Br J Cancer 1998; 78(8):1067–1075.

90. Bellmunt J, Ribas A, Eres N, et al. Carboplatin-based versus cisplatin-based chemotherapy in the treatment of surgically incurable advanced bladder carcinoma. Cancer 1997; 80(10):1966–1972.

91. Petrioli R, Frediani B, Manganelli A, et al. Comparison between a cisplatin-containing regimen and a carboplatin-containing regimen for recurrent or metastatic bladder cancer patients. A randomized phase II study. Cancer 1996; 77(2):344–351.

92. Bamias A, Aravantinos G, Deliveliotis C, et al. Docetaxel and cisplatin with granulocyte colony-stimulating factor (G-CSF) versus MVAC with G-CSF in advanced urothelial carcinoma: a multicenter, randomized, phase III study from the Hellenic Cooperative Oncology Group. J Clin Oncol 2004; 22(2):220–228.

93. Cohen MH, Rothmann M. Gemcitabine and cisplatin for advanced, metastatic bladder cancer. J Clin Oncol 2001; 19(4):1229–1231.

94. Sternberg CN, de Mulder PH, Schornagel JH, et al. Randomized phase III trial of high-dose-intensity methotrexate, vinblastine, doxorubicin, and cisplatin (MVAC) chemotherapy and recombinant human granulocyte colony-stimulating factor versus classic MVAC in advanced urothelial tract tumors: European Organization for Research and Treatment of Cancer Protocol no. 30924. J Clin Oncol 2001; 19(10):2638–2646.

95. Hainsworth JD, Meluch AA, Litchy S, et al. Paclitaxel, carboplatin, and gemcitabine in the treatment of patients with advanced transitional cell carcinoma of the urothelium. Cancer 2005; 103(11):2298–2303.

96. Dreicer R, Manola J, Roth BJ, Cohen MB, Hatfield AK, Wilding G. Phase II study of cisplatin and paclitaxel in advanced carcinoma of the urothelium: an Eastern Cooperative Oncology Group Study. J Clin Oncol 2000; 18(5):1058–1061.

97. Dreicer R, Manola J, Roth BJ, et al. Phase III trial of methotrexate, vinblastine, doxorubicin, and cisplatin versus carboplatin and paclitaxel in patients with advanced carcinoma of the urothelium. Cancer 2004; 100(8):1639–1645.

98. Bellmunt J, de Wit R, Albanell J, Baselga J. A feasibility study of carboplatin with fixed dose of gemcitabine in "unfit" patients with advanced bladder cancer. Eur J Cancer 2001; 37(17):2212–2215.

99. Carles J, Nogue M, Domenech M, et al. Carboplatin-gemcitabine treatment of patients with transitional cell carcinoma of the bladder and impaired renal function. Oncology 2000; 59(1):24–27.

100. Carles J, Nogue M. Gemcitabine/carboplatin in advanced urothelial cancer. Semin Oncol 2001; 28(3 suppl 10):19–24.

101. Friedland DM, Dakhil S, Hollen C, Gregurich MA, Asmar L. A phase II evaluation of weekly paclitaxel plus carboplatin in advanced urothelial cancer. Cancer Invest 2004; 22(3):374–382.

102. Dreicer R, Manola J, Roth BJ, et al. Phase III trial of methotrexate, vinblastine, doxorubicin, and cisplatin versus carboplatin and paclitaxel in patients with advanced carcinoma of the urothelium. Cancer 2004; 100(8):1639–1645.

103. Vaughn DJ, Manola J, Dreicer R, See W, Levitt R, Wilding G. Phase II study of paclitaxel plus carboplatin in patients with advanced carcinoma of the urothelium and renal dysfunction (E2896): a trial of the Eastern Cooperative Oncology Group. Cancer 2002; 95(5):1022–1027.

104. Redman BG, Smith DC, Flaherty L, Du W, Hussain M. Phase II trial of paclitaxel and carboplatin in the treatment of advanced urothelial carcinoma. J Clin Oncol 1998; 16(5):1844–1848.

105. Vaughn DJ, Manola J, Dreicer R, See W, Levitt R, Wilding G. Phase II study of paclitaxel plus carboplatin in patients with advanced carcinoma of the urothelium and renal dysfunction (E2896): a trial of the Eastern Cooperative Oncology Group. Cancer 2002; 95(5):1022–1027.

106. Zielinski CC, Schnack B, Grbovic M, et al. Paclitaxel and carboplatin in patients with metastatic urothelial cancer: results of a phase II trial. Br J Cancer 1998; 78(3):370–374.

107. Ardavanis A, Tryfonopoulos D, Alexopoulos A, Kandylis C, Lainakis G, Rigatos G. Gemcitabine and docetaxel as first-line treatment for advanced urothelial carcinoma: a phase II study. Br J Cancer 2005; 92(4):645–650.

108. Dreicer R, Manola J, Schneider DJ, et al. Phase II trial of gemcitabine and docetaxel in patients with advanced carcinoma of the urothelium: a trial of the Eastern Cooperative Oncology Group. Cancer 2003; 97(11):2743–2747.

109. Gitlitz BJ, Baker C, Chapman Y, et al. A phase II study of gemcitabine and docetaxel therapy in patients with advanced urothelial carcinoma. Cancer 2003; 98(9):1863–1869.

110. Kaufman DS, Carducci MA, Kuzel TM, et al. A multi-institutional phase II trial of gemcitabine plus paclitaxel in patients with locally advanced or metastatic urothelial cancer. Urol Oncol 2004; 22(5):393–397.

111. Small EJ, Lew D, Redman BG, et al. Southwest Oncology Group Study of paclitaxel and carboplatin for advanced transitional-cell carcinoma: the importance of survival as a clinical trial end point. J Clin Oncol 2000; 18(13):2537–2544.

112. Srinivas S, Guardino AE. A nonplatinum combination in metastatic transitional cell carcinoma. Am J Clin Oncol 2005; 28(2):114–118.

113. Neri B, Doni L, Fulignati C, et al. Gemcitabine plus Epi-doxorubicin as first-line chemotherapy for bladder cancer in advanced or metastatic stage: a phase II. Anticancer Res 2002; 22(5):2981–2984.

114. Ricci S, Galli L, Chioni A, et al. Gemcitabine plus epirubicin in patients with advanced urothelial carcinoma who are not eligible for platinum-based regimens. Cancer 2002; 95(7):1444–1450.

115. Sternberg CN, de Mulder PH, Schornagel JH, et al. Randomized phase III trial of high-dose-intensity methotrexate, vinblastine, doxorubicin, and cisplatin (MVAC) chemotherapy and recombinant human granulocyte colony-stimulating factor versus classic MVAC in advanced urothelial tract tumors: European Organization for Research and Treatment of Cancer Protocol no. 30924. J Clin Oncol 2001; 19(10):2638–2646.

116. Small EJ, Halabi S, Dalbagni G, et al. Overview of bladder cancer trials in the Cancer and Leukemia Group B. Cancer 2003; 97(8 suppl):2090–2098.

117. Bryan RT, Hussain SA, James ND, Jankowski JA, Wallace DM. Molecular pathways in bladder cancer: part 2. BJU Int 2005; 95(4):491–496.

118. Bryan RT, Hussain SA, James ND, Jankowski JA, Wallace DM. Molecular pathways in bladder cancer: part 1. BJU Int 2005; 95(4):485–490.

119. Young RC. Metastatic renal-cell carcinoma: what causes occasional dramatic regressions? N Engl J Med 1998; 338(18):1305–1306.

120. Aghaji AE, Odoemene CA. Renal cell carcinoma in Enugu, Nigeria. West Afr J Med 2000; 19(4):254–258.

121. Curry NS, Bissada NK. Radiologic evaluation of small and indeterminant renal masses. Urol Clin North Am 1997; 24(3):493–505.

122. Warren KS, McFarlane J. The Bosniak classification of renal cystic masses. BJU Int 2005; 95(7):939–942.

123. Israel GM, Bosniak MA. Renal imaging for diagnosis and staging of renal cell carcinoma. Urol Clin North Am 2003; 30(3):499–514.

124. Motzer RJ, Russo P, Nanus DM, Berg WJ. Renal cell carcinoma. Curr Probl Cancer 1997; 21(4):185–232.

125. Vogelzang NJ, Stadler WM. Kidney cancer. Lancet 1998; 352(9141):1691–1696.

126. Curti BD. Renal cell carcinoma. JAMA 2004; 292(1):97–100.

127. Chow WH, Devesa SS, Warren JL, Fraumeni JF Jr. Rising incidence of renal cell cancer in the United States. JAMA 1999; 281(17):1628–1631.

128. Malaeb BS, Martin DJ, Littooy FN, et al. The utility of screening renal ultrasonography: identifying renal cell carcinoma in an elderly asymptomatic population. BJU Int 2005; 95(7):977–981.

129. Mindrup SR, Pierre JS, Dahmoush L, Konety BR. The prevalence of renal cell carcinoma diagnosed at autopsy. BJU Int 2005; 95(1):31–33.

130. http://seer.cancer.gov accessed 06/28/05.

131. Calle EE, Rodriguez C, Walker-Thurmond K, Thun MJ. Overweight, obesity, and mortality from cancer in a prospectively studied cohort of U.S. adults. N Engl J Med 2003; 348(17):1625–1638.

132. George DJ, Kaelin WG Jr. The von Hippel-Lindau protein, vascular endothelial growth factor, and kidney cancer. N Engl J Med 2003; 349(5):419–421.

133. Linehan WM, Vasselli J, Srinivasan R, et al. Genetic basis of cancer of the kidney: disease-specific approaches to therapy. Clin Cancer Res 2004; 10(18 Pt 2):6282S–6289S.

134. Minervini A, Lilas L, Minervini R, Selli C. Prognostic value of nuclear grading in patients with intracapsular (pT1-pT2) renal cell carcinoma. Long-term analysis in 213 patients. Cancer 2002; 94(10):2590–2595.

135. Messing EM, Manola J, Wilding G, et al. Phase III study of interferon alfa-NL as adjuvant treatment for resectable renal cell carcinoma: an Eastern Cooperative Oncology Group/Intergroup trial. J Clin Oncol 2003; 21(7):1214–1222.

136. Kattan MW, Reuter V, Motzer RJ, Katz J, Russo P. A postoperative prognostic nomogram for renal cell carcinoma. J Urol 2001; 166(1):63–67.

137. Sultmann H, von Heydebreck A, Huber W, et al. Gene expression in kidney cancer is associated with cytogenetic abnormalities, metastasis formation, and patient survival. Clin Cancer Res 2005; 11(2 Pt 1):646–655.

138. Motzer RJ, Mazumdar M, Bacik J, Berg W, Amsterdam A, Ferrara J. Survival and prognostic stratification of 670 patients with advanced renal cell carcinoma. J Clin Oncol 1999; 17(8):2530–2540.

139. Motzer RJ, Bacik J, Mazumdar M. Prognostic factors for survival of patients with stage IV renal cell carcinoma: memorial sloan-kettering cancer center experience. Clin Cancer Res 2004; 10(18 Pt 2):6302S–6303S.

140. Atzpodien J, Royston P, Wandert T, Reitz M. Metastatic renal carcinoma comprehensive prognostic system. Br J Cancer 2003; 88(3):348–353.

141. Doherty JG, Rufer A, Bartholomew P, Beaumont DM. The presentation, treatment and outcome of renal cell carcinoma in old age. Age Ageing 1999; 28(4):359–362.

142. Damhuis RA, Blom JH. The influence of age on treatment choice and survival in 735 patients with renal carcinoma. Br J Urol 1995; 75(2):143–147.

143. Novick AC. Laparoscopic and partial nephrectomy. Clin Cancer Res 2004; 10(18 Pt 2):6322S–6327S.

144. Leibovich BC, Blute ML, Cheville JC, Lohse CM, Weaver AL, Zincke H. Nephron sparing surgery for appropriately selected renal cell carcinoma between 4 and 7 cm results in outcome similar to radical nephrectomy. J Urol 2004; 171(3):1066–1070.

145. Lau WK, Blute ML, Weaver AL, Torres VE, Zincke H. Matched comparison of radical nephrectomy vs nephron-sparing surgery in patients with unilateral renal cell carcinoma and a normal contralateral kidney. Mayo Clin Proc 2000; 75(12):1236–1242.

146. Gill IS. Laparoscopic radical nephrectomy for cancer. Urol Clin North Am 2000; 27(4):707–719.

147. Rabets JC, Kaouk J, Fergany A, Finelli A, Gill IS, Novick AC. Laparoscopic versus open cytoreductive nephrectomy for metastatic renal cell carcinoma. Urology 2004; 64(5):930–934.

148. Cobb WS, Heniford BT, Matthews BD, Carbonell AM, Kercher KW. Advanced age is not a prohibitive factor in laparoscopic nephrectomy for renal pathology. Am Surg 2004; 70(6):537–542.

149. Flanigan RC. Debulking nephrectomy in metastatic renal cancer. Clin Cancer Res 2004; 10(18 Pt 2):6335S–6341S.

150. Mickisch GH, Garin A, Van Poppel H, de Prijck L, Sylvester R. Radical nephrectomy plus interferon-alfa-based immunotherapy compared with interferon alfa alone in metastatic renal-cell carcinoma: a randomised trial. Lancet 2001; 358(9286):966–970.

151. Finelli A, Kaouk JH, Fergany AF, Abreu SC, Novick AC, Gill IS. Laparoscopic cytoreductive nephrectomy for metastatic renal cell carcinoma. BJU Int 2004; 94(3):291–294.

152. Clark JI, Atkins MB, Urba WJ, et al. Adjuvant high-dose bolus interleukin-2 for patients with high-risk renal cell carcinoma: a cytokine working group randomized trial. J Clin Oncol 2003; 21(16):3133–3140.

153. Atzpodien J, Schmitt E, Gertenbach U, et al. Adjuvant treatment with interleukin-2- and interferon-alpha2a-based chemoimmunotherapy in renal cell carcinoma post tumour nephrectomy: results of a prospectively randomised trial of the German Cooperative Renal Carcinoma Chemoimmunotherapy Group (DGCIN). Br J Cancer 2005; 92(5):843–846.

154. Rosenberg SA, Yang JC, Topalian SL, et al. Treatment of 283 consecutive patients with metastatic melanoma or renal cell cancer using high-dose bolus interleukin 2. JAMA 1994; 271(12):907–913.

155. Interferon-alpha and survival in metastatic renal carcinoma: early results of a randomised controlled trial. Medical Research Council Renal Cancer Collaborators. Lancet 1999; 353(9146):14–17.

156. Pyrhonen S, Salminen E, Ruutu M, et al. Prospective randomized trial of interferon alfa-2a plus vinblastine versus vinblastine alone in patients with advanced renal cell cancer. J Clin Oncol 1999; 17(9):2859–2867.

157. Motzer RJ, Bacik J, Murphy BA, Russo P, Mazumdar M. Interferon-alfa as a comparative treatment for clinical trials of new therapies against advanced renal cell carcinoma. J Clin Oncol 2002; 20(1):289–296.

158. Yang JC, Topalian SL, Parkinson D, et al. Randomized comparison of high-dose and low-dose intravenous interleukin-2 for the therapy of metastatic renal cell carcinoma: an interim report. J Clin Oncol 1994; 12(8):1572–1576.

159. Yang JC, Sherry RM, Steinberg SM, et al. Randomized study of high-dose and low-dose interleukin-2 in patients with metastatic renal cancer. J Clin Oncol 2003; 21(16):3127–3132.

160. Dutcher JP. Interleukin-2 based therapy for kidney cancer. Cancer Treat Res 2003; 116:155–172.

161. Schwartz RN, Stover L, Dutcher J. Managing toxicities of high-dose interleukin-2. Oncology (Williston Park) 2002; 16(11 suppl 13):11–20.

162. Yang JC, Haworth L, Sherry RM, et al. A randomized trial of bevacizumab, an antivascular endothelial growth factor antibody, for metastatic renal cancer. N Engl J Med 2003; 349(5):427–434.

163. Ahmad T, Eisen T. Kinase inhibition with BAY 43–9006 in renal cell carcinoma. Clin Cancer Res 2004; 10(18 Pt 2):6388S–6392S.

164. Hofmann HS, Neef H, Krohe K, Andreev P, Silber RE. Prognostic factors and survival after pulmonary resection of metastatic renal cell carcinoma. Eur Urol 2005; 48(1): 77–82.

165. Kavolius JP, Mastorakos DP, Pavlovich C, Russo P, Burt ME, Brady MS. Resection of metastatic renal cell carcinoma. J Clin Oncol 1998; 16(6):2261–2266.

166. Dineen MK, Pastore RD, Emrich LJ, Huben RP. Results of surgical treatment of renal cell carcinoma with solitary metastasis. J Urol 1988; 140(2):277–279.

167. Lipton A, Zheng M, Seaman J. Zoledronic acid delays the onset of skeletal-related events and progression of skeletal disease in patients with advanced renal cell carcinoma. Cancer 2003; 98(5):962–969.

17

Malignant Melanoma and Nonmelanoma Skin Cancer

Laura Kruper
Department of Surgery, University of Pennsylvania, Philadelphia, Pennsylvania, U.S.A.

Lynn M. Schuchter
Division of Hematology and Oncology, Abramson Cancer Center, University of Pennsylvania, Philadelphia, Pennsylvania, U.S.A.

MALIGNANT MELANOMAS AND NONMELANOMA SKIN CANCERS

Epidemiology of Skin Cancer

The incidence of skin cancer continues to rise rapidly and remains an important public health issue. In the United States, more than one million cases of skin cancer were expected to be newly diagnosed in 2005 (1). One in five individuals in the U.S. will develop a skin cancer during his or her lifetime, and half of all cancers diagnosed are cancers of the skin. Because the incidence of skin cancer increases with age, it can be expected that more skin cancers will occur as the U.S. population ages and life expectancy continues to improve. More than half (53%) of skin cancer–related deaths occur in individuals older than 65 years (2). In the United States, older men have the highest melanoma risk and should be the targets of screening efforts.

This chapter describes the epidemiology, early detection and prevention, clinical features, prognosis, and treatment options of the most common skin cancers: melanoma, basal cell carcinoma (BCC), and squamous cell carcinoma (SCC). Issues surrounding the management of skin cancers, particularly in the elderly, are also discussed.

Skin Cancer in the Elderly

The development of skin cancer arises from complex interactions of environmental, genetic, and other host factors. The most important environmental factor associated with the development of skin cancer is ultraviolet (UV) light (3,4). The association between UV light and skin cancer is supported by epidemiologic as well as scientific observations. Skin cancer develops more commonly in people who are sensitive to the sun and in people who live close to the equator, and typically occurs on sun-exposed areas of the skin. As shown in laboratory data, UV light can cause both direct and indirect DNA damage on a cellular level through photo-oxidative processes.

These types of DNA damage can cause mutations in tumor suppressor genes and proto-oncogenes involved in regulation and cell growth. In both BCC and SCC, mutations specifically induced by UV irradiation can be found in the p53 tumor-suppressor gene (5,6).

Certain genetic factors may predispose individuals to skin cancer such as xeroderma pigmentosum and basal cell nevus syndrome (Gorlin's syndrome), and inherited mutations in the *CDK2NA* gene (7). Regarding host factors associated with the development of skin cancer, the elderly may have a decreased capacity to repair UV-induced DNA damage, which could lead to mutated DNA with oncogenic potential (8). Also, the immune systems of the elderly have a decreased capacity to fight infection and malignancy (9). As the life expectancy of populations tends to increase, the risk of developing skin cancer also increases in individuals who are genetically predisposed to skin cancer the longer they live (10).

MELANOMA

Throughout the world, cases of melanomas are increasing at a rate of approximately 3% to 7% per year in fair-skinned populations (11). Melanoma is estimated to be the fifth and sixth most common cancer in men and women, respectively, among new cancer cases (1). In 2005, approximately 59,580 men and women in the United States were diagnosed with invasive melanoma, with an additional 46,170 diagnosed with in situ disease (1). Melanoma is the leading cause of death from cutaneous malignancies and accounts for 1% to 2% of all cancer deaths in the United States, with close to 7800 melanoma deaths estimated for 2005. During the past several decades, incidence and mortality rates from melanoma have increased substantially among all white populations. Since the 1930s, when reliable data was first recorded for melanoma, its incidence has risen more than 15-fold (12). The lifetime probability for developing melanoma is 1.72% for a man and 1.22% for a woman (13). In the younger age groups, incidence rates seem to be plateauing or decreasing. However, in the elderly, melanoma incidence and mortality rates continue to rise, particularly in men over the age of 65.

Melanoma affects adults of all ages, with a median age of 53 at diagnosis. As with many other types of cancer, the incidence of melanoma increases with age (14), with the most important trend among older men (15,16). Regarding prognosis, the survival of males and females is not equal, with men faring worse than women with the same thickness of the tumor (17). Nearly 50% of all melanoma-related deaths in the United States, Australia, and Southern Wales concern white men over 50 years of age (12). Melanoma has a more serious trend in the elderly than in younger people with the same tumor thickness; there is a significant lowering in the disease-free survival of patients older than 60 years at the time of diagnosis (15).

Risk Factors for Melanoma

Melanoma arises from the melanocyte. Malignant melanoma may arise de novo or from a precursor melanocytic nevus. Most patients with primary melanoma report preexisting pigmented lesions, though this is confirmed histologically in only about one-third of melanomas. Elderly patients tend to have fewer nevi in association with their melanomas, likely reflecting differences in the melanoma subtype prevalence, i.e., fewer superficial spreading melanomas (SSMs) relative to other histologic types

Table 1 Risk Factors for the Development of Cutaneous Melanoma

Cutaneous phenotype
  Fair skin
  Hair color—blond/red
  Eye color—blue eyes
  Freckling
Environmental
  Tendency to burn/poor tanning
  History of blistering sunburns in childhood
  Excessive sun exposure
Precursor lesions
  Dysplastic nevi
  Increased number of benign nevi
  Congenital moles
  Lentigo maligna
Other
  Personal history of melanoma
  Family history of melanoma
  Nonmelanoma skin cancers

in older individuals (18). It has also been suggested that more melanomas arise de novo with increasing age (19). Multiple factors associated with an increase in melanoma risk have been identified. These can be grouped into host factors and environmental exposures and are summarized in Table 1.

Genetics

Approximately 10% of patients with melanoma have a family history of melanoma. Some cases occur in the setting of the dysplastic nevus syndrome or the familial atypical multiple mole and melanoma syndrome (FAMM-M) (20). Persons with the FAMM-M, autosomal dominantly inherited syndrome, have a markedly increased risk of developing melanoma with estimates ranging from 55% to as high as 100%. This syndrome is defined by the presence of large numbers of moles (often greater than 50), some of which are dysplastic nevi, as well as the occurrence of melanoma in one or more first or second-degree relatives. Recent studies have shown that there are several susceptibility genes associated with the development of melanoma, the most important of these is *p16/CDKN2A*. This gene is located on chromosome 9p21 and is a member of a class of molecules that play a central role in the progression through the cell cycle. Testing for mutations in the p16/CDKN2A locus is available on a commercial basis. However, the clinical utility of genetic testing for melanoma susceptibility is limited at this time, and is therefore not recommended, unless in the setting of a clinical research trial (21).

Sun Exposure

Exposure to sunlight, or more specifically UV radiation in the UV-B range (280–320 nm), has been strongly implicated as a causative factor in the development of melanoma (22). As with BCC, a pattern of childhood sun exposure and intermittent sun exposure are strong risk factors for melanoma (4,23,24). Blistering sunburns, particularly in childhood, are associated with an increased risk of melanoma (23).

Cutaneous Phenotypes

The relationship between sun exposure and skin type and the risk of melanoma remains complex. Individuals with a tendency to burn rather than tan when exposed to sunlight have higher rates of melanoma, including those with fair complexion, blond or red hair, blue eye color, and freckles.

Precursor Lesions

Other factors linked to melanoma risk are pigmented lesions. Individuals with an increased number of typical or benign moles (melanocytic nevi) have an increased risk of melanoma. The proportion of melanomas that arise from melanocytic nevi ranges from 18% to 85%. Atypical moles or dysplastic nevi are important precursor lesions of melanoma and also serve as markers for increasing melanoma risk. Dysplastic nevi are acquired lesions of the skin and differ from common acquired nevi (moles). Unlike common moles, which are small and symmetrical with well-defined borders, dysplastic nevi are large, usually greater than 5 mm in diameter, with a flat component and a border that characteristically is ill defined or fuzzy. The presence of dysplastic nevi is associated with 6% lifetime chance of developing melanoma (25). This risk increases to as high as 80% in those individuals who have dysplastic nevi and a family history of melanoma. At least 5% of the population has at least one dysplastic nevus. Another precursor to melanoma is the congenital nevus, especially the rare giant type, which has a 6% to 7% lifetime risk of malignant transformation.

Other Risk Factors

Studies have shown that individuals with a history of basal skin cancer or squamous cell skin cancer have an increased risk of melanoma, which increases further in those individuals with both (26). Patients with a previous history of melanoma, as well as those with a family history of melanoma, are at increased risk for a second primary melanoma, particularly in the context of dysplastic nevi (27). The risk factors identified for melanoma are additive. For example, Mackie et al. of the Scottish Melanoma Group have reported that individuals who have had severe sunburns, who freckle, and who have dysplastic nevi and multiple nevi have a several 100-fold increase in the risk of melanoma (28).

Clinical Presentation

Clinically, melanoma is identified by the appearance of a new pigmented lesion or by a change in an existing mole, including change in shape, color, or surface. Early detection and recognition of melanoma is key to improving overall survival in patients with malignant melanoma. Most patients report a preexisting mole at the site of the melanoma. More than 70% of melanomas diagnosed are associated with an increase in size and change in color of the mole. The "ABCD's" used for the recognition of melanoma are useful for public education and to the clinicians to identify pigmented lesions suspicious for melanoma; A refers to asymmetry; B refers to borders that are irregular or notched; C refers to color variation: most melanomas are varying shades of brown, but black, blue, or pink may also be present; and D is for diameter greater than 6 mm (the size of a pencil eraser). Itching, burning, or pain in a pigmented lesion should increase suspicion of melanoma, although melanomas are often not associated with local discomfort. Bleeding and ulceration are signs of a more advanced melanoma. However, the most sensitive sign of melanoma is the change in color, size, or shape of a mole.

There is a stepwise tumor progression whereby a normal melanocyte passes through different stages, each stage with unique clinical and histological features, to an invasive melanoma with the ability to metastasize (29). Development of a melanoma begins with a common acquired nevus, which then progresses to a nevus with atypia and dysplasia (dysplastic nevus), to a radial growth phase melanoma, which lacks the ability to metastasize (30), to the invasive vertical growth phase with capacity for metastases, to metastatic melanoma (31). These steps of tumor progression likely represent the consequences of mutational events involving cell proliferation, invasion, migration, and metastasis.

Based upon clinical and histological features, cutaneous melanoma has been divided into four subtypes. SSM is the most common subtype, particularly between the ages of 30 and 50, and accounts for 70% of all melanomas (Fig. 1). In the elderly population, SSM is estimated to comprise 40% to 50% of cases (19). It can be located on any anatomic site but commonly occurs on the trunk and lower extremities. It has the typical clinical features described for melanoma, characterized by an asymmetric, multicolored lesion with irregular borders. Lesions are usually 1 to 2 cm in diameter and may or may not be palpable. Tan, brown, and black hues are almost always present. Pink, blue, and blue–white are also seen, the latter two hues indicating regression.

"Lentigo maligna melanoma" (LLM) (Fig. 2) accounts for 4% to 10% of all melanomas and tends to occur more commonly in older patients in areas that the chronically sun-exposed areas of the skin and is more common in women than in men. It develops in an indolent manner over the course of many years on the face, neck, backs of the hands, and rarely at other cutaneous sites. These lesions are characteristically flat, with irregular borders, and are colored by deep shades of tan, brown, and black. They are usually greater than 1 cm, and they can often be quite large in size (3–6 cm in diameter). LMM arises from a lentigo maligna, which is a slowly growing macular light brown lesion. Only 5% to 8% of lentigo malignas are estimated to evolve to invasive melanomas and this event is characterized by nodular development within the flat precursor lesion (Fig. 2). LLM may be difficult to distinguish from solar lentigo, pigmented actinic keratosis, or seborrheic keratosis.

"Nodular melanoma" (NM) (Fig. 3) accounts for 15% to 30% of melanoma and is disproportionately represented in the elderly. NMs do not resemble the other forms of the disease, but present as smooth nodules. They present as rapidly enlarging elevated or polypoid lesions, and are often blue/black in color. Some variants are amelanotic and appear as pink or flesh-toned nodules. The tumors generally arise more rapidly than other forms of melanoma, with rapid growth over weeks to

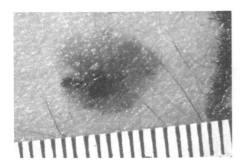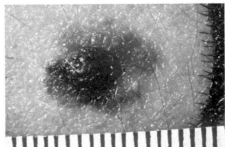

Figure 1 Superficial spreading melanoma.

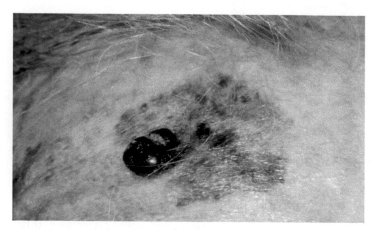

Figure 2 Lentigo maligna melanoma.

months, and most frequently develop on the trunk. NM lacks the "ABCD's" of melanoma and thus, any pigmented nodule with a history of rapid growth should raise the question of melanoma.

"Acral lentiginous melanoma" (ALM) (Fig. 4) occurs most commonly on the palms, soles, or nail beds, commonly presenting as a darkly pigmented, flat to nodular lesion. It represents only 2% to 8% of melanoma in Caucasians, but accounts for a much higher proportion (35–90%) of melanoma in African-Americans, Asians, and Hispanics. Sunlight does not seem to be involved in this subtype of melanoma. Large areas may be covered, and lesions as large as 3 cm are not uncommon. One variant is subungual (under the nail bed) melanoma, which presents as longitudinal brown/ black band within the nail plate. Irregular involvement of the skin of the posterior nail fold with tan-brown pigmentation (Hutchinson's sign) is essentially diagnostic of subungual melanoma (Fig. 5). The incidence of ALM peaks in the seventh decade and has a poorer prognosis mostly due to its association with advanced disease at diagnosis.

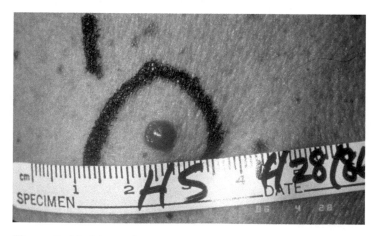

Figure 3 Nodular melanoma.

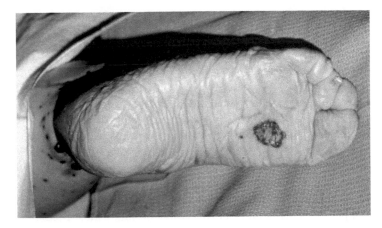

Figure 4 Acral lentigious melanoma.

Unusual subtypes of primary melanoma include desmoplastic or neurotropic melanoma, malignant blue nevus, and melanoma of soft parts (clear cell sarcoma). Together, these variants account for less than 2% of all cutaneous melanomas (32).

Diagnosis of Melanoma

Any skin lesion suspicious for melanoma should be biopsied. The proper biopsy is essential not only to establish a diagnosis, but also to allow precise histological interpretation, which will determine the prognosis and plan of therapy. Most clinically suspicious skin lesions are best biopsied by complete excision taking a 1 to 2 mm margin of normal skin including some subcutaneous fat. For lesions that are too large for complete excision, an incisional biopsy may be necessary. Shallow shave biopsies or curettage is contraindicated in lesions suspicious for melanoma as is cryosurgery, laser, and electrodessication. The differential diagnosis of a suspicious lesion resembling melanoma includes benign moles, atypical nevi, melanoma, pigmented basal cell cancer, seborrheic keratosis, blue nevi, and hemangiomas.

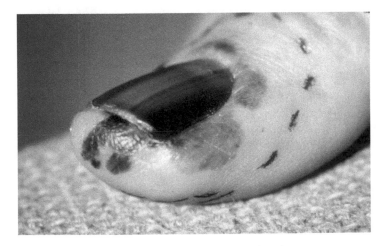

Figure 5 Hutchinson's sign with a subungual melanoma.

Prognostic Factors and Staging

To make decisions regarding treatment and therapy, it is important to be able to predict which patients are at risk for developing metastatic disease. Prognosis is based on disease stage. The most recent staging system for melanoma, revised in 2002, of the American Joint Committee on Cancer (AJCC) (33) is presented in Table 2. The AJCC system is a clinical and pathological staging system and is based on the TNM system, where T refers to tumor, N to nodes, and M to metastasis. The most recent staging system for melanoma more accurately classifies patients into groups with similar survival. Stage I and II indicates clinically localized primary melanoma and stage III melanoma indicates regional involvement (lymph nodes or in-transit metastases). Stage IV is metastatic disease beyond regional lymph nodes (i.e., lung, liver, and brain).

A number of clinical and histological features have been identified as prognostic factors, associated with a patient's probability of survival. The single most predictive factor is the depth of invasion of the original lesion (34,35), the Breslow thickness or depth, measured in millimeters from the top of the epidermis to the deepest tumor cells. Increasing thickness is associated with an increased risk for recurrence of melanoma and therefore death. In addition, the thicker the primary melanoma, the more likely there is to be microscopic lymph node involvement. Survival from melanoma depends on the stage of disease at the time of diagnosis. Elderly patients, especially men, tend to present with thicker melanomas than younger patients and women (36).

Table 2 AJCC Staging of Melanoma

Stage	TNM classification	Definition	5-year survival rate, $\% \pm SE$
IA	T1a N0 M0	≤1 mm; no ulceration (Clark level II/III)	95.3 ± 0.4
IB	T1b N0 M0	≤1 mm with ulceration or Clark level IV/V	90.9 ± 1.0
	T2a N0 M0	1.01 to 2 mm; no ulceration	89.0 ± 0.7
IIA	T2b N0 M0	1.01 to 2 mm with ulceration	77.4 ± 1.7
	T3a N0 M0	2.01 to 4 mm; no ulceration	78.7 ± 1.2
IIB	T3b N0 M0	2.01 to 4 mm with ulceration	63.0 ± 1.5
	T4a N0 M0	>4 mm; no ulceration	67.4 ± 2.4
IIC	T4b N0 M0	>4 mm with ulceration	45.1 ± 1.9
IIIA	T1-4a N1a M0	Single micro node; no ulceration	69.5 ± 3.7
	T1-4a N2a M0	2 to 3 micro nodes; no ulceration	63.3 ± 5.6
IIIB	T1-4a N1b-2c M0	1 to 3 macro nodes or in-transit mets; no ulcer	40–60
	T1-4b N1a-2a M0	1 to 3 micro nodes; ulceration	40–55
IIIC	T1-4b N1a-2b M0	1 to 3 macro nodes; ulceration	20–35
	anyT N3 M0	≥4 nodes, matted, or nodes + in-transit mets	26.7 ± 2.5
IV	AnyT anyN M1a-1b	Distant skin, SC, nodal, or lung metastasis	5–20
	AnyT anyN M1c	All visceral mets or elevated LDH with mets	9.5 ± 1.1

Abbreviations: AJCC, American Joint Committee on Cancer; TNM, tumor, node, metastases; SE, standard error; SC, subcutaneous; LDH, lactate dehydrogenase.
Source: From Ref. 33.

The age of the patient at the time of diagnosis is a prognostic factor. Older patients tend to have a worse prognosis than younger patients; however, older patients tend to present with thicker tumors and a greater percentage of ulcerated melanomas compared to younger patients (37,38). However, more recent studies suggest that age may be an independent prognostic factor, after thickness and ulceration (17). The anatomic site of the primary tumor and the gender of the patient are also clinical variables that are predictive of survival. Generally, lesions arising on the scalp, hands, and feet have a poorer prognosis than lesions arising on the extremities, arms, and legs (17,31,39). Women tend to have a better prognosis than men, although this is often confounded by the anatomic site because women more commonly have lesions on the extremities (17,31,39).

Other histologic factors associated with a poor prognosis include a high mitotic rate (>6) (31) and presence of microscopic satellites. Ulceration of the primary lesion, which is closely correlated with thickness, is associated with a worse prognosis. In the most recent AJCC staging system, thickness and ulceration are used together to determine the "T" category (33). The presence of tumor-infiltrating lymphocytes, a measure of the host immune response to the tumor, is associated with a more favorable prognosis while studies have shown that evidence of histological regression and increasing level of invasion (Clark level) are negative prognostic factors (31). The histological subtype of melanoma, such as SSM or ALM, does not confer much additional prognostic information. The presence of regional lymph node involvement is a poor prognostic sign regardless of the thickness or the level of the primary melanoma. In addition, the number of involved lymph nodes correlates with risk of distant metastatic disease and therefore survival.

Treatment

With increasing age, there is an accumulation of medical comorbidity, which can affect the overall treatment for elderly patients with melanoma. However, surgery remains the primary treatment for melanoma, and overall surgery for melanoma in the elderly is well tolerated.

The initial evaluation of a patient with melanoma includes an assessment of personal history and family history and an appropriate physical examination that includes a total skin examination and palpation of regional (draining) lymph nodes. The focus of this evaluation is to identify risk factors, signs or symptoms of metastases, dysplastic nevi, and additional melanomas. In practice, a chest X ray, liver function tests, and lactate dehydrogenase (LDH) are performed, though there are no data to support this common practice. The majority of patients who present with melanoma do not have distant metastatic disease at presentation; therefore, extensive evaluations with computerized tomography (CT) scans to search for distant metastases have an extremely low yield and consequently are not indicated in asymptomatic patients. Patients with melanoma in situ do not require screening for metastatic disease. More extensive staging evaluation with CT scans can be considered in patients with high-risk disease (thick primary melanoma >4 mm thick or node-positive disease) where the risk of distant metastatic disease is higher. The recent use of sentinel lymph node (SLN) mapping represents a powerful method for surgical staging of these patients and is discussed in detail below.

Patients with local regional disease including nodal, in-transit, and satellite metastases, and local recurrence have a risk of systemic recurrence that exceeds 50%. Despite such high incidence, staging workup with imaging studies such as

CT scans of the brain, chest, abdomen, and pelvis have a relatively low yield in detecting distant metastases in asymptomatic patients. The yield however is higher in this patient population than in patients with primary disease only, and therefore selective imaging studies may be indicated. A reasonable approach would be to include liver function tests, LDH, chest radiograph, and CT scans of the abdomen. Depending on the site of the local recurrence, CT scans of the pelvis or neck are recommended. Routine imaging of the brain in patients without symptoms is not indicated. Positron emission tomography imaging (PET) is useful in evaluating metastatic disease, but its role in screening has not been defined.

Surgery for Primary Disease

The principal treatment of primary melanoma is surgery. Tumor thickness (Breslow depth of invasion) is the predominate variable that most accurately determines prognosis and therapy. Local control of a primary melanoma requires wide excision of the tumor down to the deep fascia with a margin of clinically normal-appearing skin. Tumor thickness primarily determines the extent of the margin. For melanoma in situ, excision of the lesion with 0.5 cm border of clinically normal skin is sufficient and this should be curative. Melanomas less than or equal to 1.0 mm in thickness are treated with a 1 cm margin. If the thickness is between 1 and 2 mm, a 2 cm margin is adequate and a 1 cm margin is associated with only a 3% local recurrence rate, which has no impact on survival. For lesions thicker than 2 mm, a 2 cm margin is adequate. For lesions thicker 4.0 mm, a 3 cm margin is recommended. In cosmetically sensitive areas, such as the face, or anatomically difficult areas, such as the ear or hands, it may be difficult to achieve the desired margin. In those situations, at least a 1 cm margin should be obtained. The majority of primary cutaneous melanomas can be managed as outpatient surgical procedures with excision and primary closure. This not only achieves acceptable local control of melanoma, but also decreases morbidity for patients. The current recommendations for skin margins are based on evidence from prospective trials (40).

Surgical Management of Regional Lymph Nodes

Clinically Normal Regional Lymph Nodes. The management of clinically normal lymph nodes in patients with melanoma has been debated for decades. In about 15% to 20% of patients with melanoma who do not have clinically apparent lymph node involvement, the lymph nodes will contain occult micrometastases. SLN mapping has largely replaced elective lymph node dissections in patients with early-stage melanoma, stage I and II (41). Before wide excision, the primary tumor site is injected most commonly with both blue dye and radioactive tracer. These agents are taken up by the dermal lymphatics and drain to the one or multiple SLN. By direct visualization of the blue dye and determination of the radioactive counts by use of a hand-held gamma probe, this node or nodes can be identified and surgically removed for detailed histologic examination by a pathologist. If the SLN is negative for melanoma, no further lymph node surgery is required. If metastatic melanoma is detected in the SLN, a complete lymph node dissection is recommended. SLN mapping may be considered in patients with melanomas with a thickness of more than 1 mm, or thinner if other poor prognostic factors are present, such as Clark's level IV or the presence of ulceration (42).

SLN Biopsy in the Elderly. The SLN biopsy is best used when a patient is a candidate for adjuvant therapy. When recommending SLN biopsy to elderly patients, many issues need to be considered (10). Although the procedure is limited, it does require the use of general anesthesia and preoperative lymphoscintigraphy to identify the appropriate nodal basin. Especially in the elderly population, a patient's medical history must be reviewed to determine if the patient is stable enough to undergo adjuvant therapy. If an SLN biopsy is positive, patients and their families must consider whether they are willing to undergo complete lymph node dissection, which may cause significant morbidity, or receive interferon (IFN) therapy, which is associated with considerable toxicity. Patients must be aware that both lymph node dissection and IFN therapy may improve disease-free survival, but results for prolonging overall survival are unproven.

Clinically Enlarged Regional Lymph Nodes. Patients with clinically enlarged lymph nodes from a melanoma with no evidence of distant metastatic disease should undergo complete lymph node dissection, primarily for local control. Nodal dissection can provide long-term disease-free survival and possible cure, with 25% to 50% of patients cured by surgery.

Adjuvant Therapy

Postsurgical adjuvant therapy of melanoma is considered for patients with thick primary melanoma (>4 mm thick) or node-positive disease. These patients have at least a 50% to 75% chance of dying from melanoma. The only Food and Drug Administration (FDA)-approved treatment for this patient group is high-dose IFN administered for one year. Previous reviews have summarized the results from a series of randomized clinical trials of IFN in patients with melanoma (43). High-dose IFN alpha-2b has been shown to improve the disease-free survival compared to the observation in multiple studies, and in one study, to improve the overall survival by 10% (44,45). Prominent side effects include fatigue, fever, depression, nausea, and headache. Laboratory abnormalities include elevated hepatic transaminases, increase in triglycerides, anemia, and leukopenia. It is important to note that many of the original clinical studies of IFN excluded patients who were older than 70 years, or who had diminished performance status. The increasing medical comorbidities that arise with age may affect the clinician's decision whether to recommend adjuvant IFN; thus treatment decisions must be highly individualized. To administer IFN safely, patients must be monitored closely with appropriate dose modifications for toxicity, particularly for hepatic toxicity. Studies with low-dose IFN have not shown an improvement in disease-free or overall survival (46,47).

Vaccine therapy is a new, promising means for the treatment of melanoma, particularly in the adjuvant setting. At present, all melanoma vaccines should be considered experimental. There are relatively few side effects associated with vaccine treatment, an advantage when treating older patients.

Surveillance and Follow-Up of Patients with Melanoma

Patients with a history of melanoma should be followed regularly for evidence of local regional recurrence, distant metastatic disease, and a second primary melanoma. Generally, the frequency of follow-up is related to the tumor thickness: patients with thicker tumors, who are at greater risk for recurrence, should have more frequent follow-up examinations as part of their surveillance. Similarly, patients with regional lymph nodes involved with melanoma (stage III) should be followed more frequently. The most important component is the history and physical examination. When detailing the patient's history, it is important to ask about any new or suspicious lesions, enlarged nodes, or systemic complaints such as fatigue, cough, or headaches, because the majority of recurrences are patient detected due to symptoms. The physical examination should include a thorough skin examination, including the scalp, because the risk of second primary melanoma is increased. At least 3% of patients will develop an additional cutaneous melanoma within three years of diagnosis; this risk is higher in patients with dysplastic nevi. Regional lymph nodes should be thoroughly examined, especially in those patients without prior nodal surgery. The remainder of the examination should be comprehensive, keeping in mind frequent metastases to lung, liver, and brain.

While most follow-up evaluations include laboratory studies such as complete blood count, chemistry panel including liver function tests, and an LDH, abnormal blood tests rarely are the sole indicators of recurrence. If a patient has an elevated LDH, it is suggestive of metastatic melanoma. Periodic chest X rays are recommended, because the lungs are the most frequent site of distant disease. The routine use of screening CT scans, magnetic resonance imaging, or bone scans is not justified for follow-up surveillance. Patient education is an extremely important component of follow-up for individuals with melanoma. This should include educating patients of the early warning signs of melanoma, on how to perform periodic skin self-examination, and on the importance of sun protection and sun avoidance.

Management of Nodal or Local Recurrence

Regional node is the most common site of metastases. The risk for regional node metastasis increases as the thickness of the melanoma increases. Any palpable lymph node, particularly in the regional lymph node basin, should be further evaluated, first by fine needle aspiration (FNA). If either the FNA or the lymph node biopsy is positive for metastatic melanoma, patients should undergo a complete lymph node dissection, if they are medically stable. The goal of nodal dissection is to provide long-term disease-free survival and possibly cure and/or to provide optimum local regional control of disease.

In-transit metastases are local regional metastases that involve the dermal and subdermal lymphatics. These metastases arise between the primary tumor (more than 2.0 cm from the primary tumor) and the regional lymph node basin, with most occurrence within three years of definitive surgical therapy. In more than 50% of patients, regional lymph nodes are involved. Treatment is generally local with surgical excision with 1 to 3 cm margins depending on the anatomic site. Elderly patients with lower-extremity melanoma seem be at increased risk for this type of melanoma recurrence. At times, the disease can be quite indolent. For patients with multiple lesions or multiply recurrent in-transit disease, isolated limb perfusion (ILP) can be considered. In a study by Noorda et al., no significant differences in response rate, limb toxicity, systemic toxicity, local complications, and long-term morbidity of ILP between patients younger than 75 years and those older than 75 (48) were found. These authors concluded that older age is not a contraindication for ILP.

Management of Metastatic Melanoma (Stage IV Disease)

The treatment of a patient with metastatic melanoma depends upon multiple factors including the overall condition and age of the patient, the sites and number of metastases, pace of the disease, and the patient's preferences for treatment. Currently, the goals of treatment are directed toward palliation of symptoms. There is no evidence that treatment of metastatic melanoma has any impact on prolonging the survival. The overall survival for patients with metastatic melanoma ranges from 5 to 11 months, with a median survival of 8.5 months. The estimated five-year survival rate for patients with stage IV disease is 6% to 16% (17). Metastatic melanoma can metastasize to virtually any organ in the body. The most common site of distant metastases is the lung. The skin, liver, and brain are also common sites of metastases.

The formulation of a patient's treatment plan needs to be highly individualized, especially in the elderly who may be more susceptible to the side effects of treatment. The range of options includes observation, surgical resection of solitary metastases, single-agent chemotherapy such as dacarbazine or diethyl-triazeno-imidazole carboxamide (DTIC) (the only FDA-approved chemotherapy for melanoma) or temozolomide, combination chemotherapy, or immunotherapy. Temozolomide is an analog of dacarbazine. It is easy to administer, because it is given orally, and the standard dose is 150 to 200 mg/m^2 on days 1 to 5. Courses are repeated every four weeks. The major side effect is mild to moderate myelosuppression. Mild nausea and vomiting are also common, but are readily controlled with antiemetic medications (i.e., ondansetron). Response rates of 10% to 20% have been reported for temozolomide (49). Another property of temozolomide is that it crosses the blood–brain barrier. This is an advantage, given the high incidence of brain metastases in patients with melanoma. Combination chemotherapy regimens have not been shown to be superior to single-agent chemotherapy in terms of response or overall survival (50). Immunotherapy with drugs such as interleukin (IL)-2 or IFN must be administered with great caution in the elderly, and patient selection is critical. Practical guidelines for the safe administration of high-dose IL-2 have recently been published (51). Patients receiving IL-2 should not have other major cardiac, pulmonary, renal, hepatic, or medical illness and should have good performance status. It is important to screen for occult cardiac disease, and for this reason, all patients over 50 years of age should undergo cardiac stress testing before IL-2 treatment. Evidence of ischemic heart disease is a contraindication to high-dose IL-2 treatment. Because of the complexity of treatment, high-dose IL-2 is generally administered by nurses and doctors who have received special training in its administration and are familiar with its use.

New targets for melanoma treatment have recently been identified. Constitutive activation of the receptor tyrosine kinase–mediated Ras/Raf/mitogen-activated protein kinases pathway is a frequent and early event in melanoma development. In 2002, Davies et al. reported that activating mutation in BRAF can be found in two-thirds of melanoma tumors (52). Subsequent studies have confirmed these results, establishing BRAF as the most commonly mutated oncogene in melanoma described to date. Ongoing clinical trials are evaluating the efficacy of a RAF kinase inhibitor, sorafenib (BAY 43–9006), either as a single agent or combined with chemotherapy in patients with metastatic melanoma (53). Hopefully, this new direction in melanoma treatment will lead to improvement in overall survival in patients with metastatic melanoma.

Prevention/Screening/Patient Education

Efforts at melanoma prevention have predominantly focused on the avoidance of sunburn and excessive sun exposure, ideally starting at an early age. Sun protection should be practiced at all ages, because the damaging effects of chronic UV radiation are most likely cumulative. It remains reasonable to recommend a "safe sun strategy," which includes avoiding the peak hours of the sun, wearing sunscreen on sun-exposed body sites, avoiding the use of tanning parlors, and wearing protective clothing. Sun-protective clothing includes wearing a wide-brimmed hat and tightly woven, cotton shirts and pants. Patient education should emphasize liberal sunscreen use with sunscreens with a sun protective factor (SPF) of 15 or greater and with UV-A/UV-B protection.

Screening for skin cancer whether by self-skin examination by the patient or by the health care provider is a controversial area. The third U.S. Preventive Services Task Force concluded that there was not sufficient evidence to show that general skin examination by physicians was effective in reducing morbidity or mortality from melanoma (54). However, the report called for further studies to help clinicians identify individuals, particularly older patients, who are at higher risk for developing melanoma. In addition, the Institute of Medicine reached similar conclusions regarding general screening recommendations, but also indicated "clinicians and patients should continue to be alert to the common signs of skin cancer, with particular emphasis on older white males and on melanoma" (55). The purpose of screening individuals at high risk is to remove or closely monitor potential precursors of melanoma and to diagnose melanoma at an early stage. It has been shown that, in high-risk individuals, screening for melanoma results in the detection of thinner melanomas (56). One important study has shown that subjects who performed skin self-examinations had significantly reduced incidences of melanoma and lower risks of progression to advanced disease or death after diagnosis, reducing death from melanoma by an estimated 63% (57).

Unfortunately, when compared with younger individuals, older individuals are less likely to perform skin self-examination (58). Also when compared with younger individuals, individuals older than 50 years rarely report itching or changes in elevation or color of a mole; however, they do report ulceration more frequently—a feature associated with a poorer prognosis (59). Older patients have also been shown to have greater difficulty in detecting changes in melanoma in the photographs of pigmented lesions (59).

There are multiple factors that contribute to the poorer prognosis of melanoma in the elderly. Elderly individuals tend to have other comorbidities that may prevent them from performing skin self-examination. Decreased mobility and poor visual acuity can contribute to prevent an older individual from performing an adequate self-examination. The fact that many elderly people live alone might also prevent the early recognition of changing pigmented lesions. Also, the elderly tend to have other dermatologic lesions such as actinic keratosis, seborrheic keratosis, and lentinges, which may make it difficult to identify melanoma (10).

NONMELANOMA SKIN CANCERS: BASAL AND SQUAMOUS CELL SKIN CANCER

Nonmelanoma skin cancer is the most common malignancy in the United States. Although national statistics are imprecise, approximately 1.2 million nonmelanoma skin cancers are diagnosed annually in the United States. Basal cell carcinoma (BCC) is the most common skin cancer with more than one million new cases detected in 2000, with squamous cell carcinoma (SCC) comprising 20% of the nonmelanoma skin cancers (60). With the ability to metastasize, SCC is associated with a higher absolute mortality; the majority of the 2300 annual deaths from nonmelanoma skin cancer in the United States arise from this tumor.

Epidemiology

Overall, skin cancer incidence rates are increasing due to several factors including increased recreational sun exposure, increased life expectancy, and depletion of the ozone layer. The incidence of skin cancers has been rising by approximately 5% each year (60). Over 99% of nonmelanoma skin cancers occur in Caucasians. These skin cancers are most commonly seen in the elderly, especially those with fair complexions and long-standing sun exposure. However, increasingly, nonmelanoma skin cancers are seen in younger people, in their 30s and 40s.

Pathogenesis and Risk Factors

The cause of BCC and SCC is multifactorial, with environmental, genetic, and host factors contributing to their development (Tables 3 and 4). The most important risk factor is exposure to UV radiation from sunlight. Most dangerous is UV-B radiation, but increasing evidence suggests that UV-A is probably carcinogenic as well. The timing and pattern of sun exposure are associated with different types of skin cancer. In general, nonmelanoma skin cancers are associated with cumulative sun exposure and occur most frequently in areas maximally exposed to the sun (e.g., the face, back of hands, and forearms). Intermittent, intense exposure to the sun, particularly in childhood, is associated with an increased risk of BCC while cumulative sun exposure seems to be related to the development of SCC. Farmers, fishermen, and other individuals working primarily outdoors during the day are at particularly high risk for SCC. Individuals who have fair skin, light-colored eyes, red hair, a tendency to burn rather than tan, and a history of severe sunburns are at increased risk for nonmelanoma skin cancers.

Table 3 Risk Factors for the Development of BCC

Host factors
  Age
  Fair skin
  Hair color—blond/red
  Eye color—blue eyes
Environmental
  History of blistering sunburns
  Childhood sun exposure
  Intermittent sun exposure
  Arsenic exposure
  Radiation
Genetic
  Basal cell nevus syndrome
  Albinism
  Xeroderma pigmentosum
Other
  Personal history of BCC
  Family history of skin cancer
  Immunosuppression

Abbreviation: BCC, basal cell carcinoma.

Table 4 Risk Factors for the Development of SCC

Host factors
  Age
  Fair skin
  Hair color—blond/red
  Eye color—blue eyes
Environmental
  Chronic sun exposure
  Arsenic exposure
  Radiation
  PUVA therapy
  Genetic
Other
  Immunosuppression
  HPV infection

Abbreviations: HPV, human papillomavirus; SCC, squamous cell carcinoma; UV, ultraviolet; PUVA, psoralen plus UV-A.

Patients receiving immunosuppression after organ transplantation or for other reasons are particularly prone to SCC. Other risk factors are chronic inflammatory conditions such as chronic ulcers, or the use of psoralen plus UV-A (PUVA), a treatment for psoriasis and other diseases, which can increase one's risk of SCC 10-fold (61). The risk of lip or oral SCC is increased with cigarette smoking. For the elderly, other risk factors, particularly for SCC, include exposures that occurred during youth, such as arsenic exposure from well water or industrial sources and therapeutic radiation. Up until the 1950s, superficial ionizing radiation was used to treat tinea capitis and acne, and has been associated with an increased risk of nonmelanoma skin cancers (62). The majority of cases in African-American patients are associated with scarring or burns rather than UV exposure. Human papillomavirus infection has also been implicated in some SCCs, particularly in the autosomal dominant disorder "epidermodysplasia verruciformis" (63).

BCC

BCC can be seen in association with several conditions including the "basal cell nevus syndrome" (also called "nevoid BCC syndrome" or "Gorlin's syndrome"), albinism, and xeroderma pigmentosum. The basal cell nevus syndrome is a rare autosomal dominant disorder that is due to germline mutations in the patched gene (PTCH), a tumor suppressor gene in the hedgehog pathway. Acquired mutations in PTCH have also been identified in sporadic BCC. Sporadic BCCs are also associated with mutations in the genes encoding p53 and ras.

SCC

Often, SCC is derived from actinic keratoses, a precursor that appears as a rough, scaly, often erythematous papule that is frequently more easily palpated than seen. Estimates of the likelihood of progression of actinic keratoses to SCC range from 0.025% to as high as 20%. Mutations in the gene encoding the p53 protein and in the ras oncogene have been found in both actinic keratoses and SCCs. Mutations in p16 have also been reported in SCCs.

Prevention and Screening

The recommendations outlined previously regarding prevention of melanoma also apply to nonmelanoma skin cancers: primary prevention strategies are aimed at reducing chronic sun exposure. Public education and patient education should encourage the regular use of sunscreens with an SPF of 15 or greater, especially in childhood, and to wear sun-protective clothing. Avoidance of tanning parlors and minimizing total sun exposure, especially the midday sun (10 A.M. – 2 P.M.), is recommended. The use of sunscreen is strongly recommended in all patients with a history of cancer from exposure to the sun because studies have shown that individuals who use sunscreen regularly develop less actinic keratoses and SCC (64,65). Regarding the prevention of nonmelanoma skin cancers, efforts to preserve the ozone layer are important because the thinning of the ozone layer has been linked to increased UV radiation at the earth's surface and increases in the incidence of BCC and SCC.

Topical and systemic retinoids have been used for preventive purposes; however, chemoprevention of skin cancer has not yet been achieved. Retinoids have been used mainly in patients with xeroderma pigmentosum and in transplant patients with multiple SCC (38). These agents seem to alter the promotion of skin cancer in the early stages; however, the results are not long lasting. Whenever the use of retinoids is discontinued (there are many side effects with these agents), the skin cancers begin to grow again. Recommendations regarding the value of screening for nonmelanoma skin cancers vary depending upon the organization. Currently, evidence that total body skin examination by clinicians is effective in reducing mortality or morbidity from nonmelanoma skin cancer is lacking.

Diagnosis: Clinical Characteristics

BCC

Most BCCs occur on sun-exposed areas such as the face, neck, ears, scalp, and arms, with the nose being the most common site. Approximately 20% of these cancers arise on sites that are not typically sun exposed (66,67). BCC is a malignancy arising from the epidermal basal cells residing in the hair follicles (68). There are four clinicopathological variants of BCC: nodular, superficial, pigmented, and morpheaform. The most common is nodular, or noduloulcerative, commonly occurring on the head and neck. This subtype begins as a shiny, skin-colored or pink translucent nodule with a "pearly" rolled border, often with small telangiectatic vessels on its surface. The nodule grows slowly and its center may become ulcerated and bleed, although there is usually no associated pain or tenderness. Most are diagnosed when the tumors are 1 to 2 cm in diameter.

Superficial BCCs are more commonly found on the trunk and extremities; however, the head and neck may also be affected. These lesions present as one or several flat, erythematous plaques that slowly enlarge. The surface of these plaques may be scaly or crusted and can mimic benign inflammatory dermatoses such as psoriasis or nummular eczema. Pigmented BCCs share many of the same features with nodular BCCs, but have a heavier accumulation of melanin, often appearing as blue or black lesions. These lesions may be mistaken for melanoma or vascular proliferation. The morpheaform variant typically presents as a flat or slightly depressed, whitish or yellowish plaque with indistinct borders. This subtype has a greater potential for extensive subclinical spread and can be quite aggressive.

BCC rarely metastasizes and is usually curable with a variety of treatment approaches. Although the mortality is low, these cancers may result in significant morbidity due to invasive local growth with potential disfigurement and destruction of skin, bone, and cartilage.

SCC

SCC of the skin is a malignancy of epidermal keratinocytes. This type of skin cancer usually appears on the areas of skin that are heavily damaged by sun exposure. The most common sites include the head or neck, lip, back, forearms, and dorsum of the hand. Mucosal lesions, especially oral mucosa, tend to be more aggressive. The four clinical variants of SCC are actinic keratosis, Bowen's disease, keratoacanthoma, and invasive SCC. Actinic keratosis is at one end of the clinical spectrum, considered to be a premalignant form of SCC. Clinically, these lesions present as flat, scaly, pink papules with a rough texture, which are often difficult to visualize. There is some potential for these lesions to develop into invasive SCC. "Bowen's disease," or SCC in situ, typically presents as a solitary erythematous scaling plaque, which may develop into invasive SCC in up to 20% of cases. "Keratoacanthoma" is a variant that is characterized by rapid growth and a crateriform appearance with a central plug. These lesions can be locally aggressive and may cause significant scarring if spontaneous regression occurs. Invasive SCC usually presents as a discrete scaly erythematous papule on an indurated base. The lesion may grow over time and become ulcerated, itchy, and painful, or bleed. When SCC arises in burn scars or sites of trauma, the lesions are referred to as "Marjolin's ulcers."

The natural history of SCC depends on both tumor and host characteristics. Untreated SCC may cause significant local destruction. However, unlike BCC, SCC carries a 5% to 10% risk of metastasis. Higher-risk lesions are lesions that are larger than 2 cm, poorly or moderately differentiated, lesions on the ear or on the lip, lesions arising in scars, tumors with perineural involvement, and tumors in immunosuppressed patients. Regional lymph nodes are the most common site of metastasis, although other sites include lung, liver, brain, skin, and bone. For patients with lymph node metastases, the five-year survival rate is less than 50%.

The diagnosis of BCC as well as SCC is frequently suspected on inspection alone, but histologic confirmation is usually indicated. Either a shave or a punch biopsy technique is acceptable. Care should be taken to include the base of the lesion if using a shave biopsy technique.

Treatment

BCC

There are several different treatment options for BCC. The best method depends upon physician's expertise, the patient's medical status as well as personal preference, and characteristics of the tumor. Commonly used approaches include surgical excision, cryosurgery (liquid nitrogen), electrodessication and curettage (ED&C), and radiation therapy. The technique with the lowest recurrence rate is Mohs micrographic surgery, which utilizes frozen tissue mapping of the resection margins in stages to locate residual tumor. Mohs microsurgery should be considered when treating recurrent cases; microscopically aggressive forms such as the morpheaform subtype; lesions larger than 2 cm in greatest diameter; and tumors of the ears, eyelids, nose, nasolabial folds, and lips. This approach minimizes tissue loss while maximizing cure rates.

ED&C is a method of definitive treatment for selected low-risk BCC and SCC tumors. It is a rapid technique, performed under local anesthesia. One of the disadvantages of this technique is that wound healing occurs by granulation, which may take four to six weeks, and may leave a scar that is less cosmetically desirable than one from surgical excision. There is also no histologic evaluation of the margins with this method.

Radiation therapy can be curative; however, the recurrence rate is higher than with Mohs or surgical excision. It is useful in patients who are not good surgical candidates and as an adjunct to surgery for high-risk tumors. However, multiple visits are required, which may impose significant inconvenience for the elderly. Younger patients are not good candidates for radiation therapy because of the long-term sequelae of radiation, such as tumor recurrence and chronic radiation dermatitis.

Other treatment methods for BCC include the use of retinoids, IFN alpha, topical 5-fluorouracil (5-FU), and imiquinod and photodynamic therapy. Cure rates for BCC range between 90% and 99%.

SCC

SCC can be cured by several techniques, which include surgical excision, cryosurgery (liquid nitrogen), ED&C, and radiation therapy. Surgical excision is the most common treatment method for SCC. As with BCC, Mohs micrographic surgery provides the lowest recurrence rate of standard treatment modalities. Cure rates are greater than 90%. In particular, Mohs microsurgery should be considered with recurrent tumors or lesions that have an increased risk of metastasis as outlined above. Topical 5-FU, photodynamic therapy, or imiquimod may have a role in the management of in situ squamous cell cancers. Topical 5-FU can yield excellent results in the treatment of actinic keratoses (69). After the medication is applied to affected areas, the lesions become edematous, painful, and inflamed before resolving. This treatment modality requires high compliance and tolerance of discomfort for several weeks. One advantage is that lesions that are barely visible clinically are treated nonsurgically.

Follow-Up

Patients with BCC and SCC require ongoing follow-up to detect local recurrence and to recognize new skin cancers. The likelihood of developing a second BCC or SCC is about 40% over a period of three years (70). In addition, these patients have an increased risk for developing cutaneous melanoma. Shared risk factors and common etiologic exposure account for the increased risk. Patient education regarding modification of risk factors (i.e., sun exposure) is an important component of follow-up as discussed above.

REFERENCES

1. Jemal A, Murray T, Ward E, et al. Cancer statistics 2005. CA Cancer J Clin 2005; 55(1):10–30.
2. Weinstock MA. Death from skin cancer among the elderly: epidemiological patterns. Arch Dermatol 1997; 133:1207–1209.

3. Armstrong B, Kricker A. Epidemiology of sun exposure and skin cancer. Cancer Surv 1996; 26:133–153.
4. Grob J, Stern R, Mackie R, et al. Epidemiology, Causes, and Prevention of Skin Diseases. Cambridge: Blackwell Sciences, 1997.
5. Brash D, Rudolph J, Simon J, et al. A role for sunlight in skin cancer: UV induced p53 mutations in squamous cell carcinoma. Proc Natl Acad Sci USA 1991; 88:10124–10128.
6. Brash D, Ziegler A, Jonason A, et al. Sunlight and sunburn in human skin cancer: p53 apoptosis, and tumor promotion. J Invest Dermatol Symptom Proc 1996; 1:136–142.
7. Tsao H. Update on familial cancer syndromes and the skin. J Am Acad Dermatol 2000; 42:939–969.
8. Morris BT, Sober AJ. Cutaneous malignant melanoma in the older patient. Clin Geriatr Med 1989; 5:171–181.
9. Sunderkrotter C, Kalde H, Luger T. Aging and the skin immune system. Arch Dermatol 1997; 133:1256–1262.
10. Sachs DL, Marghoob AA, Halpern A. Skin cancer in the elderly. Clin Geriatric Med 2001; 17(4):715–738.
11. Marks R. Epidemiology of melanoma. Clin Exp Dermatol 2000; 25:459–463.
12. Howe HL, Wingo PA, Thun MJ, et al. Annual report to the nation on the status of cancer (1973–1998), featuring cancers and recent increasing trends. J Natl Cancer Inst 2001; 93:824–842.
13. Jemal A, Thomas A, Murray T, et al. Cancer statistics 2002. CA Cancer J Clin 2002; 52:23–47.
14. Crawford JC, Cohen HJ. Aging and neoplasia. Annu Rev Gerontol Geriatr 1984; 4:3–32.
15. Mackie RM, Hole DJ, Hunter JAA, et al. Cutaneous melanoma in Scotland. Incidence and mortality 1979–94. Br Med J 1997; 315:1117–1121.
16. Kelly JW. Melanoma in the elderly—a neglected public health challenge. Med J Aust 1998; 19:403–404.
17. Balch CM, Soong SJ, Gershenwald JE, et al. Prognostic factors analysis of 17,600 melanoma patients: validation of the American Joint Committee on Cancer melanoma staging system. J Clin Oncol 2001; 19(16):3622–3634.
18. Tsao H, Bevone C, Goggins W, et al. The transformation rate of moles (melanocytic nevi) into cutaneous melanoma: a population based estimate. Arch Dermatol 2003; 139: 223–238.
19. Swetter SM, Geller AC, Kirkwood JM. Melanoma in the older person. Oncology 2004; 18:1187–1196.
20. Green A, Bain C, McLennan R, et al. Risk factors for cutaneous melanoma in Queensland. Recent Results Cancer Res 1986; 102:76–97.
21. Kefford R, Bishop JN, Tucker M, et al. Melanoma genetics consortium. Reflection and reaction: genetic testing for melanoma. Lancet Oncol 2002; 3(11):653–654.
22. Beitner H, Noreel SE, Ringborg U, Moon TE. Malignant melanoma: aetiological importance of individual pigmentation and sun exposure. Br J Dermatol 1990; 122:43–51.
23. Elwood JM, Jopson J. Melanoma and sun exposure: an overview of published studies. Int J cancer 1997; 73:198–203.
24. Scotto J, Frears T. The association of solar ultraviolet and skin melanoma incidence among Caucasians in the United States. Cancer Invest 1987; 5:275–283.
25. Tucker MA, Halpern A, Holly EA, et al. Clinically recognized dysplastic nevi: a central risk factor for cutaneous melanoma [see comments]. JAMA 1997; 277:139–1444.
26. Marghoob A, Slade J, Kopf A, et al. Risk of developing multiple primary cutaneous melanomas in patients with the classic atypical-mole syndrome: a case-control study. Br J Dermatol 1996; 135:704–711.
27. Slingluff CL, Vollmer RT, Seigler HF. Multiple primary melanoma: incidence and risk factors in 283 patients. Surgery 1993; 113:330.
28. MacKie RM, Freudenberger T, Aitchison TC. Person risk-factor chart for cutaneous melanoma. Lancet 1989; 2:487.

29. Clark WH, Elder DE, Guerry D, et al. A study of tumor progression: the precursor lesions of superficial spreading and nodular melanoma. Human Pathol 1984; 15(12):1147–1165.
30. Guerry D, Synnestvedt M, Elder DE, et al. Lessons learned from tumor progression: the invasive radial growth phase of melanoma is common, incapable of metastasis, and indolent. J Invest Dermatol 1993; 100:342S–345S.
31. Clark WH, Elder DE, Guerry D IV, et al. Model predicting survival in stage I melanoma based on tumor progression. J Natl Cancer Inst 1989; 81:1893–1904.
32. Skelton HG, Smith KJ, Laskin WB, et al. Desmoplastic malignant melanoma. J Am Acad Dermatol 1995; 32:717.
33. Balch CM, Buzaid AC, Soong SJ, et al. Final version of the American Joint Committee on Cancer staging system for cutaneous melanoma. J Clin Oncol 2001; 19(16):3635–3648.
34. Balch C, Soong S, Murand T, et al. A multifactorial analysis of melanoma: II. Prognostic factors in patients with stage I (localized) melanoma. Surgery 1979; 86:343–351.
35. Breslow A. Prognostic factors in the treatment of cutaneous melanoma. J Cutan Pathol 1979; 6:208–212.
36. Hanrahan P, Hersey P, D'Este C. Factors involved in the presentation of older people with thick melanoma. Med J Aust 1998; 169:410–411.
37. Austin PF, Cruse W, Lyman G, et al. Age as a prognostic factor in the malignant melanoma population. Ann Surg Oncol 1994; 1:487–494.
38. Levine N. Role of retinoids in skin cancer treatment and prevention. J Am Acad Dermatol 1998; 39(suppl):62–66.
39. Schuchter L, Schultz DJ, Synnestvedt M, et al. A prognostic model for predicting 10-year survival in patients with primary melanoma. Ann Intern Med 1996; 125(5):369–375.
40. Houghton A, Coit D, Bloomer W, Buzaid A, et al. NCCN melanoma practice guidelines. National Comprehensive Cancer Network. Oncology (Huntingt) 1998; 12(7A):153–177.
41. Morton D, Wen D, Foshag L, et al. Technical details of intraoperative lymphatic mapping for early-stage melanoma. Arch Surg 1992; 127:392–399.
42. National Comprehensive Cancer Network. Melanoma: clinical practice guidelines in oncology.v.1.2005. Available at http://www.nccn.org/professionals/physician_gls/PDF/melanoma.pdf.
43. Pawlik TM, Sondak VK. Malignant melanoma: current state of primary and adjuvant treatment. Crit Rev Oncol Hematol 2003; 43:245–264.
44. Kirkwood JM, Strawderman MH, Ernstoff MS, et al. Interferon alpha-2b adjuvant therapy of high-risk resected cutaneous melanoma: the Eastern Cooperative Oncology Groups trial EST 1684. J Clin Oncol 1996; 14:7–17.
45. Kirkwood JM, Ibrahim JG, Sosman JA, et al. High-dose interferon alpha-2b significantly prolongs relapse free and overall survival compared with the GM2–KLH/QS21 vaccine in E1694/S9512/C509801. J Clin Oncol 2001; 19:2370–2380.
46. Cascinelli N, Belli F, MacKie RM, et al. Effect of long-term adjuvant therapy with interferon alpha-2a in patients with regional node metastases from cutaneous melanoma: a randomized trial. Lancet 2001; 358:866–869.
47. Hancock BW, Wheatley K, Harris S, et al. Adjuvant interferon in high-risk melanoma: the AIM HIGH Study—United Kingdom Coordinating Committee on Cancer Research randomized study of adjuvant low-dose extended-duration interferon alpha-2a in high-risk resected malignant melanoma. J Clin Oncol 2004; 22(1):53–61.
48. Noorda EM, Vrouenraets BC, Nieweg OE, et al. Safety and efficacy of isolated limb perfusion in elderly melanoma patients. Ann Surg Oncol 2002; 9:968–974.
49. Bleehen NM, Newlands SM, Thatcher LN, et al. Cancer research campaign phase II trial of temozolomide in metastatic melanoma. J Clin Oncol 1995; 13:910–913.
50. Chapman PB, Einhorn LH, Meyers ML, et al. Phase III multicenter randomized trial of the Dartmouth regimen versus dacarbazine in patients with metastatic melanoma. J Clin Oncol 1999; 17(9):2745–2751.
51. Schwartzentruber DJ. Guidelines for the safe administration of high dose interleukin-2. J Immunother 2001; 24:287.

52. Davies H, Bignell GR, Cox C, et al. Mutations of the BRAF gene in human melanoma. Nature 2002; 417:949–954.
53. Flaherty K, Brose M, Schuchter L, et al. Phase I/II trial of BAY 43–9006, carboplatin and paclitaxel demonstrate preliminary antitumor activity in the expansion cohort of patients with metastatic melanoma. Proc ASCO 2004:7507.
54. United States Preventive Services Task Force. Screening for skin cancer. Am J Prev Med 2001; 20(3S):44–46.
55. Institute of Medicine. Extending Medicare Coverage for Prevention and Other Services. Washington, D.C.: National Academics Press, 2000.
56. Marghoob A, Slade J, Salopek T, et al. Basal cell and squamous cell carcinomas are important risk factors for cutaneous malignant melanoma. Screening implications. Cancer 1995; 75:707.
57. Berwick M, Begg C, Fine J. Screening for cutaneous melanoma by skin self-examination. J Natl Cancer Inst 1996; 88:17–23.
58. Oliveria S, Christos P, Halpern A, et al. Evaluation of factors associated with skin self-examination. Cancer Epidemiol Biomarkers Prev 1999; 8:971–978.
59. Christos PJ, Oliveria SA, Berwick M, et al. Signs and symptoms of melanoma in older populations. J Clin Epidemiol 2000; 53:1044–1053.
60. American Cancer Society. Cancer Facts and Figures—2000. Atlanta, GA: American Cancer Society, 2000.
61. Stern R, Liebman E. Risk of squamous cell carcinoma methoxsalen (psoralen) and UV-A radiation (PUVA). A meta-analysis. Arch Dermatol 1998; 134:1582–1585.
62. Modan B, Alfondary E, Shapio D, et al. Factors affecting the development of skin cancer after scalp irradiation. Radiat Res 1993; 134:125–128.
63. McGregor J, Proby C. The role of papillomaviruses in human non-melanoma skin cancer. Cancer Surv 1996; 26:219–236.
64. Green A, Williams G, Neale R, et al. Daily sunscreen application and betacarotene supplementation in prevention of basal-cell and squamous-cell carcinomas of the skin: a randomized controlled trial. Lancet 1999; 354:723–729.
65. Thompson S, Jolley D, Marks R. Reduction of solar keratoses by regular sunscreen use. N Engl J Med 1993; 329:1147–1151.
66. Francheschi S, Levi F, Randimbison L, et al. Site distribution of different types of skin cancer: new aetological clues. Int J Cancer 1996; 67:24–28.
67. Gallagher R, Hill G, Bajdik C, et al. Sunlight exposure, pigmentary factors, and risk of nonmelanocytic skin cancer: I. Basal cell carcinoma. Arch Dermatol 1995; 131:157–163.
68. Taylor G, Lehrer M, Jensen P, et al. Involvement of follicular stem cells in forming not only the follicle but also the epidermis. Cell 2000; 102:451–461.
69. Goette D. Topical chemotherapy with 5-fluorouracil. J Am Acad Dermatol 1981; 4: 633–649.
70. Marcil I, Stern RS. Risk of developing a subsequent nonmelanoma skin cancer in patients with a history of nonmelanoma skin cancer: a critical review of the literature and meta-analysis. Arch Dermatol 2000; 136(12):1524–1530.

18
Head and Neck

William J. Brundage
Department of Surgery (Otolaryngology), University of Vermont College of Medicine, Burlington, Vermont, U.S.A.

INTRODUCTION

Head and neck cancer involves a broad range of cell types in a very anatomically complex and important area of the human body. The head and neck contain the organs of sight, hearing, taste, smell, and voice production. The mouth and throat are critical areas because the digestive process begins there. The nose and mouth warm and filter air. The voice, facial muscles, and eyes convey emotion and are critical for communication. The neck houses the blood supply to the brain, the neural communication from the brain to the body, and the endocrine organs that regulate overall body metabolism and calcium metabolism at the cellular level. While appearance and voice conspicuously reflect advanced age, there are age-related anatomic and physiologic changes throughout the head and neck. These complex and integrated functions make treating cancers in this region very challenging, especially in older patients among whom they are most common. No one chapter could adequately cover all aspects of head and neck cancer diagnosis and treatment in the elderly. The majority of patients with head and neck cancers are 60 years and older. The goal of this chapter is to provide an overview with a focus on issues relevant to older patients.

Most head and neck cancers are squamous cell carcinomas (SCC) of the mucosa of the upper aerodigestive tract. Other cancers arise from major and minor salivary glands and the thyroid gland. Skin cancers, lymphomas, and sarcomas occur in the head and neck but will be covered elsewhere in this book. This chapter will not address rare malignancies such as malignant odontogenic tumors, neuroendocrine carcinoma, malignant parathyroid tumors, and mucosal melanoma.

According to The American Cancer Society, there will likely be 64,940 new cancers of the oral cavity, pharynx, larynx, and thyroid gland diagnosed in 2005, which is 4.7% of all new cancers diagnosed in the United States. There will be 12,580 deaths related to tumors at these sites in 2005, 2.2% of all cancer deaths. Men will account for 69% of the new cases and 71% of the deaths from cancers of the oral cavity, pharynx, and larynx. Men will account for 25% of the new cases of thyroid cancer, but 42% of thyroid cancer–related deaths. With the exception of thyroid cancer, patients over the age of 65 account for approximately one-half of the new head and neck tumors and approximately 60% of the head and neck cancer–related deaths (Table 1). While only a very small percentage of thyroid cancers occur in older patients, they account for a large percentage of thyroid cancer–related deaths owing to the more aggressive nature of thyroid cancer in this group (2).

Head and neck tumors are staged using the T-primary tumor, N-regional nodes, M-distant metastasis (TNM) staging system of the American Joint Committee on Cancer (AJCC). One must evaluate the primary tumor and the regional lymph nodes, and exclude distant metastases or a synchronous primary tumor. T-stage, N-stage, and stage groupings in the head and neck are unique to each tumor site. For a detailed description of staging by site, readers should consult the latest edition (sixth at the time of this writing) of the AJCC cancer staging manual.

Normal Physiology with Aging

The nose and mouth humidify and warm the air entering the lungs. The larynx protects the airway during swallowing and allows one to speak by passing air from the lungs through nearly closed vocal folds producing sound waves. Pitch changes when the vocal folds are lengthened or shortened. The structures of the oral cavity, pharynx, and nose modulate this sound to produce voice. As anyone who has successfully estimated someone's age by voice alone knows, there are specific characteristics associated with an aging voice. Anatomic and histologic changes in the vocal cords include fibrosis and loss of elastic fibers, atrophy of submucous glands with less lubrication, degenerative changes within the cricoarytenoid joint, and replacement of cartilage with bone in the laryngeal framework (3,4). These changes cause the altered pitch, roughness, breathiness, weakness, hoarseness, and tremulousness we associate with an aging voice (5).

Eating requires fine control of structures in the oral cavity, pharynx, larynx, and esophagus to reduce food to a consistency appropriate for swallowing and to propel the resulting bolus to the stomach. This requires lubrication from salivary glands, and coordination of the muscles of the lip and cheek, jaw, pharynx, larynx, and upper esophagus. Changes with aging can include less saliva, muscle atrophy, loss of teeth and alveolar bone, change in the relative position of the structures of the neck from lordosis of the cervical spine, reduced esophageal peristalsis, and increased cricopharyngeus tone (6). Older patients with either Parkinson's disease or strokes, or who are on multiple medications with anticholinergic side effects can have additional underlying swallowing problems. Older patients are more likely to have cognitive problems, hearing loss, visual loss, vascular disease, degenerative joint disease, and periodontal disease than younger patients.

These age-related changes pose challenges in head and neck cancer management. Symptoms of voice change or dysphagia may be incorrectly attributed to

Table 1 SEER Data 1998–2002

	Percent new cancers in patients over 65 years	Percent cancer deaths in patients over 65 years
All sites	56.2	80.7
Oral cavity and pharynx	46	59
Larynx	53	63
Thyroid	17.5	71

Source: From Ref. 1.

aging, which delays diagnosis. Additional impairment from cancer and its treatment makes older patients more susceptible to problems with communication, dysphagia, and aspiration.

Treatment

The goal of treatment of head and neck cancer at every site in patients of all ages is to cure the cancer with the least possible long-term morbidity while minimizing short-term side effects. Treatment needs to address the primary cancer site, regional lymph nodes, and distant metastases. Where cancer cannot be cured, the goal must be to provide humane palliative care. Great strides have been made in surgery, radiation therapy, and chemotherapy, but all come with morbidities that can be greater in older patients. New treatment modalities show promise in maximizing tumoricidal effects while minimizing toxic effects for the patient. Teams consisting of a head and neck surgeon, radiation oncologist, medical oncologist, primary care physician or gerontologist, dentist, speech therapist, physical therapist, nutritionist, and psychologist/counselor help educate patients and their families and facilitate decision making, treatment, and convalescence.

Surgery remains a mainstay of head and neck cancer treatment. It is often used alone in early cancers and in combination with radiation or chemoradiation in advanced disease.

New techniques have lowered the long-term morbidity and improved the quality of life (QOL) for surgical patients. Partial laryngectomy procedures allow voice production and swallowing without long-term tracheostomies in even some advanced laryngeal tumors. Tracheoesophageal puncture prostheses allow hands-free voice after total laryngectomy. Modified neck dissection techniques can spare normal structures. Free flaps often provide better cosmesis and function than local and regional flaps after head and neck surgery and have been used successfully in older patients (7).

While conventional wisdom may suggest that older patients do not tolerate major surgery well, several studies contradict this for head and neck procedures. Head and neck surgery in older patients has an equal complication rate and surgical mortality as in younger patients (8–10). The complication rate in head and neck surgery increases with longer operative time and hospital stay in all age groups (10). Several reasons are suggested for the better tolerance of head and neck surgery than other major operations, by older patients. Fewer physiologic disruptions occur than in other major procedures. Patients have less pain and respiratory compromise, and fewer thromboembolic events than with procedures outside the head and neck (11). Comorbidities such as cardiovascular disease, diabetes, chronic lung disease, malnutrition, and prior radiation therapy correlate with perioperative morbidity and complications rather than age (12,13).

Radiation therapy is commonly used for the primary and postoperative treatment of head and neck cancer. It can be used with sensitizing chemotherapy. Dosing schedules such as hyperfractionation and delivery schemes such as intensity-modulated radiation therapy show promise in maximizing the tumoricidal effects of radiation while minimizing toxicity to adjacent structures. There is limited information on how older patients tolerate head and neck radiation therapy. Chin et al., in a review of 104 patients with oropharyngeal cancer, found that an older age did not predict greater acute toxicity and that age alone was not a factor in a patient's ability to complete a radical course of radiotherapy. Age was not a risk factor for loco-regional recurrence or poor survival. Continued smoking during treatment correlated best with treatment interruptions (14). Pignon et al., in a review of 1589 patients with head and neck cancer enrolled in the European Organization for Research and Treatment of Cancer trials, showed no difference in acute mucosal reactions, weight loss, late toxicity, or survival among older patients. However, older patients were shown to have more severe functional acute toxicity, with worse subjective symptoms during treatment than younger patients (15).

Head and neck squamous cell carcinomas (HNSCC) and some salivary gland neoplasms have shown a good local response to chemotherapy agents including traditional cytotoxic drugs such as methotrexate, cisplatin, carboplatin, bleomycin, and 5-fluorouracil (5-FU). The current "standard" is combination therapy with cisplatinum and 5-FU (16). Newer studies show encouraging results for taxanes (paclitaxel and docetaxel). Combination regimens with cisplatinum and paclitaxel have shown similar response rates, survival times, and QOL measures compared with platinum 5-FU combinations, but with lower toxicity (17). Combined regimens with radiation therapy are used in nasopharyngeal cancer, in organ-sparing strategies, and for postoperative treatment in advanced disease, but may come at a cost of significantly increased acute and chronic mucositis and severe muscular fibrosis when compared to radiation therapy alone. Chemotherapy also causes hematologic and gastrointestinal side effects.

There are little data regarding the benefit or side effects of combined chemotherapy and radiation therapy specific to older patients with head and neck cancer. There are more data in patients treated with combined therapy for lung cancer, but with conflicting results. A recent trial, Radiation Therapy Oncology Group (RTOG) 9410, showed increased acute toxicity including esophagitis, and more frequent severe (grade >3) neutropenia in older patients treated with combined radiation and chemotherapy than with radiation alone in locally advanced non–small cell lung cancer, but also demonstrated longer median survival (18).

New modalities are available now and will also emerge in the near future to treat head and neck cancer. Photodynamic therapy has been actively investigated in Phase III clinical trials since 1988 and is currently approved in the United States for managing obstructing esophageal and endobronchial tumors. It has shown great promise in head and neck tumors, especially SCC in the oral cavity, pharynx, and larynx. This process involves administration of a photosensitizing agent, which is concentrated in neoplastic tissues. This agent is then activated by application of a specific wavelength of light, usually by a laser. This results in tumor necrosis via several mechanisms including oxygen radical production (19). Along with avoiding surgery or radiation therapy, this therapy offers the potential advantages of no tumor resistance, cell-cycle dependence, or genetic resistance as well as the ability to repeat therapy. Problems include complex strategies for light delivery and several weeks of significant photosensitivity after therapy. Initial results have been very promising in superficial lesions and trials are underway in advanced head and neck cancers (19). There are no apparent barriers to the use of this therapy in older patients.

Early results with gene therapy have shown promise in patients who have failed to respond to conventional therapy for head and neck tumors. Gene therapy uses a vector, commonly a virus from which the virulent genes have been removed and the desired gene has been inserted, to deliver a DNA sequence into cancer cells. This DNA gets incorporated into the cellular DNA of cancer cells and codes for a protein that is toxic to the cancer cells, but not to surrounding normal tissue (20). There also has been an explosion in research on molecularly targeted agents in cancer. Many of these are being evaluated in head and neck cancer (21).

Any treatment regimen must take into account QOL issues considering both acute and long-term complications of treatment to assure that improved survival is not outweighed by significant impairment (22). This is more important in an elderly patient for whom the short-term control of the tumor with better QOL may be paramount. Side effects of any treatment for head and neck cancer can include altered appearance, xerostomia, dysphagia, aspiration, alteration in taste and smell, voice problems, airway obstruction, shoulder immobility related to accessory nerve sacrifice, hypothyroidism, lymphedema, sexual dysfunction, and depression. These aggressive regimens may require a gastrostomy feeding tube or tracheostomy, which can transform an independent elder into a nursing home patient. Current data are sparse relating to QOL outcomes by treatment modality for head and neck cancer in not only elderly patients, but in all patient populations. Hopefully, as we refine our treatment strategies, we will minimize these adverse effects.

In patients with incurable cancer, the main goal of palliative care is to improve QOL at all disease stages. This will sometimes conflict with management strategies for maximal tumor response and prolonged survival. Argiris et al. looked at the outcomes of elderly patients undergoing palliative chemotherapy for head and neck cancer in two phase III randomized trials. Elderly patients had similar response rates and survival outcomes, but at the cost of a significantly higher occurrence of severe side effects (17). Compassionate competent care of the dying patient is an obligation of every physician dealing with cancer. Physicians dealing with elderly terminal head and neck cancer patients face the challenges of pain, disfigurement, bleeding, airway obstruction, and dysphagia as well as the increased side effects of palliative therapy. Early discussions with patients and their families and advanced directives should address issues such as the necessity for tracheostomy, feeding tubes, etc. and the possibility of catastrophic bleeding.

HEAD AND NECK SCC

SCC comprises the majority of noncutaneous head and neck malignancies. These tumors arise from the mucosa of the upper aerodigestive tract and often metastasize to regional cervical lymph nodes. The most common site for distant metastases is the lungs. SCC are divided into keratinizing and nonkeratinizing types and are described based on their degree of differentiation. There also are several other less common forms of SCC. Verrucous carcinoma is a highly differentiated form of SCC that is locally destructive but has a very low risk of metastasis. These most commonly occur in the sixth or the seventh decade of life. Surgery is the mainstay of treatment for verrucous carcinoma. Spindle cell squamous carcinoma (carcinosarcoma) is a tumor comprised of conventional in situ or invasive SCC and a malignant spindle cell stromal component. These occur predominantly in men in the sixth to eighth decades of life. In general, these are aggressive lesions and require surgical therapy although radiation may be used as well. Basaloid SCC is a highly aggressive tumor, which is commonly multifocal and deeply invasive with early metastases. Histologically, these tumors contain a predominant malignant basaloid cell component with associated malignant squamous cells. These tumors are more common in men than women and occur most frequently in the sixth and seventh decades of life. Lymphoepithelioma arises predominantly from the mucosa-covered lymphatic tissue of the Waldeyer's ring. It can present at any age, but more advanced age carries a poorer prognosis. These tumors are most commonly found in the nasopharynx (23).

The mucosa of the upper aerodigestive tract is divided into separate anatomic regions including the lip, oral cavity, pharynx, larynx, sinuses, and nasal cavity. The neck is divided into separate levels to characterize the location of lymph nodes. This has prognostic significance in patients with head and neck cancer. Level I includes the submandibular and submental triangles. It is bounded by the posterior belly of the digastric muscle, hyoid bone, and mandible. Levels II, III, and IV represent the jugular lymph nodes. Level II extends from the skull base to the level of the hyoid bone and includes nodes posterior to the posterior belly of the digastric and anterior to the posterior border of the sternocleidomastoid muscle. Level III extends inferiorly from the hyoid level to the cricoid cartilage. Level IV extends below this to the clavicle. Level V lies posterior to the sternocleidomastoid muscle (SCM), anterior to the trapezius muscle, and superior to the clavicle. The postero-inferior one-half of this area is known as the supraclavicular fossa. Level VI is the anterior central compartment and contains nodes between the medial borders of the carotid sheaths and extends from the hyoid superiorly to the suprasternal notch. Level VII contains the upper mediastinal nodes (24).

Risk Factors

The association of tobacco and alcohol use with HNSCC is well known, although tumors of the nasopharynx, sinuses, and nose appear to be less smoking related (25). Day et al. have estimated that the combined effects of tobacco and alcohol are responsible for 73% of oral and pharyngeal cancers in non-Hispanic whites and 83% of these cancers in African-Americans (26). Case-controlled studies have demonstrated that smokers have a 3- to 12-fold higher risk of developing HNSCC than nonsmokers (27). Smoking may not be as prevalent among older head and neck cancer patients as in younger patients. A study of 161 older adult patients with laryngeal SCC showed that patients older than 70 were less likely to use tobacco and alcohol and more likely to be women than their younger counterparts (28). In a study of head and neck SCC patients treated at Johns Hopkins Hospital between 1988 and 1993, 59.5% of patients over 70 years of age were smokers and 37% over 70 had a significant alcohol consumption history compared to 89% and 69%, respectively, in the younger control group. This suggests that age itself plays a role in development of this malignancy (8).

Besides smoking and alcohol, there are other factors related to specific cell types and sites for head and neck cancer. We are just beginning to investigate genetic factors relating to head and neck cancer. Epstein–Barr virus (EBV) is associated with nasopharyngeal cancer, and human papilloma virus (HPV) may play a role in some SCC of the larynx and oropharynx. Chronic reflux and other inflammatory conditions such as lichen planus have been linked to HNSCC. Diets high in vitamins and carotenoids found in fruits and vegetables have been shown to lower the risk of HNSCC, while patients with HNSCC have been shown to have lower levels of some of these nutrients compared to controls, even after accounting for alcohol and tobacco use (29).

Prevention and Screening

The mainstay of prevention of HNSCC includes making correct lifestyle choices, most importantly not using tobacco. Chemoprevention, or the pharmacological use of natural or synthetic compounds to suppress, reverse, or delay the progression to invasive cancer, has been studied extensively in patients with premalignant lesions and evidence of "condemned mucosa," as well as in the prevention of second primary malignancies. Retenoids have been most extensively studied, but the list of potential agents is long and includes cyclo-oxygenase inhibitors, lipo-oxygenase inhibitors, vitamin D analogues, epidermal growth factor–receptor inhibitors, protease inhibitors, antioxidants, and demethylating agents. Retenoids have been shown to shrink oral premalignant lesions and decrease second primary tumors, but only at high doses. This high-dose therapy is associated with significant toxicity, however, and benefits are not sustained after stopping the medication (30). There is much potential benefit to be obtained from future research in this area.

Any patient with a history of tobacco use should undergo a screening history and examination for HNSCC with their regular medical and dental care. Older patients often get less regular dental care, which puts a greater burden on the primary care provider. A screening history for HNSCC should include questions about hoarseness, dysphagia, odynophagia, hemoptysis, throat pain, ear pain, weight loss, oral lesions, or neck masses. One should also remember that loose teeth, nasal obstruction, epistaxis, serous otitis, or diplopia can be symptoms of sinonasal or nasopharyngeal malignancies. Screening examinations for HNSCC should include careful systematic inspection of all accessible mucosal surfaces in the nasal cavity, oral cavity, and oropharynx, as well as careful palpation of the neck. Any worrisome symptoms or lesions should be referred to a specialist who can do indirect mirror examination or office endoscopy of the upper aerodigestive tract and evaluate any worrisome lesions. In the future, we may be able to obtain a screening saliva sample in at-risk patients for genetic studies or tumor markers, but currently, a high index of suspicion and careful examination are the best screening tools available.

Evaluation

Many tools are available to accurately stage HNSCC. Suspicious or malignant lesions in the head and neck are frequently evaluated and sampled with rigid endoscopy of the upper aerodigestive tract with the patient under general anesthesia. Fine-needle aspiration (FNA) is used extensively in the office for the cytologic evaluation of neck masses. Computerized axial tomography scans and magnetic resonance imaging (MRI) are used for the evaluation of primary tumors and regional disease in HNSCC. Ultrasound can be used to evaluate and follow neck masses and guide FNAs. Positron emission tomography (PET) and PET/computerized tomography (CT) scans help evaluate local, regional, and distant disease. Laboratory studies are of limited benefit in evaluating HNSCC, but provide important information regarding comorbitities that, when considered with performance status, impact treatment choice. One must also be aware of the possibility of a second synchronous primary tumor involving the upper aerodigestive tract, esophagus, or lungs. In one retrospective review of 851 patients with HNSCC, 66 (7.8%) had other synchronous primary tumors (31).

T-stage criteria are unique to each primary tumor site. In general, T1 tumors are small or involve only one subsite of the involved area. T2 tumors are larger or involve adjacent subsites. T3 tumors involve adjacent structures or, in the case of the larynx and hypopharynx, cause vocal cord fixation. T4a tumors invade either the bones or structures outside the aerodigestive tract but are resectable, while T4b tumors are unresectable due invasion of vital structures. N-stage criteria are consistent throughout the head and neck except for tumors of the nasopharynx and thyroid gland. In general, the N1 stage has a single ipsilateral node measuring 3 cm or less in its greatest dimension. The N2a stage has a single ipsilateral node measuring more than 3 but less than 6 cm. N2b signifies multiple ipsilateral nodes, none of which are more than 6 cm. N2c signifies bilateral or contralateral adenopathy, none of which are more than 6 cm. N3 stage describes any node measuring more than 6 cm (24).

Treatment

Tumor factors, patient factors, and physician factors influence the choice of treatment in HNSCC. The first tumor-related factors are the size and location of the primary tumor. In general, early stage (T1,2) HNSCC is treated with single modality therapy. Radiation therapy and surgery offer similar cure rates in these lesions at most sites. Primary surgical treatment offers some advantages. Treatment is accomplished in one session. Pathologists can accurately stage cancers and evaluate margins, tumor thickness, and perineural and perivascular invasion. Patients can undergo further surgery if necessary. Disadvantages include cosmetic and functional problems, the need for hospitalization, and the risk of complications associated with a surgical procedure. Also, postoperative radiation may be required based on pathologic findings such as positive margins or neck nodes for a tumor that could have been treated with radiation alone. Radiation offers outpatient treatment without surgery and can simultaneously address the primary site of the tumor as well as the neck disease. A typical course of radiation in the head and neck usually takes five or six weeks to complete and causes both short- and long-term problems including mucositis and xerostomia. There is a risk of osteoradionecrosis with radiation to the mandible, especially in oral cavity or oropharynx lesions. Location of the lesion is very important. A T2 cancer of the lip or anterior tongue, for example, is often a good candidate for primary surgical treatment. These tumors are easily accessible and surgical excision usually causes minimal morbidity. In contrast, surgical excision of a T2 cancer of the soft palate can cause significant long-term problems in voice production and swallowing. These tumors are frequently superficial and respond well to primary radiation therapy, without these long-term problems.

More advanced tumors usually require combined modality therapy. Until recently, the standard combined therapy included surgery with pre- or postoperative radiation therapy. Chemotherapy now plays an expanding role. In 1998, a European study was published comparing concurrent chemoradiation therapy to radiation therapy alone for stage 3 and 4 HNSCC including all the sites. The three-year survival was 48% for the combined group versus 24% for the radiation therapy group alone, but this study has been criticized for its scheduled 11-day treatment breaks in the radiation-alone group (32). Two multi-institutional studies published in 2004 have shown that for advanced tumors, or those with poor prognostic findings after excision, combined postoperative radiation and concurrent cisplatinum offers better local and regional control and disease-free survival, but at the cost of increased adverse effects (33,34). One of these two studies also demonstrated improved survival with concomitant therapy (34). With encouraging data for chemoradiation in larynx preservation, in postoperative treatment as well as in unresectable lesions, there is great interest in the use of chemoradiation therapy for primary treatment of advanced HNSCC outside the larynx. The optimal treatment regimens have yet to be defined, however, and the definitive studies comparing outcome and morbidity from primary chemoradiation and more traditional primary surgical treatment have yet to be done for these sites.

Another tumor-related factor that influences the choice of treatment is the status of the lymph node involvement in the neck. For small tumors without lymphadenopathy (N0) that, based on size or thickness, present a low risk of occult nodal disease, careful follow-up may be all that is required after surgical excision of the primary tumor. In N0 necks with less favorable primary tumors, the lymph nodes should be sampled, or treated empirically with radiation therapy if that is the method chosen to treat the primary cancer. There is controversy in the management of N+ neck disease. For surgery, authors differ as to what constitutes adequate surgical extirpation in the treatment of pathologic lymph nodes. "Radical" neck dissections remove both lymphatic-bearing and normal tissue. "Modified" neck dissections preserve nonlymphatic tissue such as the spinal accessory nerve, the internal jugular vein, and the sternocleidomastoid muscle. "Selective" neck dissections remove only the most at-risk lymph node groups based on the location of the primary tumor and the predictable drainage pattern of the lymphatics in the neck. Obvious adverse pathologic findings such as extracapsular spread of disease and multilevel lymphadenopathy usually necessitate adjuvant radiation or concomitant chemoradiation to the neck. For less obvious findings such as the presence of two small positive nodes without extracapsular spread, the type of neck dissection performed, issues related to the treatment of the primary tumor, and the judgment of the treating physician help determine if additional treatment is necessary.

Opinions vary as to the number and size of nodes that can adequately be treated with radiation therapy alone. Many authors concur that single pathologic nodes less than 3 cm (N1) can be sterilized with radiation alone. The ability of radiation to adequately treat N2 disease is less clear. Comparison of these lesions is complicated by the broad array of neck disease in this group. A neck staged N2b can have two small first-echelon metastatic lymph nodes, while N2a can represent a 6-cm node with extracapsular spread and N2c disease can represent bilateral adenopathy up to 6 cm. In general, more advanced neck diseases treated with primary radiation therapy should also have posttreatment neck dissection of some type, but opinions vary here as to what constitutes advanced disease and one does not have the benefit of pathologic evaluation of the specimen. Combined chemoradiation regimens and more sensitive posttreatment imaging studies such as PET/CT will play an important, but yet ill-defined role in this debate.

The presence of distant metastases profoundly impacts treatment decisions in HNSCC. Although prolonged remission is possible, cure is unlikely. Chemotherapy usually plays a central role, although radiation and surgery can still be used to control local and regional disease.

Patient and physician factors play a major role in the treatment choice as well. Patients' comorbidities (other diseases, illnesses, or conditions such as alcoholism, stroke, heart disease, diabetes, poorly controlled hypertension, or malnutrition), performance status, physiologic age, independence, and preferences impact treatment decisions. Expertise among head and neck surgeons, oncologists, and radiation oncologists as well as the facilities available determine what treatments are possible.

Patients with HNSCC have a significant risk of developing a second primary malignancy in the future. This may influence the choice of treatment for the first lesion, especially if it is an early lesion with a favorable prognosis and different treatment options.

In a retrospective review, Schwartz et al. found that the probability of developing a second metachronous cancer five years after undergoing treatment for the initial HNSCC was 22% overall, with a higher risk in patients who continued to smoke and consume alcohol (31). While it seems logical that younger patients with a longer life expectancy have a higher risk of developing second primary malignancies, the opposite may be true. Two studies have shown up to a twofold increase in the occurrence of second primary malignancies in patients over 65 years compared to younger controls. Some of this disparity may be due to higher rates of continued smoking and alcohol use in the older population, however (35,36).

Prognostic Factors

There are many prognostic factors for SCC, foremost of which are the tumor stage and primary site location. There are other characteristics of the disease that significantly impact loco-regional control, metastases, and survival but are not included in the staging system. Margin status after resection of the primary tumor, tumor grade, host immune response, and presence of perineural and vascular invasion have prognostic significance. The total volume and depth of invasion of the primary tumor are also significant. The actual size of the metastatic nodes may have less significance for survival than their location or the presence of extracapsular spread of the tumor. Metastatic nodes outside the primary drainage area of the tumor or "sentinel node" regions and extracapsular spread (tumor spread through the lymph node capsule) are independent predictors of distant metastases and poor survival (37).

While alcohol and tobacco exposure are well-known risk factors for developing HNSCC, a history of alcohol use as well as the continuing use of alcohol and tobacco are associated with poor outcomes as well. This is likely due to nutritional factors, poor treatment tolerance, immunosuppression, decreased tissue oxygenation, and increased risk of second primary malignancies. Comorbidities are significant independent predictors for both treatment-related complications and survival (37).

Demographic parameters also have an impact on the prognosis. There is conflicting data on the role of age in outcomes. In some studies, age has been found to be a covariable, and does not seem an independent predictor of cause-specific survival or tumor behavior when corrected for TNM stage and the presence of comorbidities (28,35,38). One recent study of 591 patients with advanced (stage 3 or 4) HNSCC and a retrospective review of 1030 patients with HNSCC of the larynx, oral cavity, and pharynx suggest age is a significant independent predictor of poor survival (35,36). Head and neck SCC behaves similarly in men and women. African-American patients are more likely to present with advanced stage cancer of the head and neck than age-matched white patients, but tumor behavior is similar in both races when controlled for stage and comorbidities (37).

Special Considerations: Lip and Oral Cavity

The oral cavity extends from the skin–vermillion junction of the lips to the junction of the hard and soft palate superiorly and the circumvallate papilla on the posterior tongue. Structures of the lip and oral cavity include: mucosa of the lip, buccal area, alveolar ridge, retromolar trigone, floor of mouth, hard palate and the anterior two-thirds of the tongue. Many of these areas lie in close proximity to the bone of the mandible and maxilla. The most common sites for oral cavity SCC are the saliva-bathed areas of the lateral and undersurface of the tongue and the floor of mouth. First echelon lymph node drainage from the lip and oral cavity includes the submental, submandibular, and upper jugular nodes (level I, II).

In 2005, the most recent year for which estimates are available, the American Cancer Society estimates that more than 20,000 new cases of lip and oral cavity cancer will be diagnosed in the United States (2). Tumors in this area can be ulcerated, exophytic, or hyperkeratotic. Common symptoms include a nonhealing ulcer, bleeding, or pain.

A review of five-year disease-specific survival for oral cavity HNSCC by stage at Memorial Sloan-Kettering Cancer Center from 1986 to 1995 shows stage 1 at 90%, stage 2 at 80%, stage 3 at 65% and stage 4 at approximately 58% (39).

Special Considerations: Pharynx

The pharynx is divided into three separate regions: nasopharynx, oropharynx, and hypopharynx. According to the latest American Cancer Society estimates, there will be 8590 new cases of pharyngeal cancer and 1890 deaths from pharyngeal cancer in 2005 (2).

Nasopharynx

The nasopharynx is bordered anteriorly by the choanae, posteriorly by the posterior pharyngeal wall, and inferiorly by an artificial line at the free border of the soft palate.

The nasopharynx contains the posterior margins of the choanal orifices and nasal septum, the mucosa covering the eustachian tube orifice, and the superior surface of the soft palate. It also contains the lymphatic tissue of the adenoids. Carcinomas that arise from the lymph-bearing regions in the nasopharynx are a distinct entity known as nasopharyngeal carcinomas (NPCs) owing to the unique risk factors of genetic susceptibility, EBV exposure, and environmental cofactors (40). Smoking and alcohol consumption play a less significant role in the nasopharynx than in other sites in the head and neck. NPC is relatively rare worldwide with an age-standardized annual incidence rate less than one per 100,000 individuals. In populations of southern China (especially Guangdong Province), Hong Kong, and parts of Southeast Asia, however, rates are 10 to 30 times higher than for the world population as a whole. NPC is also prevalent among Alaskan Eskimos (40). In the United States, the median age at diagnosis for NPC is 53, which is 10 years younger than the median age at diagnosis for oral cavity and pharynx as a whole. The median age of death from NPC is 62, which is six years younger than for patients with oral cavity and pharynx cancer as a group (1).

The World Health Organization has classified NPC into three different types. Type 1 is SCC. Type 2 is nonkeratinizing carcinoma with or without lymphoid stroma. Type 3 is undifferentiated carcinoma with or without lymphoid stroma. The lymphocytic stroma is neither neoplastic nor integral to the carcinoma (41). Type 3 has the strongest association with EBV. The link between nasopharyngeal cancer and EBV was first observed in 1966, when the sera of patients with the malignancy were found to manifest precipitating antibodies against cells infected with the virus (42). Since then, it has been demonstrated that essentially all cases of undifferentiated NPC contain the EBV genome. Exposure to EBV is extremely common throughout the world both in groups at high risk and low risk for NPC, however. This implicates genetic or environmental cofactors as critical in the pathogenesis of NPC (41).

NPC produces few symptoms early in the course of the tumor. The most common symptom of NPC at presentation is a neck mass. This is followed by unilateral hearing loss due to an obstructed eustachian tube, bloody rhinorrhea, nasal obstruction, and cranial nerve deficits causing double vision or paresthesias of the lower two-thirds of the face.

Lymph node involvement in NPC is staged differently than other HNSCC owing to the differing distribution and prognostic impact of nodes in NPC. All ipsilateral involved lymph nodes that are less than 6 cm and above the supraclavicular fossa are N1. Bilateral nodes of the same dimension and location are N2. N3a includes nodes larger than 6 cm and N3b includes extension to the supraclavicular fossa (24).

Traditionally, radiation has been the main modality of treatment of NPC. This has been in part because of the difficulty in obtaining surgical access and margins around these tumors, which commonly present at an advanced stage. Although surgical approaches to the nasopharynx have been described and are used, surgery is commonly reserved for failures in the neck when there has been a complete response of the primary tumor.

Relatively high rates of local failure and distant metastases with radiotherapy for advanced lesions have prompted early investigation into combined treatment with chemotherapy and radiation therapy for NPC. Initial trials with adjuvant and neoadjuvant chemotherapy have shown significant toxicities with limited overall benefit. Concurrent administration of cisplatin with radiation, however, has been shown by the intergroup study 00–99 to significantly reduce local recurrences and distant metastases as well as improve survival, and has become the standard treatment in the United States for advanced disease (43,44). Although a recent study from Europe has shown survival benefit with postoperative chemoradiotherapy in HNSCC, these intergroup and subsequent data for NPC are the best evidence thus far of improved survival with the addition of any chemotherapy at any site within the head and neck.

For patients with T1 and T2 tumors treated with high-dose radiation therapy alone, five-year local failure-free survival is around 80% with one study showing local control rates as high as 93% for T1 lesions (45,46). In the intergroup study of stage 3 and 4 lesions that demonstrated significant benefit to combined therapy, the overall five-year survival in the combined treatment group was 67% (43,44).

Oropharynx

The oropharynx continues inferiorly from the posterior margin of the soft palate to the level of the hyoid bone or the floor of the vallecula. The oropharynx contains the base of tongue, inferior surface of the soft palate, uvula, tonsillar pillars, and sulci as well as the pharyngeal tonsils and posterior and lateral pharyngeal walls.

Tumors arising in the lymphatic tissue of the pharyngeal tonsil and base of tongue behave differently than tumors of the nonlymphatic mucosa. The median age of tonsil cancer patients at diagnosis is 57 compared to 63 years for the oropharynx overall. The median age of cancer patients at death is 63 for the tonsil and 67 for the oropharynx (1). T1 tonsil and tongue base cancers have been reported to have up to a 70% incidence of positive lymph nodes at presentation compared to less than 10% for T1 cancers of the soft palate and 25% for T1 cancers of the oropharyngeal wall (47). Lymph node metastasis from the tonsil and tongue base cancers can be cystic and are often mistaken for benign lesions such as branchial cleft cysts, even after imaging studies and cytologic testing.

There appears to be a subset of tonsillar carcinomas that are HPV-related. While HPV, much like EBV is ubiquitous, there is a strong association between the high-risk subtypes (e.g., HPV-16) and these distinctive oropharyngeal carcinomas with molecular characteristics indicative of viral oncogene functions. These cancers occur in younger patients than non-HPV HNSCC and there is less correlation with smoking and alcohol consumption. These tumors have better overall survival rates, which may be due in part to increased sensitivity to radiation therapy (48). Identification of HPV expression in oropharynx malignancies may have implications in the future relating to choice of therapy.

A review of five-year observed survival by the AJCC staging for SCC of the oropharynx in more than 7000 patients from 1985 to 1991 shows stage 1 survival of 50% with a near-linear reduction in survival to 26% for stage 4 disease (2). SEER data for oral cavity and pharynx as a whole have shown improved relative survival rates from the late 1980s to the last half of the 1990s (54.4% vs. 59.4%) (1).

Hypopharynx

The hypopharynx extends from below the floor of the vallecula or hyoid bone to the inferior border of the cricoid cartilage, but excludes the structures of the larynx.

The hypopharynx contains the left and right piriform sinuses, postcricoid region and posterior and lateral walls of the hypopharynx and is contiguous with the cervical esophagus inferiorly.

Likely owing to the paucity of symptoms at an early stage, hypopharynx tumors commonly present at an advanced stage as large primary tumors with extensive submucosal spread or with bulky adenopathy. These advanced tumors commonly cause dysphagia that, when combined with alcohol use, causes malnutrition at presentation in many of these patients. Surgical treatment of these lesions often includes a total laryngectomy, but combined chemoradiation therapy is used as well. The median age of hypopharynx cancer patients at diagnosis, based on estimates from select areas of the United States, is 66 years (1).

Outcomes for hypopharynx cancer are poor. Five-year observed survival by combined AJCC staging from 1985 to 1991 is approximately 35% in stage 1, 2, and 3 disease, and less than 20% in stage 4 disease. Of the approximately 3000 patients, more than half were stage 4 (2). Other studies involving fewer patients have shown better survival rates in early stage disease treated with external beam radiation therapy.

Available data for HNSCC often group oral cavity and pharyngeal malignancies together. The American Cancer Society estimates that there will be 29,370 new cases of oral cavity and pharynx cancer in 2005, the latest year for which estimates are available. Of these cancers, 19,100 will occur in men and 10,270 will occur in women (2). SEER data suggest the lifetime risk of dying from oral cavity and pharyngeal cancer to be 0.38%. The peak incidence of oral cavity and pharyngeal cancer is from the age of 75 to the age of 79 with 43.8 cases per 100,000 individuals. In contrast, the incidence in the 50- to 54-year-old population is 18.3 per 100,000 individuals. Five-year relative survival rates are 64% for patients under 65 years, but only 52% for patients over 65 years old. Overall trends for the five-year survival rate show a 6% to 7% improvement for oral and pharyngeal cancers diagnosed in 1997, compared to those diagnosed in 1977 (1,2).

Special Considerations: Larynx

The larynx begins superiorly at the tip of the epiglottis and extends inferiorly to the lower border of the cricoid cartilage. Its posterior border is made up of the aryepiglottic folds, arytenoids, interarytenoid area, and mucosa along the inner aspect of the posterior cricoid cartilage. The larynx can be divided into three regions. The supraglottis lies above a line drawn through the junction of the lateral aspect of the true vocal cord and the laryngeal ventricle. The glottis extends inferiorly for 1 cm from this line. Below this, the subglottis extends to the lower border of the cricoid cartilage. The supraglottis contains the epiglottis, aryepiglottic folds, arytenoids, and false vocal cords. The glottis is composed of the superior and inferior surfaces of the true vocal cords, including the anterior and posterior commissures. The subglottis includes the area from 1 cm below the lateral margin of the ventricle to the lower margin of the cricoid cartilage.

The American Cancer Society estimates that there will be 10,270 new cases of larynx cancer in 2004. Of these, 8060 will be in men and 2210 will be in women. According to SEER data, the median age of laryngeal cancer patients at diagnosis is 65. The median age of cancer patients at death is 69 (1,2).

Supraglottic SCC frequently presents with throat pain or referred ear pain owing to the rich sensory innervation of this area. Voice problems usually suggest advanced local disease. Tumors in this location commonly present with adenopathy, and bilateral disease is not uncommon. The most common site for regional metastases are the deep jugular lymph nodes (levels II, III, and IV). Primary glottic cancers frequently present with hoarsenenss. Pain and airway obstruction are signs of advanced disease. In contrast to the supraglottic larynx, the glottic larynx has few lymphatics and early regional metastases from glottic cancers are uncommon. Regional metastases from advanced glottic cancers may spread to either the jugular lymph nodes, or the pre- or paratracheal nodes. Primary subglottic tumors typically present late with voice or airway problems. Lymph node involvement in subglottic tumors usually follows extra laryngeal spread of the primary and is to the pretracheal, paratracheal and lower jugular nodes.

Early stage (T1–T2) cancers of the larynx are usually treated with a single-modality therapy—either external beam radiation therapy or surgery—with excellent results. Actual five-year survival rates for T1 glottic and supraglottic carcinoma are around 80% with higher local control. T2 carcinomas of the glottis have a somewhat better five-year survival than their supraglottic neighbors (77% vs. 60%) (49). Surgery consists of open partial laryngectomy or endoscopic laser excision for small lesions, combined with neck dissection for at-risk lymph nodes. Often, the voice result with radiation therapy is superior to that obtained with surgical treatment, but this is balanced by the shorter treatment time, less xerostomia, and slightly lower rates of salvage laryngectomy for recurrence with surgery than with radiation. Treatment for advanced laryngeal cancer has changed dramatically in the past 15 years. Advanced (T3–T4) cancers have traditionally been treated with combined total laryngectomy, neck dissection, and radiation therapy, which remains a viable treatment option. While this approach offers reasonable control rates and survival, and predictably good QOL, it leaves patients with a permanent tracheostome and a suboptimal alaryngeal voice. The landmark Department of Veteran's Affairs (VA) laryngeal preservation study was published in 1991. In that study, 332 patients with advanced laryngeal cancer (stage 3, 4) were randomized to receive either the traditional total laryngectomy and radiation therapy or three cycles of induction chemotherapy with cisplatin and fluorouracil, followed by radiation therapy. Patients in this latter group were evaluated after two cycles of chemotherapy, and if they demonstrated a partial or complete response they continued with the third cycle and planned radiation with the intent to preserve their larynges. If they demonstrated a less than partial response, they went on to total laryngectomy followed by radiation.

Sixty-four percent of the patients in the induction chemotherapy group were able to preserve their larynges and there was no difference in survival between the two groups on follow-up of almost three years (50). This sparked great interest in organ-preservation treatment strategies in advanced laryngeal cancer, which now extends to other sites within the head and neck.

The same year that the VA study was published, the RTOG began enrolling patients with locally advanced laryngeal cancer into a study with three arms. The first arm was similar to the VA organ-preservation group with induction chemotherapy. The second group received concurrent chemoradiation therapy and the last group received radiation therapy alone. There was no surgery arm in this study. The results, published in 2003, showed a larynx preservation rate of 72% in the induction arm, which was similar to the VA study, but the concurrent group achieved an 84% larynx preservation rate (51). Interestingly, the radiation-alone group achieved a 67% larynx preservation rate, which was not different from the induction group. Survival rates were similar, but acute toxicities were increased with any chemotherapy, and the rate for the use of permanent tracheostomies and gastric tubes is unknown (51). One major criticism of the RTOG study was that a large number of patients enrolled would have been candidates for organ-preservation surgery (52).

While the role of nonsurgical management of laryngeal cancers has been evolving, surgeons in the United States and Europe have been expanding the envelope of partial (organ-preservation) laryngectomy. Endoscopic laser resections are now done for more advanced cancers, which, when combined with neck dissections, offer similar cure rates to radical surgery or chemoradiation. Open partial laryngectomies offer complete resection of many moderately advanced (T2, T3) laryngeal malignancies without the need for permanent stomas and with serviceable voice. Patients need to have adequate pulmonary reserve to tolerate some degree of aspiration, however, which may exclude some older patients, especially those with chronic lung disease.

Special Considerations: Nasal Cavity and Sinus

The nasal and sinus cavities are bordered by the skull base, orbits, nasopharynx, and oral cavity. There are paired maxillary, ethmoid, sphenoid, and frontal sinuses. The nasal cavity contains the turbinates, septum, nasal floor, and olfactory areas. Tumors in this area are rare.

The structures involved have a thin respiratory epithelium covering the bony skeleton. Nonsquamous malignancies occur with the same frequency as SCC. These include inverting papilloma, a locally aggressive lesion without propensity for metastasis, minor salivary gland malignancies, adenocarcinoma, sinonasal undifferentiated carcinoma, small cell carcinoma, esthesioneuroblastoma, natural killer T-cell lymphoma, sarcoma, plasmacytoma, and lymphoma. Management of these malignancies is difficult because they typically present at an advanced stage and because of the close proximity and frequent involvement of the skull base and orbital structures. The most common site for tumors in this region is the maxillary sinus followed by the nasal cavity and ethmoid sinus. Tumors of the sphenoid sinus and frontal sinus are very rare. Lymph node metastases are rare with these lesions, but when they do occur they can be to facial, submandibular, upper jugular, parotid, and retropharyngeal nodes and are associated with poor outcomes. Because of the varied drainage, regional disease does not lend itself well to surgical control. Tobacco and alcohol exposure are less important in the etiology of these tumors than in tumors of the larynx or oral cavity. Occupational exposure to wood dust and nickel dust has been shown to be a risk factor for ethmoid sinus tumors, primarily adenocarcinoma (53). The age of the patient at presentation is dependant on the cell type, but most patients present in their 60s.

Nasal and sinus malignancies can present with nasal drainage, obstruction, or pain, but commonly present at an advanced stage with symptoms related to invasion of adjacent structures, such as tearing, double vision, loose teeth, or facial numbness.

It is difficult to summarize treatment strategies or outcomes given the broad range of cell types and locations for sinonasal cancer. Surgery is usually the preferred method of treatment for nasal cavity and maxillary and ethmoid sinus tumors and can include local resection, maxillectomy with orbital exenteration, or craniofacial resection with removal of the involved dura. Induction chemotherapy, concurrent chemoradiation, and radiation therapy also play an ever-increasing role. Outcomes vary widely based on cell type, stage, and treatment modality.

Special Considerations: Unknown Primary

Occasionally, patients will present with neck metastases diagnosed on FNA and no evident primary lesion, despite a thorough office examination of the entire mucosa of the upper aerodigestive tract, careful inspection of skin, and appropriate scans of the upper airway and chest. These patients should undergo careful rigid endoscopic examination under general anesthesia with careful attention to the nasopharynx, oropharynx, and hypopharynx, and biopsy of any suspicious lesions. Some authors recommend routine ipsilateral tonsillectomy due to rates of up to 32% occult primary tonsil lesions reported in some series (54). Some authors also suggest random biopsies of the nasopharynx and the tongue base to try to identify the primary lesion. While the yield with random biopsies is low, identifying the primary site offers a benefit by decreasing the fields and the morbidity associated with high-dose radiation treatment of the upper aerodigestive tract mucosa (55). New imaging techniques such as PET/CT, improved resolution with CT and MRI, and better endoscopes for office and operative evaluation should make the finding of small primary tumors easier than it has been in the past.

The traditional therapy has been neck dissection followed by external beam radiation therapy to potential mucosal sites, including the entire mucosa of the Waldeyer's ring. However, in cases where neck dissection has been the only treatment, the incidence of delayed presentation of a primary tumor is quite low (16% in one series compared with 9–10% for patients treated with radiation therapy), which questions the need for extended treatment fields (56). One could argue that minimal nodal disease could be treated with surgery or radiation therapy alone to the neck with careful surveillance for a primary neoplasm. With advanced neck disease, recent data support the use of concurrent chemoradiation therapy after surgery (22,23).

Supraclavicular adenopathy carries with it a much worse prognosis than disease elsewhere in the neck with a five-year survival less than 10% (57). Overall, N-stage appears to predict survival with N1 rates in the 75% range, and N2 and N3 survival rates approximately in the range of 50% to 25%, respectively (58).

SALIVARY GLAND MALIGNANCIES

Although rare overall, salivary gland malignancies represent a broad range of tumors with varying behavior and response to treatment. Unlike mucosal sites within the head and neck, SCC is rare among primary neoplasms of major salivary glands.

There are three paired major salivary glands. The largest is the parotid gland, followed by the submandibular (or submaxillary) gland. The smallest of the major salivary glands is the sublingual gland. Overall the average daily production of saliva in normal individuals is approximately 1 to 1.5 L. The percentage of tumors that are malignant in each gland is inversely proportional to the size of the gland. While reports vary, approximately 25% of primary parotid neoplasms are malignant. About half of the submandibular gland neoplasms are malignant and 75% of sublingual gland neoplasms are malignant. There are minor salivary glands throughout the mucosa of the upper aerodigestive tract. While most minor salivary gland malignancies present in the oral cavity, they can occur anywhere, including the nasal and sinus cavities and larynx.

The parotid gland lies deep to the cheek skin anterior and inferior to the ear canal. It is a unilobular gland surrounded by fascia and lies in the preauricular and infra-auricular region. The facial nerve enters the posterior deep portion of the gland and divides into approximately five main branches within the substance of the gland. Each of these branches exits at the anterior border of the gland. The majority of the gland lies superficial to this nerve. This portion is referred to as the supraneural or superficial lobe of the gland, while the parotid tissue deep to the nerve is referred to as the infraneural or deep lobe. The deep lobe extends into the parapharyngeal space. There are multiple lymph nodes within the parotid gland, most of which are in the superficial lobe. These constitute the primary drainage area for the ear, scalp, and area around the eye; metastatic skin cancer is common in the parotid gland in older individuals. The acinar cells of the parotid gland are primarily serous and increase the production of thin saliva in response to parasympathetic stimulation by food. The saliva passes through the Stenson's duct and enters the oral cavity through the buccal mucosa opposite the second molar.

The submandibular glands lie in the submandibular triangles of the upper neck. In older patients, they frequently are ptotic and can be seen and felt below the mandible. They contain a mixture of mucinous and serous acinar cells. The submandibular glands are responsible for a major part of the saliva production between meals. The saliva leaves the submandibular glands via the Wharton's ducts and enters the oral cavity just lateral to the lingual frenulum in the floor of the mouth.

The sublingual glands lie just below the mucosa of the floor of the mouth. They contain mostly mucinous acinar cells. The saliva from the sublingual glands enters the mouth from multiple small ducts that lie in the floor of the mouth.

There are many different malignancies that arise from the salivary glands (Table 2). This broad range of malignancies reflects their origins from different cell types within the salivary unit. The most common malignancy of the major salivary glands is the mucoepidermoid carcinoma. Most of these occur in the parotid gland. They are divided into low-grade and high-grade lesions based on their degree of differentiation. Their behavior correlates well with their degree of differentiation, with high-grade lesions akin to poorly differentiated SCC. These lesions can occur at any age and are the most common salivary gland malignancies in children. Most series show a marked female predominance.

Adenoid cystic carcinomas are the most common malignancies of all but the parotid glands. These locally aggressive tumors have a slow relentless course and a high propensity for perineural spread. Metastases from adenoid cystic carcinomas spread hematologically rather than via lymphatic channels.

Acinic cell carcinomas are low-grade malignancies which tend to recur locally but metastasize rarely. They occur most commonly in women and in middle-aged

Table 2 Types of Salivary Gland Carcinomas

Mucoepidermoid carcinoma
Adenoid cystic carcinoma
Acinic cell carcinoma
Malignant mixed tumor
Polymorphous low-grade adenocarcinoma
Epithelial–myoepithelial carcinoma
Salivary duct carcinoma
Mucinous adenocarcinoma
Papillary cystadenocarcinoma
Adenocarcinoma
Sebaceous carcinoma
Oncocytic carcinoma
Myoepithelial carcinoma
Squamous cell carcinoma
Small cell carcinoma
Undifferentiated carcinoma

Source: From Ref. 59.

and elderly patients. These tumors can occur bilaterally. Malignant mixed tumor, or carcinoma ex-pleomorphic adenoma usually reflects cancer arising within a benign lesion. There is also a form that is a carcinosarcoma with both primary malignant elements.

Unlike in HNSCC, smoking and alcohol are not major risk factors in salivary gland malignancies. Overall, the etiologic agents are poorly understood, although low-dose radiation therapy for other conditions may increase the risk of salivary gland neoplasms.

The median age of salivary gland cancer patients at diagnosis is 63, the same as for HNSCC of the oral cavity and pharynx. The median age of salivary gland patients at death is 74, however, which is six years older than for oral cavity and pharynx malignancies (1). Given the small number of these lesions and the broad range of cell types, it is difficult to make generalizations. Overall, low-grade or locally aggressive malignancies occur most commonly in younger patients, while high-grade tumors such as high-grade mucoepidermoid carcinoma, SCC, and adeno-carcinoma are more common in older patients.

Most of these lesions present as a painless mass within the gland. Symptoms of pain, facial nerve paralysis, or lymphadenopathy signal an aggressive lesion. Open biopsy of salivary gland masses should be avoided because of the high incidence of recurrence following open biopsies of benign lesions despite definitive surgery. FNA has been used extensively with salivary gland masses but some still advocate complete excision of the lesion and the surrounding gland as the primary diagnostic and therapeutic procedure. Imaging studies including CT, MRI, PET/CT, and ultrasound help determine the extent of a primary lesion and evaluate regional lymph nodes.

Given the rarity of these tumors and the poorly understood risk factors, the only logical screening exercise is a careful history, inspection, and palpation of the salivary glands and oral mucosa.

The primary treatment for salivary gland malignancies is surgical. Gross involvement of the facial nerve requires resection and possible grafting of the involved portion of the nerve. The role of neck dissection as well as postoperative treatment with radiation therapy or chemoradiation depends on the behavior of the specific tumor.

Outcomes vary widely based on cell type. Even with aggressive surgery and radiation, some high-grade tumors show poor survival rates while low-grade lesions can be cured with surgical excision alone. For locally aggressive lesions such as adenoid cystic carcinoma, three- or five-year survival statistics look good, but most patients remain alive with disease. Fifteen-year cures are very rare.

In older patients, one needs to consider the natural course of the disease in conjunction with the patient's physiologic age when deciding on the treatment. Xerostomia is frequent in older patients who are on multiple medications. Salivary gland excision and/or radiation can further decrease saliva production. Facial nerve weakness or paralysis, in addition to cosmetic and communication problems, can make manipulation of an oral food bolus more difficult and compound other age-related swallowing problems.

THYROID MALIGNANCIES

Thyroid cancers are much more common in women than in men, and in younger patients than in old. When they occur in men or in older patients, they are more lethal, however. From American Cancer Society estimates, men will account for only 25% of the new cases of thyroid cancer in 2005, but 42% of thyroid cancer–related deaths. Thyroid is the only head and neck site at which age is taken into account in the staging system owing to its negative impact on outcomes. The median age of patients diagnosed with thyroid malignancy is 46, while the median age of thyroid cancer patients at death is 74 (1,2). In older patients not only are thyroid cancers more likely to exist in more lethal forms, but also well-differentiated cancers behave more aggressively.

The thyroid gland is ordinarily comprised of a right and left lobe with a midline isthmus connecting the two lobes, overlying the upper trachea and esophagus. Occasionally there is a pyramidal lobe extending upwards in the midline to the thyroid cartilage. There are commonly four parathyroid glands adjacent to the thyroid gland. The recurrent laryngeal nerves lie in the tracheoesophageal grooves just posterior to the thyroid gland. These nerves contain fibers that control both abduction and adduction of the vocal folds.

The common forms of thyroid cancer are divided into well-differentiated, medullary, and anaplastic types based on the behavior of the tumors. Well-differentiated tumors include papillary carcinoma, follicular carcinoma, and Hurthle-cell carcinoma. These types arise from the thyroid follicular cells. While overall, outcomes with well-differentiated thyroid cancer are excellent, it has long been recognized that certain criteria—most notably age—carry with them a worse prognosis (60). Reflecting these clinical factors, which are associated with poorer outcomes in well-differentiated thyroid cancer, criteria have been developed to help stratify risk in these tumors and help identify those that require aggressive management. AMES (age, metastases, extent, and size), AGES (age, grade, extent, and size), and MACIS (metastases, age, completeness of surgery, invasiveness, and size) are three of the most common criteria groups used (61–63). In a review comparing 339 patients between the ages of 20 and 40, to 154 patients from 60 to 80 years of age with well-differentiated thyroid cancer, there were only four deaths (1.2%) in the younger group but 48 (31%) in the older group with the disease. Of those patients who died, the median time from diagnosis to death was nine years in the younger group but only five years in the older group. The younger group had excellent survival despite multiple positive nodes, tumors greater than 4 cm, extrathyroidal spread, and even residual gross disease after surgery. Each of these factors was predictive of significantly poorer outcomes in older patients, however (60). Incidental papillary carcinomas measuring less than 1 cm are a relatively common finding (6–13%) in pathological and autopsy studies (64,65). These are felt by some authors to have little biologic significance, and rarely metastasize. We have yet to know which small tumors in elderly patients will grow and act aggressively and which will follow a benign indolent course.

Medullary carcinoma of the thyroid occurs both sporadically and in association with three familial syndromes: multiple endocrine neoplasia syndrome type IIa and type IIb, and familial medullary thyroid carcinoma. The sporadic type accounts for 60% to 70% of cases overall and represents most of the tumors in older patients. Medullary carcinoma arises from the parafollicular or C cells of the thyroid gland, which are involved in calcium metabolism regulation through the production of calcitonin. Basal and stimulated calcitonin levels are important markers of medullary carcinoma and are used in the follow-up as a marker of persistent or recurrent disease. Overall survival rates are good for medullary carcinoma, but advanced age and tumor stage are predictors of poor survival (66).

Anaplastic carcinoma occurs more commonly in women with a peak incidence in the seventh decade of life. This is a highly aggressive lethal form of thyroid cancer with survival typically measured in months. These tumors frequently arise in thyroid glands that had either a goiter or a well-differentiated thyroid disease previously. Patients present with a rapidly enlarging mass and frequently have airway obstruction symptoms or dysphagia due to local invasion of the recurrent laryngeal nerves, trachea, or esophagus. These patients can also present with Horner's syndrome due to sympathetic chain involvement, which suggests possible carotid artery invasion. Anaplastic carcinomas can metastasize early, most commonly to the lungs (67). The AJCC considers all anaplastic carcinomas as T4 and stage 4 (24).

Thyroid lymphoma also occurs and represents up to 5% of thyroid malignancies. These tumors are more common in women and arise most commonly in the sixth decade of life. These tumors have a good prognosis when the disease is confined to the thyroid gland. They are primarily treated with radiation or combined therapy. Thyroid lymphoma is almost always associated with clinical and histological evidence of chronic lymphocytic thyroiditis (68,69).

Family history of thyroid cancer and exposure to low-dose radiation therapy are the known risk factors for developing thyroid malignancy. While most thyroid cancers present as painless masses within the thyroid gland, most thyroid masses are benign. Ultrasound and FNA are the two diagnostic tools used most frequently in the evaluation of thyroid masses. While ultrasound cannot reliably distinguish benign from malignant disease, it can examine the presence, size, and structure of nodules within the thyroid gland and aid in the accurate sampling of lesions by FNA. Certain ultrasound characteristics, such as microcalcification in papillary carcinoma, suggest diagnoses and identify at-risk lesions. Borderline lesions can be accurately followed for enlargement with serial ultrasound. FNA can frequently distinguish benign from malignant disease. Papillary carcinoma is identified on FNA by identifying typical nuclear features. Although follicular lesions can be identified on FNA, it is usually not possible to discern well-differentiated follicular cancer from adenomas. This requires careful pathologic evaluation of the surgical specimen for capsular or vascular invasion. Medullary carcinoma can be diagnosed with FNA by typical cytologic features and specific stains for calcitonin on the aspirate. FNA plays an important role in identifying tumors for which surgery is often not the first-line treatment such as anaplastic carcinoma and lymphoma.

Nodal staging is unique to thyroid cancer. N1 reflects all nodal spread of any size with N1a involving level VI nodes and N1b involving other cervical or mediastinal lymph nodes (24).

Surgery is the initial treatment for most well-differentiated and medullary cancers. While medullary cancer requires total thyroidectomy with lymph node dissection, the extent of surgery required for well-differentiated carcinoma is controversial. Total thyroidectomy addresses potential multifocal disease and, by removing all normal functional thyroid tissue, allows the evaluation and treatment of distant disease with radioactive iodine. Serum thyroglobulin can be followed to monitor for recurrent disease after total thyroidectomy as well. Total thyroidectomy carries with it, however, a higher incidence of complications such as recurrent laryngeal nerve injury and hypoparathyroidism, and requires long-term thyroid replacement therapy. Proponents of partial thyroid surgery for well-differentiated disease cite excellent outcomes and lower complications in low-risk patients. Older patients, however, rarely fit into this low-risk category.

Patients with high-risk or metastatic well-differentiated thyroid cancers are often treated with ^{131}I after total thyroidectomy to ablate residual disease. The exact role of external beam radiation therapy is controversial. It is usually reserved for cancers that invade outside the thyroid capsule, are surgically unresectable, or in high-risk (e.g., older) patients with advanced local and regional disease. External beam radiation can also be used for persistent disease that does not take up radioactive iodine. Chemotherapy plays a limited role in differentiated thyroid cancer and is used primarily for palliation in disseminated disease.

The treatment goals for anaplastic thyroid cancer are often palliative at the outset. Initial goals should be airway protection and nutritional support. Overall outcomes with this disease are very poor with survival rates of 10% to 15%. Effective palliation in some patients as well as rare long-term survival on using surgery and radiation therapy has led some authors to recommend aggressive treatment in amenable tumors despite poor overall survival rates (70,71). Anaplastic tumors have shown a response to concomitant radiation therapy and chemotherapy as well as to using cisplatin and fluorouracil. Newer chemotherapeutic agents such as paclitaxel and manumycin also hold promise in treating this disease (72,73).

SUMMARY

Head and neck cancer is common among older patients. Its management is complex due to the important structures it involves and their profound role in our function and appearance. While the cumulative effects of tobacco and alcohol use are greater in the older population, there is evidence to suggest that age itself is a risk factor for some head and neck cancers. Age also appears to be a predictor of worse outcome in patients with these tumors. While older patients may have less reserve in their ability to tolerate certain treatments for head and neck carcinoma due to the common physiologic changes that occur with aging, studies show that healthy older adults tolerate surgery and radiation therapy well. These ideas contradict the conventional wisdom that older patients should receive less aggressive treatments to manage their head and neck malignancies than their younger counterparts.

More information on how current treatments affect older patients in particular is critical to designing regimens that aggressively treat head and neck tumors in older patients and minimize the morbidity in this group. The development of new, less toxic drugs and treatment modalities will be of great benefit to older patients.

REFERENCES

1. http://seer.cancer.gov/csr/1975_2002/ (accessed June 2005).
2. http://www.cancer.org/downloads/STT/CAFF2005f4PWSecured.pdf (accessed June 2005).
3. Paulsen F, Tillmann B. Degenerative changes in the human cricoarytenoid joint. Arch Otolaryngol Head Neck Surg 1998; 124:903–906.
4. Kahane JC. Connective tissue changes in the larynx and their effects on voice. J Voice 1987; 1:27–30.
5. Kent RD, Burkard R. Changes in the acoustic correlates of speech production. In: Beasley DS, Davis GA, eds. Aging, Communication Process and Disorders. New York: Grune and Stratton, 1981:47–62.
6. Logemann J. Effects of aging on the swallowing mechanism. Oto Clin North Am 1990; 23(6):1045–1055.
7. Bridger AG, O'Brien CJ, Lee KK. Advanced patient age should not preclude the use of free-flap reconstruction for head and neck cancer. Am J Surg 1994; 168:425–428.
8. McGuirt WF, Davis SP III. Demographic portrayal and outcome analysis of head and neck cancer surgery in the elderly. Arch Otolaryngol Head Neck Surg 1995; 121:150–154.
9. Harries M, Lund VJ. Head and neck surgery in the elderly: a maturing problem. J Laryngol Otol 1989; 103:306–309.
10. Barzan L, Veronesi A, Caruso G, et al. Head and neck cancer and ageing: a retrospective study in 438 patients. J Laryngol Otol 1990; 104:634–640.
11. Robinson DS. Head and neck considerations in the elderly patient. Surg Clin North Am 1994; 74(2):431–439.
12. Koch WM, Patel H, Brennan J, et al. Squamous cell carcinoma of the head and neck in the elderly. Arch Otolaryngol Head Neck Surg 1995; 121:262–265.
13. Jones AS, Husband D, Rowley H. Radical radiotherapy for squamous cell carcinoma of the larynx, oropharynx, and hypopharynx: patterns of recurrence, treatment and survival. Clin Otolaryngol 1998; 23:496–511.
14. Chin R, Fisher RJ, Smee RI, et al. Oropharyngeal cancer in the elderly. Int J Radiat Oncol Biol Phys 1995; 32:1007–1016.
15. Pignon T, Horiot, JC, Venden Bogaert W, et al. No age limit for radical radiotherapy in head and neck tumours. Euro J Cancer 1996; 32(A)12:2075–2081.
16. Lu C, Kies, M. Systemic therapy for recurrent and metastatic diseases. In: Harrison LB, Sessions RB, Hong WK, eds. Head and Neck Cancer, a Multidisiplinary Approach. 2d ed. Philadelphia: Lippincott Williams and Wilkins, 2004:919–928.
17. Argiris A, Li Y, Murphy BA, Langer CJ, Forastiere AA. Outcome of elderly patients with recurrent of metastatic head and neck cancer treated with cisplatin-based chemotherapy. J Clin Oncol 2004; 22(2):262–268.
18. Langer CJ, Hsu C, Curran W, et al. Do elderly patients withlocally advanced non-small cell lung cancer benefit from combined modality therapy? Int J Radiat Oncol Biol Phys 2001; 51:20–21.
19. Biel M. Photodynamic therapy and the treatment of head and neck neoplasia. Laryngoscope 1998; 108:1259–1268.
20. Gleich L. Gene therapy for head and neck cancer. Laryngoscope 2000; 110:708–725.
21. Cohen E. Novel therapeutic targets in squamous cell carcinoma of the head and neck. Semin Oncol 2004; 31(6):755–768.

22. List M, Bilir S. Evaluations of quality of life and organ function. Semin Oncol 2004; 31(6):827–835.
23. Wenig BM, Cohen JM. General principles of head and neck pathology. In: Harrison LB, Sessions RB, Hong WK, eds. Head and Neck Cancer, a Multidisiplinary Approach. 2d ed. Philadelphia: Lippincott Williams and Wilkins, 2004:11–48.
24. Greene FL, Page DL, Fleming ID, et al., eds. AJCC Cancer Staging Manual. 6th ed. Philadelphia: Lippincott Williams and Wilkins, 2002.
25. Zhu K, Levine RS, Brann EA, et al. Case-control study evaluating the homogeneity and heterogeneity of risk factors between sinonasal and nasopharyngeal cancers. Int J Cancer 2002; 99:119–123.
26. Day GL, Blot WJ, Austin DF, et al. Racial differences in risk of ral and pharyngeal cancer: alcohol, tobacco, and other determinants. J Natl Cancer Inst 1993; 85:465–473.
27. Sturgis EM, Wei Q, Spitz M. Descriptive epidemiology and risk factors for head and neck cancer. Semin Oncol 2004; 31(6):726–733.
28. Leon X, Quer M, Agudelo D, et al. Influence of age on laryngeal carcinoma. Ann Otol Rhinol Laryngol 1998; 107:164–169.
29. Nomura AM, Ziegler RG, Stemmermann GN, et al. Serum micronutrients and upper aerodigestive tract cancer. Cancer Epidemiol Biomarkers Prev 1997; 6(6):407–412.
30. Gustin DM. Chemoprevention of head and neck cancer. Semin Oncol 2004; 31(6):827–835.
31. Schwartz LH, Ozsahin M, Zhang GN, et al. Synchronous and metachronous head and neck carcinomas. Cancer 1994; 74(7):1933–1938.
32. Wendt TG, Grabenbauer GG, Rodel CM, et al. Simultaneous radiochemotherapy versus radiotherapy alone in advanced head and neck cancer: a randomized multicenter study. J Clin Oncol 1998; 16(4):1318–1324.
33. Cooper JS, Pajak TF, Forastiere AA, et al. Postoperative concurrent radiotherapy and chemotherapy for high-risk squamous-cell carcinoma of the head and neck. N Engl J Med 2004; 350:1937–1944.
34. Bernier J, Domenge C, Ozsahin M, et al. Postoperative irradiation with or without concomitant chemotherapy for locally advanced head and neck cancer. N Engl J Med 2004; 350:1945–1952.
35. Verschurr HP, Irish JC, O'Sullivan B, et al. A matched control study of treatment outcome in young patients with squamous cell carcinoma of the head and neck. Laryngoscope 1999; 109:249–258.
36. Lacy PD, Piccirillo JF, Merritt MG, et al. Head and neck squamous cell carcinoma: better to be young. Otolaryngol Head Neck Surg 2000; 122:253–258.
37. Smith BD, Haffty BG. Prognostic factors in patients with head and neck cancer. In: Harrison LB, Sessions RB, Hong WK, eds. Head and Neck Cancer, a Multidisiplinary Approach. 2d ed. Philadelphia: Lippincott Williams and Wilkins, 2004:49–73.
38. Siegelmann-Danieli N, Hanlon A, Ridge JA, et al. Oral tongue cancer in patients less than 45 years old: institutional experience and comparison with older patients. J Clin Oncol 1998; 16:745–753.
39. Shah JP, Zelefsky MJ. Cancer of the oral cavity. In: Harrison LB, Sessions RB, Hong WK, eds. Head and Neck Cancer, a Multidisiplinary Approach. 2d ed. Philadelphia: Lippincott Williams and Wilkins, 2004:266–305.
40. Chan AT, Teo PM, Huang DP. Pathogenesis and treatment of nasopharyngeal carcinoma. Semin Oncol 2004; 31(6):794–801.
41. Peters LJ, Rischin D, Corry J, et al. Cancer of the nasopharynx. In: Harrison LB, Sessions RB, Hong WK, eds. Head and Neck Cancer, a Multidisiplinary Approach. 2d ed. Philadelphia: Lippincott Williams and Wilkins, 2004:529–559.
42. Old LJ, Boyse EA, Oettgen HE, et al. Precipitating antibodies in human serum to an antigen present in cultured Burkitt's lymphoa cells. Proc Natl Acad Sci USA 1966; 56:1699.
43. Al-Sarraf M, LeBlanc M, Giri P, et al. Chemoradiotherapy versus radiotherapy in patients with advanced nasopharyngeal cancer: phase III randomized Intergoup study 0099. J Clin Oncol 1998; 16:1310–1317.

44. Al Sarraf M, LeBlanc M, Giri P, et al. Superiority of five year survival with chemora-diotherapy vs radiotherapy in patients with locally advanced nasopharyngeal cancer. NPC Intergroup 0099. Proc Am Soc Clin Oncol 2001; 20:905.

45. Lee AW, Law SC, Foo W, et al. Nasopharyngeal carcinoma: local control by megavol-tage irradiation. Br J Radiol 1993; 66:528–536.

46. Sanguineti G, Geara FB, Garden AS, et al. Carcinoma of the nasopharynx treated by radiotherapy alone: determinants of local and regional control. Int J Radiat Oncol Biol Phys 1997; 37:985–996.

47. Lindberg R. Distribution of cervical lymph node metastases from squamous cell carci-noma of the upper respiratory and digestive tracts. Cancer 1972; 29:1446–1449.

48. Gillson ML. Human papillomavirus—associated head and neck cancer is a distinct epi-demiologic, clinical, and molecular entity. Semin Oncol 2004; 31(6):744–754.

49. Mendenhall WM, Sulica L, Sessions RB. Early stage cancer of the larynx. In: Harrison LB, Sessions RB, Hong WK, eds. Head and Neck Cancer, a Multidisiplinary Approach. 2d ed. Philadelphia: Lippincott Williams and Wilkins, 2004:352–380.

50. Wolf et al. Induction chemotherapy plus radiation compared with surgery plus radiation in patients with advanced laryngeal cancer. The Department of Veterans Affairs Laryn-geal Cancer Study Group. N Engl J Med 1991; 324:1685–1690.

51. Forastiere AA, Goepfert H, Maor M, et al. Concurrent chemotherapy and radiotherapy for organ preservation in advanced laryngeal cancer. N Engl J Med 2003; 349:2091–2098.

52. Weinstein GS. Organ preservation surgery for laryngeal cancer: the evolving role of the surgeon in the multidisciplinary head and neck cancer team. Operative Tech Otolaryngol Head Neck Surgery 2003; 14(1):1–2.

53. Jiang GL, Morrison WH, Garden AS, et al. Ethmoid sinus carcinomas: natural history and treatment results. Radiother Oncol 1998; 49:21–27.

54. Righi P, Sofferman RA. Screening unilateral tonsillectomy in the unknown primary. Laryngoscope 1995; 105:548–550.

55. Lee D, Rostock RA, Harris A, et al. Clinical evaluation of patients with metastatic squa-mous cell carcinoma of the neck with occult primary tumor. South Med J 1986; 79:979–983.

56. Fu KK. Neck node metastases from unknown primary. Front Radiat Ther Oncol 1994; 28:66–78.

57. Glynne-Jones RG, Anand AK, Young TE, et al. Metastatic carcinoma in the cervical lymph nodes from an occult primary: a conservative approach to the role of radio-therapy. Int J Radiat Oncol Biol Phys 1990; 18:289–294.

58. Davidson BJ, Harter KW. Metastatic cancer to the neck from an unknown primary site. In: Harrison LB, Sessions RB, Hong WK, eds. Head and Neck Cancer, a Multidisipli-nary Approach. 2d ed. Philadelphia: Lippincott Williams and Wilkins, 2004:245–265.

59. Luna MA. Pathology of tumors of the salivary glands. In: Thawley SE, Panje WR, Batsakis JG, et al., eds. Comprehensive Management of Head and Neck Tumors. 2d ed. Philadelphia: W.B. Saunders, 1999:1106–1146.

60. Cady B. Presidential address: beyond risk groups—a new look at differentiated thyroid cancer. Surgery 1998; 124(6):947–957.

61. Cady B, Rossi R. An expanded review of risk-group definition in differentiated thyroid cancer. Surgery 1988; 104(6):947–953.

62. Hay ID, Taylor WF, McConahey WM. A prognostic score for prediciting outcome in papillary thyroid carcinoma. Endocrinology 1986; 119:T15.

63. Hay ID, Bergstralh EJ, Goellner JR, et al. Predicting outcome in papillary thyroid car-cinoma: development of a reliable prognostic scoring system in a cohort of 1,779 patients surgically treated at one institution during 1940–1989. Surgery 1993; 114(6): 1050–1057.

64. Sampson RJ, Woolner LB, Bahn RC, et al. Occult thyroid carcinoma in Olmestead County Minnesota: revalence at autopsy compared with that in Hiroshima and Nagasaki, Japan. Cancer 1974; 34(6):2072–2076.

65. Ludwig G, Nishiyama RH. The prevalence of occult papillary thyroid cancer in 100 consecutive autopsies in an American population. Lab Invest 1976; 34:320–324.
66. Modigliani E, Cohen R, Campos JM, et al. Prognostic factors for survival and for biochemical cure in medullary thyroid carcinoma: results in 899 patients. The GETC Study Group. Groupe D'etude des tumeurs a calcitonine. Clin Endocrinol (Oxf) 1998; 48(3):265–273.
67. Venkatesh YSS, Ordonez NG, Schultz PN, et al. Anaplastic carcinoma of the thyroid: a clinicopathologic study of 121 cases. Cancer 1990; 66(2):321–330.
68. Anscome AM, Wright DH. Primary malignant lymphoma of the thyroid: a tumor of mucosa-associated lymphoid tissue: review of seventy-six cases. Histopathology 1985; 9(1):81–97.
69. Hamburger JL, Miller JM, Kini SR. Lymphoma of the thyroid. Ann Intern Med 1983; 99(5):685–693.
70. Demeter JG, De Jong SA, Lawrence AM, et al. Anaplastic thyroid carcinoma: risk factors and outcome. Surgery 1991; 110(6):956–961.
71. Voutilainen PE, Multanen M, Haapiainen RK, et al. Anaplastic thyroid carcinoma survival. World J Surg 1999; 23(9):975–979.
72. Simpson WJ. Anaplastic thyroid carcinoma: a new approach. Can J Surg 1980; 23(1):25–27.
73. Yeung SC, Xu G, Pan J, et al. Manumycin enhances the cytotoxic effect of paclitaxel on anaplastic thyroid carcinoma cells. Cancer Res 2000; 60(3):650–656.

19
Soft Tissue Sarcomas

Vadim Gushchin
SUNY at Buffalo School of Medicine, Roswell Park Cancer Institute,
Buffalo, New York, U.S.A.

John M. Kane III and William G. Kraybill
Department of Breast and Soft Tissue Surgery, SUNY at Buffalo School of Medicine,
Roswell Park Cancer Institute, Buffalo, New York, U.S.A.

Michael K. K. Wong
Department of Medicine, SUNY at Buffalo School of Medicine, Roswell Park Cancer
Institute, Buffalo, New York, U.S.A.

INTRODUCTION

Soft tissue sarcomas (STS) are malignant tumors of mesenchymal origin. It is estimated that 9420 new cases of STS will be diagnosed in the United States in 2005,
and of these 3490 patients will die because of disease-related causes (1). It has been
difficult to study STS behavior and the effectiveness of treatment for these biologically diverse tumors because of their rarity, owing to the fact that they represent less
than 1% of all adult tumors. Management guidelines for STS are based upon few
randomized prospective trials and the clinical experience of specialized centers that
manage comparatively large numbers of sarcomas. In light of this, most treatment
recommendations are practice-based.

Management of the elderly patient with STS can be especially challenging and
difficult. A methodical approach to this complex issue can be obtained by analyzing
three critical components: the expected tumor biology, patient factors (including
medical comorbidities/functionality), and alternative treatment modalities. STS
biology defines the expected tumor behavior and the anticipated response to treatment. Thus, a low-grade STS of the leg typically has an indolent behavior and rarely
invades the bone or neurovascular bundle. As a consequence, an elderly patient with
a low-grade STS not amenable to a negative margin resection may be better served
with a microscopically positive margin resection and, possibly, intraoperative radiation therapy rather than radical amputation. Although there is still a risk of
recurrence even with perioperative radiation, the recurrence usually develops slowly
and could possibly be treated with re-resection. Amputation is a sound oncological
procedure, but the immobile elderly patient would then be at a high risk for developing a life-threatening complication. In contrast to a low-grade STS, an intentional

microscopically positive resection would be ill-advised in the case of a more aggressive high-grade STS.

Several "patient-related" factors make caring for the elderly unique. Advanced age should alert the clinician to diminished functional reserve, where relatively insignificant untoward events might lead to postoperative complications or even mortality. Life charts are useful for estimating the patient's life expectancy and make overall survival assessments more accurate. Comorbidities and the functional status are important in decision-making and should be comprehensively assessed during the initial STS evaluation. The degree to which they impact upon treatment will vary according to the severity of the comorbidities and the proposed therapy. A patient undergoing resection of a retroperitoneal sarcoma will inherently have more difficulty with postoperative recovery compared to a patient being treated for a small extremity STS. The social support structure is also an integral part of the patient evaluation. For example, when considering radiation as part of the treatment, it is imperative to determine beforehand if the patient will be able to adhere to the rigors of a daily treatment schedule. Finally, the patient's expectations and goals should be sought early in the development of the therapeutic plan. Treatment would hardly be considered "successful" should the patient become a permanent nursing home resident against his or her wishes. The social worker and clinical psychologist may help to address these important issues before treatment begins.

Although STS treatment principles are not fundamentally different for the elderly, it is frequently useful to consider less morbid alternatives to the "standard of care." Multidisciplinary discussions by dedicated physicians with an interest in and experience with STS (particularly surgical oncologists, radiation oncologists, medical oncologists, pathologists, orthopedic oncologists, and skilled plastic/ reconstructive surgeons) are highly desirable. Consider an 80-year-old patient with an STS of the buttock. Hemipelvectomy may be the oncological treatment of choice, but an experienced radiation oncologist might suggest primary radiation therapy as a reasonable alternative (2,3). When one realizes that the average general surgeon and orthopedist will see very few STS in their careers, it becomes apparent why these patients would be better served at specialty centers with a specific interest in this problem (4). Although a European study identified a trend toward not referring elderly patients with sarcomas to specialized centers (5), we think that older patients with STS would benefit greatly from a multidisciplinary approach.

DIAGNOSIS, STAGING, AND WORK-UP

The clinical evaluation of elderly STS patients should accomplish two major goals: adequate staging of the tumor and assessment of comorbidities/functional status. In regard to staging, the type of STS, the extent of the disease, and its expected behavior should be determined. The principles of the STS staging work-up are similar in younger and older patients. The work-up should address the major components of the staging system: size of the tumor, its location in relation to investing fascia, its histopathological type, the tumor grade, and the presence or absence of distant or nodal metastases (American Joint Committee on Cancer staging ref.). Tumor grade and histology should be assessed by a pathologist with special expertise in these uncommon tumors. If there is any question concerning the diagnosis or tumor grade, a second opinion should be sought (6,7).

Clinical suspicion of STS is paramount in the patient presenting with a mass or symptoms of mass effect and should trigger a diagnostic imaging evaluation prior to biopsy. Computerized tomography (CT) is the imaging modality of choice for patients with tumors of the body wall and retroperitoneum. Given that intravenous contrast is frequently employed in most CT protocols, it is advisable to take measures to protect the renal function in the elderly because it is frequently compromised. This consists of adequate hydration and the use of N-acetylcysteine or sodium bicarbonate (8). Magnetic resonance imaging (MRI) is more frequently used to image extremity STS. MRI can delineate the relationship between the tumor and the surrounding structures such as vessels, nerves, bone, or fascial planes. It can also display the anatomy in multiple different planes. Some tumors (e.g., lipomas, hemangiomas, schwannomas, neurofibromas, and intramuscular myxomas) have a characteristic MRI appearance that may help in the differential diagnosis (9). Overall, MRI is a sensitive and specific modality for the assessment of bone invasion by STS (10). However, older patients frequently have implanted hardware, which may be a contraindication to MRI (10,11). Consequently, other imaging modalities such as extremity CT scan or CT angiography or ultrasound (US) may need to be considered. MRI and US can also be useful in the follow-up setting and for guiding the biopsy of potential recurrent disease (10,12). Finally, there is some data available on the role fluorodeoxyglucose positron emission tomography (FDG-PET) imaging for the diagnosis and staging of STS of the extremities and retroperitoneum. According to one report, FDG-PET had a sensitivity of 100% in differentiating benign tumors from primary high- and intermediate-grade STS. FDG-PET, in conjunction with CT or MRI, was also useful in diagnosing recurrent sarcomas (13). As a developing diagnostic modality, the ultimate role of FDG-PET in the pretreatment evaluation of STS remains to be defined.

All suspicious soft tissue masses should have a definitive pathologic diagnosis before final treatment planning. In experienced hands, core needle biopsies have been highly successful for this purpose (14). In addition, image guidance allows for sampling of the most suspicious areas of a tumor or safe biopsy of nonpalpable masses. Adequate tissue for special studies can also be obtained by multiple core needle biopsies. Incisional biopsy provides more tissue with less sampling error and a higher probability of accurate grading. However, incisional biopsies can result in significant complications or adverse long-term treatment outcomes (such as tumor seeding) when improperly done. Strict adherence to well-described principles of biopsy for STS is mandatory and it is advisable that the biopsy be directed by the surgeon who will be performing the curative operation for the tumor (9).

Age greater than 50 has been reported as a negative prognostic factor for STS recurrence (both local and distant) as well as for disease-free survival (15). This may be related to a different distribution of histological types of sarcoma in the elderly. Malignant fibrous histiocytomas and liposarcomas are more frequent in patients older than 65 years in a Roswell Park Cancer Institute series (Table 1), which is consistent with other reports (16). An STS prognostic model had been developed at the Memorial Sloan Kettering Cancer Center for patients undergoing surgery with a curative intent (17). The nomogram has also been validated with a series from another institution, but only for the extremity location (18). Commonly available clinical variables (such as age, tumor size, grade, histological subtype, tumor depth, and location) are used to estimate the disease-specific survival at 4, 8, and 12 years. This information is invaluable when assessing the risk-to-benefit ratio for a particular patient with an operable STS.[a]

---

[a] Online or software versions of the nomogram are available at www.nomograms.org or www.mskcc.org/mskcc/html/6181.cfm.

Table 1 Histological Types of Sarcoma and Age

Sarcoma type	Age < 65, $n = 449$ (%)	Age > 65, $n = 139$ (%)
Malignant fibrous histiocytoma	84 (19)	52 (38)
Liposarcoma	110 (24)	36 (26)
Leiomyosarcoma	63 (14)	25 (18)
Synovial sarcoma	35 (8)	3 (2)
Rhabdomyosarcoma	21 (5)	3 (2)
Fibrosarcoma	20 (5)	1 (1)
Hemangiopericytoma	20 (5)	1 (1)
Spindle cell sarcoma	16 (4)	1 (1)
Malignant schwannoma	11 (2)	2 (1)
Clear cell sarcoma	6 (1)	0
Chondrosarcoma	6 (1)	0
Angiosarcoma	4 (1)	3 (2)
Unclassified	24 (5)	5 (4)
Others	29 (6)	6 (4)

History and physical examination are central to the assessment of comorbidities and the functional status of an elderly STS patient. Appropriate cardiac work-up as well as evaluation of other organ systems according to the patient's comorbidities is essential. A cardiology consultation is frequently obtained for patients older than 75 years of age who are being considered for surgical treatment. The comorbidity assessment should be done in collaboration with the patient's primary care physician (PCP). It is also important to communicate to the PCP the overall objectives of the work-up. Finally, the physicians responsible for the patient's overall care, including the PCP, should consider potential treatment-related complications. For example, nausea and vomiting following radiation treatments or surgery for a retroperitoneal sarcoma should be promptly evaluated with the diagnosis of intestinal obstruction in mind. An elderly patient with this condition and a limited reserve can quickly become dehydrated, and intestinal ischemia may develop without classical symptoms. As a result of this global assessment of comorbidities and functionality, a particular patient may choose to avoid an oncologically optimal treatment with significant potential morbidity in favor of another less morbid treatment plan. Therefore, we cannot stress enough the importance of a multidisciplinary approach where specialists from all branches of oncology with expertise in STS weigh in on different therapeutic strategies. The patient's comorbidities may become one of the most important deciding factors in these discussions and significantly limit the available treatment options.

Another important but frequently underappreciated component of the work-up of an elderly STS patient is an understanding of his/her expectations, goals, and psychosocial support system. For example, an older patient may not be able to keep frequent radiation therapy appointments, which may preclude this modality from the treatment plan. Unfortunately, lack of family support and financial restrictions commonly surface in the rehabilitation phase of treatment and may ultimately negate the outcome of a "state-of-the-art" treatment. The patient's social history should be actively taken into account when formulating the treatment plan. It is always prudent to make sure that the patient, family members, and referring physicians are cognizant of the realistic expectations for the proposed treatment.

TREATMENT

Extremity and Truncal STS

General Treatment Guidelines

Standard treatment for STS depends heavily upon the tumor stage. Small (<5 cm), low- or high-grade tumors, resectable with widely negative margins are treated surgically. In general, radiation does not improve local control in small, low-grade STS (19). Therefore, adjuvant radiation therapy should only be considered if the margins are less than 1 cm and re-resection is not possible. Large (≥5 cm), low-grade tumors are often treated with surgical resection as well as neoadjuvant or adjuvant external beam radiation therapy (EBRT) (19). If adequate margins can be achieved and the morbidity of adjuvant radiation therapy is estimated to be significant, consideration could be given to treating these patients with surgery alone. Large, high-grade STS are treated with a multimodality therapy consisting of neoadjuvant or adjuvant radiation combined with surgery. Neoadjuvant or adjuvant chemotherapy may be considered in selected patients, but only in the setting of a clinical trial because this is an area of significant controversy. Extremely high-risk deep, large high-grade tumors or marginally resectable STS should be treated with surgery and radiation. In these situations, many sarcoma experts would strongly consider preoperative radiation or combined chemo-radiation followed by surgery. Although an attempt at limb preservation through multimodality therapy is usually the treatment plan of choice, there are still some extremity STS that require amputation.

Local Therapy for STS in the Elderly

Local therapy for STS in the elderly follows the general treatment plan as outlined above with some notable exceptions. Surgical resection with negative margins is still the primary surgical goal. However, the rationale for limb salvage therapy is not only to preserve the extremity, but also to maintain its function by leaving major neurovascular structures and essential muscle groups intact. Although a poorly functioning limb acting as a "bioprosthesis" may be acceptable in a young patient, the extra energy necessary for ambulation may exceed the cardiopulmonary reserve of an older patient. Therefore, though difficult, an effort should be made to estimate the ultimate functional outcome following treatment. A major concern following the wide excision of nerves and tendons in elderly patients is also the rehabilitation necessary to overcome the functional difficulties. Hence, inclusion of physiatrists and physical therapists on the STS multidisciplinary team is key to a good outcome (20).

Sometimes close or microscopically positive margins result from this "functional" strategy and adjuvant radiation becomes a good therapeutic option (21). We often see previously resected, elderly, low-grade STS patients with positive margins on the final pathological examination. The standard of care for these patients should be wide re-excision of the tumor bed, if possible. Although radiation is not a substitute for inadequate surgery (22), adjuvant radiation alone may be considered when re-excision is not feasible (due to anatomical considerations or patient comorbidities). It is also important to remember that radiation may improve local control but has no impact upon overall survival (19). Therefore, in an attempt to reduce treatment-related morbidity in an elderly patient, one may accept microscopically positive or close resection margins in low-grade tumors with a consequentially higher local recurrence rate. Low-grade STS generally have an indolent behavior, recur locally, and are often amenable to multiple local excisions with or without radiation therapy, over a span of many years. This should be kept in mind as a viable option in the treatment of selected elderly patients with low-grade STS.

For larger STS and even some small high-grade tumors, surgical resection is supplemented with neoadjuvant and/or adjuvant radiation. Radiation modalities include EBRT, brachytherapy, or a combination of the two. Adjuvant EBRT can be used to improve local control after limb-sparing surgery at the expense of late complications such as joint stiffness and muscle weakness (19). These complications may be of particular clinical significance in elderly patients because they negatively affect mobility and balance, which may lead to further unwanted events such as decubitus ulcers, falls resulting in bone fractures, etc. Postoperative radiation is also associated with other long-term complications such as soft tissue necrosis and bone fractures, which are very difficult to treat (23). One STS study showed that women older than 55 years who underwent high-dose (60–66 Gy) postoperative radiation to the thigh appear to have a particularly high risk for developing long bone fractures, including fractures at multiple locations (24). Older patients also frequently require additional time to recuperate from surgery, especially if they develop postoperative complications. In this case, adjuvant radiation may need to be postponed for several months. Despite this delay, an increased dose of radiation is not necessary (25). Given the potential side effects in the elderly, radiation therapy may be avoided if the tumor is primary and resected with more than a 1-cm margin in all directions. However, this should be discussed in a multidisciplinary setting. Should a recurrence occur, it can often be treated with salvage surgery and/or radiation therapy.

Preoperative EBRT typically employs a lower total dose of radiation (usually 50–54 Gy) over a smaller area, as compared to postoperative radiation. Consequently, it is favored by many STS centers. Preoperative versus postoperative radiation approaches for high-grade STS are similar in regard to local control, but the complication profiles are somewhat different. The problems with postoperative EBRT are outlined above. In contrast, given that surgery follows radiation, preoperative EBRT is associated with increased perioperative wound complications, especially in the lower extremity (26). In one study, age greater than 40 years was found to be a risk factor for developing wound complications in patients treated with preoperative radiation (27). These authors also advocated extra caution in planning radiation treatment near joints in elderly STS patients owing to the development of arterial aneurysms and avascular bone necrosis in addition to the other treatment-related toxicities. Potential wound healing problems in the elderly must be weighed against the advantages of significantly lower doses and smaller fields, when using preoperative EBRT. Conversely, there is some evidence to suggest that preoperative radiation may result in better long-term functional outcomes (26). Myocutaneous and free flaps may also help to avoid the wound complications associated with preoperative radiation therapy (28). Soft tissue reconstruction should always be an important therapeutic consideration in all patients undergoing limb-sparing resection for extremity or truncal STS. At the same time, the reconstructive part of the operation may significantly increase the magnitude of surgical stress on the elderly patient.

Brachytherapy with iridium-192 implants is another radiation modality used to improve local control in patients with high-grade STS of the extremity and trunk by delivering high doses in a very limited area. Given that it is frequently administered over a short period of time in the immediate postoperative setting, there is an associated increase in wound-related complications (29). However, it may be very convenient for older patients because it is delivered over four to six days and the entire STS treatment (surgery and radiation) is completed in two weeks. As compared to EBRT, it may also limit the total dose of radiation delivered to vital organs such as the lungs, heart, or kidneys. This would be important for older patients with preexisting cardiopulmonary or renal dysfunction. Perioperative radiation, including brachytherapy, does not seem to affect healing after soft tissue flap reconstruction, even in older patients (30–32).

Amputation remains an effective treatment for selected extremity STS patients and should be considered in patients with rapidly growing tumors not amenable to functional limb salvage resections as well as in chronically bedridden older patients who do not use their extremity effectively (e.g., extremity contracture, neurological deficits, etc.). Amputation might also be a reasonable palliative intervention for the patient with a symptomatic extremity sarcoma who is not a candidate for curative surgery. For example, a patient with a recurrence in a previously irradiated limb may have painful, ulcerated lesions with little or no hope for successful wound healing. Quality of life in this setting may be significantly improved with amputation (33). Unrelieved pain is one of the most feared sequelae of advanced tumors. Many patients worry more about experiencing pain than their eventual death from cancer (34). Major amputation for STS in a palliative setting has been shown to significantly alleviate patient discomfort and improve overall well-being (35). Palliative amputations, including forequarter and hindquarter resections, are feasible, safe, and worth performing even in low-performance status patients suffering from locally advanced disease. It is reasonable to expect an improvement in the quality of life and even the performance status in severely ill and elderly patients following the control of symptoms with palliative amputation (33,36,37).

Local resections without a curative intent may also have a role in the palliation of elderly patients who are truly high-risk surgical candidates or for patients who would not accept the functional outcomes of an aggressive resection/amputation. Patients who are not candidates for surgical treatment of their STS or those who choose not to have surgery may also be considered for definitive radiation treatment with or without chemotherapy (3,38). If this is not feasible or is judged as unlikely to be effective, consultations with pain experts and a hospice are viable options to improve quality of life.

Chemotherapy for STS in the Elderly

At present, there is no clear consensus amongst STS specialists regarding the benefit of adjuvant chemotherapy. In the elderly, the data are even more limited because most randomized STS chemotherapy studies have excluded patients over the age of 75. In addition, the best results have been obtained in studies using dose-intensive regimens (39,40), which are difficult to administer in older patients secondary to their increased susceptibility to the associated toxicities in normal tissues. Finally, a large meta-analysis showed that adjuvant chemotherapy improves relapse-free survival in resectable sarcomas, but not overall survival, thus tempering the enthusiasm for this treatment modality (41).

Doxorubicin, dacarbazine, and ifosfamide possess the highest activities against STS. Given the potential toxicity of chemotherapeutic drugs, one must strongly consider the baseline heart or kidney dysfunction in older patients prior to administering these agents. Even in the absence of documented cardiac comorbidities and normal multiple gated acquisition scans (MUGA-scan), cardiotoxicity is not uncommon in the elderly. Therefore, older patients usually receive a dose-reduced course of doxorubicin and/or ifosfamide. Neutropenia is another serious concern because it occurs more frequently in the elderly and can have dire consequences. Therefore, granulocyte-stimulating factors are commonly employed, even on the first cycle. Despite these risks, regimens containing these drugs have been successfully administered to older patients. Some large series examining neoadjuvant/adjuvant chemotherapy for STS have included patients up to the age of 90 in the doxorubicin group and the age of 81 in the ifosfamide group (42). Unfortunately, these studies also showed that the improvements in disease-free and overall survival were small.

We suggest that decisions regarding adjuvant chemotherapy should be made on a case-by-case basis. Age alone should not be an absolute contraindication to chemotherapy because the patient's comorbidities and functional status are also major deciding factors. Generally, we may consider neoadjuvant/adjuvant chemotherapy for older patients with large high-grade extremity STS, tumors having a marginal resectability due to their close proximity to critical structures, or positive margins after maximal surgical therapy. However, we do not advocate the routine use of high-dose, "aggressive" neoadjuvant or adjuvant chemotherapeutic regimens off-protocol. More often than not, we decide not to utilize chemotherapy in elderly patients and look for less toxic treatment alternatives.

Retroperitoneal Sarcomas

The biology of retroperitoneal sarcomas (RPS) is characterized by a high rate of local recurrence and subsequent poor prognosis. Reported five-year local control and overall survival rates are 15% to 71% and 29% to 56%, respectively (43–45). In contrast to extremity STS, it is the local recurrence and not the distant metastases that is the main cause of mortality from RPS. Therefore, the completeness of resection is an important prognostic factor for RPS. The ability to achieve a negative margin resection reflects the extent of disease and the biological behavior of the RPS, as well as the surgeon's technical ability in removing the tumor. Local invasion of adjacent organs, viscera, or major vascular structures is not uncommon in primary tumors, as well as in recurrent disease. Complete resection of a primary RPS is possible in only 40% to 65% of cases and decreases to 30% to 45% for recurrent tumors (46,47). Patients treated at tertiary referral centers tend to have higher rates of complete resection and, therefore, fewer local recurrences (48).

Complete surgical resection with negative margins is the most effective therapy for RPS. Unfortunately, it may be an almost unachievable goal in large high-grade tumors. These operations frequently involve the resection of adjacent organs and can be very physiologically demanding on elderly patients. Preoperative cardiac assessment along with evaluation of other organ systems as directed by the patient's medical history helps to select the most appropriate therapy for an individual patient. If possible, chronic medical problems should be well compensated with known effective perioperative strategies such as beta blockade in high–cardiac risk patients or aggressive blood glucose management in diabetics. When nephrectomy is anticipated as part of the surgical plan, a preoperative renal scan is useful to estimate the function of the contralateral kidney.

Radiation therapy might be considered for RPS and can be delivered preoperatively, intraoperatively, and/or postoperatively (45). Preoperative radiation is an attractive option because a smaller treatment field is employed (minimizing exposure of adjacent organs) and may potentially make the resection easier. Its effectiveness is currently being evaluated in a phase III clinical trial (49). Serious treatment-related complications attributed to radiation therapy include intestinal obstruction (18%), intestinal fistula (9%), and peripheral neuropathy (6%) (50).

Systemic chemotherapy does not have a proven role in the management of RPS (51) and we do not routinely recommend it. If there are contraindications to surgery because of patient comorbidities or the extent of tumor, palliative nonoperative care may be considered. Therefore, in the setting of unresectable symptomatic tumors, a less toxic regimen with gemcitabine and docetaxel might be a reasonable option (52). When administering chemotherapy to the elderly patient with an unresectable RPS, we follow the same precautions as described earlier for adjuvant therapy. Primary radiation therapy appears to have little benefit in the treatment of RPS.

Historically, patients who present with symptoms related to their RPS have tumors that are less likely to be completely resectable. Palliative resection without an initial intent to cure may be the only option in symptomatic patients with these difficult presentations, especially those with more indolent tumors such as liposarcomas. A recent review of this liposarcoma subgroup demonstrated that incomplete resection can achieve successful palliation of symptoms in 75% of patients as well as an overall survival benefit, irrespective of age (46,53). Patient symptoms consisted mainly of abdominal or flank pain, consequences of intestinal and ureteral obstruction, neural invasion, and dyspnea. It is important to emphasize that the patients in this report had liposarcomas. Patients with rapidly progressing, undifferentiated RPS are unlikely to benefit from palliative resection.

Except when there is an obvious invasion of major vascular structures, it is often difficult to preoperatively determine that a RPS is conclusively unresectable. Therefore, it is frequently during the operation that the surgeon is faced with dilemma of whether to perform an incomplete palliative resection or abandon attempts at removing the bulk of the tumor. In this setting, our advice is to make an attempt to remove as much tumor as is safely possible. However, in patients identified preoperatively as truly being unresectable and without symptoms amenable to palliation, the decision not to attempt resection is often the correct one. Intuitively, it seems that debulking might prevent or at least delay morbidity from intestinal obstruction, caval or ureteral compressive syndromes, or respiratory embarrassment. But the patient with multiple RPS recurrences has a lower survival and, as a rule, often has a "hostile abdomen" due to previous procedures and sometimes even extended field radiation. The potential for complications is enormous and it goes without saying that leaving a patient in a condition worse than the preoperative state has done the patient no service at all. Consequently, a higher level surgical judgment must be relied upon when contemplating complex resections in the incurable patient. Estimates of survival and quality of life, with or without intervention, and other treatment options are factored into the decision to operate upon a patient with no hope for cure. Given that no prospective information is available, once again, surgical judgment is paramount.

Metastatic STS in the Elderly

Extremity or truncal STS preferentially metastasize to the lung, while RPS may spread to the liver or peritoneal cavity (sarcomatosis). Less common metastatic sites for STS include the central nervous system and lymph nodes. Once metastatic disease develops, median survival is fairly short at 12 months (54,55). Elderly patients with an anticipated short survival and no symptoms attributable to their metastases can be managed expectantly because it is difficult to improve the asymptomatic patient.

However, there is a potential curative role for the resection of isolated metastatic disease in selected STS patients. It has been shown that hepatic resection of metastases, even in patients up to the age of 74, can prolong survival provided that the primary tumor is controlled (56). Depending upon the extent of disease, ablative therapies such as radiofrequency ablation (RFA) can also be used to achieve local control of liver metastases. RFA is often amenable to less invasive percutaneous or laparoscopic approaches that may be ideal in the older patient who is at an increased risk for surgical morbidity (57). Similarly, selected patients with isolated pulmonary metastases can be treated by wedge resections using video-assisted thoracoscopic surgery. This can be readily accomplished in elderly patients with marginal pulmonary function and may even lead to an appreciable survival benefit.

Chemotherapy is a potential treatment option for older patients with metastatic disease, especially rapidly growing tumors. We suggest the same considerations and precautions as previously discussed, including an up-front dose reduction and the use of colony-stimulating growth factors. Single agent therapy with liposomal doxorubicin has a reasonable risk/benefit ratio in the elderly owing to its decreased toxicity (58). There is also a growing experience with less toxic regimens such as gemcitabine and docetaxel (52).

CONCLUSIONS

The management of any STS patient is very complex, but it can be especially challenging in the elderly. An overall decline in vital organ functions with age may preclude standard treatment options such as radiation and even surgery. In addition, the outcome expectations are often different for the older patient as compared to a younger population. Conversely, many elderly STS patients are actually very healthy with a reasonable long-term life expectancy. Therefore, decision making should stem from the perceived tumor biology (indolent vs. aggressive, resectable vs. unresectable, localized vs. metastatic, etc.) and the patient's comorbid conditions/functional status, and not just advanced age per se. The experience of the treatment team (e.g., expertise in brachytherapy, availability of intraoperative radiotherapy, etc.), the availability of less toxic chemotherapy regimens, and the integration of plastic/reconstructive surgery can make a significant difference in the outcome in elderly STS patients. A collaborative, multidisciplinary approach is essential and effective for formulating the optimal, individualized treatment plan based upon both the standard of care and its alternatives.

REFERENCES

1. Jemal A, Murray T, Ward E, et al. Cancer statistics, 2005. CA Cancer J Clin 2005; 55:10–30.
2. Schwarz R, Krull A, Lessel A, et al. European results of neutron therapy in soft tissue sarcomas. Recent Results Cancer Res. 1998; 150:100–112.
3. Slater JD, McNeese MD, Peters LJ. Radiation therapy for unresectable soft tissue sarcomas. Int J Radiat Oncol Biol Phys 1986; 12:1729–1734.
4. Rosenthal TC, Kraybill W. Soft tissue sarcomas: integrating primary care recognition with tertiary care center treatment. Am Fam Phys 1999; 60:567–572.
5. Nijhuis PH, Schaapveld M, Otter R, et al. Soft tissue sarcoma—compliance with guidelines. Cancer 2001; 91:2186–2195.

6. Alvegard TA, Berg NO. Histopathology peer review of high-grade soft tissue sarcoma: the Scandinavian Sarcoma Group experience. J Clin Oncol 1989; 7:1845–1851.

7. Cooper TM, Sheehan M, Collins D, et al. Soft tissue sarcoma of the extremity. Ann R Coll Surg Engl 1996; 78:453–456.

8. Merten GJ, Burgess WP, Gray LV, et al. Prevention of contrast-induced nephropathy with sodium bicarbonate: a randomized controlled trial. JAMA 2004; 291:2328–2334.

9. Cormier JN, Pollock RE. Soft tissue sarcomas. CA Cancer J Clin 2004; 54:94–109.

10. Elias DA, White LM, Simpson DJ, et al. Osseous invasion by soft-tissue sarcoma: assessment with MR imaging. Radiology 2003; 229:145–152.

11. Shellock FG. Reference Manual for Magnetic Resonance Safety. W.B. Saunders Company, 2002.

12. Choi H, Varma DG, Fornage BD, et al. Soft-tissue sarcoma: MR imaging vs. sonography for detection of local recurrence after surgery. AJR Am J Roentgenol 1991; 157:353–358.

13. Trovik CS, Bauer HC, Brosjo O, et al. Fine needle aspiration (FNA) cytology in the diagnosis of recurrent soft tissue sarcoma. Cytopathology 1998; 9:320–328.

14. Heslin MJ, Lewis JJ, Woodruff JM, et al. Core needle biopsy for diagnosis of extremity soft tissue sarcoma. Ann Surg Oncol 1997; 4:425–431.

15. Weitz J, Antonescu CR, Brennan MF. Localized extremity soft tissue sarcoma: improved knowledge with unchanged survival over time. J Clin Oncol 2003; 21:2719–2725.

16. Brennan MF, Singer S, et al. Sarcomas of the soft tissues and bone: Section 1: Soft tissue sarcoma. In: Devita VT, Hellman S, Rosenberg SA, eds. Cancer: Principles and Practice of Oncology. Lippincott Williams & Wilkins, 2004.

17. Kattan MW, Leung DH, Brennan MF. Postoperative nomogram for 12-year sarcoma-specific death. J Clin Oncol 2002; 20:791–796.

18. Mariani L, Miceli R, Kattan MW, et al. Validation and adaptation of a nomogram for predicting the survival of patients with extremity soft tissue sarcoma using a three-grade system. Cancer 2005; 103:402–408.

19. Yang JC, Chang AE, Baker AR, et al. Randomized prospective study of the benefit of adjuvant radiation therapy in the treatment of soft tissue sarcomas of the extremity. J Clin Oncol 1998; 16:197–203.

20. Popov P, Tukiainen E, Asko-Seljavaara S, et al. Soft-tissue sarcomas of the upper extremity: surgical treatment and outcome. Plast Reconstr Surg 2004; 113:222–230.

21. Choong PF, Petersen IA, Nascimento AG, et al. Is radiotherapy important for low-grade soft tissue sarcoma of the extremity? Clin Orthop Relat Res 2001; 387:191–199.

22. Zagars GK, Ballo MT, Pisters PW, et al. Surgical margins and reresection in the management of patients with soft tissue sarcoma using conservative surgery and radiation therapy. Cancer 2003; 97:2544–2553.

23. Zagars GK, Ballo MT, Pisters PW, et al. Preoperative vs. postoperative radiation therapy for soft tissue sarcoma: a retrospective comparative evaluation of disease outcome. Int J Radiat Oncol Biol Phys 2003; 56:482–488.

24. Holt GE, Griffin AM, Pintilie M, et al. Fractures following radiotherapy and limb-salvage surgery for lower extremity soft-tissue sarcomas. A comparison of high-dose and low-dose radiotherapy. J Bone Joint Surg Am 2005; 87-A:315–319.

25. Ballo MT, Zagars GK, Cormier JN, et al. Interval between surgery and radiotherapy: effect on local control of soft tissue sarcoma. Int J Radiat Oncol Biol Phys 2004; 58:1461–1467.

26. O'Sullivan B, Davis AM, Turcotte R, et al. Preoperative versus postoperative radiotherapy in soft-tissue sarcoma of the limbs: a randomised trial. Lancet 2002; 359:2235–2241.

27. Kunisada T, Ngan SY, Powell G, et al. Wound complications following pre-operative radiotherapy for soft tissue sarcoma. Eur J Surg Oncol 2002; 28:75–79.

28. Kane JM, III, Gibbs JF, McGrath BE, et al. Large, deep high-grade extremity sarcomas: when is a myocutaneous flap reconstruction necessary? Surg Oncol 1999; 8:205–210.

29. Pisters PW, Harrison LB, Leung DH, et al. Long-term results of a prospective randomized trial of adjuvant brachytherapy in soft tissue sarcoma. J Clin Oncol 1996; 14:859–868.

30. Kim JY, Youssef A, Subramanian V, et al. Upper extremity reconstruction following resection of soft tissue sarcomas: a functional outcomes analysis. Ann Surg Oncol 2004; 11:921–927.

31. Lee HY, Cordeiro PG, Mehrara BJ, et al. Reconstruction after soft tissue sarcoma resection in the setting of brachytherapy: a 10-year experience. Ann Plast Surg 2004; 52:486–491.

32. Spierer MM, Alektiar KM, Zelefsky MJ, et al. Tolerance of tissue transfers to adjuvant radiation therapy in primary soft tissue sarcoma of the extremity. Int J Radiat Oncol Biol Phys 2003; 56:1112–1116.

33. Malawer MM, Buch RG, Thompson WE, et al. Major amputations done with palliative intent in the treatment of local bony complications associated with advanced cancer. J Surg Oncol 1991; 47:121–130.

34. McCahill L, Ferrell B. Palliative surgery for cancer pain. West J Med 2002; 176:107–110.

35. Clark MA, Thomas JM. Major amputation for soft-tissue sarcoma. Br J Surg 2003; 90:102–107.

36. Merimsky O, Kollender Y, Inbar M, et al. Is forequarter amputation justified for palliation of intractable cancer symptoms? Oncology 2001; 60:55–59.

37. Merimsky O, Kollender Y, Inbar M, et al. Palliative major amputation and quality of life in cancer patients. Acta Oncol 1997; 36:151–157.

38. Rhomberg W, Hassenstein EO, Gefeller D. Radiotherapy vs. radiotherapy and razoxane in the treatment of soft tissue sarcomas: final results of a randomized study. Int J Radiat Oncol Biol Phys 1996; 36:1077–1084.

39. Bramwell VH. Adjuvant chemotherapy for adult soft tissue sarcoma: Is there a standard of care? J Clin Oncol 2001; 19:1235–1237.

40. Frustaci S, Gherlinzoni F, De Paoli A, et al. Adjuvant chemotherapy for adult soft tissue sarcomas of the extremities and girdles: results of the Italian randomized cooperative trial. J Clin Oncol 2001; 19:1238–1247.

41. Adjuvant chemotherapy for localised resectable soft-tissue sarcoma of adults: meta-analysis of individual data. Sarcoma Meta-analysis Collaboration. Lancet 1997; 350: 1647–1654.

42. Eilber FC, Eilber FR, Eckardt J, et al. The impact of chemotherapy on the survival of patients with high-grade primary extremity liposarcoma. Ann Surg 2004; 240:686–695.

43. Alvarenga JC, Ball AB, Fisher C, et al. Limitations of surgery in the treatment of retroperitoneal sarcoma. Br J Surg 1991; 78:912–916.

44. Youssef E, Fontanesi J, Mott M, et al. Long-term outcome of combined modality therapy in retroperitoneal and deep-trunk soft-tissue sarcoma: analysis of prognostic factors. Int J Radiat Oncol Biol Phys 2002; 54:514–519.

45. Sindelar WF, Kinsella TJ, Chen PW, et al. Intraoperative radiotherapy in retroperitoneal sarcomas. Final results of a prospective, randomized, clinical trial. Arch Surg 1993; 128:402–410.

46. Jaques DP, Coit DG, Hajdu SI, et al. Management of primary and recurrent soft-tissue sarcoma of the retroperitoneum. Ann Surg 1990; 212:51–59.

47. Storm FK, Mahvi DM. Diagnosis and management of retroperitoneal soft-tissue sarcoma. Ann Surg 1991; 214:2–10.

48. van Dalen T, Hennipman A, van Coevorden F, et al. Evaluation of a clinically applicable post-surgical classification system for primary retroperitoneal soft-tissue sarcoma. Ann Surg Oncol 2004; 11:483–490.

49. Windham TC, Pisters PW. Retroperitoneal sarcomas. Cancer Control 2005; 12:36–43.

50. Alektiar KM, Hu K, Anderson L, et al. High-dose-rate intraoperative radiation therapy (HDR-IORT) for retroperitoneal sarcomas. Int J Radiat Oncol Biol Phys 2000; 47:157–163.

51. Pirayesh A, Chee Y, Helliwell TR, et al. The management of retroperitoneal soft tissue sarcoma: a single institution experience with a review of the literature. Eur J Surg Oncol 2001; 27:491–497.

52. Hensley ML, Maki R, Venkatraman E, et al. Gemcitabine and docetaxel in patients with unresectable leiomyosarcoma: results of a phase II trial. J Clin Oncol 2002; 20:2824–2831.

53. Shibata D, Lewis JJ, Leung DH, et al. Is there a role for incomplete resection in the management of retroperitoneal liposarcomas? J Am Coll Surg 2001; 193:373–379.
54. Blay JY, van Glabbeke M, Verweij J, et al. Advanced soft-tissue sarcoma: a disease that is potentially curable for a subset of patients treated with chemotherapy. Eur J Cancer 2003; 39:64–69.
55. Kostler WJ, Brodowicz T, Attems Y, et al. Docetaxel as rescue medication in anthracycline- and ifosfamide-resistant locally advanced or metastatic soft tissue sarcoma: results of a phase II trial. Ann Oncol 2001; 12:1281–1288.
56. DeMatteo RP, Shah A, Fong Y, et al. Results of hepatic resection for sarcoma metastatic to liver. Ann Surg 2001; 234:540–547.
57. Siperstein A, Garland A, Engle K, et al. Local recurrence after laparoscopic radiofrequency thermal ablation of hepatic tumors. Ann Surg Oncol 2000; 7:106–113.
58. Judson I, Radford JA, Harris M, et al. Randomised phase II trial of pegylated liposomal doxorubicin (DOXIL/CAELYX) versus doxorubicin in the treatment of advanced or metastatic soft tissue sarcoma: a study by the EORTC Soft Tissue and Bone Sarcoma Group. Eur J Cancer 2001; 37:870–877.

20

Assessment of Health Status and Outcomes in the Older Cancer Patient: QOL and Geriatric Assessment

Arash Naeim, Patricia A. Ganz, David B. Reuben, and Homayoon Sanati
UCLA Department of Medicine, Los Angeles, California, U.S.A.

INTRODUCTION

Historically, most clinical trials in oncology have used tumor shrinkage, time to disease progression, treatment-related toxicities, and survival as their main study end points. However, over the past three decades, quality of life (QOL) has emerged as an important end point in the field of oncology as well as other fields of medicine. QOL considerations have been brought to the forefront of health care research as a result of the convergence of several important factors. These include (i) prolonged life expectancy, from the eradication of many infectious diseases and the successful treatment of other conditions (e.g., diabetes and kidney failure); (ii) the appearance of many new chronic diseases (e.g., arthritis, heart disease, cancer, and HIV infection); (iii) the increasing cost and toxicities of some treatments; and (iv) the concern about health outcomes beyond mortality. Coincident with these circumstances has been a rapidly growing science of outcomes assessment, which borrows extensively from concurrent methodological advances in the social sciences, enabling the quantification and evaluation of the QOL outcomes of diseases and their treatments (1). In this chapter, we will have an opportunity to examine the intersection of these events from the perspective of cancer in the elderly.

In parallel with the developments in the measurement of subjective well-being and QOL assessment, the field of geriatrics has been rapidly expanding and systematizing the approach to the evaluation of the older person. There are many parallels between geriatric assessment and QOL assessment, in that they are multidimensional and broad. Both utilize standardized instruments that frequently rely on patient perceptions and other "biologically soft" measures. Nevertheless, they focus on issues that are among the most important to older persons, particularly the ability to function fully in social roles and participate in activities consistent with their desires. On the other hand, some differences between the two constructs illustrate that the two are not synonymous. For example, QOL is best assessed by the patient, whereas functional status and other dimensions of geriatric assessment may be better assessed by clinicians or proxies such as family members.

There are considerable opportunities to integrate many of the components of QOL assessment with geriatric assessment. Knowledge about both of these disciplines will facilitate better care of the older cancer patient and has great promise for improving the quality of cancer research conducted with older patients. In this chapter, we provide an introduction to both of these approaches to evaluation of health status and outcomes, as well as propose strategies for integrating the two methods of assessment in practice with the older cancer patient.

There are numerous textbooks, reviews, and internet sites that devote considerable time to the examination of QOL assessment (2–16). This chapter cannot cover all of the important topics that a reader may be interested in, and therefore, reference will be made to more detailed resources, but it will provide sufficient information to allow discussion of critical issues relevant to older persons with cancer. We will review the following topics: the definition and conceptualization of QOL; methods of measuring QOL; the role of QOL assessment in the elderly cancer patient; special aspects of QOL in the elderly; and future directions for research and application.

QOL ASSESSMENT IN THE CANCER PATIENT

Definition and Conceptualization of QOL

Definition and History

Although most of us intuitively understand what the phrase "quality of life" connotes, it has been exceedingly difficult for social scientists, health services researchers, and clinicians to define precisely. Often "quality of life" is used by the authors of scientific papers without explicit definition and several variables are used as measures of QOL (from physiologic indicators such as weight loss to standardized psychologic measures of emotional distress) (17). "Quality of life" has been a frequently abused catch phrase. Currently, there is no standard definition of QOL that is appropriate for both practice and research. Numerous definitions of QOL can be found in the literature. Here are some examples:

- QOL is the state of well-being that is a composite of two components: the ability to perform everyday activities that reflect physical, psychological, and social well-being; and patient satisfaction with levels of functioning and control of the disease (18).
- QOL is the subjective evaluation of the good and satisfactory character of life as a whole (19).
- QOL is the gap between the patient's expectations and achievements. The smaller the gap, the higher the QOL (20).
- QOL represents the functional effect of an illness and its consequent therapy upon the patient as perceived by the patient (21).
- QOL is defined as individual's overall satisfaction with life and general sense of well-being (22).
- QOL is patients' perceptions of their position in life in the context of the culture and value systems in which they live and in relation to their goals, expectations, standards, and concerns (23).
- QOL refers to patients' appraisal of and satisfaction with their current level of functioning compared to what they perceive to be possible or ideal (24).
- QOL is the subjective perception of satisfaction or happiness with life in domains of importance to the individual (25).

These definitions include concepts like well-being, satisfaction, happiness, and physical functioning, which are included in various instruments to measure the QOL. The concept of QOL has a broad, general meaning based on its roots in ancient philosophical works (26). Contemporary definitions of QOL and measurement strategies derive from historical efforts designed to measure the well-being of the population using social indicators such as general satisfaction and happiness, as well as satisfaction with housing, employment, income, etc. (27–29). The World Health Organization (WHO) definition of health as a "state of complete physical, mental, and social well-being and not merely the absence of disease" (30) is central to current work designed to measure health-related QOL (HRQOL) outcomes. Although the WHO definition was considered impossible to operationalize and measure at the time of its publication, contemporary QOL assessment tools focus on these three critical dimensions (physical, mental, and social) of health and QOL. Current conceptualization of QOL as measured in relationship to disease and treatment is called HRQOL, because it tends to limit the focus to dimensions of QOL that are directly affected by health and/or disease states (31,32).

In oncology practice, the Karnofsky performance status scale (scored 0–100 in 10 point increments where 0 is dead and 100 is completely normal) (33) was one of the earliest tools used to measure the functional performance of cancer patients. The scale was developed by clinicians primarily to collect and record information that was thought to be important for diagnosis, treatment, and clinical response. Another commonly used scale for measuring performance status has been developed by Eastern Cooperative Oncology Group-Performance Status, ECOG-PS (scored 0–5 in 1 point increments where 0 is fully active and 5 is dead) (34). The ECOG performance score is commonly used by oncologists because of its simplicity. Like the Karnofsky scale, the ECOG performance score has been found to correlate well with survival duration (35) and response to treatment (36). In one study, Buccheri et al. compared ECOG and Karnofsky performance scores in 537 patients with lung cancer. ECOG score was found to be better than Karnosky score in predicting patient's prognosis (37). Both Karnofsky and ECOG performance scores correlate highly with the physical functioning dimension of QOL questionnaires in some studies, but they do not seem to correlate well with overall measures of QOL in cancer patients (38). Both Karnofsky and ECOG performance measures are limited because they are rated by the "clinician" rather than the "patient." However, they have the advantage of being brief and acceptable in the clinical setting and having a clear relationship to other important clinical variables such as mortality (33,35).

Early in the 1980s, Spitzer et al. developed a tool specifically to evaluate the QOL of cancer patients (39). This instrument contains a uniscale for the global evaluation of QOL, along with separate components that evaluate the physical and emotional aspects of QOL. This latter 10-point scale is appealing because of its simplicity as well as the ease with which it can be rated by an observer. For this reason, it was extensively used in cancer research during the 1980s (e.g., the National Hospice Study). However, over the past decade, there has been growing consensus that QOL should be rated by the patient rather than by a clinician or proxy (40). Thus, many new tools have been developed to capture the patient's own assessment of QOL.

In the last decade of the 20th century, many instruments were developed to measure the QOL in cancer patients. European Organization for the Research and Treatment of Cancer (EORTC) has developed QOL Questionnaire Core Module (EORTC QLQ-C30) (41) to measure the QOL of patients enrolling in international clinical trials. Functional Assessment of Cancer Therapy (FACT)—general (42), which is a commonly used instrument in cancer patients, has been developed by Cella et al. The National Cancer Institute conducted two workshops (1990 and 1995) on the topic of QOL assessment in clinical trials (43), and now each of the clinical trials cooperative groups has clinical investigators and staff devoted to the consideration of inclusion of QOL end points in clinical treatment trials. In addition, many pharmaceutical companies are routinely including QOL measures as part of the evaluation of new drugs. Recently, improvements in QOL (including pain and symptom relief) have been acknowledged as being relevant end points in the new drug approval process.

Multidimensionality of QOL

Most experts in this field perceive QOL as a multidimensional construct that includes several key dimensions (6,8,31,44). These include *physical functioning* (performance of self-care activities, functional status, mobility, physical activities, and role activities such as work or household responsibilities); *disease- and treatment-related symptoms* (specific symptoms from the disease such as pain or shortness of breath, or side effects of drug therapy such as nausea, hair loss, impotence, or sedation); *psychological functioning* (anxiety or depression that may be secondary to the disease or its treatment); and *social functioning* (disruptions in normal social activities). Additional considerations in the evaluation of QOL may include spiritual or existential concerns, sexual functioning and body image, and satisfaction with health care.

Whenever possible, HRQOL should be assessed by the patient (17,45) and should reflect the evaluation of a number of dimensions affecting the patient's life at that moment. Although ratings on specific dimensions at any point in time may vary, the individual's overall QOL may in fact remain stable or change depending on how these dimensions fluctuate and interact. For this reason, some have argued that both the component dimensions of QOL as well as a global assessment should be considered (46). Therefore, in the research or clinical setting, one should always ask what specific dimensions of QOL are likely to be affected and choose a QOL tool based on its content relevance to the questions of interest.

Measurement of QOL

Data Collection Methods

Although there is consensus that the patient should assess QOL, there are a variety of ways in which this information can be obtained. The clinical interview (using structured questions from a validated instrument) is the most comprehensive approach in that it allows participation of the greatest number of individuals (e.g., those who cannot read or write and those with visual impairment or frailty). However, the personal interview is more costly in terms of the number of personnel and time and there may be some bias introduced through in-person interaction. Interviews can be conducted in person or by telephone and can assure less missing data. For geriatric research, the clinical interview is a standard approach for a variety of reasons, but often because of the frailty of the target population. However, geriatric assessment relies heavily on self-administered questionnaires (especially in healthier older persons) and performance-based measures, in addition to the clinical interview.

In contrast, most of the research on QOL with cancer patients has focused on self-administered questionnaires. This has occurred primarily because of an interest in the inclusion of QOL assessments in clinical trials where a large number of personnel are unavailable for conduct of interviews. The advantages of the self-administered format include limited need for personnel to collect data, more accurate responses for sensitive information, and administration at a time and place convenient for the patient. However, there are important limitations to self-administered instruments, which include a requirement for literacy and language translation, familiarity with completion of pencil and paper tests, and the increased likelihood of missing data (47). A study in a geriatric population has showed that about 20% of the elderly and 50% of the nursing home residents were unable or unwilling to participate in QOL assessments themselves (48). In addition, very ill patients (e.g., Karnofsky score less than 60) may have difficulty completing more than the briefest scales (49).

Ideally, a combination of these two approaches should be used in the assessment of QOL in cancer patients. One can start with the self-administered format and reserve the structured research interview for those patients who are unable to complete the written form without assistance. Even when a self-administered format is used, however, it is important to review all questionnaires for missing data. Thus, the combination of the two approaches can lead to the greatest efficiency in terms of data completeness and personnel time. In the Medical Outcomes Study, which included a sizeable portion of outpatients over 65 years of age, their fairly lengthy survey was self-administered by the majority of subjects, with telephone interview required in the remainder (50). While in general, results from self-report and telephone interviews are similar, there can be some variation, especially on sensitive topics, and researchers should track the mode of administration. In research studies with older cancer patients, an attempt should be made to collect the data in a single systematic format. If resources permit, the interview may be the best approach to ensure inclusion of all eligible older patients.

Quality-Adjusted Life Years

HRQOL is commonly expressed in terms of quality-adjusted life years (QALYs) or quality-adjusted time without symptoms or toxicity (Q-TWiST). QALY concept has been developed by health economists as an aid to make health policy decisions. QALY is a utility approach to measure QOL (51). QALY measurement adjusts QOL estimates of the utilities valued from 0.0 to 1.0. For example, if a patient gives a utility a score of 0.5 and spends one year in that state, the state would have an equal value as half of the year in perfect health. This type of measurement has limitations and is often controversial when used to analyze the cost effectiveness of different health care interventions (52). Q-TWiST has been developed to estimate costs and benefits in the field of oncology. Q-TWiST divides survival in areas with and areas without symptoms or toxicity (53). By comparing durations of health states, Q-TWiST has been useful to compare treatments in oncology trials.

Choice of Instruments

Over the past two decades, a large number of QOL instruments were been developed. None of these instruments, however, can measure HRQOL across all domains, populations, diseases, or treatments (54). The choice of the instrument mostly depends on the objectives of the measurement. Many of the QOL instruments were not specifically designed for the elderly population, and validity of the instrument needs to be demonstrated in the geriatric population (55).

In the field of QOL assessment there is a tension between using instruments that are highly specific to the research or clinical question at hand (e.g., a unique toxicity for a treatment) versus use of a tool that has been widely used with other samples of cancer patients or patients with other chronic conditions (e.g., diabetes, arthritis, and heart disease). One issue is the use of generic measures versus cancer-specific/cancer site- and phase-specific tools (Table 1).

In considering the geriatric cancer patient, one must also consider a whole body of geriatric assessment tools [e.g., Mini-mental Status Exam (66), the Geriatric Depression Scale (GDS) (67)], and these will be discussed later in this chapter. However, for the purpose of this discussion, we will focus on QOL instruments that have been used in a broad range of populations.

Generic instruments such as the Rand Corporation measures (50,57,58), the Dartmouth Care Cooperative Information Project charts (61), and the Duke scales (68) have considerable value if one wishes to compare the general impact of differing diseases/conditions on HRQOL. From a policy standpoint, this may be important in terms of preventing discrimination against cancer patients, because their functional status and QOL may exceed that of patients with other chronic conditions (69). On the other hand, the information obtained from these scales often lacks the sensitivity to detect impairments directly resulting from cancer treatments (70,71).

In contrast, the cancer-specific QOL instruments (e.g., EORTC or FACT) that have been developed during the past decade have high reliability and validity and are responsive to changes from treatments (72). In addition, they are more likely to capture the known toxicities and concerns related to cancer treatment. Therefore, they should be a preferred choice in the comparative evaluation of cancer treatments. However, each of these "generic" cancer-specific instruments may need to be supplemented with disease-specific modules (e.g., for breast cancer, prostate cancer,

Table 1   Examples of HRQOL Instruments Used with Cancer Patients

---

Generic health status measures
Sickness Impact Profile (56)
RAND Health Insurance Experiment Measures (50,57)
Medical Outcomes Study instruments (58)
Nottingham Health Profile (59)
Psychosocial Adjustment to Illness Scale (60)
Dartmouth COOP charts (61)
Generic cancer-specific instruments
QOL Index (39)
QOL Index (62)
Functional Living Index—Cancer (44)
EORTC QOL Questionnaire (41)
Cancer Rehabilitation Evaluation System (63)
FACT (42)
Cancer site–specific instruments
Breast Cancer Chemotherapy Questionnaire (64)
Linear Analogue Self-Assessment for Breast Cancer (65)
Site-specific modules for the FACT and the EORTC-QLQ

Abbreviations: COOP, Care Cooperative Information Project; EORTC-QOL, European Organization for Research and Treatment of Cancer Quality of Life; FACT, Functional Assessment of Cancer Therapy; HRQOL, health-related QOL; QOL, quality of life.

leukemia, etc.) or condition-specific QOL issues (e.g., pain, nausea, sexual functioning, etc.). Thus, in selecting a QOL assessment, one must carefully define the expected impacts of the disease and its treatment on QOL and use a battery of assessment tools that are likely to reflect these effects.

With the growing number of multinational trials and increasing diversity of the United States, there is a need for standard guidelines to convert a validated QOL measurement for use in different languages and cultures. When choosing a QOL instrument, cultural and language barriers must be considered. Most HRQOL instruments have been developed in English and may need to be modified for use in another language to maintain the content and validity of the instrument. Standard guidelines for cross-cultural adaptations for measurements of HRQOL have been proposed based on research in psychology and sociology (73,74). These guidelines include steps for translation (including semantic, idiomatic, experimental, and conceptual equivalences), back-translation, expert committee review, pretesting, and reexamination techniques.

When considering how to assess QOL in the geriatric cancer patient, special issues may arise in very frail elderly samples, especially those who are not routinely included in clinical trials because of other exclusion criteria. Relatively little research has been conducted with this group of cancer patients and it is unclear whether other chronic conditions (e.g., arthritis, heart disease, and pulmonary disease) will overwhelm any specific contribution made by the cancer. This is clearly an area ripe for further research and is beginning to receive attention from several investigators (75,76).

Role of QOL Assessment in Cancer Treatment

QOL assessment can be used for a variety of purposes: to describe the impact of cancer and its treatment on patients; to compare the outcome of different treatments in clinical trials; to identify unanticipated benefits or toxicities of treatment; and to inform future treatment planning through modification of aspects that detract from QOL. Information gained from prior QOL research can help inform treatment decisions. For example, multiple studies have shown that overall QOL, and most of its dimensions, differ little among women who choose mastectomy over lumpectomy in the primary treatment of breast cancer (77). Therefore, a woman who is considering alternative surgical treatments for breast cancer can be reassured that her subsequent adjustment will not be dependent on the type of surgery she receives; however, because research has shown that in some dimensions, such as body image, there is more disruption from mastectomy compared to lumpectomy (78). Consequently, a woman who expresses concerns about her body image should be encouraged to consider a lumpectomy.

Several studies have also demonstrated that QOL is an important prognostic factor for survival (49,79). Thus, assessing patient-rated QOL may help physicians frame discussions about the aggressiveness of cancer therapy. In this regard, there is mounting evidence that physicians sometimes do not consider the advance directives or expressed wishes of patients regarding end-of-life support (80). Regular evaluation of a patient's QOL over time can capture functional deterioration, which physicians may overlook (45). Physicians may be reluctant to engage in QOL discussions with seriously ill patients, instead substituting more objective and quantified measures of outcome. Although these issues are relevant to all cancer patients, they are particularly salient for the elderly in whom the majority of cancer deaths occur.

Special Relevance of QOL in the Geriatric Cancer Patient

Often there have been assumptions made about the QOL impact of cancer and its treatment on older patients. These include the belief that older patients suffer more side effects from treatment or have more difficulty adjusting to a cancer diagnosis. As indicated earlier, the elderly are quite heterogeneous and one cannot assume that chronological age is the primary factor affecting functioning or well-being. In one study (81), 300 matched pairs of adult patients with cancer and their physicians were interviewed concerning the effects of disease and treatment on the patients' QOL. The physicians overestimated the problems of the elderly cancer patients, while younger patients reported more difficulties. These authors suggest that physicians need to become more sensitized to the individualized, personal nature of their patients' QOL and the factors that may shape or modify it (81). Thus, it is critical that health care providers assess the individual patient's QOL; there is no room for paternalistic decision-making for older adults simply because of their age.

When side effects of cancer treatment have been examined (e.g., nausea and vomiting), older patients often fare better than younger patients, requiring less antiemetic therapy (82). Nevertheless, some side effects such as diarrhea (and resultant dehydration) may be more of a problem in the older cancer patient receiving chemotherapy. Pain is an important symptom that may detract from QOL (83,84), and care should be given to provide adequate education and treatment for this problem. Even though older persons with cancer are the majority of those cared for in hospice programs, pain research specific to the elderly is sparse (85,86).

Several studies have documented better mental health in the elderly in general, with consistent findings among older cancer patients (69). Life experiences as well as familiarity with the health care setting allow older cancer patients to cope with a cancer diagnosis with more resiliencies. With greater awareness of this disease experience from their peers, older cancer patients often are not as distressed as younger cancer patients. A specific issue for the elderly, however, may be their need for assistance of various types. In a detailed study of determinants of need and unmet need among cancer patients residing at home, physiological factors (metastases, disease stage, and functional status) were associated with the need for assistance in the areas of personal care, instrumental tasks, and transportation (87). Also, older age (over 65) and low income predicted need for help with personal care, and women were more likely than men to report illness-related need for assistance with instrumental tasks and transportation. Unmet need was primarily associated with the patients' social support system (87). There may be considerable variation in the degree of social support among elderly cancer patients, and this may influence the patient's functioning and well-being. Health care providers should include evaluation of social support when considering treatment decisions as well as the patient's subjective assessment of well-being. Geriatric assessment, described in the following section, is critical to the translation of information from QOL assessment into active interventions for the older cancer patient.

FEATURES OF GERIATRIC ASSESSMENT

History and Definition of Geriatric Assessment

Geriatric assessment has been described as the "heart and soul" of the geriatrics (88). Pioneers in the field of geriatrics developed the framework of geriatric assessment in the early 1970s. Williams et al. first used geriatric assessment in an out-patient setting for nursing home placement screening (89). In the early 1980s, Rubenstein et al. showed the effectiveness of geriatric assessment in a randomized clinical trial (90). The elderly patients who got screened and treated in the geriatric unit were more likely to regain their functional status and less likely to be discharged to a nursing home. Over the past three decades, geriatric assessment has gained increasing attention in the field of oncology. Cancer centers in the United States and Europe have started to use geriatric assessment tools to identify common geriatric syndromes that can complicate the cancer treatments.

The National Institutes of Health consensus conference on geriatric assessment methods in 1987 defined geriatric assessment as "a multidisciplinary evaluation in which multiple problems of older persons are uncovered, described, and explained, if possible, and in which resources and strength of the person are catalogued, need for services assessed, and a coordinated care plan developed to focus on interventions on the person's problems" (91). Geriatric assessment extends beyond the traditional medical evaluation of older persons' health to include assessment of cognitive, affective, functional, social, economic, and environmental status, as well as a discussion of patient preferences regarding advance directives (Table 2).

For younger and healthier seniors, simple probes for the presence of common geriatric problems may suffice. Those who are frail or at high risk for functional decline or nursing home placement should receive more extensive evaluation conducted by individual practitioners or by a multidisciplinary team of health care professionals (comprehensive geriatric assessment). For the oncologist, referral for comprehensive geriatric assessment might be considered when an elderly patient's cancer is well controlled but the patient is failing to thrive.

Assessment instruments can be used to guide these brief evaluations but must be interpreted in the context of their limitations. They are rarely, if ever, diagnostic tests. Rather they indicate the need for further evaluation. Nor do they substitute for good clinical skills and judgment, including the skill of eliciting important items from the patient's history and physical examination. However, information obtained from assessment instruments can be used to quickly direct the clinician's attention to issues that are particularly relevant to an individual patient. The clinician must also be able to act on the information obtained by seeking additional diagnostic tests, by implementing therapy for problems detected, or by referring patients to appropriate professionals for additional evaluation and management. Although detailed discussion of management of problems identified through assessment instruments is beyond the scope of this article, possible referral resources are indicated in Table 2. The remaining part of this article will focus on the initial multidimensional assessment on the assumption that the oncologist is the primary care physician.

Assesment for Geriatric Conditions

Medical Assessment

Regardless of whether the oncologist serves as a consultant or primary care physician for an elderly patient, nutritional and gait and balance assessments should be performed, and a medication review should be conducted.

Malnutrition/weight Loss: Among oncology patients, the most common nutritional disorder is energy undernutrition (including protein energy undernutrition). Causes of malnutrition could include decreased food intake, malabsorption (mostly

Table 2 Assessment of the Elderly Oncology Patient

Dimension	Brief screening test	Potential referral resource
Medical		
Nutrition	BMI, serum albumin and cholesterol	Dietitian
Mobility/balance	Time Up & Go (92), office-based maneuvers (93)	Physical therapist
Visual impairment	Snellen eye chart, ADVS (94)	Optician, ophthalmologist
Hearing impairment	Whispered test, Audioscope, hearing handicap Inventory for the Elderly-Screening Version (95), or Brief Scale to Detect Hearing Loss Screener (96)	Audiologist
Urinary incontinence	Two questions, PVR measurement	Geriatrician, urologist, gynecologist
Osteoporosis	Bone density scan (DEXA scan)	
Cognitive		
Dementia	Three item recall, Mini-mental State Examination (66)	Geriatrician, psychiatrist, neurologist
Delirium	CAM (97)	
Affective	GDS (67,98)	Geriatrician, psychiatrist
Functional status	BADL (99), IADL (100), AADL (96), questions	Geriatrician, social worker, physical therapist, occupational therapist
Social assessment		
Social support	Specific questions	Social worker
Caregiver burden	CRA (101)	Social worker
Economic status	Specific questions	Social worker
Environment	Home safety checklist	Physical therapist, home health nurse, social worker
Advance directive	Specific questions	Social worker
Elder abuse	Specific questions and observations	Social worker, adult protective agency

Abbreviations: ADVS, activities of daily vision scale; BMI, body mass index; BADL, basic activities of daily living; CAM, Confusion Assessment Method; IADL, instrumental or intermediate activities of daily living; AADL, advanced activities of daily living; CRA, caregiver reaction assessment; GDS, Geriatric Depression Scale; PVR, postvoid residual; DEXA, dual-energy X-ray absorptiometry.

in gasterointestinal cancers), and increased caloric consumption secondary to tumor burden. Decreased food intake can occur due to problems with mastication, alteration in taste, cancer-related anorexia, nausea/vomiting, depression, and cognitive impairment. New patients can be asked on a previsit questionnaire about weight loss within the previous six months and all patients should be weighed at every office visit. Height should also be measured on the initial visit to allow calculation of body mass index (BMI) and if possible yearly, because of changes in height due to thinning of vertebral disks with age and possible changes due to vertebral compression fractures. Healthy older adults should have a BMI between 18.5 and 25 kg/m^2 (102). An involuntary weight loss of more than 5% in one month, 7% in three months, and 10% in six months requires nutritional evaluation (103).

Energy undernutrition states include adult marasmus (energy undernutrition) and adult Kwashiorkor (protein energy undernutrition). Protein energy undernutrition is defined by the presence of clinical (physical signs such as wasting and low BMI) and biochemical (albumin or other protein) evidence of insufficient intake. The importance of low serum albumin and low cholesterol as prognostic factors for mortality in community-dwelling older persons has been demonstrated (104,105). It is probably appropriate to order these tests as baseline and screening tests for oncology patients (92), particularly those for whom chemotherapy, radiation therapy, or surgery are being considered. Additional evaluation may be needed if albumin level is below 3.5 g/L (104) and total cholesterol level is below 160 mg/dL (103). Prealbumin may also be used to monitor the effect of nutritional interventions. Prealbumin has a shorter half-life (approximately 48 hours) than albumin (approximately 18–21 days) and can reflect acute changes in the nutritional status.

Mobility and Balance Disorders/Fall Risk. As a result of other age-related diseases and the burden of their malignancy and associated treatments, older persons cared for by oncologists may be at high risk for falling and subsequent consequences (e.g., hematomas and hip fractures). Accordingly, the assessment of falls risk by assessing balance, gait, lower extremity strength, and a history about previous falls is quite valuable. A question about falls may be included on a previsit questionnaire. A positive response to the question "During the past 12 months have you fallen all the way to the ground or fallen and hit something like a chair or stair?" should prompt subsequent questions by the clinician, such as those that assess the likelihood of injurious falls (e.g., loss of consciousness, long lie of five minutes or more before arising, or frequent falls). Balance and gait disorders are best assessed by observing a patient perform tasks. The timed "Up & Go" test is a timed measure of the patient's ability to rise from an arm chair, walk 3 m (10 ft), turn, walk back, and sit down again; those who take longer than 20 seconds to complete the test merit further evaluation (93). It can be administered by office staff prior to the clinicians visit. The Performance-Oriented Assessment of Mobility instrument is a standardized instrument that measures gait and balance (106) and has been used in research and some clinical settings.

All clinicians should learn to conduct a basic evaluation of gait and balance, which requires little time and provides an excellent assessment of the patient's mobility and risk of falling. Once trained, the alert clinician can perform a gait evaluation while the patient is entering or leaving the examining room. Several tests of balance and mobility can also be performed quickly in the office and provide substantial clinical information. These include the ability to maintain a tandem or semitandem stand for 10 seconds, resistance to a sternal nudge, and observation of a 360° turn. Quadriceps strength can be briefly assessed by observing an older person arising from a hard armless chair without the use of the hands. Additional diagnostic evaluations or physical therapy referrals may be required if a problem with gait or imbalance has been identified.

Polypharmacy. Because older persons often receive care from multiple providers who may not communicate with each other and because they may fill prescriptions at several pharmacies, each patient should be told to bring all their current medications to each visit. This is particularly important when the oncologist comanages a patient with another primary care physician. Office personnel can check these against the medication list in the medical record and discrepancies can be brought to the clinician's attention at the time of the patient encounter. With the popularity of alternative medicine, there are increasing numbers of patients who are taking herbal or alternative medications (107,108). Patients often take over-the-counter medications without informing their doctors. Office staff must include alternative and over-the-counter medications in the list of medications. Several drug interaction programs are commercially available to check for potential drug–drug interactions.

Visual and Hearing Impairment. When the oncologist is the primary care physician, several other dimensions of the medical assessment need to be included. Visual impairments can lead to increased morbidity (109–111) and can affect the QOL of the elderly by restricting their activities and independence (112). Impaired vision can increase the risk of imbalance and falls. Hearing impairment can impact social function and QOL of elderly patients (94,113).

Screening for visual impairments can be done using a Snellen chart or Activities of Daily Vision Scale (ADVS) instrument (114). Office staff should be trained to test visual acuity using a Snellen eye chart, which requires the patient to stand 20 ft from the chart and read letters, using their best-corrected vision. Patients who are unable to read all the letters on the 20/40 line should be referred to an ophthalmologist or optometrist for further evaluation. ADVS is a reliable and validated instrument that can help to detect visual disabilities that could have been missed by routine screening. ADVS uses five subscales each scored from 0 (not able to perform activity due to impaired vision) to 100 (no disability). These subscales include near vision, distance vision, glare disabilities, daytime driving, and nighttime driving. ADVS has been used to assess the fall risk in elderly patients with visual impairment (95).

Several methods to screen for hearing loss are available, which can be administered by office staff or can be included on a questionnaire. The most accurate of these is the Welch Allyn Audioscope™ (Welch Allyn, Inc., Skaneateles Falls, New York, U.S.A.), a hand-held otoscope with a built-in audiometer. The audioscope can be set at several different levels of intensity, but should be set at 40 dB to evaluate hearing in older persons. A pretone at 60 dB is delivered and then four tones (500, 1000, 2000, and 4000 Hz) at 40 dB are delivered. Patients fail the screen if they are unable to hear either the 1000- or 2000-Hz frequency in both ears or both the 1000- and 2000-Hz frequencies in one ear (115).

Office staff can also administer the whispered voice test by whispering three to six random words (numbers, words, or letters) at a set distance (6, 8, 12, or 24 in.) from the person's ear and then asking the patient to repeat the words. The examiner should be behind the person to prevent speech reading and the opposite ear should be occluded during the examination. Further evaluation is indicated for those who cannot repeat 50% of the whispered words correctly (115).

Specific instruments can be used to screen for hearing impairment. A self-administered test of emotional and social problems associated with impaired hearing, the Hearing Handicap Inventory for the Elderly—Screening Version, can be included as part of a questionnaire. However, it is less accurate than the audioscope (115). The Brief Scale to Detect Hearing Loss Screener is another instrument that can be used to detect hearing loss (116). This instrument consists of seven questions. A score of 3 out of eight possible points is considered positive.

Urinary Incontinence. The impact of urinary incontinence on the patient's QOL is usually underestimated. Incidence of incontinence in the community-dwelling elderly has been reported from 15% to 30%, and it rises to 50% to 60% in a nursing home (117). Cancer or its treatment can cause or exacerbate urinary incontinence. Metastatic disease to the central nervous system may impair micturation pathways (118,119). Fluids and diuretics are commonly given with chemotherapy treatments, which can exacerbate symptoms of urinary incontinence. Impaired immune system after chemotherapy treatments makes patients more prone to urinary tract infections that can present as urinary incontinence.

Urinary incontinence is usually thought as a normal part of aging by the patients, and some patients are embarrassed to spontaneously report that they have incontinence. This problem can be uncovered by inclusion of two questions on a previsit questionnaire: (i)"In the last year, have you ever lost your urine and gotten wet?" and (ii)"Have you lost urine at least six separate days?" Answering "yes" to both questions indicates a potential problem with urinary incontinence that needs further investigation by the clinician (120).

Additional evaluations may include a postvoid residual (PVR) measurement via catheterization or ultrasound. A PVR of greater than 200 cc suggests detrusser muscle weakness or bladder outlet obstruction, and a PVR less than 100 cc indicates stress or urge incontinence.

Osteoporosis.   A common problem found among elderly women is osteoporosis. About one-third of women aged over 65 have had at least one vertebral fracture due to osteoporosis. Elderly men who have a history of hypogonadism, alcoholism, or malnutrition or those who are receiving corticosteroids for more than one month are also at increased risk for osteoporosis. Many cancer treatments can increase the risk of osteoporosis (121). Hypogonadism can occur with certain hormonal chemotherapy, or radiation treatments. The issue of osteoporosis becomes more relevant for breast cancer patients. With the increasing use of aromatase inhibitors for the treatment of breast cancer, screening for osteoporosis has become important in postmenopausal women with breast cancer (122).

Screening for osteoporosis is commonly done by measuring bone mineral density. Dual-energy X-ray absorptiometry (DEXA) is used to measure bone mineral density, which is reported as a T-score (number of standard deviations above or below the mean value in young women). According to the WHO definition of osteoporosis, patients with T-scores of less than -2.5 are diagnosed with osteoporosis (123). DEXA scan may also report the results as a less commonly used Z-score (the number of standard deviations above or below the mean value in age-matched population) (124). Patients with Z-scores less than -1.5 are considered to have osteoporosis.

Cognitive Assessment

Dementia.   Evaluation of cognitive function in elderly cancer is an important issue because it has implications in decision-making in regard to cancer treatment. Often cognitive impairment in cancer patients is unrecognized (125). Screening for cognitive impairment is necessary because cancer treatments can exacerbate the underlying cognitive dysfunction. This has been seen in patients who received postoperative adjuvant chemotherapy for breast cancer (126).

Because the prevalence of Alzheimer's disease and other dementia rises considerably with advancing age, the yield of screening for cognitive impairment will be highest in the 85 years and older age group. The most commonly used screen is the Mini-mental State Examination (66), a 30-item interviewer-administered assessment of several dimensions of cognitive function (127). Several shorter screens have also been validated, including recall of three items at one minute, the clock drawing test, and the serial sevens test (patients are asked to subtract 7 from 100 five times), as well as combinations of these tasks (128). Although normal results on these tests vastly reduce the probability of dementia and abnormal results increase the odds of dementia, these tests are neither diagnostic for dementia nor do normal results exclude the possibility of this disorder. Shortcomings include their lack of relevance to functional activities of daily life and their failure to account for educational level, languages other than English, and cultural differences.

Delirium: Delirium is an acute onset impairment of attention and cognitive changes that have a fluctuating course. Delirium can go unrecognized or be confused with dementia. In one study, the prevalence of delirium has been reported to be about 10% in elderly patients who presented to the emergency room (97). Delirium usually occurs in an inpatient setting or among patients who will require hospitalization.

Delirium can be rapidly detected by the Confusion Assessment Method (CAM), which has been widely used and validated for screening of delirium (129). CAM is an algorithmic test that evaluates four features of delirium. Feature 1 is an acute onset or fluctuating course; feature 2 is inattention; feature 3 is disorganized thinking; and feature 4 is altered level of consciousness. Diagnosis of delirium is made if there is abnormal rating in feature 1 and 2 and either 3 or 4. By definition, delirium has a physical or medical cause, especially medication, infections, and metabolic disturbances.

Affective Assessment

Affective assessment is particularly important in oncology patients because the complications of malignant diseases, particularly those that are incurable, may lead to depressive symptoms. For example, increased dependency or the anticipation of reduced life expectancy may precipitate adjustment disorders or major depression. Many symptoms of depression such as decreased appetite, weight loss, and loss of energy are similar to cancer symptoms. Thus, depression may be unrecognized by clinicians. Depressed elderly patients are at increased risk for completed suicides (98,130).

Many screening tools for depression have been developed. In 1982, Yesavage et al. developed a 30-item questionnaire to screen for depression (67). This GDS was simplified to 15 questions by Sheikh and Yesavage in 1986. A shorter version of GDS has been recently developed, which uses five questions and has accuracy comparable to the 15-item GDS (131).

Older patients can be asked about depression on a previsit questionnaire using the question "Do you often feel sad or depressed?" (99). This single question, however, tends to be overly sensitive and may be better used in tandem with a second screen such as GDS (67).

Assessment of Function

Measurement of functional status is a cardinal component of assessment of older persons. Fortunately, the importance of functional status has been recognized by oncologists for decades and has been used to provide prognostic information. It has been increasingly regarded as an important outcome measure, particularly because survival may not be prolonged in this age group. In many respects, the patient's ability to function is among the most important measures of the overall impact of diseases and disorders. From a clinical perspective, the major shift for the oncologist is not only to measure functional status for prognostic or outcome purposes but also to attempt to remediate functional impairment as part of the management plan. As such, changes in functional status may prompt further diagnostic evaluation and intervention, monitoring of response to treatment, and suggest a prognosis and plan for long-term care.

Functional status can be assessed at three levels: basic activities of daily living (BADLs) (100), instrumental or intermediate activities of daily living (IADLs) (96), and advanced activities of daily living (AADLs) (132). BADLs assess the ability of the patient to complete basic self-care tasks (e.g., bathing, dressing, toileting, continence, feeding, and transferring). IADLs measure the patient's ability to maintain an independent household (e.g., shopping for groceries, driving or using public transportation, using the telephone, meal preparation, housework, handyman work, laundry, taking medications, and handling finances). AADLs measure the patient's ability to fulfill societal, community, and family roles as well as participate in recreational or occupational tasks. These advanced activities vary considerably from individual to individual but may be exceptionally valuable in monitoring functional status prior to the development of disability.

Questions about specific BADL and IADL function can be incorporated into a previsit questionnaire. Some AADLs (e.g., exercise and leisure time physical activity) can also be ascertained in this manner, but open-ended questions about how older persons spend their days may provide a better assessment of function in healthier older persons.

The relationship of Karnofsky and ECOG performance scores to BADL and IADL has been evaluated in a number of studies. In one study, Karnofsky performance status showed strong association with both BADL and IADL. Karnofsky performance score, performing equally well or better than BADL and IADL, was also highly predictive of outcome (133). ECOG scores also show moderate correlation between BADL and IADL (134). However, BADL and IADL are more sensitive than ECOG performance status in the older cancer patients (13).

In a study of about 800 newly diagnosed elderly cancer patients, presence of functional impairments combined with insufficient social support has deleterious effect on the care of these patients (135). Early assessment and prompt interventions are important in the care of elderly cancer patients.

Social Assessment

Social Support. The older patient's family structure can be assessed by a few questions on a previsit questionnaire; however, the quality of these relationships must be assessed by the clinician during the patient encounter. Many larger oncology clinics have nurse clinicians or social workers who routinely assess for potential problems in this domain. In smaller practices, it becomes incumbent upon the physician or office staff to probe systematically into the adequacy of social support. For very frail older persons, the availability of assistance from family and friends is frequently the determining factor of whether a functionally dependent older person remains at home or is institutionalized. If dependency is noted during functional assessment, the clinician should inquire as to who provides help for specific BADL and IADL functions and whether these persons are paid or voluntary help. Even in healthier older persons, it is often valuable to raise the question of who would be available to help if the patient becomes ill; early identification of problems with social support may prompt planning to develop resources should the necessity arise.

Caregiver Burden. Providing care for elderly cancer patients at home is a challenging and sometimes an overwhelming task for the caregivers. Most elderly patients are cared for by their family members at home. One study found that family caregivers spent an average of 4.7 hours per day providing care for cancer patients at home (101). Family caregivers may provide assistance in medication, transportation for clinic visits, help with activities of daily living, and emotional support. Often family caregivers need to quit or change their jobs to accommodate these responsibilities. Worsening of functional status of the patient adds additional burden on the caregiver, and inability of caregivers to meet patient's needs can compromise patient care.

There are instruments that can screen for caregiver overburden and prompt the needed social support. Caregiver reaction assessment (CRA) is an instrument that evaluates reactions of family members caring for patients with physical impairment, Alzheimer's disease, and cancer (136). The instrument consists of 24 questions assessing five domains of caregiver reactions (disrupted schedule, financial problems, lack of family support, caregiver's health problems, and caregiver's self-esteem). CRA has been found to be a reliable and valid instrument for assessing both negative and positive reactions from caregivers of cancer patients (137).

Environmental Assessment

Environmental assessment encompasses two dimensions—the safety of the home environment and the adequacy of the patient's access to needed personal and medical services. Particularly among the frail and those with mobility and balance problems, the home environment should be assessed for safety. Although most physicians do not personally conduct environmental assessments, the National Safety Council has developed a Home Safety Checklist that patients and their families can complete. For those at high risk of recurrent falls, home health agencies can send health professionals to inspect homes for safety and can recommend installation of adaptive devices (e.g., shower bars and raised toilet seats). In addition, home health agencies can make home safety inspections.

Older persons who begin to develop IADL dependencies should be evaluated for the geographic proximity of necessary services (e.g., grocery shopping and banking), their need for use of such services, and their ability to utilize these services in their current living situations. Transportation needs may be exceptionally important among oncology patients who may need frequent medical visits for radiation therapy or injections (e.g., chemotherapy).

Advance Directives

Although important in all practices of medicine, discussions of advance directives are particularly important for oncology patients who have life-threatening tumors. When treating cancer patients in ambulatory settings, the oncologist needs to begin early on to discuss the patient's goals and preferences for care should the patient become unable to communicate because of progressive cognitive impairment or acute illness. The durable power of attorney for health care, which asks the patient to designate a surrogate to make medical decisions if the patient loses decision-making capacity, is often less emotionally laden than specifying treatments that the patient may or may not want.

Although it is often difficult to find time to discuss advance directives in detail during the initial office visit, a previsit questionnaire can determine whether the patient already has such a directive and patients can be given information to read at home in preparation for subsequent discussions.

Oncologists must also be careful not to equate these preferences for advance directives with preferences for aggressiveness of treatment of the tumor. These are separate issues and it should be made clear that discussions of advance directives should not be interpreted by patients or oncologists as "giving up on a patient."

For example, a patient may want all available treatment for a cancer yet may not want to be resuscitated should a cardiac arrest occur. As such, discussions about advance directives should not be reserved for the days when death is imminent but rather be addressed early on. These should be reassessed as more medical information becomes available and as patients may revise their thoughts about the benefits of treatment.

Elder Abuse

Elder abuse can be in the forms of physical abuse, psychological abuse, sexual abuse, neglect, or material and financial exploitation. Clinicians must be aware of the signs and symptoms of elder abuse. These signs can include unexplained anxiety and fearfulness in the presence of the caregiver, poor eye contact, hesitation to speak openly, poor hygiene, bruises, hematomas, or multiple fractures at different stages of healing.

Pain Assessment

Pain, now considered as the fifth vital sign, is a common symptom associated with cancer. Elderly patients are less likely to report pain leading to under treatment of cancer pain. Assessment of pain can be done by various methods (Table 3).

A numeric, visual, or categorical scale may be used for unidimensional pain measurement. The numeric scale, which is the most commonly used scale, rates the intensity of pain on a scale of 1 (least amount of pain) to 10 (worst pain ever). The visual analog scale incorporates a similar concept but uses a 10 cm line on which patient points the amount of pain on the scale. The categorical pain scale uses four categories to measure pain (none, mild, moderate, and severe).

To assess pain at a multidimensional level, other instruments have been used. The McGill pain questionnaire measures sensory, affective, and evaluative component of pain (138). Memorial Pain Assessment Card has been developed for rapid evaluation of cancer pain. It has three visual scales—pain intensity, pain relief, and mood (139). The Wisconsin Brief Pain Questionnaire is another instrument that has been developed for cancer patients. The questionnaire contains a human figure on which patients can mark the location of the pain, a numeric scale for pain intensity and relief, and categorical scale to measure how much pain interferes with mood, relationships, walking ability, sleep, normal work, and enjoyment of life (140).

Table 3 Symptom Assessment

Symptoms	Instruments
Pain assessment	Unidimensional: numeric, visual, or categoric pain scales
	Multidimensional
	McGill pain questionnaire (138)
	Memorial pain assessment card (139)
	Wisconsin brief pain questionnaire (140)
Insomnia	Jenkins Sleep Evaluation Questionnaire (141)
Symptoms distress	Symptoms distress scale (142)
Nausea	Morrow assessment of nausea and emesis (143)
Fatigue	Brief fatigue inventory (144), Cancer-Related Fatigue Distress Scale (145)

Symptom Distress

Elderly cancer patients can experience a number of symptoms associated with the cancer, its treatment, or other comorbid conditions. Management and palliating these symptoms are very important because they can affect the QOL significantly. An instrument for evaluating symptom distress, the Symptom Distress Scale (142), is a 13-item questionnaire that measures patients' degree of discomfort in 11 symptoms. These symptoms include nausea, loss of appetite, insomnia, pain, difficulty in breathing, cough, change in bowel movement patterns, loss of concentration, change in outlook, and change in appearance.

Insomnia

Sleep disorders are common among elderly patients. Approximately 50% of the elderly report sleeping problems, 30% of which are chronic. Many newly-diagnosed cancer patients report difficulty sleeping and at comparable rates (146). Sleep disruption can worsen cancer-related complications like fatigue or functional impairment and can affect the QOL. Although insomnia is a common symptom of depression, a new diagnosis of cancer and its treatment is often the precipitating factor for sleep disorders. Cancer pain is also a common cause of insomnia in oncology patients (147). Postchemotherapy nausea and vomiting, or treatment of these symptoms with drugs (e.g., dexamethasone or granisteron) can cause insomnia (148).

Assessment of insomnia should be done routinely. Clinicians must review sleep habits and exacerbating factors, and if a specific pathology like obstructive sleep apnea is suspected, referral for a nocturnal polysomnography must be made (149).

Special Relevance of Geriatric Assessment to the Cancer Patient

Older persons account for approximately 40% of visits to internists' offices. Although specific estimates for oncologists are not available, there is ample support for the importance of older persons in the oncologist's practice. For example, the probability that a man 60 to 79 years of age will develop an invasive cancer is one in three; for women it is one in four (150). For both genders, cancer is among the top two causes of deaths (heart disease is the other) among persons 55 years of age or older. The three leading causes of cancer death in this age group are lung, colorectal, and breast (in women) carcinomas. Moreover, this proportion of oncology practice that will focus on older persons will increase as demographic trends indicate substantial growth in the elderly population, particularly after the year 2010.

Clinicians caring for older persons must recognize the heterogeneity of the elderly population and focus the assessment and care plan accordingly. For those older patients who are younger and are in good health or have few chronic conditions, the focus is geared towards preventive geriatrics (i.e., lifestyle modifications, chemoprophylaxis, immunizations, and screening for diseases) and brief screening for potential geriatric problems. In contrast, for those above the age of 85 and those with multiple complex health and social problems, a more extensive assessment is indicated.

For the patient with advanced cancer or with whom cancer is the major health problem, the oncologist frequently becomes the primary care physician. It should be noted that the medical and functional impairments caused by many systemic cancers and their treatments precipitate typical geriatric problems. Thus, the oncologist needs to be more familiar than most specialists with the multidimensional components of the assessment of the older patient. In other cases, the care of the patient is shared with a primary care physician who may occasionally be a geriatrician. This primary care physician will likely attend to the geriatric aspects of the patient. Regardless of which role the oncologist plays for a particular patient, the oncologist's responsibilities should be delineated clearly early in the relationship.

Information obtained from assessment instruments (Table 2) can be used to quickly direct the clinician's attention to issues that are particularly relevant to an individual patient. The clinician must also be able to act on the information obtained by seeking additional diagnostic tests, by implementing therapy for problems detected, or by referring patients to appropriate professionals for additional evaluation and management.

STRATEGIES FOR COMBINING QOL AND GERIATRIC ASSESSMENT APPROACHES IN THE FUTURE

In summary, cancers are particularly common among older persons. As the population and percentage of elderly people increases, the oncologist's role in caring for older persons will assume increasing importance. Unfortunately, many of the health problems associated with aging are precipitated earlier and are amplified by malignancies and their treatment. By broadening the oncologist's assessment skills to include domains that are beyond traditional internal medicine and oncology training, the profession can better serve their older cancer patients.

Although the majority of cancer patients are over the age of 60, the elderly are not always adequately represented in clinical trials or QOL research. In particular, patients with comorbid conditions or physiologic abnormalities of aging (e.g., decreased renal function) usually are excluded from clinical treatment trials. Therefore, it may be difficult to extrapolate information obtained in clinical trials to the general elderly population. There is increasing awareness of the need for effectiveness studies (examination of what clinical practices work in the real world) to determine which treatments are best for the general community of older cancer patients. Similarly, QOL studies in older cancer patients should be conducted under these circumstances to better understand their values and estimation of QOL. These studies are particularly necessary because survival and disease-free survival may have less meaning than QOL in older patients. Observation and community-based studies of elderly cancer patients will be critical for increasing our understanding of the specific needs of this population.

From our vantage point there seems to be considerable promise in beginning to integrate some of the formal aspects of geriatric assessment into the management of the older cancer patient. In particular, oncologists could adapt some of components of geriatric assessment in their evaluation of newly-diagnosed older patients. This can provide more accurate information on the hardiness of patients who are planning to undergo treatment, as well as to identify concomitant geriatric problems that should be attended to (e.g., cognitive problems, functional limitations, social support), which would enhance the likelihood of successful cancer treatment. This approach could also be used to screen patients for eligibility for cancer treatment trials to ensure that representative numbers of older cancer patients are treated to inform clinical practice in the future. It would seem that the time is ripe for more active collaboration among oncologists and geriatricians to merge their skills and common interests in the older patient with cancer.

REFERENCES

1. Ellwood PM. Shattuck lecture—outcomes management. A technology of patient experience. N Engl J Med 1988; 318(23):1549–1556.
2. Aaronson NK, Beckmann J. The Quality of Life of Cancer Patients. New York: Raven Press, 1987.
3. McDowell I, Newell C. Measuring Health: A Guide to Rating Scales and Questionnaires. New York: Oxford University Press, 1987.
4. Osoba D. Effect of Cancer on Quality of Life. Boca Raton: CRC Press, 1991.
5. de Haes JC. Quality of Life: Conceptual and Theoretical Considerations. Psychosocial Oncology. Pergamon Press, 1988.
6. Aaronson NK. Quality of life: what is it? How should it be measured? Oncology (Huntingt) 1988; 2(5):69–76, 64.
7. Cella DF, Tulsky DS. Quality of life in cancer: definition, purpose, and method of measurement. Cancer Invest 1993; 11(3):327–336.
8. de Haes JC, van Knippenberg FC. The quality of life of cancer patients: a review of the literature. Soc Sci Med 1985; 20(8):809–817.
9. Bottomley A. The cancer patient and quality of life. Oncologist 2002; 7(2):120–125.
10. Di Maio M, Perrone F. Quality of life in elderly patients with cancer. Health Qual Life Outcomes 2003; 1(1):44.
11. Michael M, Tannock IF. Measuring health-related quality of life in clinical trials that evaluate the role of chemotherapy in cancer treatment. CMAJ 1998; 158(13):1727–1734.
12. Pais-Ribeiro JL. Quality of life is a primary end-point in clinical settings. Clin Nutr 2004; 23(1):121–130.
13. Repetto L, Comandini D, Mammoliti S. Life expectancy, comorbidity and quality of life: the treatment equation in the older cancer patients. Crit Rev Oncol Hematol 2001; 37(2):147–152.
14. Sprangers MA. Quality-of-life assessment in oncology. Achievements and challenges. Acta Oncol 2002; 41(3):229–237.
15. Mapi Research Inst. The patient-reported outcome and quality of life instruments database, 2001.
16. Pennifer E. OLGA: The On-line Guide to Quality of Life Assessment, 1988.
17. Hollandsworth JG Jr. Evaluating the impact of medical treatment on the quality of life: a 5-year update. Soc Sci Med 1988; 26(4):425–434.
18. Gotay CC, et al. Quality-of-life assessment in cancer treatment protocols: research issues in protocol development. J Natl Cancer Inst 1992; 84(8):575–579.
19. van Knippenberg FC, de Haes JC. Measuring the quality of life of cancer patients: psychometric properties of instruments. J Clin Epidemiol 1988; 41(11):1043–1053.
20. Calman KC. Quality of life in cancer patients—an hypothesis. J Med Ethics 1984; 10(3):124–127.
21. Schipper H, Clinch J. Assessment of treatment of cancer. Measuring Health: A Practical Approach. New York: Wiley & Sons, 1988.
22. Schumacher M, Olschewski M, Schulgen G. Assessment of quality of life in clinical trials. Stat Med 1991; 10(12):1915–1930.
23. Study protocol for the World Health Organization project to develop a Quality of Life assessment instrument (WHOQOL). Qual Life Res 1993; 2(2):153–159.
24. Cella DF, Cherin EA. Quality of life during and after cancer treatment. Compr Ther 1988; 14(5):69–75.
25. Leidy N, Revicki D, Geneste B. Recommendations for evaluating the validity of quality of life claims for labeling and promotions. Value Health 1999; 2:113–127.
26. Aristotle, Ethics. Harmondsworth. England: Penguin Books, 1976.
27. Andrews F, Withey S. Social Indicators of Well Being: Americans' Perception of Life Quality. New York: Plenum, 1976.
28. Campbell A. Subjective measures of well-being. Am Psychol 1976; 31(2):117–124.

29. Campbell A. The Sense of Well-being in America: Recent Patterns and Trends. New York: McGraw-Hill, 1981.

30. WHO. Constitution in Basic Documents. Geneva, 1948.

31. Ware JJ. Conceptualizing disease impact and treatment outcomes. Cancer 1984; 53(suppl):2316–2323.

32. Guyatt GH, Feeny DH, Patrick DL. Measuring health-related quality of life. Ann Intern Med 1993; 118(8):622–629.

33. Karnofsky D, Burchenal J. The clinical evaluation of chemotherapeutic agents in cancer. In: Evaluation of Chemotherapeutic Agents. New York: Columbia University Press, 1949:199–205.

34. Oken MM, et al. Toxicity and response criteria of the Eastern Cooperative Oncology Group. Am J Clin Oncol 1982; 5(6):649–655.

35. Albain KS, et al. Survival determinants in extensive-stage non-small-cell lung cancer: the Southwest Oncology Group experience. J Clin Oncol 1991; 9(9):1618–1626.

36. Sengelov L, et al. Predictive factors of response to cisplatin-based chemotherapy and the relation of response to survival in patients with metastatic urothelial cancer. Cancer Chemother Pharmacol 2000; 46(5):357–364.

37. Buccheri G, Ferrigno D, Tamburini M. Karnofsky and ECOG performance status scoring in lung cancer: a prospective, longitudinal study of 536 patients from a single institution. Eur J Cancer 1996; 32A(7):1135–1141.

38. Adams A, et al. Relative contribution of the Karnofsky Performance Status scale in a multi-measure assessment of quality of life in cancer patients. Psycho-Oncology 1995; 4:239–246.

39. Spitzer WO, et al. Measuring the quality of life of cancer patients: a concise QL-index for use by physicians. J Chronic Dis 1981; 34(12):585–597.

40. Moinpour CM, et al. Quality of life assessment in Southwest Oncology Group trials. Oncology (Huntingt) 1990; 4(5):79–84, 89; discussion 104.

41. Aaronson NK, et al. The European Organization for Research and Treatment of Cancer QLQ-C30: a quality-of-life instrument for use in international clinical trials in oncology. J Natl Cancer Inst 1993; 85(5):365–376.

42. Cella DF, et al. The Functional Assessment of Cancer Therapy scale: development and validation of the general measure. J Clin Oncol 1993; 11(3):570–579.

43. Nayfield S, Hailey B. Quality of Life Assessment in Cancer Clinical Trials. Report of the Workshop on Quality of Life Research in Clinical Trials. U.S. Dept. of Health & Human Services, Public Health Service, NIH, Bethesda, Maryland, July 16–17, 1990.

44. Schipper H, et al. Measuring the quality of life of cancer patients: the Functional Living Index-Cancer: development and validation. J Clin Oncol 1984; 2(5):472–483.

45. Slevin ML, et al. Who should measure quality of life, the doctor or the patient? Br J Cancer 1988; 57(1):109–112.

46. de Haes JC, van Knippenberg F. Quality of life instruments for cancer patients: "Babel's Tower revisited". J Clin Epidemiol 1989; 42(12):1239–1241.

47. Bernhard J, et al. Missing quality of life data in cancer clinical trials: serious problems and challenges. Stat Med 1998; 17(5–7):517–532.

48. Magaziner J. The use of proxy responders in health studies of the aged. In: The Epidemiologic Study of the Elderly. New York: Oxford University Press, 1992:120–129.

49. Ganz PA, et al. Estimating the quality of life in a clinical trial of patients with metastatic lung cancer using the Karnofsky performance status and the Functional Living Index—Cancer. Cancer 1988; 61(4):849–856.

50. Stewart A, Ware J. Measuring function and well-being. In: The Medical Outcomes Study Approach. Durham: Duke University Press, 1992.

51. Torrance GW. Measurement of health state utilities for economic appraisal. J Health Econ 1986; 5(1):1–30.

52. Fallowfield L. Quality of life: a new perspective for cancer patients. Nat Rev Cancer 2002; 2(11):873–879.

53. Gelber R, et al. The Q-TWiST method. Quality of Life and Pharmacoeconomics in Clinical Trials. Philadelphia: Lippincott-Raven, 1996:437–444.

54. Revicki DA, et al. Recommendations on health-related quality of life research to support labeling and promotional claims in the United States. Qual Life Res 2000; 9(8):887–900.

55. Dempster M, Donnelly M. How well do elderly people complete individualized quality of life measures: an explanatory study. Qual Life Res 2000; 9:369–375.

56. Bergner M, et al. The Sickness Impact Profile: development and final revision of a health status measure. Med Care 1981; 19(8):787–805.

57. Ware JE Jr, Sherbourne CD. The MOS 36–item short-form health survey (SF-36). I. Conceptual framework and item selection. Med Care 1992; 30(6):473–483.

58. Hays RD, Sherbourne CD, Mazel RM. The RAND 36–Item Health Survey 1.0. Health Econ 1993; 2(3):217–227.

59. Hunt SM, et al. The Nottingham Health Profile: subjective health status and medical consultations. Soc Sci Med A 1981; 15(3 Pt 1):221–229.

60. Morrow GR, Chiarello RJ, Derogatis LR. A new scale for assessing patients' psychosocial adjustment to medical illness. Psychol Med 1978; 8(4):605–610.

61. Nelson E, et al. Assessment of function in routine clinical practice: description of the COOP Chart method and preliminary findings. J Chronic Dis 1987; 40(suppl 1): 55S–69S.

62. Padilla GV, et al. Quality of life index for patients with cancer. Res Nurs Health 1983; 6(3):117–126.

63. Schag CA, Heinrich RL. Development of a comprehensive quality of life measurement tool: CARES. Oncology (Huntingt) 1990; 4(5):135–138; discussion 147.

64. Levine MN, et al. Quality of life in stage II breast cancer: an instrument for clinical trials. J Clin Oncol 1988; 6(12):1798–1810.

65. Selby PJ, et al. The development of a method for assessing the quality of life of cancer patients. Br J Cancer 1984; 50(1):13–22.

66. Folstein MF, Folstein SE, McHugh PR. "Mini-mental state". A practical method for grading the cognitive state of patients for the clinician. J Psychiatr Res 1975; 12(3): 189–198.

67. Yesavage JA, et al. Development and validation of a geriatric depression screening scale: a preliminary report. J Psychiatr Res 1982; 17(1):37–49.

68. Parkerson GR Jr, Broadhead WE, Tse CK. The Duke Health Profile. A 17-item measure of health and dysfunction. Med Care 1990; 28(11):1056–1072.

69. Cassileth BR, et al. Psychosocial status in chronic illness. A comparative analysis of six diagnostic groups. N Engl J Med 1984; 311(8):506–511.

70. Litwin MS, et al. Quality-of-life outcomes in men treated for localized prostate cancer. JAMA 1995; 273(2):129–135.

71. Ganz PA, et al. Breast cancer survivors: psychosocial concerns and quality of life. Breast Cancer Res Treat 1996; 38(2):183–199.

72. Cella DF, Bonomi AE. Measuring quality of life: 1995 update. Oncology (Huntingt) 1995; 9(suppl 11):47–60.

73. Guillemin F, Bombardier C, Beaton D. Cross-cultural adaptation of health-related quality of life measures: literature review and proposed guidelines. J Clin Epidemiol 1993; 46(12):1417–1432.

74. Beaton DE, et al. Guidelines for the process of cross-cultural adaptation of self-report measures. Spine 2000; 25(24):3186–3191.

75. Silliman RA, et al. Breast cancer care in old age: what we know, don't know, and do. J Natl Cancer Inst 1993; 85(3):190–199.

76. Goodwin JS, Hunt WC, Samet JM. Determinants of cancer therapy in elderly patients. Cancer 1993; 72(2):594–601.

77. Kiebert GM, de Haes JC, van de Velde CJ. The impact of breast-conserving treatment and mastectomy on the quality of life of early-stage breast cancer patients: a review. J Clin Oncol 1991; 9(6):1059–1070.

78. Ganz PA, et al. Breast conservation versus mastectomy. Is there a difference in psychological adjustment or quality of life in the year after surgery? Cancer 1992; 69(7): 1729–1738.

79. Coates A, et al. Improving the quality of life during chemotherapy for advanced breast cancer. A comparison of intermittent and continuous treatment strategies. N Engl J Med 1987; 317(24):1490–1495.

80. A controlled trial to improve care for seriously ill hospitalized patients. The study to understand prognoses and preferences for outcomes and risks of treatments (SUPPORT). The SUPPORT Principal Investigators. JAMA 1995; 274(20):1591–1598.

81. Kahn SB, Houts PS, Harding SP. Quality of life and patients with cancer: a comparative study of patient versus physician perceptions and its implications for cancer education. J Cancer Educ 1992; 7(3):241–249.

82. Nerenz DR, et al. Psychosocial consequences of cancer chemotherapy for elderly patients. Health Serv Res 1986; 20(6 Pt 2):961–976.

83. Hillier R. Control of pain in terminal cancer. Br Med Bull 1990; 46(1):279–291.

84. Stein WM, Miech RP. Cancer pain in the elderly hospice patient. J Pain Symptom Manage 1993; 8(7):474–882.

85. Portenoy RK. Pain management in the older cancer patient. Oncology (Huntingt) 1992; 6(suppl 2):86–98.

86. Ferrell BR, et al. Pain management for elderly patients with cancer at home. Cancer 1994; 74(suppl 7):2139–2146.

87. Mor V, et al. Determinants of need and unmet need among cancer patients residing at home. Health Serv Res 1992; 27(3):337–360.

88. Soloman D. In: Osterweil D, Brummel-Smith K, Beck J, eds. Comprehensive Geriatric Assessment. New York: Mc-Graw Hill, 2000.

89. Williams TF, et al. Appropriate placement of the chronically ill and aged. A successful approach by evaluation. JAMA 1973; 226(11):1332–1335.

90. Rubenstein LZ, et al. Effectiveness of a geriatric evaluation unit. A randomized clinical trial. N Engl J Med 1984; 311(26):1664–1670.

91. NIHCS: National Institute of Health Consensus Statement. Geriatric Assessment Methods for Clinical Decision Making, 1987:1–21.

92. Reuben DB, Greendale GA, Harrison GG. Nutrition screening in older persons. J Am Geriatr Soc 1995; 43(4):415–425.

93. Podsiadlo D, Richardson S. The timed "Up & Go": a test of basic functional mobility for frail elderly persons. J Am Geriatr Soc 1991; 39(2):142–148.

94. Mulrow CD, et al. Quality-of-life changes and hearing impairment. A randomized trial. Ann Intern Med 1990; 113(3):188–194.

95. Kamel HK, Guro-Razuman S, Shareeff M. The activities of daily vision scale: a useful tool to assess fall risk in older adults with vision impairment. J Am Geriatr Soc 2000; 48(11):1474–1477.

96. Lawton MP, Brody EM. Assessment of older people: self-maintaining and instrumental activities of daily living. Gerontologist 1969; 9(3):179–186.

97. Lewis LM, et al. Unrecognized delirium in ED geriatric patients. Am J Emerg Med 1995; 13(2):142–145.

98. Zubenko GS, et al. Mortality of elderly patients with psychiatric disorders. Am J Psychiatr 1997; 154(10):1360–1368.

99. Lachs MS, et al. A simple procedure for general screening for functional disability in elderly patients. Ann Intern Med 1990; 112(9):699–706.

100. Katz S, et al. Studies of illness in the aged. The index of Adl: a standardized measure of biological and psychosocial function. JAMA 1963; 185:914–919.

101. Stommel M, Given CW, Given BA. The cost of cancer home care to families. Cancer 1993; 71(5):1867–1874.

102. NIH. Clinical guidelines on the identification, evaluation, and treatment of overweight and obesity in adults, 1998.

103. Tchekmedyian NS, et al. Assessment and maintenance of nutrition in older cancer patients. Oncology (Huntingt) 1992; 6(suppl 2):105–111.
104. Corti MC, et al. Serum albumin level and physical disability as predictors of mortality in older persons. JAMA 1994; 272(13):1036–1042.
105. Noel MA, Smith TK, Ettinger WH. Characteristics and outcomes of hospitalized older patients who develop hypocholesterolemia. J Am Geriatr Soc 1991; 39(5):455–461.
106. Tinetti ME. Performance-oriented assessment of mobility problems in elderly patients. J Am Geriatr Soc 1986; 34(2):119–126.
107. Eisenberg DM, et al. Trends in alternative medicine use in the United States, 1990–1997: results of a follow-up national survey. JAMA 1998; 280(18):1569–1575.
108. Tindle HA, et al. Trends in use of complementary and alternative medicine by US adults: 1997–2002. Altern Ther Health Med 2005; 11(1):42–49.
109. Lord SR, Dayhew J. Visual risk factors for falls in older people. J Am Geriatr Soc 2001; 49(5):508–515.
110. Nevitt MC, et al. Risk factors for recurrent nonsyncopal falls. A prospective study. JAMA 1989; 261(18):2663–2668.
111. Rovner BW, Zisselman PM, Shmuely-Dulitzki Y. Depression and disability in older people with impaired vision: a follow-up study. J Am Geriatr Soc 1996; 44(2):181–184.
112. Rubin GS, et al. Visual impairment and disability in older adults. Optom Vis Sci 1994; 71(12):750–760.
113. Weinstein BE, Ventry IM. Hearing impairment and social isolation in the elderly. J Speech Hear Res 1982; 25(4):593–599.
114. Mangione CM, et al. Development of the "Activities of Daily Vision Scale". A measure of visual functional status. Med Care 1992; 30(12):1111–1126.
115. Mulrow CD, Lichtenstein MJ. Screening for hearing impairment in the elderly: rationale and strategy. J Gen Intern Med 1991; 6(3):249–258.
116. Reuben DB, et al. Hearing loss in community-dwelling older persons: national prevalence data and identification using simple questions. J Am Geriatr Soc 1998; 46(8):1008–1011.
117. Fultz NH, Herzog AR. Epidemiology of urinary symptoms in the geriatric population. Urol Clin North Am 1996; 23(1):1–10.
118. Ehrlich RM, Walsh GO. Urinary incontinence secondary to brain neoplasm. Urology 1973; 1(3):249–250.
119. Voigt JC, Kenefick JS. Sacrococcygeal chordoma presenting with stress incontinence of urine. S Afr Med J 1971; 45(20):557.
120. Diokno AC, et al. Clinical and cystometric characteristics of continent and incontinent noninstitutionalized elderly. J Urol 1988; 140(3):567–571.
121. Pfeilschifter J, Diel IJ. Osteoporosis due to cancer treatment: pathogenesis and management. J Clin Oncol 2000; 18(7):1570–1593.
122. Mackey JR, Joy AA. Skeletal health in postmenopausal survivors of early breast cancer. Int J Cancer 2005.
123. Kanis JA. Diagnosis of osteoporosis and assessment of fracture risk. Lancet 2002; 359(9321):1929–1936.
124. Genant HK, et al. Noninvasive assessment of bone mineral and structure: state of the art. J Bone Miner Res 1996; 11(6):707–730.
125. Davis BD, et al. Diagnosis of dementia in cancer patients. Cognitive impairment in these patients can go unrecognized. Psychosomatics 1987; 28(4):175–179.
126. Schagen SB, et al. Cognitive deficits after postoperative adjuvant chemotherapy for breast carcinoma. Cancer 1999; 85(3):640–650.
127. Tombaugh TN, McIntyre NJ. The mini-mental state examination: a comprehensive review. J Am Geriatr Soc 1992; 40(9):922–935.
128. Siu AL. Screening for dementia and investigating its causes. Ann Intern Med 1991; 115(2):122–132.

129. Inouye SK, et al. Clarifying confusion: the confusion assessment method. A new method for detection of delirium. Ann Intern Med 1990; 113(12):941–948.

130. Lebowitz BD, et al. Diagnosis and treatment of depression in late life. Consensus statement update. JAMA 1997; 278(14):1186–1190.

131. Hoyl MT, et al. Development and testing of a five-item version of the Geriatric Depression Scale. J Am Geriatr Soc 1999; 47(7):873–878.

132. Reuben D, Wieland D, Rubenstein L. Functional status assessment of older persons: concepts and implications. Facts Res Gerontol 1993; 7:231–240.

133. Crooks V, et al. The use of the Karnofsky performance scale in determining outcomes and risk in geriatric outpatients. J Gerontol 1991; 46(4):M139–M144.

134. Extermann M, et al. Comorbidity and functional status are independent in older cancer patients. J Clin Oncol 1998; 16(4):1582–1587.

135. Goodwin JS, Hunt WC, Samet JM. A population-based study of functional status and social support networks of elderly patients newly diagnosed with cancer. Arch Intern Med 1991; 151(2):366–370.

136. Given CW, et al. The caregiver reaction assessment (CRA) for caregivers to persons with chronic physical and mental impairments. Res Nurs Health 1992; 15(4):271–283.

137. Nijboer C, et al. Measuring both negative and positive reactions to giving care to cancer patients: psychometric qualities of the Caregiver Reaction Assessment (CRA). Soc Sci Med 1999; 48(9):1259–1269.

138. Melzack R. The McGill Pain Questionnaire: major properties and scoring methods. Pain 1975; 1(3):277–299.

139. Fishman B, et al. The Memorial Pain Assessment Card. A valid instrument for the evaluation of cancer pain. Cancer 1987; 60(5):1151–1158.

140. Daut RL, Cleeland CS, Flanery RC. Development of the Wisconsin Brief Pain Questionnaire to assess pain in cancer and other diseases. Pain 1983; 17(2):197–210.

141. Jenkins CD, et al. A scale for the estimation of sleep problems in clinical research. J Clin Epidemiol 1988; 41(4):313–321.

142. McCorkle R, Young K. Development of a symptom distress scale. Cancer Nurs 1978; 1(5):373–378.

143. Morrow GR. A patient report measure for the quantification of chemotherapy induced nausea and emesis: psychometric properties of the Morrow assessment of nausea and emesis (MANE). Br J Cancer Suppl 1992; 19:S72–S74.

144. Mendoza TR, et al. The rapid assessment of fatigue severity in cancer patients: use of the Brief Fatigue Inventory. Cancer 1999; 85(5):1186–1196.

145. Holley SK. Evaluating patient distress from cancer-related fatigue: an instrument development study. Oncol Nurs Forum 2000; 7(9):1425–1431.

146. Savard J, Morin CM. Insomnia in the context of cancer: a review of a neglected problem. J Clin Oncol 2001; 19(3):895–908.

147. Dorrepaal KL, Aaronson NK, van Dam FS. Pain experience and pain management among hospitalized cancer patients. A clinical study. Cancer 1989; 63(3):593–598.

148. Osoba D, et al. Effect of postchemotherapy nausea and vomiting on health-related quality of life. The Quality of Life and Symptom Control Committees of the National Cancer Institute of Canada Clinical Trials Group. Support Care Cancer 1997; 5(4):307–313.

149. Sateia MJ, et al. Evaluation of chronic insomnia. An American Academy of Sleep Medicine review. Sleep 2000; 23(2):243–308.

150. Parker SL, et al. Cancer statistics 1997. CA Cancer J Clin 1997; 47(1):5–27.

21

Opportunities and Challenges for Appropriate Nutrition of the Elderly Cancer Patient

Susan S. Percival
Department of Food Science and Human Nutrition, University of Florida, Gainesville, Florida, U.S.A.

Karen A. Johnson
Breast and Gynecologic Cancer Research Group, Division of Cancer Prevention, National Cancer Institute, Bethesda, Maryland, U.S.A.

John A. Milner
Nutritional Science Research Group, Division of Cancer Prevention, National Cancer Institute, National Institutes of Health, Rockville, Maryland, U.S.A.

INTRODUCTION

Appropriate nutrition is fundamental to the health and functioning of elderly individuals. Unfortunately, the elderly are particularly susceptible to inappropriate nutrition, independent of whether or not they are hospitalized. Depletion of nutritional reserves and significant weight loss can precipitate an increased risk of morbidity, reduced chemotherapy response, and shorter survival in patients with cancer.

The negative consequences of malnutrition in the elderly necessitate that health care professionals and providers be particularly vigilant in promoting nutritional health, particularly in cancer patients. Physiological, psychological, and economic changes in the later years can be particularly challenging to the elderly cancer patient and may require multifaceted interventions to overcome the factors contributing to suboptimal nutrient intakes (1). The magnitude of the problem is illustrated by recent findings from Spain where 52% of 781 patients with various types of cancer were malnourished at a moderate or severe level, and over 90% required nutritional intervention or counseling (2).

A deterioration in the nutritional status can markedly influence a patient's quality of life (QOL) and psychosocial well-being (3,4). Likewise, impairment in the nutritional status can increase the risk of infection and promote sepsis (5), change the phenotypic expression of neoplasms (6), and increase mortality risk (7,8). It is becoming increasingly apparent that one's nutritional status can be compromised as a result of tumor-induced changes in metabolism. Enhanced metabolism of fats, proteins, and carbohydrates is relatively common in cancer patients. These perturbations in bioenergetics may ultimately manifest as cachexia, which is characterized by involuntary weight loss, muscle wasting, and reduced QOL. Extreme weight loss related to the presence of a tumor is frequently observed in end-stage cancer where the tumor burden is high. Cachexia is most often observed in patients with lung, pancreatic, and upper gastrointestinal tract cancers, and somewhat less frequently observed in patients with breast cancer or lower gastrointestinal cancer. Multiple factors may mediate a change in metabolism in the cancer patient, including cytokines, neuropeptides, neurotransmitters, and tumor-derived factors. Substances arising from host tissue, which may partially account for the catabolic state, include tumor necrosis factor-α, interleukin-1, interleukin-6, and interferon-γ. Likewise, tumor products with direct catabolic effects such as lipid-mobilizing factor and proteolysis-inducing factor may influence the degree of cachexia. Although anorexia is relatively widespread in cancer patients, several studies provide evidence that the wasting phenomenon is not simply corrected by increased caloric intake, which is unlikely to reverse the overall catabolic state. Consequently, this chapter will emphasize opportunities for nutritional management early in the disease process, for which evidence indicates the potential for clinical benefit.

NUTRITIONAL ASSESSMENT AT DIAGNOSIS

Risk factors for inadequate nutritional intake associated with malnutrition include diagnostic category, functional disabilities, inadequate or inappropriate food intake, poor dentition or difficulty swallowing, polypharmacy, alcoholism, depression, and a poor socioeconomic status. Patients with any of these risk factors need to be identified, and nutritional screening should be a routine part of their medical care. No single measurement exists for monitoring the nutritional status of an individual. Thus, an assessment must build upon a comprehensive evaluation, including for example, anthropometric and biochemical evaluations (Table 1). Nutritional screening should be the first step in developing a nutritional care program that can be targeted to the specific individual (9,10). New screening tools that can be verified for the assessment of muscle weakness (11), immune system status (12), and alterations that may occur in the structure and function of the gastrointestinal system are needed (13).

Poor nutritional status is considered a contributor to death in as many as 80% of cancer patients (14). Assessment tools are aimed at identifying those who need nutritional care, and developing planned intervention strategies. Successful assessment, however, requires standardization of definitions, validated assessment tools, clear criteria for nutritional intervention, and appropriate end points for outcomes—a feat that has not yet been achieved in cancer management (15,16).

Given the multiplicity of types of nutritional data and assessment methods, many approaches are possible. It is most appropriate to select one that systematically organizes nutritional information along four lines; for example, (i) nutritional history, (ii) physical examination and anthropometric data, (iii) comprehensive clinical assessment profiles, and (iv) biochemical tests. Starting with the nutritional history, at the time the elderly oncology patient is interviewed, information should be collected about the patient's appetite, dietary intake including content and pattern; bowel activity, and symptoms related to digestion as well as food aversions, intolerance, and allergies. Other parts of the medical history that have a bearing on

Table 1 Assessing Nutritional Status at the Time of Diagnosis

Anthropometrics	Height, weight, arm and calf circumference	Can be used with minimal training
Biochemical measurements	Blood, plasma, serum, and urine	Requires trained technical assistance
MNA	18 items on anthropometry, geriatric assessment, dietary intakes, and self-assessment of health	Can be used with minimal training
NRI	Serum albumin and recent weight loss	Requires blood draw
SGA and Scored PG-SGA	16 items on weight changes, dietary changes, and GI symptoms, functional capacity, medical status, and physical assessment	Requires trained health care provider

Abbreviations: MNA, Mini-Nutrition Assessment; NRI, Nutritional Risk Assessment; PG-SGA, Patient Generated–Subjective Global Assessment; SGA, Subjective Global Assessment.

nutritional status include items such as activity level, smoking history, and medications. As part of the standard physical examination, height and weight are usually measured; and to these, skinfold thickness and waist and hip diameters may be added. From physical measurements like height and weight, anthropometric parameters such as body mass index (BMI) can be calculated, or specialized anthropometric measures such as body fat versus muscle content can be determined using impedance measurements. Anthropometric measurements quantify the body compartments and are compared with values from age- and sex-matched normal populations to estimate body muscle and fat mass. For this discussion, BMI will serve as the primary example of anthropometric assessment.

Instead of relying only on a medical history and physical examination, which is not standardized with regard to nutritional information, investigators have sought to develop overarching tools that rely on a limited number of data points for a comprehensive indication of the nutritional status (15). Examples of nutritional tools that profile patients and offer some standardized and reliable results include the Subjective Global Assessment (SGA), the Nutritional Risk Index (NRI), and the Mini-Nutrition Assessment (MNA). These tools will be described in more detail below. For the future, we are hopeful that biochemical markers from the serum, urine, or tissues may offer a simplified approach to nutritional assessment, guiding the clinician to beneficial interventions that enhance nutritional status. At present, there are only a few nutritional markers with test characteristics that suggest potential for broad clinical application and these will be described in greater detail.

Dietary Data and Food Intake

Undeniably, inadequate nutrition exists in the United States, and its prevalence is significantly associated with the income status of the elderly. Decreased food intake, a sedentary lifestyle, and reduced energy expenditure in older adults are significant risk contributors to malnutrition, especially for protein and micronutrients, and may further contribute to the decline of bodily functions and the development of chronic age-associated degenerative diseases. A recent survey of 40,000 subjects in the 88 U.S. communities included in the third National Health and Nutrition Examination Survey (NHANES) included input from about 5000 elderly participants grouped from 60 to 69 years, 70 to 79 years, and 80+ years (17). Generally, the median daily intake of total energy in elderly subjects was lower than the recommended 2300 kilocalories (kcal) for men and 1900 kcal for women. However, the contribution of caloric intake from fat in the elderly was higher than the 30% typically recommended. The survey also discovered that increasing age was associated with increased consumption of folate and vitamin B_{12}. However, elderly respondents to the NHANES survey appeared not to be consuming sufficient calcium, which contributes to the increased risk of osteoporosis and bone fracture observed in this population.

Appetite loss, or anorexia, is a frequent contributor to nutritional deterioration in end-stage cancer patients, and results from several intricately linked physiopathological mechanisms. Psychological factors such as depression can also precipitate changes in eating behavior. Several investigations have suggested that about 50% of cancer patients have some degree of altered taste and smell including an alteration in the perception of sweetness in about one-third of the patients (18,19). Changes in the perception of bitterness (which has been linked to meat aversion), sourness, and saltiness occur less frequently. These kinds of change in taste have been correlated with decreased nutrient intake, and poor prognosis (20).

Evaluation of food intake is complicated not only by changes in eating behaviors among elderly cancer patients, but also with the rather widespread use of dietary supplements. Increased use of dietary supplements is correlated with more health conscious strategies among the elderly (21). Table 2 reflects the current dietary reference intake values for the elderly (22). The Consumer Health Products Association (http://www.chpa-info.org/Web/index.aspx) suggests that ailments such as arthritis, insomnia, and constipation, which become more prevalent with advancing age, are responsible for the increased use of dietary supplements among elderly persons.

Anthropometric Assessment

Of the anthropometric measures related to nutritional status, BMI is a highly convenient indicator of adiposity. Because height is fairly stable and weight is routinely measured in oncology practice, oncologists usually have the means for assessing weight change in their patients. Although it would be possible to follow weight alone, BMI is preferable because it adjusts weight according to height and allows interpretation in the context of medical literature for patient subsets and circumstances of known clinical relevance. The BMI is calculated as the weight of the patient in kilograms divided by the square of the patient's height in meters. Consequently, for a woman who weighs 150 pounds and measures 5 ft 6 in. in height, the calculated value of BMI would be close to 24. Similarly for a 175-pound man with a height of 5 ft 11 in., the BMI calculation gives a result just over 24, near the top of the normal range. A BMI from 18.5 to 24.9 is considered normal (23). By this convention, an underweight status is assigned to individuals with a BMI less than 18.5. Although a BMI between 25 and 30 corresponds to being overweight, frank obesity is defined as having a BMI of 30 or more.

Although an individual can be classified and monitored for change, it is hard to infer clinical significance to BMI measurements without reference to large study populations of subjects who are like the patient of interest. Nevertheless, a few

Table 2 DRI for Adults 50 to 70 Years Old and > 70 Years Old

	DRI (per day)	Recommendation for elderly cancer patient (per day)	Notes
Energy	25–30 kcal/kg	30–35 kcal/kg	
Protein	1.0 g/kg	1.5 g/kg	
Carbohydrate			
Fat			No specifications for the elderly: 30% of calories from fat and 10% from saturated fat
Fiber	21–39 g		Decreased from recommendations for younger adults
Fluid	30 mL/kg	More may be required in case of fever, infections, or use of medications such as diuretics or laxatives	Volume requirements decrease with age
Calcium	1200 mg	Increase frequency of calcium intake to offset reduction in absorption	200 mg increase over recommendations for younger adults
Vitamin D	50–70 yr 10 μg > 70 yr 15 μg	To be taken with calcium	5 μg increase from recommendations for younger adults
Phosphorus	700 mg		NC
Sodium	50–70 yr 1.3 mg > 70 yr 1.2 mg		Decreased from recommendations for younger adults (1.5 mg)
Magnesium	320–420 mg[a]		NC
Manganese	1.8–2.3 mg		NC
Fluoride	3–4 mg		NC
Thiamin	1.1–1.2 mg	Increase to meet increased caloric intake	NC
Riboflavin	1.1–1.3 mg		NC
Niacin	14–16 mg		NC
Vitamin B_6	1.5–1.6 mg	Increase to meet increased protein requirements	Increased from recommendations for younger adults
Folate	400 μg		NC
Vitamin B_{12}	2.4 μg		NC
Pantothenic acid	5 mg		NC
Biotin	30 μg		NC
Choline	425–550 mg		NC
Vitamin C	75–90 mg		NC
α Tocopherol	15 mg		NC
Selenium	55 μg	Increase	NC
Vitamin K	90–120 μg		NC
Zinc	8–11 mg	Increase	
Iron	8–18 mg		Postmenopausal women 8 mg /day
Iodine	150 μg		NC
Vitamin A	700–900 μg		NC

Recommendations for the elderly cancer patient.
NC: Did not change from recommendations made for younger adults.
[a]The two numbers reflect requirements for women and men, respectively.
Abbreviation: DRI, dietary reference intake.
Source: From Ref. 22.

generalizations can be made. The relationship between mortality and weight follows a U- or a J-shaped curve with the observation of increased mortality for individuals of low BMI as well as high BMI in comparison with individuals of normal BMI (24). An association between mortality and low BMI may be of particular relevance to elderly patients as exemplified by findings from NHANES I, where men aged 65 and older experienced a 24% increase in mortality for a BMI less than 22 compared with men aged 45 to 54 years, in whom there was no excess mortality for low BMI (25). On the other hand, summary data from a meta-analysis of studies that included individuals aged 65 and above, suggested that the detrimental mortality effect of obesity is relaxed for elderly individuals. When overweight BMI was compared with BMI in the low range (22.5–24.9), the relative risk of mortality for older adults was 0.97 compared with a relative risk of 1.24 for the general population (26). And finally, another consideration in interpreting BMI data involves smoking history. It appears that BMI data is most reliable for nonsmokers and for cancers that are not smoking related. For example, in one study of survival after breast cancer, an association of increased mortality with increased BMI at diagnosis was seen only in nonsmokers (27). In another study, the association of BMI with mortality was complicated by competing effects in individuals with smoking-related cancers (i.e., mortality trend as a function of BMI vs. the opposing effect of smoking on BMI and cancer) (28). The authors indicated their belief that BMI data is most useful when it comes from studies of individuals who have never smoked.

Comprehensive Nutritional Profile Assessment

Screening is the initial step in delivering appropriate nutritional therapy. There is no single best parameter for screening. While some may consider a full nutritional assessment to be time and resource consuming relative to other procedures, it is not. Far too often, nutritional needs in the elderly go unrecognized because of the belief that the time and cost of nutritional assessment are excessive. A useful guide to nutritional assessment has been developed by the American Dietetic Association (29).

The SGA is one of the most frequently used tools for nutritional assessment. It is performed by a trained independent health care provider using a standard form including questions about food intake and symptoms such as vomiting, diarrhea, and loss of weight. Responses to these questions generate a score that is used to classify patients into one of three categories of nutritional status: A: well nourished, B: moderately malnourished, or C: severely malnourished (30). The SGA defines nutritional and functional status of patients with the aim of identifying those who could benefit from a nutritional intervention (31). In several studies, the SGA was not sensitive for detecting the beginning stages of malnutrition. Nevertheless, Raguso et al. (32) reported that its specificity and predictive validity were demonstrable in several clinical situations associated with malnutrition including kidney disease, AIDS, and cancer.

The Patient Generated-SGA (scored PG-SGA) questionnaire (PG-SGA) is an adaptation of the validated SGA (30). The PG-SGA has specifically been used in a cancer population (33), and easily allows for a quick identification and prioritization of malnutrition issues in less than 30 minutes (34). The PG-SGA score has been found to correlate with a variety of objective parameters including BMI, handgrip strength, and mortality (35,36). Isenring et al. (37) reported a linear trend for change in PG-SGA score between those patients whose nutritional status improved (5%), remained stable (56.7%), or deteriorated (33.3%). A similar trend was observed for the global QOL. Overall, their study revealed that the scored PG-SGA is a viable nutrition assessment tool that helps identify poor nutritional status and predict changes in the QOL of ambulatory oncology patients receiving radiotherapy.

NRI is a simple equation that uses serum albumin and recent weight loss. NRI = (1.489 × serum albumin, g/L) + 41.7 × (present weight/usual weight) to define nutritional status. Typically, an NRI > 100 indicates that the patient is adequately nourished; 97.5 to 100 indicates mild malnourishment, 83.5 to less than 97.5 indicates moderate malnourishment and less than 83.5 indicates severe malnourishment (38).

The MNA is another tool that has been used to evaluate the frail elderly patient and complement other screening tools, such as the SGA (39). The MNA collects 18 objective and subjective items including simple anthropometric measures, general geriatric assessment items, a brief dietary assessment, and a self-assessment of the perception of nutritional health. With no biochemical assessment included, the MNA can be completed in about 20 minutes and does not require extensive training.

Biochemical Assessment

Serum albumin has long been used as a biochemical assessment of nutritional status. Levels less than 3.5 g/dL are indicative of malnutrition. Albumin concentration is recognized as a nonspecific but sensitive measure of disease presence and severity. A number of health-related conditions such as protein/calorie deprivation, renal disease, and other chronic or subclinical diseases characterized by inflammatory processes are associated with a reduction in serum albumin. In cancer patients, albumin concentrations below 3.0 g/dL have been proposed to be an unfavorable indicator of extensive dissemination of the tumor process (40). While albumin-binding capacity for such compounds as bilirubin has also been employed to diagnose poor nutrition early, its utility for cancer patients has not been well characterized.

Compared with albumin, measurement of prealbumin concentration may be a more sensitive and cost-effective method of assessing the severity of malnutrition in patients who have cancer (41,42). In the study of cancer patients by Guo et al. (42), half had prealbumin concentrations that were below normal, and a comparable percentage had symptoms of weight loss or anorexia. Given the low cost and ease of testing, the use of serum prealbumin concentration deserves consideration as a routine screening test to identify cancer patients with early-stage malnutrition.

Given the current limitations of albumin and its precursors, an earlier, more sensitive index of malnutrition is needed. Candidate biomarkers include insulin-like growth factor (IGF) (43,44), antioxidant status, or a combination of these. In healthy individuals, the serum concentration of IGF family members is associated with QOL. Meyerhardt et al. (4) studied colorectal cancer (CRC) patients to see if IGF proteins were associated with QOL in this setting. Lower levels of both IGF-I and IGF-II were associated with decreased QOL as reflected by individual factors like fatigue as well as a composite of factors defined by a Symptom Distress Scale score. Levels of IGF binding protein-3 were not associated with baseline QOL. These results from this study suggest that molecular biomarkers may eventually find a use in the prediction of QOL.

Free radicals and oxidative stress are recognized as having important consequences to aging and several age-related degenerative diseases. The free-radical theory of aging postulates a time-dependent shift in the antioxidant/prooxidant balance with increases in the generation of free radicals, an increase in oxidative stress, and associated dysregulation of cellular function. Dietary factors that alter this balance could alter the rates of aging and the development of age-associated diseases.

After further development, tests that measure free-radical damage or antioxidant status may give clearer diagnostic and predictive tools for cancer or even premalignant conditions. DNA damage assayed by the comet assay detects not only smoking-related exposures, but also dietary modifications (45). Lycopene supplementation, an antioxidant from tomatoes, was associated with a lowering of prostate-specific antigen in patients diagnosed with prostate adenocarcinoma, although this change did not reach statistical significance (46). In addition to lycopene, antioxidants including flavonoids, allyl sulfur, vitamin E, and vitamin C are under investigation at the U.S. National Cancer Institute for their role in cancer management. Current research can be found by searching the Human Nutrition Research Information Management system (http://hnrim.nih.gov). Biochemical markers to assess nutritional status or the impact of nutrition on cancer are needed.

NUTRITIONAL AND PHYSIOLOGICAL ISSUES IN THE ELDERLY CANCER PATIENT

Half of all new cancer cases occur in individuals over the age of 65. Weight loss and malnutrition are common in cancer patients. Some elderly patients may start at diagnosis with a nutritional disadvantage. Severe weight loss may be due to malignancy, while in some patients it may be due to inadequate dietary habits, chronic illness, or a poor socioeconomic environment.

Overnutrition

A report by Notarnicola et al. (6) has associated the development of distant metastases with elevated levels of serum lipids in CRC patients. In patients with metastases, total cholesterol (TC), low-density lipoprotein cholesterol (LDL-C), and the LDL-C/high-density lipoprotein cholesterol (HDL-C) ratio were all found to be significantly higher ($P < 0.05$) compared with the CRC patients who did not have distant metastases. These measures were independent of sex, age, and BMI. The serum lipid profile including TC, LDL-C and the LDL-C/HDL-C ratio was also predictive of QOL of CRC patients with vs. without synchronous distant metastases. It would be of interest to obtain similar data for other diagnoses.

Breast cancer is the diagnosis for which overnutrition has been most studied. Numerous observational studies are consistent with the premise that increased weight at the time of breast cancer diagnosis is a negative prognostic factor. For example, in one comprehensive review of trials from 1990 to 2001, there were 34 selected articles examining the relationship between increased body weight or BMI and outcomes such as recurrence risk or survival for women with resectable breast cancer (47). A good majority of those articles (26 out of 34) reported statistically significant results that indicated a shorter interval to breast cancer recurrence and/or reduced overall survival for the women who were overweight. Differences in study methodology did not allow for a consistent definition of mortality risk based on a single weight-related parameter. Another limitation of these studies was the absence of age-specific information.

Since the overview article of 2002 by Chlebowski et al. (47), several more recent studies have clarified aspects of the relationship between BMI and breast cancer survival. Dignam et al. (48) have provided an instructive analysis of the impact of obesity and tamoxifen use on outcomes for women with estrogen receptor (ER)-positive, early-stage breast cancer. This analysis relied on data for 3385 women participating in treatment studies conducted by the National Surgical Adjuvant Breast and Bowel

Project and has particular relevance for early-stage breast cancer patients using tamoxifen. Obesity was not associated with tamoxifen effectiveness, breast cancer recurrence, or with breast cancer mortality. However, mortality from causes other than breast cancer was increased for obese patients. The clinical trials setting was particularly useful in separating the effect of cancer-related mortality versus death due to other causes. Because the analysis was conducted with data from patients who had participated in a clinical trial, it would have been possible to examine the age group of 65 and older but this was not done. There still seems to be an opportunity in this heavily studied area to examine the effect of age on the relationship between obesity and cancer prognosis.

A second large analysis of BMI as a prognostic feature in breast cancer clinical trials was performed with data for 6792 women who participated in trials conducted by the International Breast Cancer Study Group (49). The women in these studies received chemotherapy as well as tamoxifen and other endocrine therapies. In this setting, a decrease in overall survival was associated with elevated BMI, but disease-free survival was not significantly affected. This result prompted the observation that noncancer causes of death may be responsible for decreased survival in obese patients (50).

In addition to the conclusion that weight at diagnosis is prognostic, there has also been a perception that women undergoing adjuvant chemotherapy for breast cancer could expect a change in weight as a consequence of treatment. Some specific information is available from a cohort of 445 women who were prospectively followed after surgery that led to a first-time diagnosis of breast cancer (51). One year after diagnostic surgery, reassessment confirmed that 84% of patients had gained weight. Because recalled caloric intake decreased and reported physical activity increased, neither of those study variables could be used to explain the observed gain in weight. Instead, the data from this study identified adjuvant chemotherapy with or without the onset of menopause as the two factors most associated with a gain in weight averaging 2.5 kg for chemotherapy.

Despite the number of studies that have been performed to examine the relationship between overnutrition and mortality from breast cancer, investigations looking at other diagnoses are sparse. The most convincing data for a relationship between obesity and cancer mortality comes from a study of 900,000 individuals of whom 45% were men. From an analysis of prospectively collected data, it was observed that excess body weight is related to increased cancer mortality for all cancers combined and for cancers from many individual organ sites as well (28). For BMI above 40, death rates from cancer were more than 50% higher for men and more than 60% higher for women. This report does not strictly address the influence of weight at diagnosis on prognosis, because the BMI measurement was obtained before a diagnosis of cancer was made, sometimes years in advance. Nevertheless, BMI at an earlier point in time can be considered a surrogate for the later BMI at the time of diagnosis, but a BMI at diagnosis, in addition to the one from years before, might give additional information on prognosis. Because age-adjusted death rates were used in this study, it was not possible to examine the effect of age—a drawback when age-specific information is desired.

One of the difficulties of assessing the impact of overnutrition on cancer is the apparent inconsistency of results, which is observed when subset differences or differences in methodology are not taken into consideration; for example, smoking status or differences in timing of measurements relative to cancer diagnosis, etc. An additional example of this phenomenon is provided by several disease-specific reports about kidney cancer. In two recent studies involving just over a total of

1000 patients, independent results from M.D. Anderson in the United States (52) and from the University Hospital Graz in Austria (53) suggested that increased BMI was associated with an improved prognosis for renal cell carcinoma. Although the Calle report (28) shows an increased mortality associated with obesity prior to a diagnosis of kidney cancer, this result is not necessarily inconsistent with better survival of kidney cancer patients who have a BMI over 25 at the time of diagnosis. The group of individuals in the single center reports underwent nephrectomy and consequently do not represent a wider patient population as captured in the cohort study that included everyone in the study population regardless of whether they had surgery or not.

In the quest to obtain nutritional information that will be clinically useful in the management of cancer patients, it may be that randomized clinical trials will be the approach that proves to be most forthcoming. Very few trials of this type have been done. One approach that was used to ask a nutritional question was incorporated in the Women's Intervention Nutrition Study (54). Postmenopausal women with early breast cancer were randomized to a low-fat dietary intervention for comparison with a control group that followed a regular diet. The total study population numbered 2437, ranging in age from 48 to 79 with an average age of 62. In the intervention arm, the goal was a diet where only 20% of the calories were obtained from fat in contrast to the usual diet where about 40% of calories came from fat. The primary end point of the study was to ascertain if the recurrence of breast cancer in the study population could be decreased by a low-fat diet. The women were followed for five years with the initial results reported as American Society of Clinical Oncology in the spring of 2005. The women in the intervention arm consumed an average of 33 g of fat a day compared with the control group, who consumed 51 g of fat per day. After five years, 9.8% of the women on the intervention arm had recurrence compared with 12.4% of the women in the control group, for a reduction of approximately 24% ($P = 0.034$). An interesting result of subset analysis was that the benefit seemed to occur largely in women with ER-negative breast cancers. The results mentioned here were derived from the oral meeting presentation and remain preliminary until journal publication. In the meantime, they provide food for thought about the type and number of studies that need to be done and how the results can be used to improve patient care.

Poor Nutritional Status

Table 3 provides some of the physiological characteristics of the elderly, which are linked to poor nutritional status. Decreased skeletal mass accompanied by increased body fat, particularly in the truncal area, may occur. Such conditions may be precipitated by failure to meet protein needs (0.8–1.0 g/kg body weight/day) in a diet with increased caloric intake. Poor dentition and altered taste and smell may contribute to inappropriate intakes among the elderly. Likewise, reduced absorptive capacity associated with increased age may lead to imbalances in selected nutrients.

NUTRITIONAL INTERVENTIONS TO MANAGE THERAPEUTIC SYMPTOMS IN THE ELDERLY CANCER PATIENT

Malnutrition at diagnosis is more common in cancers of the gastrointestinal tract, esophagus, stomach, and pancreas. Malnutrition is known to increase hospital stay, thereby decreasing the cost–benefit and increasing the risk–benefit ratios of anticancer treatment. Although there is some evidence that adequate nutrition is

Table 3 Physiological Characteristics and Nutritional Concerns in the Elderly

	Physiological characteristics of the elderly	Nutritional concerns in the elderly
Body composition	Decline in skeletal muscle mass sarcopenia	Protein needs may be increased from 0.8–1.0 g/kg body weight
	Increase in total body fat, particularly visceral area	Altered caloric requirements
	Decreased BMR	
Mouth and esophagus	Poor dentition	Reduced food intake
	Dry mouth	Reduced appetite
	Altered taste and smell perception	
	Modest decrease in motility of the esophagus	
Intestine	Delayed gastric emptying	Calcium absorption is decreased, may not acquire enough vitamin D
	Only modest changes in intestinal structure and function	Lactase activity may decline
	Constipation and incontinence	B_{12} absorption is impaired only in conjunction with atrophic gastritis
Other organs	Increased rigidity and thickening of the heart	
	Decreased pulmonary function	
	Decreased renal function including decreased urinary creatine and sodium concentration	
	Alterations in circulating hormone levels and actions	
	Dysregulation of immunity	

Abbreviation: BMR, basal metabolic rate.

important during treatment, not much is known regarding what should or should not be consumed by young and middle-aged individuals. Even less is known about the elderly. Some of the physiological consequences of chemotherapy and potential nutritional support are shown in Table 4.

Two evidence-based reviews suggest that nutritional support can reduce hospital stays in certain cancer patients; however neither focuses on elderly patients. Glutamine supplementation through parenteral solutions was associated with shorter hospital stays and lower incidence of positive blood cultures in bone marrow transplant patients (59). Protein and energy supplementation was associated with a lower relative risk of mortality and shorter hospital stays in older people recovering from cancer treatment or in critical care (60). Data do support preoperative tube feeding for a week or two before surgery for moderately to severely malnourished cancer patients (61).

Table 4 Physiological Characteristics and Nutritional Concerns Regarding Chemotherapy

	Physiological characteristics of chemotherapy	Nutritional concerns of chemotherapy
General side effects of chemotherapy	Anorexia	Protein increases to 1.5 g/kg/day
General side effects of chemotherapy	Nausea and/or vomiting	No known nutritional support to alleviate this symptom
General side effects of chemotherapy	Diarrhea or constipation	No known nutritional support to alleviate this symptom
Radiation, particularly head and neck, 5FU, CMF	Inflammation of the mouth—*mucositis*	Ambivalent results about glutamine and zinc. Weak and unreliable evidence regarding allopurinol mouthwash, vitamin E, immunoglobulin, or human placental extract
Metatastic cancer, radio chemotherapy	Alterations in taste and smell perception	Zinc (55)
5FU	Direct damage to rapidly proliferating intestine	Broad range of nutrients
Methotrexate	Direct damage to rapidly proliferating intestine	Broad range of nutrients
Multidrug chemotherapy	Myelosuppression, neutropenia, and leukopenia	Broad range of nutrients. Growth factor therapy. Perhaps selenium (56)
Doxorubicin or other anthracyclines	Cardiotoxicity	No demonstration that any single antioxidant is effective
Doxorubicin or other anthracyclines	Central neuropathy	No known nutritional support to alleviate this symptom
Cytarabine	Cerebellar toxicity	No known nutritional support to alleviate this symptom
Multidrug chemotherapy	Anemia	See Table 5
Paclitaxal, docetaxel, cisplatin	Peripheral neuropathy	α-Lipoic acid, weak evidence (57)
	Bone loss associated with ovarian dysfunction	Calcium, vitamin D (57)
Cisplatin	Nephrotoxicity	Selenium (58)
Multidrug chemotherapy	White blood cell numbers, Hair loss, and QOL	Selenium (56)

Abbreviations: 5FU, 5-fluorouracil; QOL, quality of life.

Ravasco et al. (62) investigated the role of dietary counseling or nutritional supplements on clinical end points for 111 CRC patients by evaluating their nutritional status, morbidity, and QOL during radiation therapy. At radiotherapy completion, caloric intake increased in those given dietary consultation compared with intake in those with no dietary counseling. Impressively, after radiotherapy and at three months, the rates of anorexia, nausea, vomiting, and diarrhea were significantly higher in those allowed ad libitum behavior over those seen in patients who had dietary consultations. Likewise, following radiotherapy, the QOL scores improved proportionally with adequate nutritional intake in those given counseling; but worsened in those eating ad libitum. Specific therapeutic nutritional intervention before and during radiotherapy may induce a radio-protective effect for healthy tissues. For example, an elemental diet composed of free amino acids, short chain polysaccharides, and small amounts of triglycerides may offer protection through various mechanisms including the attenuation of biliary and pancreatic secretions. In addition, nutritional intervention may act as a radioenhancer as has been reported for polyunsaturated fatty acids (PUFA) (63).

Nakamura et al. (64) investigated the effects of supplementation with omega-3 fatty acids and arginine on plasma biomarkers for patients undergoing major surgery for cancer. Supplementation led to an increase in the plasma levels of omega-3 fatty acids, whereas the ratio of omega-6 fatty acids to omega-3 fatty acids and thromboxane B_2 levels were lower. Inflammatory markers and cytokine receptors in the supplemented group were also lower in comparison with the control group. Dramatic decreases in polymorphonuclear leukocyte-elastase and interleukin-8 in the supplement group were found on postoperative days 1 and 3. Overall, this study provides evidence that use of an omega-3 fatty acid–containing supplement for five days before surgery may improve preoperative nutritional status as well as preoperative and postoperative inflammatory and immune responses in cancer patients.

Dietary fatty acids are known to have an important role in health and disease. Two specific types of fatty acids are generally considered to be dietary "essentials." Alpha linolenic acid is the precursor of the essential n-3 family of PUFA, with the first double bond in the molecule occurring three carbons away from the methyl terminus. Linoleic acid is the other precursor for the essential n-6 PUFA family, with the first double bond in the molecule occurring six carbons away from the methyl terminus. Because mammals lack the requisite enzymes to insert a double bond at the n-3 or n-6 position, these two fatty acids are essential dietary components. The n-3 fatty acids are particular interesting because they have been suggested to possess a wide range of beneficial effects in humans including patients with cancer (65,66). They have been implicated as factors determining membrane fluidity, blood lipid profile, eicosanoid biosynthesis, cell-signaling cascades, and gene expression profiles. Their ability to alter these or other processes has been suggested to account for the observation that they can influence the onset and progression of several disease states including cardiovascular disease and cancer. The effectiveness of radiation and of some cancer chemotherapy agents including doxorubicin, epirubicin, irinotecan hydrochloride (CPT-11), 5-fluorouracil, and tamoxifen in preclinical rodent models has been shown to be improved when the diet includes supplemental n-3 fatty acids (65). Unfortunately information in humans is not as plentiful. In a study by Bougnoux et al. (67), enhanced n-3 fatty acids intake and accompanying higher docosahexaenoic acid in breast adipose tissue from patients was associated with complete or partial remission responses to cytotoxic drugs. While data about the health benefits associated with increased n-3 intake are interesting, it is clear that not all individuals respond identically (68,69).

Opportunities to use nutritional interventions to improve response to treatment and QOL are many and varied. For example, manipulation of diet after radiotherapy may help to reduce or eliminate chronic, undesirable changes in bowel habits once they have occurred. A number of dietetic interventions such as lactose

Table 5 Causes and Solutions of Anemia

Causes	Characteristics	Potential solutions
Iron deficiency	Microcytic, hypochromic	Iron supplements
B_{12} deficiency	Macrocytic, hyporegenerative, and associated with pancytopenia	B_{12} injections
Anemia of chronic disease	Cannot mobilize iron from reticuloendothelial cells of the bone marrow; increased catabolic cytokines; and decreased erythropoietin and/or increased resistance to erythropoietin	Not clear: how to treat
Renal insufficiency	Normocytic, normochromic	Erythropoietin

restriction, fat restriction, reduced intake of motility stimulants such as caffeine and a decrease in fiber-containing foods (70) have been suggested. Further work in this area is needed. Aging is associated with changes in cytochrome P450 enzymes and Phase II conjugases, which may increase toxicity of chemotherapeutic agents. This increase in toxicity may in some cases be offset by reduced absorption of drugs in older patients. Decreased liver mass may also result in reduced drug metabolism. Nutritional approaches to compensating for these changes have not received much scientific attention.

Changes in fat, body water, and muscle mass over time may alter the distribution of drugs depending on the lipophilic and lipophobic properties of the compound. Some drugs that bind to red blood cells, such as taxanes and anthracyclines, are increased in the circulation as free (unbound) drug when anemia is present. The prevalence of anemia in the elderly is high. Anemia recognition is important as it may represent the first sign of underlying disease and is known to be associated with several morbid conditions (Table 5). The cause of anemia may be due to several factors including iron deficiency (especially if blood loss is involved), B_{12} deficiency, and renal insufficiency leading to a decreased ability to produce erythropoietin (71).

NUTRITIONAL FACTORS AS COMPONENTS OF TREATMENT

Once the diagnosis of cancer is established, patients often enter a high-risk category for occurrence of a second primary tumor. This setting may provide an opportunity for a preventive intervention of benefit to cancer patients. For example, certain vitamins or calcium supplements may reduce colorectal adenoma recurrence. Whelan et al. (72) conducted a case–control study to study the association between vitamin or calcium supplementation and the incidence of adenomatous polyps in patients with previous colonic neoplasia, who were undergoing follow-up colonoscopy. The effect of vitamin supplements (any vitamin) on adenoma recurrence was protective (odds ratio, 0.41; 95% confidence interval, 0.27–0.61). Similarly, the odds ratio for calcium supplementation was also reduced (odds ratio, 0.51; 95% confidence interval, 0.27–0.96). More research is needed in this area.

Carnitine is the generic term for a number of amino acid derivatives found in nearly all cells of the body. This class of compounds may have a role in modifying events leading to malignancy. Carnitine has a critical role in energy production by assisting with the transport of long-chain fatty acids into the mitochondria. It also assists with the transport of toxic compounds out of the mitochondria. Fatigue resulting from chemotherapy, radiation treatment, and poor nutritional status is common in cancer patients (73). In a series of 50 patients receiving cisplatin or ifosfamide, who were found to have low plasma levels of carnitine, carnitine supplementation (4 g/day for one week) restored blood levels to normal and ameliorated fatigue in 45 of the 50 as measured by the Functional Assessment of Cancer Therapy-Fatigue QOL instrument (74). In a more recent, but smaller study of 18 terminal cancer patients with fatigue, 15 were found to be carnitine deficient. Preliminary data for 13 of these individuals showed improvement in mood and quality of sleep with reduction in fatigue in response to carnitine supplementation (doses ranging from 250 mg/day to 3 g/day).

The use of herbal supplements by cancer patients is becoming increasingly prevalent (75,76). Use of these products is very high (about 80%) among patients with breast cancer (77,78). Likewise, among those with prostate cancer (79), the usage has also been significant (80). Caucasians and patients over 60 years of age predominate among users. In a study by Kumar et al. (81) involving more than 800 subjects, about 29% reported taking one or more nutritional supplements during treatment. Although 59% consumed multivitamin/mineral preparations, several patients reported taking one or more other vitamins, minerals, botanicals, and/or biologics in addition to the multivitamin/minerals. The most frequently used complementary/integrative nutritional therapies were vitamins (86.9% of the patients), followed by botanicals/biologics (43.8%) and mineral supplements (28.6%) (76).

Oncologists need to be aware of exposures that increase the likelihood of bleeding. Garlic, ginger, ginkgo, and ginseng, known as the "4 Gs," are the most popular herbal supplements used by cancer patients, and modulate coagulation. Other herbal supplements that have been demonstrated to interact with aspirin and other nonsteroidal anti-inflammatory drugs are bromelain, cayenne, chamomile, feverfew, dong quai, eleuthero/Siberian, licorice, bilberry, turmeric, meadowsweet, and willow. Those containing coumarin (chamomile, motherwort, horse chestnut, fenugreek, and red clover) and tamarind enhance the risk of bleeding.

It is likely that the response to foods and food components is dependent on the genetic background of the patient. Nutrigenomics, or the scientific study of the way genes interact with foods and their components, is an emerging science that holds promise to provide new insights into personalized nutrition. Based on a molecular approach, nutrigenomics is expected to provide logical criteria for understanding why the health consequences of eating behaviors vary from individual to individual. The promise of nutrigenomics builds on the premise (i) that diet and dietary components can alter the risk of disease development by modulating multiple processes involved with the onset, incidence, progression, and/or severity of cancer; (ii) that food components can act on the human genome, either directly or indirectly, to alter the expression of genes and gene products; and (iii) that the health consequences of a diet are dependent on the balance of health and disease states and on an individual's genetic background (82,83). The study of nutrigenomics and/or associated changes in proteomics and metabolomics will ultimately identify molecular targets that can be used for appropriate and personalized nutritional preemption. The complexity of understanding the interrelationships between genes and diet is illustrated by recent findings related to the nuclear receptors, peroxisome proliferator–activated receptors (PPARs), and dietary fatty acids. The involvement of PPARγ in regulating insulin resistance is well known. In individuals with a specific polymorphism in the PPARγ (Pro12Ala), a low polyunsaturated to saturated fat ratio has been linked with an increased BMI and higher fasting insulin concentrations. When the dietary ratio of polyunsaturated (P) to saturated (S) fats is high, the opposite is true (84). These data suggest that when the dietary P:S ratio is low, the BMI in Ala carriers is greater than that in Pro homozygotes, but, when the dietary ratio is high, the opposite is seen. As more information surfaces about the diet–gene interaction, health care professionals should be in a better position to explain the large heterogeneity in findings that has plagued clinical nutrition.

To date, few investigations have related gene expression patterns to QOL measurements. Preliminary data suggests that genetic variants affecting folate metabolism are associated with QOL indicators in patients with metastatic CRC (85).

SUMMARY: NUTRITIONAL MANAGEMENT PRINCIPLES

As illustrated in this chapter, the nutritional status of cancer patients has multiple dimensions and there is reason to believe that the approach to nutritional management should be adjusted according to age-related factors. Nevertheless, nutritional considerations also appear to vary according to the organ site of the cancer and the status of the disease as it progresses through its natural history. Unfortunately, these issues are complicated and the intersection of nutritional and oncologic research only scratches the surface of some very important questions. Although the nutritional status of the elderly is a focus of research, and the nutritional status of the cancer patient is also a focus, it is rare to find specifics related to the nutrition of elderly cancer patients. Worthwhile benefit to patients is expected when these gaps in knowledge are addressed. Until then the following need to be taken into consideration:

- Nutritional interventions need to be tailored according to diagnosis and disease status.
- Assessing nutritional status at diagnosis, throughout treatment, and after the completion of treatment is an essential part of appropriate management. At a minimum, BMI and food intake should be monitored. Weight management should be individualized.
- Dealing with nutritional issues early in the disease process rather than at the point of end-stage disease is important, as emphasized in this chapter.
- Dietary counseling is a critical component of cancer management with great potential for improving the QOL.
- Protein and energy as well as glutamine intake seem to be fairly well established to reduce hospital stays. Less well established is the idea of supplementing with omega-3 fatty acids, herbs, or carnitine.
- The elderly population and the cancer population both have nutritional issues, but nutritional studies involving elderly cancer patients are rare. The recommendations in the chapter are sometimes based on extrapolation from data for younger individuals with cancer or older individuals without cancer.
- In the future, oncologists are encouraged to pursue research in biochemical measures of nutritional status.

REFERENCES

1. Wolfe WS, Frongillo EA, Valois P. Understanding the experience of food insecurity by elders suggests ways to improve its measurement. J Nutr 2003; 133(9):2762–2769.
2. Segura A, Pardo J, Jara C, et al. An epidemiological evaluation of the prevalence of malnutrition in Spanish patients with locally advanced or metastatic cancer. Clin Nutr 2005, Jun 29 (Epub ahead of print).
3. Crogan NL, Pasvogel A. The influence of protein-calorie malnutrition on quality of life in nursing homes. J Gerontol A Biol Sci Med Sci 2003; 58(2):159–164.
4. Meyerhardt JA, Sloan JA, Sargent DJ, et al. Associations between plasma insulin-like growth factor proteins and C-peptide and quality of life in patients with metastatic colorectal cancer. Cancer Epidemiol Biomarkers Prev 2005; 14(6):1402–1410.
5. Potter J, Klipstein K, Reilly JJ, Roberts M. The nutritional status and clinical course of acute admissions to a geriatric unit. Age Ageing 1995; 24(2):131–136.
6. Notarnicola M, Altomare DF, Correale M, et al. Serum lipid profile in colorectal cancer patients with and without synchronous distant metastases. Oncology 2005; 68(46):371–374.
7. Muhlethaler R, Stuck AE, Minder CE, Frey BM. The prognostic significance of protein-energy malnutrition in geriatric patients. Age Ageing 1995; 24(3):193–197.
8. Ockenga J, Freudenreich M, Zakonsky R, Norman K, Pirlich M, Lochs H. Nutritional assessment and management in hospitalized patients: implication for DRG-based reimbursement and health care quality. Clin Nutr 2005, Jul 18 (Epub ahead of print).
9. Rasmussen HH, Kondrup J, Ladefoged K, Staun M. Clinical nutrition in Danish hospitals: a questionnaire-based investigation among doctors and nurses. Clin Nutr 1999; 18(3): 153–158.
10. Kondrup J, Johansen N, Plum LM, et al. Incidence of nutritional risk and causes of inadequate nutritional care in hospitals. Clin Nutr 2002; 21(6):461–468.
11. Arora NS, Rochester DF. Respiratory muscle strength and maximal voluntary ventilation in undernourished patients. Am Rev Respir Dis 1982; 126(1):5–8.
12. Chandra RK. Nutrition and the immune system: an introduction. Am J Clin Nutr 1997; 66(2):460S–463S.
13. Reynolds JV, O'Farrelly C, Feighery C, et al. Impaired gut barrier function in malnourished patients. Br J Surg 1996; 83(9):1288–1291.
14. Ollenschlager G, Viell B, Thomas W, et al. Tumor anorexia: causes, assessment, treatment. Recent Results Cancer Res 1991; 121:249–259.
15. Ottery FD. Definition of standardized nutritional assessment and interventional pathways in oncology. Nutrition 1996; 12(1 suppl):S15–S19.
16. Sarhill N, Mahmoud F, Walsh D, et al. Evaluation of nutritional status in advanced metastatic cancer. Support Care Cancer 2003; 11(10):652–659.
17. Chumlea WM, Sun SS. The availability of body composition reference data for the elderly. J Nutr Health Aging 2004; 8(2):76–82.
18. DeWys WD. Changes in taste sensation and feeding behaviour in cancer patients: a review. J Hum Nutr 1978; 32(6):447–453.
19. Berteretche MV, Dalix AM, d'Ornano AM, Bellisle F, Khayat D, Faurion A. Decreased taste sensitivity in cancer patients under chemotherapy. Support Care Cancer 2004; 12(8):571–576.
20. Nitenberg G, Raynard B. Nutritional support of the cancer patient: issues and dilemmas. Crit Rev Oncol Hematol 2000; 34(3):137–146.
21. Ervin RB, Wright JD, Kennedy-Stephenson J. Use of dietary supplements in the United States, 1988–94. Vital Health Stat 1999; 11:i–iii, 1–14.
22. Chernoff R. Normal aging, nutrition assessment and clinical practice. Nutr Clin Pract 2003; 18:12–20.
23. US National Institutes of Health. Clinical Guidelines for the Identification, Evaluation, and Treatment of Overweight and Obesity in Adults. Bethesda, MD: National Institutes of Health, 1998.

24. Troiano RP, Frongillo EA, Sobal J, Levitsky DA. The relationship between body weight and mortality: a quantitative analysis of combined information from existing studies. Int J Obes 1996; 20:63–75.

25. Davis MA, Neuhaus JM, Moritz DH, Lein D, Barclay JD, Murphy SP. Health behaviors and survival among middle-aged and older men and women in the NHANES I Epidemiologic Follow-up Study. Prev Med 1994; 23:369–376.

26. Katzmarzyk PT, Janssen I, Ardern CI. Physical inactivity, excess adiposity and premature mortality. Obes Rev 2003; 4:257–290.

27. Kroenke CH, Chen WY, Rosner B, Holmes MD. Weight, weight gain, and survival after breast cancer diagnosis. J Clin Oncol 2005; 23:1370–1378.

28. Calle EE, Rodriguez C, Walker-Thurmond K, Thun MJ. Overweight, obesity, and mortality from cancer in a prospectively studied cohort of U.S. adults. N Engl J Med 2003; 348:1625–1638.

29. Chanrey P, Malone A. ADA Pocket Guide to Nutrition Assessment. American Dietetic Association, 2004.

30. Detsky AS, McLaughlin JR, Baker JP, et al. What is subjective global assessment of nutritional status? JPEN 1987; 11(1):8–13.

31. Gupta D, Lammersfeld CA, Vashi PG, Burrows J, Lis CG, Grutsch JF. Prognostic significance of Subjective Global Assessment (SGA) in advanced colorectal cancer. Eur J Clin Nutr 2005; 59(1):35–40.

32. Raguso CA, Maisonneuve N, Pichard C. Subjective Global Assessment (SGA): evaluation and follow-up of nutritional state. Rev Med Suisse Romande 2004; 124(10): 607–610.

33. Ottery F. Supportive nutritional management of the patient with pancreatic cancer. Oncology 1996; 10(9 suppl):26–32.

34. Bauer J, Capra S, Ferguson M. Use of the scored Patient-Generated Subjective Global Assessment (PG-SGA) as a nutrition assessment tool in patients with cancer. Eur J Clin Nutr 2002; 56(8):779–785.

35. Persson MD, Brismar KE, Katzarski KS, Nordenstrom J, Cederholm TE. Nutritional status using mini nutritional assessment and subjective global assessment predict mortality in geriatric patients. J Am Geriatr Soc 2002; 50(12):1996–2002.

36. Ottery FD. Supportive nutrition to prevent cachexia and improve quality of life. Semin Oncol 1995; 22(2 suppl 3):98–111.

37. Isenring E, Bauer J, Capra S. The scored Patient-generated Subjective Global Assessment (PG-SGA) and its association with quality of life in ambulatory patients receiving radiotherapy. Eur J Clin Nutr 2003; 57(2):305–309.

38. Kyle UG, Schneider SM, Pirlich M, Lochs H, Hebuterne X, Pichard C. Does nutritional risk, as assessed by Nutritional Risk Index, increase during hospital stay? A multinational population-based study. Clin Nutr 2005; 24(4):516–524.

39. Thorsdottir I, Jonsson PV, Asgeirsdottir AE, Hjaltadottir I, Bjornsson S, Ramel A. Fast and simple screening for nutritional status in hospitalized, elderly people. J Hum Nutr Diet 2005; 18(1):53–60.

40. Afanas'eva AN, Evtushenko VA. Conformation changes in albumin molecule as a marker of dissemination of the tumor process. Bull Exp Biol Med 2004; 138(2):177–178.

41. Mears E. Outcomes of continuous process improvement of a nutritional care program incorporating serum pre-albumin measurements. Nutrition 1996; 12:479–484.

42. Guo Y, Palmer JL, Kaur G, Hainley S, Young B, Bruera E. Nutritional status of cancer patients and its relationship to function in an inpatient rehabilitation setting. Support Care Cancer 2005; 13(3):169–175.

43. Goodwin PJ, Ennis M, Pritchard KI, et al. Insulin-like growth factor binding proteins 1 and 3 and breast cancer outcomes. Breast Cancer Res Treat 2002; 74:65–76.

44. Kumar N, Allen KA, Riccardi D, et al. Fatigue, weight gain, lethargy and amenorrhea in breast cancer patients on chemotherapy: is subclinical hypothyroidism the culprit? Breast Cancer Res Treat 2004; 83:149–159.

45. Glei M, Habermann N, Osswald K, et al. Assessment of DNA damage and its modulation by dietary and genetic factors in smokers using the Comet assay: a biomarker model. Biomarkers 2005; 10(2–3):203–217.

46. Kucuk O, Sarkar FH, Sakr W, et al. Phase II Randomized Clinical Trial of lycopene supplementation before radical prostatectomy. Cancer Epidemiol Biomarkers Prev 2001; 10:861–868.

47. Chlebowski RT, Aiello E, McTiernan A. Weight loss in breast cancer patient management. J Clin Oncol 2002; 20:1128–1143.

48. Dignam JJ, Wieand K, Johnson KA, Fisher B, Xu L, Mamounas EP. Obesity, tamoxifen use, and outcomes in women with estrogen receptor-positive early-stage breast cancer. J Natl Cancer Inst 2003; 95:1467–1476.

49. Berclaz G, Lil S, Price KN, et al. On behalf of the International Breast Cancer Study Group. Body Mass Index as a prognostic feature in operable breast cancer: The International Breast Cancer Study Group experience. Ann Oncol 2004; 15:875–884.

50. Dignam JJ, Mamounas EP. Obesity and breast cancer prognosis: an expanding body of evidence. Ann Oncol 2004; 15:850–851.

51. Goodwin PJ, Ennis M, Pritchard KI, et al. Adjuvant treatment and onset of menopause predict weight gain after breast cancer diagnosis. J Clin Oncol 1999; 17:120–129.

52. Kamat AM, Shock RP, Naya Y, Rosser CJ, Slaton JW, Pisters LL. Prognostic value of Body Mass Index in patients undergoing nephrectomy for localized renal tumors. Urology 2004; 63:46–50.

53. Schips L, Lipsky K, Zigeuner R, et al. Does overweight impact on the prognosis of patients with renal cell carcinoma: a single center experience of 683 patients. J Surg Oncol 2004; 88:57–62.

54. Chlebowski RT, Blackburn GL, Elashoff RE, et al. Dietary fat reduction in postmenopausal women with primary breast cancer: Phase III Women's Intervention Nutrition Study (WINS). J Clin Oncol 2005; 16:S3.

55. Ripamonti C, Zecca E, Brunelli C, et al. A randomized, controlled clinical trial to evaluate the effects of zinc sulfate on cancer patients with taste alterations caused by head and neck irradiation. Cancer 1998; 82(10):1938–1945.

56. Sieja K, Talerczyk M. Selenium as an element in the treatment of ovarian cancer in women receiving chemotherapy. Gynecol Oncol 2004; 93(2):320–327.

57. Rock E, DeMichele A. Nutritional approaches to late toxicities of adjuvant chemotherapy in breast cancer survivors. J Nutr 2003; 133(11 suppl 1):3785S–3793S.

58. Hu YJ, Chen Y, Zhang YQ, et al. The protective role of selenium on the toxicity of cisplatin-contained chemotherapy regimen in cancer patients. Biol Trace Elem Res 1997; 56(3):331–341.

59. Murray SM, Pindoria S. Nutrition support for bone marrow transplant patients. Cochrane Database Syst Rev 2002(2):CD002920.

60. Milne AC, Potter J, Avenell A. Protein and energy supplementation in elderly people at risk from malnutrition. Cochrane Database Syst Rev 2002; (3):CD003288. Review. Update in: Cochrane Database Syst Rev 2005; (2):CD003288.

61. Barrera R. Nutritional support in cancer patients. J Parenter Enteral Nutr 2002; 26(5 suppl):S63–S71.

62. Ravasco P, Monteiro-Grillo I, Vidal PM, Camilo ME. Dietary counseling improves patient outcomes: a prospective, randomized, controlled trial in colorectal cancer patients undergoing radiotherapy. J Clin Oncol 2005; 23(7):1431–1438.

63. Conklin KA. Dietary polyunsaturated fatty acids: impact on cancer chemotherapy and radiation. Altern Med Rev 2002; 7(1):4–21.

64. Nakamura K, Kariyazono H, Komokata T, Hamada N, Sakata R, Yamada K. Influence of preoperative administration of omega-3 fatty acid-enriched supplement on inflammatory and immune responses in patients undergoing major surgery for cancer. Nutrition 2005; 21(6):639–649.

65. Hardman WE. (n-3) fatty acids and cancer therapy. J Nutr 2004; 134(12 suppl):3427S–3430S.

66. Terry PD, Terry JB, Rohan TE. Long-chain (n-3) fatty acid intake and risk of cancers of the breast and the prostate: recent epidemiological studies, biological mechanisms, and directions for future research. J Nutr 2004; 134(12 suppl):3412S–3420S.
67. Bougnoux P, Chajes V, Germain E, et al. Cytotoxic drug efficacy correlates with adipose tissue docosahexaenoic acid level in locally advanced breast carcinoma. Lipids 1999; 34(suppl):S109.
68. Shahidi F, Miraliakbari H. Omega-3 (n-3) fatty acids in health and disease: part 1—cardiovascular disease and cancer. J Med Food 2004; 7(4):387–401.
69. Ma DW, Seo J, Switzer KC, et al. n-3 PUFA and membrane microdomains: a new frontier in bioactive lipid research. J Nutr Biochem 2004; 15(11):700–706.
70. Classen J, Belka C, Paulsen F, Budach W, Hoffmann W, Bamberg M. Radiation-induced gastrointestinal toxicity. Pathophysiology, approaches to treatment and prophylaxis. Strahlenther Onkol 1998; N174(suppl 3):82–84.
71. Balducci L. Anemia, cancer, and aging. Cancer Control 2003; 10(6):478–486.
72. Whelan RL, Horvath KD, Gleason NR, et al. Vitamin and calcium supplement use is associated with decreased adenoma recurrence in patients with a previous history of neoplasia. Dis Colon Rectum 1999; 42(2):212–217.
73. Cruciani RA, Dvorkin E, Homel P, et al. L-carnitine supplementation for the treatment of fatigue and depressed mood in cancer patients with carnitine deficiency: a preliminary analysis. Ann NY Acad Sci 2004; 1033:168–716.
74. Graziano F, Bisonni R, Catalano V, et al. Potential role of levocarnitine supplementation for the treatment of chemotherapy-induced fatigue in non-anemic cancer patients. Br J Cancer 2002; 86:1854–1857.
75. Piersen CE. Phytoestrogens in botanical dietary supplements: implications for cancer. Integr Cancer Ther 2003; 2(2):120–138.
76. Kumar NB, Allen K, Bell H. Perioperative herbal supplement use in cancer patients: potential implications and recommendations for presurgical screening. Cancer Control 2005; 12(3):149–157.
77. Newman V, Rock CL, Faerber S, Flatt SW, Wright FA, Pierce JP. Dietary supplement use by women at risk for breast cancer recurrence. The Women's Healthy Eating and Living Study Group. J Am Diet Assoc 1998; 98(3):285–292.
78. Morris KT, Johnson N, Homer L, Walts D. A comparison of complementary therapy use between breast cancer patients and patients with other primary tumor sites. Am J Surg 2000; 179(5):407–411.
79. Lippert MC, McClain R, Boyd JC, Theodorescu D. Alternative medicine use in patients with localized prostate carcinoma treated with curative intent. Cancer 1999; 86(12):2642–2648.
80. Burstein HJ, Gelber S, Guadagnoli E, Weeks JC. Use of alternative medicine by women with early-stage breast cancer. N Engl J Med 1999; 340(22):1733–1739.
81. Kumar NB, Hopkins K, Allen K, Riccardi D, Besterman-Dahan K, Moyers S. Use of complementary/integrative nutritional therapies during cancer treatment: implications in clinical practice. Cancer Control 2002; 9(3):236–243.
82. Davis CD, Milner J. Frontiers in nutrigenomics, proteomics, metabolomics and cancer prevention. Mutat Res 2004; 551(1–2):51–64.
83. Kaput J, Rodriguez RL. Nutritional genomics: the next frontier in the postgenomic era. Physiol Genomics 2004; 16:166–177.
84. Luan J, Browne PO, Harding AH, et al. Evidence for gene-nutrient interaction at the PPARgamma locus. Diabetes 2001; 50:686–689.
85. Sloan JA, McLeod H, Sargent D, et al. Preliminary evidence of relationship between genetic markers and oncology patient quality of life (QOL). Proc Meet Am Soc Clin Oncol 2004:23.

22

Comorbidity and Cancer Treatment in Older Populations

William A. Satariano
School of Public Health, University of California, Berkeley, California, U.S.A.

Rebecca A. Silliman and Timothy L. Lash
Boston University Schools of Medicine and Public Health,
Boston, Massachusetts, U.S.A.

INTRODUCTION

There has been a sustained interest during the past three decades on the effects of comorbidity on cancer treatment in older populations (1–4). This interest is reflected in a growing number of research papers on the topic, the selection of comorbidity as a plenary topic at scientific and professional meetings, and the convening of scientific working groups to establish research and practice agendas in the area.

Comorbidity is defined as the presence of one or more health conditions in people diagnosed with an index condition, in this case, cancer (1). The clinical and public health interest in comorbidity has been motivated, in large part, by the aging of the population and, more significantly, the aging of the cancer population (5,6). Older cancer patients are more likely than younger patients to present with concurrent, comorbid conditions (5,6). These comorbid conditions, in turn, complicate the diagnosis, treatment, and management of cancer in older populations (2,4,7). There are two consistent findings from the research on comorbidity and cancer. First, cancer patients with comorbidity have poorer duration and quality of life than patients without comorbidity, after taking into account other prognostic indicators. Second, patients with comorbidity are typically administered less intensive forms of therapy, especially radiation therapy and chemotherapy, than are patients without comorbidity, again, taking into account relevant covariates. One common interpretation of this finding is that physicians are concerned that standard cancer therapy may be too risky because of the presence of other conditions. The magnitude and severity of comorbidity are thus viewed as important indicators of physiologic age and reserve.

Research focusing on the intersection of aging, cancer, and comorbidity has been based in large part on work done in clinical epidemiology and health services research (8). However, there is a growing interest in the field of geriatric oncology to develop more appropriate and effective approaches to treatment among older adults who have a range of comorbid illnesses and conditions (4,9–12). Our purpose here is to review current research on comorbidity and consider its implications for cancer treatment in older populations. In particular, we will examine two types of research currently conducted on comorbidity. "Applied research" includes the evaluation of measures of comorbidity to characterize the overall physiologic capacity of patients and thus more appropriately tailor specific treatments to specific patients. In contrast, "basic research" examines the biological and behavioral mechanisms that explain the temporal interactions between comorbidity and health outcomes, such as quality and duration of survival. This research, in turn, has implications for the design of new approaches to treatment.

BACKGROUND

There have been a number of comprehensive reviews of the research on comorbidity (3,4,8,13,14). In this section, we will focus specifically on three measures of comorbidity that are currently used in studies of cancer in older populations. Together, these three measures highlight the different ways in which the extent and severity of comorbidity have been summarized. We will also review different sources of data for work in this area.

CHARLSON INDEX

This index, clearly the most commonly used comorbidity measure, provides an overall score based on a composite of values weighted by level of severity and assigned for any of 19 selected conditions (15). Many versions of the Charlson index have been developed for use with medical records, administrative databases, and personal interviews. The score for each condition is based on the results of a preliminary study of the one-year, age-adjusted relative risks of death for hospitalized patients with selected conditions. In its original version, a score of 1 was assigned to those conditions with an age-adjusted relative risk of 1.2 to 1.5 (e.g., myocardial infarction); a score of 2 was assigned to those conditions with an age-adjusted relative risk of 1.5 to 2.5 (e.g., diabetes with end organ damage); and a score of 3 was assigned to those conditions with age-adjusted relative risks of 2.5 to 6.0 (e.g., moderate or severe liver disease). A score of 6 was assigned to two conditions (acquired immunodeficiency syndrome and other metastatic cancer) with an age-adjusted relative risk of 6 or more. Conditions with a relative risk of less than 1.2 were not included. Scores for most conditions ranged from 1 to 3. Using these severity weights, the overall comorbidity score is based on the sum of the scores for the individual conditions. Charlson et al. developed a later version of this instrument, which included chronological age in the final calculation of the severity score (16).

CUMULATIVE ILLNESS RATING SCALE

The cumulative illness rating scale (CIRS) was originally developed to provide a general measure of health (13,14,17). Rather than focusing on individual diagnosed conditions, as was done with the Charlson index, the CIRS is based on a systematic assessment of separate organ systems. Each of the organ systems is rated on a scale from 0 to 4 in the following manner—no disease, mild, moderate, severe, or very severe/life threatening. The score for each organ system is based on the score for the most severe health condition within that category. The organ systems are (a) cardiac; (b) vascular; (c) respiratory; (d) eyes, ears, nose, throat; and larynx; (e) upper gastrointestinal (GI); (f) lower GI;

(g) liver; (h) renal, or genitourinary; (i) musculoskeletal; (j) neurological; (k) psychiatric; and (l) endocrine-metabolic. The total score is based on the summation of scores across the organ systems. This is an example of a standard measure of overall health that has been used to assess comorbidity. This measure is being used increasingly in studies of comorbidity and cancer (13,14).

ADULT COMORBIDITY EVALUATION (ACE-27)

This is a new measure that was designed specifically to assess comorbidity among cancer patients (18). The presence and severity of 27 health diagnoses and conditions are rated within 11 different categories. The 27 conditions consist of both regular diagnoses such as myocardial infarction and end-stage renal disease, and conditions or states such as alcohol levels and obesity. The categories include the cardiovascular, respiratory, GI, endocrine, neurological, psychiatric, rheumatologic, immunological, and malignancy, as well as substance abuse and body weight. Each category is rated in terms of the severity of the most serous condition within that category. Severity is measured by three grades: mild, moderate, and severe "decompensation." The overall comorbidity score is based on the highest-ranked single condition within a category and summarized on a four-point scale (none: 0, mild: 1, moderate: 2, and severe: 3). If two or more grade 2 conditions are found in one or more of the categories, the overall comorbidity score is assigned the most severe category of 3. The measure has been shown to independently predict survival among patients diagnosed with head and neck cancer (19). To our knowledge, the prognostic utility of this instrument has not been compared to either the Charlson or CIRS indices.

SUMMARY

Each of the three instruments provides a summary score that reflects the overall severity of conditions for subjects with an index condition of cancer. The more severe the level of comorbidity, the greater the risk of dying. All three measures assume an additive relationship among the health conditions. This means that the overall "comorbidity burden" experienced by a patient is based on the summation of the levels of severity for each individual condition or category. The possibility of multiplicative or synergistic relationships among conditions is not considered. In addition, none of the three measures includes information about the date of the onset of the conditions. In other words, the temporal ordering of conditions, i.e., when they were first diagnosed and treated, is not included in the calculation of the final severity score. It makes no difference in the scoring of the instruments whether an individual health condition preceded or followed another. In all cases, researchers adapt the instrument by deleting the index condition from the list of health conditions to avoid double counting. For example, the index cancer is not included in the calculation of the overall comorbidity score. However, other past and current primary cancers would be included. Despite the similarities among the instruments, there are also differences. The overall scores for the CIRS and ACE-27 are based, for the most part, on the individual's most severe condition or state within a category. In contrast, the Charlson index is derived from a total of the values for each individual health condition, severity value being based on the risk of death associated with each condition. Finally, unlike the Charlson index and the CIRS, information about treatment is included in the calculation of severity for the ACE-27. Conditions that require current medical management are considered to be more severe than those that are managed without medications.

This review represents only a brief summary of the similarities and differences among three leading comorbidity measures. The reader is referred to more detailed reviews and comparison of these and other measures (3,4,13,14,20).

SOURCES OF DATA

Medical records, administrative databases, and personal interviews are the three major sources of information on comorbidity. We will consider each source in turn.

Medical records have been the most common source of data for measures of comorbidity, especially in epidemiological studies (8,14,15,17). Although it is possible that comorbid conditions may be antecedent, concurrent, or subsequent to the index cancer, data on comorbidity are typically based on medical records from the hospitalization associated with the first cancer treatment. While medical records represent the most common source of data on comorbidity, concerns about selection bias have been raised. Differences in the number and types of comorbidity may reflect the number of physician visits and hospitalizations rather than actual health differences among people. A person who has had more physician visits and hospitalizations has a greater chance of having a comorbid condition identified. An additional concern is that a review of medical records may be too time consuming and costly for large cohorts of patients. Finally, reductions in hospital use and lengths of stay mean that hospitalization-based data are likely to be incomplete because they do not often include information contained in records from the ambulatory care setting, further exacerbating problems of accessibility and cost.

It should be noted that there are systems in place to access medical records for studies of comorbidity and cancer, more efficiently. For example, the National Institute on Aging/National Cancer Institute Comorbidity Study demonstrated that it was feasible for cancer registrars to collect information on comorbidity from the medical record as part of their regular cancer case identification process (21,22). In this case, data on comorbidity were obtained from a review of medical records, primarily physicians' notes, anesthesia notes, nursing notes, discharge summaries, and radiology and laboratory reports. As another example, the ACE-27 was designed to be used by cancer registrars as part of regular cancer surveillance (18). In fact, Piccirillo and colleagues developed and evaluated detailed instructional methods for cancer registrars in the use of the ACE-27 (23).

Electronic administrative databases have been evaluated as a more efficient source of data (24). The size and complexity of the databases range from computerized discharge summaries of individual hospitals to the computerized records of the Medicare and Medicaid populations in the United States. Comorbidity data are based on the diagnostic code fields associated with a hospitalization or visit. Although at least five comorbidity indices have been adapted for use with administrative data, there are potential challenges. As an example, in 1993, Deyo et al. (25) adapted and evaluated the Charlson index for an outcome study of Medicare beneficiaries who underwent lumbar spine surgery. Later, Romano et al. (26), although acknowledging the prognostic significance of the Charlson index, expressed reservations about the translation between the items in the Charlson index and the International Classification of Disease (ICD-9-CM) administrative data. They also argued that the Charlson index, based on an examination of a hospitalized population in New York, may not be completely generalizable to other patients with other conditions, a concern also expressed by others. Later comparisons found no significant difference between the Romano and Deyo adaptations (27). Finally, there is also growing evidence that the comprehensiveness and generalizability of administrative databases are variable and can be improved by including records from both inpatient and outpatient care. In one national study, for example, less than 10% of elderly prostate and breast cancer patients had comorbid conditions, as summarized by a Charlson index, when data were obtained from Part A Medicare hospital claims. However, the percentage of patients with comorbid conditions increased to approximately 25% when data from physician claims data also were used (28).

Personal interviews have also been used as a source of information on comorbidity, especially in studies that are designed to estimate the prevalence of comorbid conditions in the general population (29,30). Katz et al. (31) have developed an interview-based version of the Charlson index. Although personal interviews have been used in general population surveys, they are less likely to be used in studies of comorbidity in cancer patients. The use of interviews as a source of comorbidity data has several advantages. First, it is an efficient and less costly procedure than a review of medical records. Second, in a case–control study, it ensures that data on comorbidity are obtained in the same manner for both cancer patients and controls. Third, it provides an opportunity to obtain alternative data on severity. Unlike an index such as the Charlson measure, which uses the risk of death as the sole measure of severity, an interview-based system may also use the subject's reported functional limitations to establish severity. Although comorbidity measures such as the Greenfield index (32) include functional data from the medical record, there is concern that functional data, typically found only in nurses' notes, are not consistently available. Finally, personal interviews may provide a more comprehensive view of health by including information on the prevalence of reported symptoms, in addition to diagnosed conditions. Despite these strengths, there are weaknesses. As with medical records and administrative databases, the personal interview may not completely ascertain all of a patient's past and current health conditions. Further, patients, especially elderly patients, may not know or accurately recall all diagnoses.

Multiple sources of data can be used together to provide a more complete picture of a patient's level of comorbidity (33). The multiple informant approach is ideally suited for circumstances in which multiple measures of a concept are available, but none is comprehensive or without missing data. As such, this approach merges parallel streams of information from all measures into a unified regression model, allowing for use of all available information. Using this approach, the multiple informant regression was superior to regression models that included only one measure of comorbidity (33).

COMORBIDITY AND CANCER MANAGEMENT

In general, older cancer patients with comorbid conditions are less likely than younger patients with comorbid conditions to receive standard definitive therapies (34–39). One of the important questions is whether these variations in care result in the best outcomes for older patients with comorbid conditions. Research to identify the most effective treatment approaches that take into account reduced physiologic reserve associated with comorbidity have been based on case studies, observational studies, and decision analyses (40–45). Decision analysis is a method for the incorporation of data from a variety of clinical and epidemiologic sources to model and compare different approaches to treatment (46). Although these studies have proved useful in understanding the effects of comorbidity on cancer management, there is general agreement that clinical trials will provide the most definitive information about the effects of comorbidity on cancer treatment efficacy. Unfortunately, as is well known, older people are less likely than younger people to be recruited for and enrolled in clinical trials (47–49). One of the reasons for this enrollment difference is that older people are less likely than younger people to meet physiologic and functional inclusion criteria. In addition, one study of breast cancer patients found that physicians' perceptions of age and tolerance of toxicity were the most significant predictors of invitations to participate in clinical trials (48). In general, the exclusion of older people with comorbidity from clinical trials serves to maintain the "internal validity" of the trial (absence of extraneous variables, clarity of design, and ease of administration) at the expense of its "external validity" (representativeness of the sample subjects and generalizability of results to the population of interest).

APPLIED COMORBIDITY RESEARCH

One of the primary objectives of geriatric oncology is to develop treatment plans that are tailored to the physiologic capacity of older patients (4,10,50). Comprehensive geriatric assessment (CGA) is one strategy to individualize cancer treatment to meet the special needs of older cancer patients. CGA is defined as "a multidimensional, interdisciplinary process that identifies medical, functional, and psychosocial problems and helps to develop a comprehensive management and care plan" (4, p. 149). One function of CGA is to identify three categories of older cancer patients (51). First, there are patients who are functionally independent and without comorbidity. These patients are candidates for most standard cancer treatments, with bone marrow transplants being an example of an exception. Second, there are complexly ill patients who are most appropriately candidates for a palliative care approach. Finally, there is a heterogeneous group of older patients between these robust and sick groups who will benefit from a tailored approach that takes into account individual vulnerabilities.

Although the approach to CGA varies, it typically includes assessments of physical functional status, cognition, emotional status, social support, nutrition, medications, and, important for our considerations here, comorbidity (50). Recent work is considering comorbidity, both in terms of measures of overall severity and in terms of the number of individual conditions, within the broader context of evaluations of the CGA strategy. There are several reasons for this approach. First, comorbidity and other factors such as physical function independently predict future life expectancy (52–54). For example, Walter et al. (53) developed and validated a prognostic index to predict one-year mortality in older adults after hospitalization. The prognostic index was derived from an examination of survival among 1495 patients aged 70 and older who were treated by a general medical service at a tertiary care hospital. The index was later validated in a cohort of patients discharged from a community teaching hospital. The original set of variables included measures of overall cognitive function, modified versions of Activities of Daily Living and Instrumental Activities of Daily Living, laboratory values, and the Charlson index, described previously. In these cohorts, measures of function predicted survival, independent of comorbidity. However, only two of the medical diagnoses from the Charlson index (congestive heart failure and cancer) predicted subsequent one-year survival. These results suggest that while comorbidity is important, it is only one of several factors that should be taken into account in developing cancer treatment plans for older patients. Second, in addition to a more refined calculation of life expectancy, the inclusion of comorbid conditions may result in more effective overall management of the older cancer patient when the comorbid condition can be more effectively addressed.

This point was underscored in the recent report of the National Comprehensive Cancer Network that presented an algorithm for the development of management plans for older cancer patients (55). The algorithm consists of three stages: screening, assessment, and findings. The screening stage is designed to assess the patient's future life expectancy. Following from the previously noted work of Walter et al. (53), life expectancy is based on functional status and comorbidity. If life expectancy is judged to be less than the life expectancy for someone with the specific type and stage of cancer, then the older patient is a candidate for symptom management and supportive care. If, however, the patient is expected to die of cancer or experience complications within the patients' estimated lifetime, then an evaluation should be done to determine the extent of functional dependency and comorbidity. This assessment includes the detection and correction of reversible conditions that may complicate treatment.

Although CGA has been shown to reduce pain and improve mental health of older cancer patients (56), there have been relatively few systematic assessments of its effectiveness. Moreover, even if CGA were shown to be effective, its feasibility in clinical practice is questionable (5). As Misra et al. (5, p. 458) report:

> Geriatric assessment in the evaluation of older cancer patients is an area of active research. Such an assessment may help the oncologist get a sense of the patient's biological age and identify patients at risk for functional decline or treatment toxicity. However, this is a time-consuming process, expensive and labor intensive. Therefore, CGA is often not feasible in a clinical setting.

BASIC COMORBIDITY RESEARCH

Basic comorbidity research examines the temporal interaction among such key variables as aging, comorbidity conditions, and functional status. This research includes investigation of possible multiplicative associations among variables. In applied research, as noted previously, the objective is to identify the most parsimonious set of factors such as comorbidity and physical and cognitive functioning to best characterize physiologic age and best predict subsequent life expectancy. In basic research, the task is to understand the mechanisms and causal patterns among those variables. To date, basic comorbidity research has not focused on cancer as an index condition. As outlined by Albert et al. (57), physiological changes of aging, such as sarcopenia and hypometabolism, may independently, or in conjunction with single and multiple conditions, affect the risk of disability (Fig. 1).

Moreover, as Verbrugge and Jette (58) note, the timing and scope of the disablement process are also affected by a variety of behavioral, social, and environmental factors.

Research in this area may lead to a clearer understanding of the physiologic mechanism associated with comorbidity. For example, there is a growing body of research on "allostatic load," a measure of dysregulation across multiple organ systems that has been associated longitudinally with functional decline and death

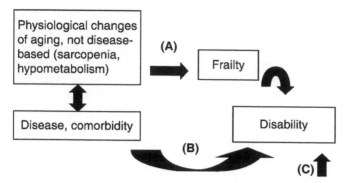

Figure 1 Three pathways to disability: (**A**) senescence leading to frailty; (**B**) disease; and (**C**) environmental, psychological, and social factors. *Source*: From Ref. 57.

(59). Indeed, Seeman et al. (59) point to comorbidity as a clinical manifestation of cumulative physiological burden:

> No single form of comorbidity occurs with high frequency, but rather a multiplicity of diverse combinations are observed (e.g., osteoarthritis and diabetes, colon cancer, coronary heart disease, depression, and hypertension). This diversity underscores the need for an early warning system of biomarkers that can signal early signs of dysregulation across multiple physiological systems.

Although research on allostatic load and its implications for basic research in comorbidity is promising, criticisms have been raised (60). First, there is concern over the fact that only a small number of indicators of dysregulation have been available for examination. As a result, it has not been possible to examine a full complement of possible biological systems. Second, there are concerns that the measurements of these systems are based on resting levels and may not accurately reflect the actual allostatic process—a process that may be better reflected in a setting based on an environmental challenge.

There has also been discussion about the interrelationship among comorbidity, frailty, and disability (61). While some researchers tend to see these concepts as overlapping, Fried et al. (61) view frailty as a summary physiologic pathway between comorbidity and disability. The task is to explain how and under what circumstances comorbidity, in conjunction with other factors, leads to frailty, which in turn affects functional limitations and disability. Work in this area will depend on refinements in the conceptualization and measurement of both frailty and comorbidity.

Basic research also requires a reconsideration of the diagnosed condition, as the primary unit of comorbidity. The unit of comorbidity may be expanded to include "pre-clinical conditions" on the one hand and disease symptoms on the other. Unlike applied research, basic research is not restricted to data that are readily available to most practitioners. It is reasonable to assume that studies in this area will require large clinical and population-based epidemiologic studies.

In conclusion, it is important to realize that while applied research and basic research have distinct research agendas, their activities are related in important ways. First, applied comorbidity research reminds us that one of the key objectives of all cancer research is to improve the likelihood of survival and the quality of life of cancer patients. Second, basic research should lead ultimately to better understanding of the mechanisms of the associations among cancer, comorbidity, function, and survival. This knowledge, in turn, should contribute to more effective applied research and practice.

RECOMMENDATIONS

1. More refined measures of comorbidity should be developed for future work in this area. First, it necessary to examine the independent effects of individual comorbid conditions in combination with specific forms of cancer on the duration and quality of life. Second, it is necessary to determine whether the nature of those prognostic effects varies by age, gender, race, socioeconomic status, tumor type, and tumor biology. Disease algorithms should be developed for the clear and consistent identification of individual comorbidities as well as assessment of potential risks, including side effects, associated with strategies to treat the index cancer. The objective should be to determine the additive and, as noted previously, the multiplicative effects of specific combinations of conditions in older adults, as well as overall summary measures of comorbidity. In other words, it should be possible to move from the assessment of individual conditions, to combinations of conditions, to overall summary measures of comorbidity.

2. An assessment of patterns of comorbidity and cancer should include an examination of the extent to which the diagnosis of an index cancer affects the treatment and course of a pre-existing comorbid condition. This will provide a more complete picture of the constellation of conditions that may be affecting a patient over time.

3. The independent, prognostic significance of new measures of comorbidity should be assessed, in conjunction with other measures such as physical function.

4. Clinical trials in representative populations of older people with cancer are needed to better establish the efficacy of CGA in this context. Moreover, determining which components are most useful in specific groups of patients is also critically needed.

5. Basic research in comorbidity should be encouraged. Specifically, more attention should be given to the mechanisms and pathways that connect comorbidity, cancer, disability, and death. Perhaps, research on multiple physiological systems such as allostatic load will contribute important information about the interface of comorbidity, functional status, and tumor biology.

6. Special effort should be made to support methodological studies to enhance both applied and basic comorbidity research. This research agenda should include comparisons of the utility and validity of different indices, different data sources, and different analytic techniques. The utility of multiple informant regression as an alternative approach ought to be compared with the implementation of just a single index from one data source, identified at the outset of study to be the optimal choice.

7. The epidemiology of comorbidity needs to be more fully developed. For example, is there a common set of risk factors that underlie multiple conditions? This research agenda will include the examination of genetic, behavioral, social, and environmental factors associated with specific patterns of comorbid conditions among older people diagnosed with cancer.

8. There is need to develop a new generation of clinical trials. Following the development of more refined measures of physiologic age, it may be possible to establish more sophisticated designs for clinical trials. It may be possible, for example, to stratify by different levels of physiologic capacity. Subjects could then be randomly assigned to different treatment protocols within each level of capacity. Not only will this design enable researchers to better assess the relationship between individual reserve and treatment outcomes, but it will also provide an opportunity to more effectively generalize the results of the trial to a wider population of older cancer patients. In many ways, the development of a new generation of clinical trials will represent the convergence of basic and applied comorbidity research, facilitating the optimization of patient care.

REFERENCES

1. Feinstein AR. The pre-therapeutic classification of co-morbidity in chronic diseases. J Chron Dis 1970; 23:455–469.
2. Piccirillo JF, Feinstein AR. Clinical symptoms and comorbidity: significance for prognostic classification of cancer. Cancer 1996; 77:834–842.
3. Satariano WA. Comorbidities and cancer. In: Hunter CP, Johnson KA, Muss HB, eds. Cancer in the Elderly. New York: Marcel Dekker, 2000:477–499.
4. Rao AV, Seo PH, Cohen HJ. Geriatric assessment and comorbidity. Semin Oncol 2004; 31:149–159.
5. Misra D, Seo PH, Cohen HJ. Aging and cancer. Clin Adv Hematol Oncol 2004; 2:457–465.
6. Yancik R, Havlik RJ, Wesley MN, et al. Cancer and comorbidity in older patients: a descriptive profile. Ann Epidemiol 1996:399–412.
7. Satariano WA, Silliman RA. Comorbidity: implications for research and practice in geriatric oncology. Crit Rev Oncol Hematol 2003; 48:239–248.
8. Gijsen R, Hoeymans N, Schellevis FG, Ruwaard D, Satariano WA, van den Bos GA. Causes and consequences of comorbidity: a review. J Clin Epidemiol 2001; 54:661–674.
9. Yates JW. Comorbidity considerations in geriatric oncology research. CA J Clin 2001; 51:329–336.
10. Repetto L, Venturino A, Fratino L, et al. Geriatric oncology: a clinical approach to the older patient with cancer. Eur J Cancer 2003; 39:870–880.
11. Lichtman SM. Guidelines for treatment of elderly cancer patients. Cancer Control 2003; 10:445–453.
12. Yancik R, Ganz PA, Varricchio CG, Conley B. Perspectives on comorbidity and cancer in older patients: approaches to expand the knowledge base. J Clin Oncol 2001; 19: 1147–1151.
13. Extermann M. Measurement and impact of comorbidity in older cancer patients. Crit Rev Oncol Hematol 2000; 35:181–200.
14. Extermann M. Measuring comorbidity in older cancer patients. Eur J Cancer 2000; 36:453–471.
15. Charlson ME, Pompei P, Alex KL, Mackenzie CR. A new method of classifying prognostic comorbidity in longitudinal studies: development and validation. J Chron Dis 1987; 40:373–383.
16. Charlson ME, Szatrowski TP, Peterson J, Gold J. Validation of a combined comorbidity index. J Clin Epidemiol 1994; 47:1245–1251.
17. Linn BS, Linn MW, Gurel L. Cumulative illness rating scale. J Am Geriatr Soc 1968; 16: 622–626.
18. Piccirillo JF, Creech C, Zequeira R, Anderson S, Johnston AS. Inclusion of comorbidity into oncology data registries. J Reg Man 1999; 26:66–70.

19. Piccirillo JF. The impact of comorbidity in head and neck cancer. J Reg Man 2001; 28:173–176.

20. DeGroot V, Beckerman J, Lankhourst GJ, Bouter LM. How to measure comorbidity: a critical review of available methods. J Clin Epidemiol 2003; 56:221–229.

21. Yancik R, Wesley MN, Ries LA, et al. Comorbidity and age as predictors of risk for early mortality of male and female colon carcinoma patients: a population-based study. Cancer 1998; 82:2123–2134.

22. Yancik R, Wesley MN, Ries LA, Havlik RJ, Edwards BK, Yates JW. Effect of age and comorbidity in postmenopausal breast cancer patients aged 55 years and older. JAMA 2001; 285:885–892.

23. Johnston AS, Piccirillo JF, Creech C, Littenberg B, Jeffe J, Spitznagel EL. Validation of a comorbidity education program. J Reg Man 2001; 26:66–70.

24. Klabunde CN, Warren J, Legler JM. Assessing comorbidity using claims data: an overview. Med Care 2002; 40(8 suppl):IV-26–IV-35.

25. Deyo RA, Cherkin DC, Clol MA. Adapting a clinical comorbidity index for use with ICD-9-CM administrative databases. J Clin Epidemiol 1992; 45:613–619.

26. Romano PS, Roos LL, Jollis JG. Adapting a clinical comorbidity index for use with ICD-9-CM administrative data: differing perspectives. J Clin Epidemiol 1993; 46:1075–1079.

27. Ghali WA, Hall RE, Rosen AK, Ash AS, Moskowitz MA. Searching for an improved comorbidity index for use with ICD-9-CM administrative data. J Clin Epidemiol 1996; 49:273–278.

28. Klabunde CN, Potosky AL, Legler JM, Warren JL. Development of a comorbidity index using physician claims data. J Clin Epidemiol 2000; 53:1258–1267.

29. Seeman TE, Guralnik JM, Kaplan GA, Knudsen L, Cohen R. The health consequences of multiple morbidity in the elderly: the Alameda County Study. J Aging Health 1989; 1:50–66.

30. Guralnik JM, LaCroix AZ, Everett DF, Kovar MG. Aging in the Eighties: The Prevalence of Comorbidity and Its Association with Disability, Vol. 170. Hyattsville, MD: Advanced Data from Vital and Health Statistics, National Center for Health Statistics, 1989.

31. Katz JN, Change LC, Sangha O, Fossel AH, Bates DW. Can comorbidity be measured by questionnaire rather than medical record review? Med Care 1996; 34:73–84.

32. Greenfield S, Blanco DM, Elashoff RM, Ganz PA. Patterns of care related to age of breast cancer patients. JAMA 1987; 257:2766–2770.

33. Lash TL, Thwin SS, Horton NJ, Guadagnoli E, Silliman RA. Multiple informants: a new method to assess breast cancer patients' comorbidity. Am J Epidemiol 2003; 157:249–257.

34. Samet J, Key C, Hunt W, Goodwin JS. Choice of cancer therapy varies with age of the patient. JAMA 1986; 255:3385–3390.

35. Guadagnoli E, Weitberg A, Mor V, Silliman RA, Glicksman AS, Cummings FJ. The influence of patient age on the diagnosis and treatment of lung and colorectal cancer. Arch Intern Med 1990; 150:1485–1490.

36. Audisio RA, Ramesch H, Longo WE, Zbar AP, Pope D. Preoperative assessment of surgical risk in oncogeriatric patients. Oncologist 2005; 10:262–268.

37. Lemmens VEPP, Janssen-Heignen MLG, Verheij CDGW, Houterman S, Repelaer van Driel OJ, Coebergh JWW. Co-morbidity leads to altered treatment and worse survival of elderly patients with colorectal cancer. Br J Surg 2005; 92:615–623.

38. Louwman WJ, Janssen-Heignen MLG, Houterman S, et al. Less extensive treatment and inferior prognosis for breast cancer patient with comorbidity: a population-based study. Eur J Cancer 2005; 41:779–785.

39. Truong PT, Kader HA, Lacy B, et al. The effects of age and comorbidity on treatment and outcomes in women with endometrial cancer. Am J Clin Oncol 2005; 28:157–164.

40. Robinson BE, Balducci L. Breast lump in an 85-year-old women with dementia: a decision analysis. J Am Geriatr Soc 1995; 43:282–285.

41. Ravdin PM. A computer program to assist in making breast cancer adjuvant therapy decision analysis. J Am Geriatr Soc 1995; 43:282–285.

42. Katton MW, Carven ME, Miles BJ. A decision analysis for treatment of clinically localized prostate cancer. J Gen Intern Med 1997; 12:299–305.

43. Mandelblatt JS, Wheat ME, Monane M. Breast cancer screening for elderly women: with and without Comorbid conditions: a decision model. Ann Intern Med 1992; 116:772–730.

44. Extermann M. Decision analysis for cancer prevention and cancer treatment in the elderly. Cancer Treat Res 2005; 124:223–232.

45. Cohen J, Britten N. Who decides about prostate cancer treatment? A qualitative study. Fam Pract 2005; 20:724–729.

46. Pauker SG, Kassirer JP. Decision analysis. N Engl J Med 1987; 316:250–258.

47. Applegate WB, Curb JD. Designing and executing randomized clinical trials involved elderly persons. J Am Geriatr Soc 1990; 38:943–950.

48. Kemeny MM, Peterson BL, Kornblith AB, et al. Barriers to clinical trial participation by older women with breast cancer. J Clin Oncol 2003:2268–2275.

49. Aapro MS, Kohne C-H, Cohen HJ, Extermann M. Never too old? Age should not be a barrier to enrollment in cancer clinical trials. Oncologist 2005; 10:198–204.

50. Repetto L, Balducci L. A case for geriatric oncology. Lancet Oncol 2002; 3:289–297.

51. Balducci L, Extermann M. Management of cancer in the older person: a practical approach. Oncologist 2000; 5:224–237.

52. Extermann M, Overcash J, Lyman GH, Parr J, Balducci L. Comorbidity and functional status are independent in older cancer patients. J Clin Oncol 1998; 16:1582–1587.

53. Walter LC, Brand RJ, Counsell SR, et al. Development and validation of a prognostic index for 1-year mortality in older adults after hospitalization. JAMA 2001; 285:2987–2994.

54. Walter LC, Covinsky KE. Cancer screening in elderly patients: a framework for individualized decision making. JAMA 2001; 285:2750–2756.

55. Clinical Practice Guidelines in Oncology—Vol. 1. National Comprehensive Cancer Network, 2005.

56. Rao AV, Hsieh F, Feussner JR, Cohen HJ. Geriatric evaluation and management units in the care of the frail elderly cancer patient. J Geront Med Sci 2005; 60A:798–803.

57. Albert SM, Im A, Raveis VH. Public health and the second 50 years of life. Am J Public Health 2002; 92:1214–1216.

58. Verbrugge LM, Jette AM. The disablement process. Soc Sci Med 1994; 38:1–14.

59. Seeman TE, McEwen BS, Rowe JW, Singer BH. Allostatic load as a marker of cumulative biological risk: Macarthur studies of successful aging. PNAS 2001; 98:4770–4775.

60. Satariano WA. Epidemiology of Aging: An Ecological Approach. Sudbury, Massachusetts: Jones & Bartlett, 2006:52–53.

61. Fried LP, Ferrucci L, Darer J, Williamson JD, Anderson G. Untangling the concepts of disability, frailty, and comorbidity: implications for improved targeting and care. J Geront Med Sci 2004; 59:255–263.

23

Exercise and Physical Fitness in Older Cancer Survivors

Kerry S. Courneya, Margaret L. McNeely, Kristina H. Karvinen, and Christopher M. Sellar
Faculty of Physical Education and Recreation, University of Alberta, Edmonton, Alberta, Canada

INTRODUCTION

Exercise is considered a foundational behavior for human health and well-being in almost all populations including older adults (≥ 65 years of age) and most chronic disease populations. Cancer is one chronic disease, however, where the benefits and risks of exercise are only beginning to be described. Moreover, what little is known about exercise in cancer survivors is derived largely from research on middle-aged and younger survivors despite the fact that the majority of people diagnosed with cancer are older adults. In the present chapter, we review the potential role of exercise in attenuating the effects of cancer and its treatments in older cancer survivors.

We begin by defining some of the key terms in the field of kinesiology and reviewing the literature on functional decline associated with aging. We then review several recent systematic reviews on exercise in cancer survivors, noting that very few studies have focused on older adults. Given this state of affairs, we conduct a supplementary literature review of exercise in older adults in general. Following these reviews, we provide general exercise screening, testing, and prescription guidelines for older cancer survivors. After that, we discuss the issue of exercise motivation and adherence in older cancer survivors. Finally, we offer future research directions to move this emerging field of research and practice forward. We conclude that although there is limited direct evidence on the benefits of exercise in older cancer survivors, there is convincing evidence of the benefits of exercise in other older adult populations and promising evidence for the benefits of exercise in middle-aged and younger cancer survivors. This evidence makes us cautiously optimistic that exercise will be an effective supportive care and rehabilitation therapy for older cancer survivors both during and after treatments.

KEY DEFINITIONS IN THE FIELD OF KINESIOLOGY

Kinesiology is the study of human movement. By human movement, we mean any bodily movement that is produced by the skeletal muscles and results in an energy expenditure that exceeds resting levels. From a health perspective, four key kinesiology -related terms are "physical activity," "leisure-time physical activity," "exercise," and "physical fitness." Bouchard and Shephard (1) have provided consensus definitions of these terms. Physical activity is defined as human movement that results in a *substantial* increase in energy expenditure over resting levels. While the term "substantial" is not explicitly defined, we take it to mean human movement of at least a moderate intensity (e.g., brisk walking). Leisure-time physical activity is defined as physical activity undertaken during discretionary time, with the key element being personal choice. This form of physical activity is often contrasted with occupational and household physical activity. While all types of physical activity are believed to contribute to health, most behavior-change interventions are, by necessity, directed toward leisure-time physical activity. Exercise is defined as a form of leisure-time physical activity that is usually performed on a repeated basis over an extended period of time with the intention of improving fitness, performance, or health. An exercise training prescription usually includes activity mode (e.g., walking, swimming), volume (i.e., frequency, intensity, and duration), progression, or periodization (i.e., increase or variability over time), and context (i.e., physical and social environment). Physical fitness is defined as the ability to perform muscular work satisfactorily and commonly includes the components of cardiorespiratory fitness, muscular fitness, flexibility, agility/balance, and body composition.

DECLINES IN PHYSICAL FUNCTIONING WITH AGE

It is well known that aging is associated with declines in physical functioning. One significant physical change with aging is the development of sarcopenia, which is defined as the loss of skeletal muscle mass, strength, and quality (2,3). It is estimated that individuals begin to lose muscle mass between 30 and 40 years of age (4). Older adults may also experience compromised bone density (low bone mass) that may ultimately lead to osteoporosis. Decreased bone mass may substantially affect an individual's capacity to perform activities of daily living and is associated with frailty in the elderly (5).

Research has also documented the loss of flexibility with age. The inability to perform movements with the full range of motion may be associated with difficulty climbing stairs and getting out of bed, and with the use of a walking aid (6). Functional capacity also declines with age. Maximal oxygen consumption declines approximately 10% per decade (7). It appears that these declines begin in the third decade of life. In older adults, it is expected that over half of their functional capacity has been lost, thus compromising their ability to execute common activities of daily living due to an inadequate cardiovascular system (8). Taken together, declines in muscle function, bone density, flexibility, postural control, and functional capacity all contribute to a decrease in the functional well-being and quality of life (QOL) of older adults. Moreover, as noted in other chapters in this book, almost all of these declines are exacerbated by cancer and its treatments.

EXERCISE BENEFITS IN OLDER CANCER SURVIVORS

An important question is whether exercise might offset some of the declines in functioning and QOL that occur with cancer treatments in older adults. There have been four recent systematic reviews of exercise in cancer survivors (9–12) and one narrative review that has adopted an older adult perspective (13). Given the plethora of recent reviews on this topic, we have elected to summarize these reviews rather than provide details of the original studies. The reader is referred to these reviews for more details of individual studies.

Stevinson et al. (9) completed a systematic review of 33 controlled trials (25 randomized) that examined the effects of exercise in any cancer survivor group. Thirteen (39%) of the trials focused exclusively on breast cancer survivors while another 11 (33%) included breast cancer survivors. Interestingly, the ages of the participants were not even reported in this review. Nineteen (58%) of the trials tested aerobic exercise interventions (mainly walking and biking) while another 10 (30%) combined aerobic and resistance exercise. Most trials compared an exercise intervention to usual care. Only 17 (52%) trials tested an exercise intervention that lasted 10 weeks or longer. The results from this review showed that exercise is an effective intervention for improving physical function in cancer survivors both during and after treatments without exacerbating fatigue or increasing the incidence of adverse events. The evidence for other outcomes such as QOL was considered to be insufficient to make even tentative conclusions. Moreover, the overall methodological quality of the trials was considered modest.

Galvao and Newton (10) reviewed 26 published exercise interventions that examined the effects of exercise in any cancer survivor group either during or after treatment. Eighteen (69%) of the studies were conducted during treatments, while the other eight (31%) were conducted after treatments. Twelve (46%) of the studies focused exclusively on breast cancer survivors while another five (19%) included breast cancer survivors. Only one study (4%) reported a mean age of ≥65 years and only 10 studies (38%) reported an age range that included survivors ≥65 years of age. Eighteen (69%) of the studies focused exclusively on aerobic exercise while another six (23%) tested a combined aerobic and resistance exercise intervention. The authors concluded that, despite some methodological concerns and small sample sizes, a majority of studies have shown physiological and psychological benefits for cancer survivors both during and after treatment.

Schmitz et al. (11) completed a systematic review and meta-analysis of 32 controlled exercise trials (27 randomized) in cancer survivors either during or after treatment. Twenty (63%) of the studies examined exercise during treatments while 12 (37%) focused on the post-treatment time period. Breast cancer survivors were the exclusive or primary group in 23 (72%) of the studies and the mean sample size of the studies was 54. The majority of the interventions consisted of aerobic exercise of moderate-to-vigorous intensity, three to five days per week, for 20 to 30 minutes each day. The length of the interventions was three months or less in 25 (79%) of the studies. Again, the ages in the study samples were not reported. The results showed that exercise was effective in improving cardiorespiratory fitness during and after cancer treatments, symptoms and physiologic effects during treatment, and vigor post-treatment. Other outcomes were deemed insufficient to make conclusions.

McNeely et al. (12) performed a meta-analysis of randomized controlled trials (RCTs) examining the benefits of exercise for breast cancer survivors.

The meta-analysis included 14 relevant studies involving 715 participants ranging in age from 35 to 72 years, with no study having an average age of over 65 years. Six studies focused exclusively on aerobic exercise training, one focused exclusively on resistance training, one study with three forms compared aerobic training and resistance training to a control condition, and one study examined the effect of Tai Chi Chuan. The pooled data from included studies showed significant positive effects of exercise on QOL, cardiorespiratory fitness, and physical functioning. The pooled data also demonstrated a statistically significant effect of exercise on symptoms of fatigue. The benefit was both statistically and clinically significant following cancer treatment; however, the evidence suggested a potentially small effect of exercise on fatigue during adjuvant treatment. There was also no evidence of significant benefit of exercise in reducing body weight. The authors concluded that future research would benefit from larger sample sizes, increased attention to study quality, and examination of long-term effects.

Courneya et al. (13) have recently reviewed 50 studies of exercise in cancer survivors from an older adult perspective. They reported that of the 48 studies that provided data on the age of the sample, 10 actually used age as an exclusion criterion. Except for one study that focused on children, the upper age restriction was 60 in three studies, 65 in two studies, and 70 in four studies. Consequently, similar to cancer treatment trials, some exercise trials have also excluded older adults based on age. Moreover, the mean age of the 48 samples was 48 ± 9 and the median age was 50. In fact, only two studies had samples with a mean age above 65 years and only two additional studies had a mean age above 60 years. Finally, of the 22 studies that reported the age range of their sample, very few even had an upper age range that would include a substantial number of older cancer survivors. Specifically, only one study had an age range above 80 years, and only one additional study had an age range above 75 years. It is clear from this review that no exercise studies have specifically targeted older cancer survivors for recruitment and, consequently, most exercise studies have attracted younger cancer survivors.

To partially address this issue, Courneya et al. (13) reported ancillary sub-analyses based on age for two of their previously published trials: the Rehabilitation Exercise for Health After Breast Cancer (REHAB) trial (14,15) and the Group Psychotherapy and Home-Based Physical Exercise (GROUP-HOPE) trial (16–18). The REHAB trial was an RCT that examined the effects of supervised aerobic exercise training on cardiopulmonary, QOL, and biologic outcomes in postmenopausal breast cancer survivors with or without current hormone therapy use. Fifty-three breast cancer survivors were randomly assigned to an exercise ($n = 25$) or control ($n = 28$) group. The exercise group trained on a cycle ergometer three times per week at a moderate intensity, progressing from 15 to 35 minutes over a 15-week period. The main results showed statistically significant and clinically meaningful changes in peak oxygen consumption and overall QOL in favor of the exercise group (15). The sub-analysis of these data based on age [<60 years of age ($n = 35$) and ≥60 years of age ($n = 17$)] revealed that there was no age-by-group interaction for either QOL or peak oxygen consumption. The authors noted that the study was underpowered to detect such a difference; but, at least it provided some assurance that older cancer survivors may respond equally well to an exercise intervention.

The GROUP-HOPE trial was an RCT that examined if a home-based exercise program could improve QOL in cancer survivors beyond the benefits of group psychotherapy (16–18). About 44% of the participants were receiving adjuvant therapy at the time of the intervention. Twenty-two group psychotherapy classes consisting of 108 cancer survivors were randomly assigned to group psychotherapy alone (11 classes; $n = 48$) or group psychotherapy plus exercise (11 classes; $n = 60$). The exercise group was asked to exercise independently three to five times per week for 10 weeks (the length of the classes) at a moderate intensity for at least 20 to 30 minutes each time. The main results showed significant effects in favor of the exercise group for functional well-being, fatigue, and sum of skin-folds (17). Once again, the sub-analysis of these data based on age [<60 years of age ($n = 77$) vs. $\geq$60 years of age ($n = 18$)] revealed that there was no age-by-group interactions for functional well-being, fatigue, or sum of skin-folds. These data suggest that there were no differences in how younger and older cancer survivors responded to the exercise intervention, although it is important to point out that the study was underpowered to detect such differences.

The previous reviews indicate that exercise may be an effective intervention to enhance physical function, fatigue, and some aspects of QOL in middle-aged and younger cancer survivors. Unfortunately, no studies have been conducted on the effects of exercise training in older cancer survivors (i.e., $\geq$65 years). Given this fact, we turn our attention to the much more developed literature on exercise training in older adults without cancer. Our purpose here is to provide an overview of the general findings of this literature rather than provide a comprehensive and systematic review.

EFFECTS OF EXERCISE ON FUNCTIONING IN OLDER ADULTS

A large volume of research has revealed that regular exercise training in older adults ($\geq$65 years) can attenuate or even improve some of the age-associated declines in physical and mental functioning (19). One important finding is that exercise has been shown to attenuate the age-related decline in muscle mass and strength, which can greatly affect an older adult's ability to carry out activities of daily living (20). Hurley and Roth (6) reviewed 10 studies of exercise and muscle mass in older adults and concluded that exercise results in a moderate to large increase in muscle mass. In addition to improving muscle mass, exercise can also increase muscle strength in older adults. A recent review by Skelton and Beyer (21) of 11 studies showed that muscle strength and power may be improved by resistance training even in very old adults.

Regular aerobic exercise has been shown to attenuate the decline in maximal aerobic capacity and exercise tolerance, and thus assist the maintenance of functional capacity (19). The mechanisms for this positive change can be attributed to improved function in both central (cardiac output) and peripheral (endothelium) circulation (20). It is important to note that older adults have been shown to experience improvements similar to younger adults in exercise capacity following endurance training (20).

Exercise also attenuates the accumulation of body fat that tends to accompany the aging process. Toth et al. (22) conducted a meta-analysis and found that participation in both aerobic and resistance exercise seems to have a positive effect on body composition in terms of fat reduction. Exercise has also been associated with improved bone mineral density (23) and diminished levels of osteoporosis-related fractures in older adults (24). A review by Gregg et al. (24) examined 33 prospective and case–control studies on physical activity and osteoporotic fractures. Results indicated that exercise might improve bone mineral density by 2% to 5% and result in a reduced rate of bone loss, consequently reducing the risk of osteoporosis and slowing its progression. Resistance training may also result in improvements, or at least attenuation of the age-related decline of bone mineral density in older adults.

Another important benefit of participation in regular physical activity for older adults appears to be a reduced risk of falls. A review of 13 studies by Chang et al. (25) revealed that exercise interventions significantly reduced the risk of falling and monthly fall rate. This reduced rate of falling and the subsequent reduction in injuries or severity of injuries following exercise training may be a result of a number of factors. Improved functional ability, coordination, balance, reaction time, muscular strength and power, and improvements in or delayed loss of bone mineral density may all contribute to lower incidence of falls and injuries in the elderly (21).

Mazzeo et al. (26) suggest that depression and perceptions of control or self-efficacy often decline as part of the aging process. A recent review by Taylor et al. (20) suggests that exercise interventions may be a means to improve mental health, emotional, cognitive, social function, and self-efficacy, and to reduce the many physical symptoms associated with aging, including decreased joint pain and fatigue.

EFFECTS OF EXERCISE ON CHRONIC DISEASE PREVENTION AND MANAGEMENT IN OLDER ADULTS

Older cancer survivors often have other chronic diseases at the time of their cancer diagnosis and are also at greater risk for developing and dying from these other chronic diseases after their cancer treatments. Consequently, the role of exercise in the prevention and management of other chronic diseases in older cancer survivors may be particularly important.

Exercise has been shown to reduce the incidence of many cardiovascular diseases including coronary artery disease (CAD), chronic heart failure, stroke, and hypertension (27–29). A scientific report from the American Heart Association (28) stated that the research evidence clearly shows that physical activity reduces the risk of CAD. This protective effect of regular exercise in reducing the incidence of cardiovascular diseases is primarily attributed to the improvement of the risk factors associated with the diseases. These include improved cholesterol and lipid profiles, heart and endothelial function, glucose tolerance and insulin sensitivity, decreased blood pressure, and prevention of obesity (28).

Exercise rehabilitation for patients suffering from cardiovascular diseases is recommended for the management of CAD, heart failure, peripheral arterial disease, and stroke (28,29). The cardioprotective mechanisms of physical activity that slow the progression of existing cardiovascular disease are similar to the positive effects on risk factors as described above for exercise as primary prevention. These include improvements in exercise tolerance, endothelial function, insulin sensitivity, and glucose tolerance, and reductions in inflammation (C-reactive protein), serum triglycerides, body weight, and adiposity (27,28). A review by Ades (30) summarizes the beneficial effects of exercise rehabilitation in patients over 65 years with cardiovascular diseases as improved functional capacity, decreased symptoms, and reduced disease-specific and all-cause mortality. Also, research has shown that the benefits of cardiac rehabilitation are not limited to younger patients, with older adults in the ninth decade of life experiencing significant improvements from exercise rehabilitation without adverse events (31).

Regular exercise has also been shown to be effective in reducing the incidence of type 2 diabetes. A large RCT of 3234 participants at high risk of developing type 2 diabetes revealed that a lifestyle intervention (exercise and diet) was effective in reducing the incidence of diabetes, even more so than a drug (metformin) intervention (32). The main mechanisms of this positive effect of exercise include improved glucose tolerance and insulin sensitivity. Further benefits of regular exercise on risk factors for diabetes include improved body composition (especially reduced central adiposity), lipid profile, and weight loss (33,34).

As with cardiovascular diseases, regular exercise is recommended for the management of type 2 diabetes. In a recent position statement, Zinman et al. (33) stated that the benefits of exercise in type 2 diabetics include improved glycemic control and lipid profiles, and decreased hypertension. This is supported by a meta-analysis (35) that found that supervised exercise training in type 2 diabetics induced a clinically significant effect on glycemic control without a significant decrease in weight. The insulin resistance syndrome (high insulin and glucose concentrations, poor lipid profile, high blood pressure) in type 2 diabetics appears to be a risk factor for cardiovascular disease, with improvement in insulin sensitivity being related to many of the protective effects of exercise on cardiovascular disease risk (34).

Chronic pulmonary diseases can initiate a number of limiting symptoms that lead to a cycle of decreased physical activity, deconditioning, and increasing severity of exercise-limiting symptoms (36). Pulmonary rehabilitation can halt this cycle by improving exercise capacity/functional ability and QOL, and reducing dyspnea (37). The official statement on pulmonary rehabilitation by the American Thoracic Society (38) is that exercise training is the foundation of pulmonary rehabilitation and is the only component of rehabilitation that has demonstrated a significant ability to enhance pulmonary outcomes in controlled clinical trials.

Osteoarthritis is the most prevalent chronic condition in adults over the age of 65, affecting over half of individuals in this age group (19). Exercise interventions are an effective means of primary prevention and management of osteoarthritis (19). A consensus statement by the American Geriatric Society Panel on Exercise and Osteoarthritis (39) suggests that exercise interventions are an effective means to reduce pain and improve function, without exacerbating disease progression or joint pain. The beneficial effects of exercise for those individuals with osteoarthritis include improvements in overall functional capacity, aerobic capacity, muscular strength and endurance, and postural and gait stability, which can possibly reduce the risk of falls (19,39).

Aerobic exercise interventions also appear to reverse the aging process on the brain and enhance the performance of cognitive tasks (40). This finding is supported by Colcombe and Kramer (41) who completed a meta-analysis of 18 studies, which showed that fitness training increased cognitive performance regardless of type of cognitive task, type of exercise training, or subject characteristics. The mechanisms responsible for these improvements are not known, but may include increased neuronal number and interconnections (40).

Regular physical activity also appears to have a protective effect on the development of Alzheimer's disease (42). This is supported by a large cohort study of 6434 older adults (≥65 years old) followed for five years (43). In this population, regular physical activity was associated with a reduced risk of Alzheimer's disease. The reasons for this protective effect of exercise are still unclear, but may include increased cerebral blood flow and neural capacity, reduced obesity and hypertension, or favorable changes in lipid profile, hormone and insulin concentrations, and the immune system (43).

Participation in leisure activities has been associated with a reduced risk of dementia (44). A large cohort study of 469 subjects greater than 75 years of age followed for a median of five years supported a significant protective effect of physical activity on risk of developing dementia (44). Again, the mechanisms of this effect are unclear but may include an increase in cognitive reserve and slower progression of the disease.

It is currently unclear whether physical activity reduces the risk of developing Parkinson's disease (45). The results from Chen et al. (45), who prospectively followed a large cohort of nearly 50,000 men, suggest that high levels of physical activity may lower the risk of Parkinson's disease. Physical activity may also be beneficial in the management of individuals with Parkinson's disease. Sixteen weeks of aerobic exercise was found to improve aerobic capacity and movement initiation in individuals with Parkinson's disease, suggesting that exercise may reduce the negative effects of neuromuscular slowing associated with Parkinson's disease (46).

EXERCISE SCREENING, TESTING, AND PRESCRIPTION GUIDELINES FOR OLDER CANCER SURVIVORS

The previous review stresses the need for all older adults, even those diagnosed with cancer, to include regular physical activity in their daily lives regardless of age or current health status. Nevertheless, the older adult's decision to undergo exercise testing and/or participate in an exercise program during or following cancer treatment should be made with qualified medical advice. A medical evaluation is necessary to identify the frail older individual, to rule out any potential contraindications to exercise (Table 1), and to identify any acute or chronic impairments related to cancer and/or its treatment (Table 2). The evaluation must also include an assessment of risk factors for, and/or symptoms of, cardiovascular, pulmonary, and metabolic diseases. As well, possible effects of medications on exercise and other existing conditions such as osteoarthritis or osteoporosis must be considered.

The overall goal of medical screening is to ensure that participation in a given exercise program results in improved health and QOL. The Physical Activity Readiness Medical Examination (PARmed-X) is a comprehensive screening tool developed by the Canadian Society for Exercise Physiology (CSEP) [available through CSEP's web site (47)]. The PARmed-X is a four-page physical activity–specific checklist to convey clearance for exercise participation and is completed by the individual's physician prior to initiating any exercise testing or program. The PARmed-X was not developed for a clinical population and as such cannot replace a complete history and physical; however, it is valuable as an additional tool to identify individuals for whom physical activity might be inappropriate, unsafe, or require medical supervision.

Table 1 Contraindications to Exercise Testing and Participation in the Older Adult

Absolute contraindications	Relative contraindications
Recent ECG changes or MI	Elevated blood pressure
Unstable angina	Cardiomyopathy
Uncontrolled arrhythmias	Valvular heart disease
Third degree heart block	Complex ventricular ectopy
Acute congestive heart failure	Uncontrolled metabolic diseases

Abbreviations: ECG, electrocardiogram; MI, myocardial infarction.

Table 2 Contraindications and Precautions for Exercise During Cancer Treatment

Considerations	Contraindications/precautions for exercise
Factors related to cancer treatment	No exercise on days of intravenous chemotherapy or within 24 hrs of treatment No exercise prior to blood draw Caution if on treatments that affect lungs and/or heart or if at risk of heart disease Severe tissue reaction to radiation therapy Mouth sores/ulcerations: avoid mouthpieces for maximal testing; use facemasks
Hematologic (laboratory values)	Platelets <50,000 White blood cells <3000 Hemoglobin <10 g/dL Absolute granulocyte count <2500/mm^3
Musculoskeletal	Bone, back, or neck pain of recent origin Unusual muscular weakness Any pain or cramping Severe cachexia Unusual/extreme fatigue Poor functional status: avoid exercise testing if Karnofsky performance status score ≤60% Avoid high-impact exercise if at risk of fracture
Systemic	Acute infections Febrile illness: fever >100°F (38°C) General malaise
Gastrointestinal	Nausea Vomiting or diarrhea within previous 24 to 36 hrs Dehydration Poor nutrition: inadequate or compromised fluid and/or food intake
Cardiovascular	Chest pain Resting pulse >100 b/min or <50 b/min Resting blood pressure >145 mm Hg systolic and >95 mmHg diastolic[a] Resting blood pressure <85 mm Hg systolic Irregular pulse Swelling of ankles Lymphedema: wear compression garment on limb when exercising If on any medication that alters heart rate, excercise prescription based on heart rate reserve may not be appropriate; do not overexert
Pulmonary	Dyspnea Cough Wheezing Chest pain increased by deep breath

(Continued)

Table 2 Contraindications and Precautions for Exercise During Cancer Treatment
(*Continued*)

Considerations	Contraindications/precautions for exercise
Neurological	Dizziness/lightheaded
	Disorientation
	Blurred vision
	Peripheral sensory neuropathy
	Ataxia

[a]Physician clearance required if resting blood pressure (systolic or diastolic) exceeds these cut points.

We recommend that the full form be completed with signed medical clearance prior to initiating any exercise and/or exercise testing in older cancer survivors.

Prior to performing exercise testing, information must be collected on important diagnostic and treatment variables such as the type and stage of disease, type of cancer treatment, and any known or suspected side effects of treatments (48). The decision concerning the appropriate mode of exercise to use for testing will depend on the limitations and impairments imposed by the cancer treatment combination, and the general health of the older adult. The current American College of Sports Medicine (ACSM) Guidelines for Exercise and Physical Activity for Older Adults (26) advise medical supervision of older adults undergoing exercise testing due to the high prevalence of symptomatic and asymptomatic cardiovascular disease. While maximal testing is desirable, it is of questionable value for older adults simply wishing to increase daily physical activity. The test, whether maximal or submaximal, must, however, stress the individual to at least the level of the proposed exercise regimen so that any symptoms that might be experienced are identified under the supervised environment (48).

At present, there are no published exercise guidelines explicitly for older adults with cancer. While numerous exercise guidelines have been published for the cancer population in general, none of these guidelines are considered evidence based (49). As a result, the most beneficial exercise regimen in terms of type, frequency, duration, or intensity for cancer survivors of any age is currently not known (49). Even if known, the optimal exercise prescription would likely vary depending on the cancer type, stage of disease, and prescribed cancer treatment, and require some modification for the older adult (49). Nevertheless, some general exercise guidelines can be drawn from the literature on exercise and cancer (49–51) and the literature on older adults with other chronic diseases [ACSM guidelines for older adults (26)].

The exercise prescription involves four key components: cardiorespiratory fitness, muscular strength, postural stability, and flexibility (Table 3). This exercise prescription may need to be modified based on current fitness level, existing comorbidities, and specific symptoms and side effects resulting from cancer treatment. Exercise prescription will also vary depending on the goals of the treatment program and treatment trajectory. Exercise may be prescribed to prevent or attenuate functional decline during treatment, to rehabilitate treatment-specific problems, or to optimize general health in the recovery period following cancer treatment (48).

The exercise program should be structured to include a warm-up, the exercise phase, and a cool-down phase (52). In older individuals, it is important to do a slow, prolonged warm-up period to prepare the cardiopulmonary and musculoskeletal systems for exercise (52). The exercise prescription should consider the lifestyle needs

Table 3 General Exercise Recommendations for Otherwise Healthy Older Adults with Cancer

Components of exercise program	Parameter	Recommendation	Comment
Cardiorespiratory fitness (aerobic exercise training)	Mode	Exercises involving large muscle groups such as walking and cycling	The exercise prescription may need to be modified based on acute or chronic effects from cancer treatment and other co-morbidities
	Frequency	Three to five days per week	For the very deconditioned or fatigued survivor, exercise may need to be broken into 5 min bouts. Exercise can then be progressed each week by 1–2 min per bout as the training effect occurs
	Intensity	40–60% of heart rate reserve or 11–13 RPE on the Borg scale	Monitoring of heart rate, perceived exertion, and blood pressure before, during, and following the exercise session is advised
	Duration	20–30 min; if possible gradually progress to 45 min	Older individuals may tolerate extreme environmental conditions poorly, may need to move indoors during very hot or very cold weather
Muscular strength and endurance (resistance exercise training)	Mode	Progressive resistance exercise of the major muscle groups of the upper and lower extremities and trunk	Resistance training should follow rather than precede aerobic exercise training if performed on the same day
	Exercises	8–10 exercises of major muscle groups of upper and lower extremities and trunk	Monitor symptoms of pain and fatigue, delayed muscle soreness; reduce/ adjust workload if worsening of symptoms with exercise
	Intensity (resistance)	Start at 40% of one RM progressing to 60% of one RM	In the very deconditioned or fatigued survivor, resistance may need to start with very light weights (e.g., 2 lbs) and slowly progress over time

(Continued)

Table 3 General Exercise Recommendations for Otherwise Healthy Older Adults with Cancer (*Continued*)

Components of exercise program	Parameter	Recommendation	Comment
	Frequency	Two to three days per week	
	Repetitions	10–15 repetitions	
	Sets	1–3 sets	The first set should feel relatively easy to complete. Ideally, some muscular "tiredness" should occur in the last few repetitions of the second set
	Rest	One to two minutes between exercise stations and up to four minutes between sets	The rest period should be long enough such that the individual feels they can complete the next exercise or set
	Recovery	Minimum of 48 hrs between sessions	Older individuals may recover more slowly from an exercise session and delayed muscle soreness may require >48 hrs to resolve
Flexibility training	Mode	Slow, static stretches	
	Exercises	Individualized	Stretching of muscle groups to improve posture may include the pectorals, hip flexors, and ankle plantar flexors
	Frequency	Minimum of two days per week	Stretching exercises can be performed daily
	Repetitions	Four repetitions	
	Duration	10-30 sec per stretch	Maximal benefit of stretching for some muscle groups occurs with long stretches of one minute in length (e.g., hamstrings)
	Intensity	Gentle, low intensity stretch	The muscle or joint should be stretched to a point of tension that is still comfortable. No pain should be experienced moving into the stretch, during the stretch, or when returning to the start position (release from the stretch)

(*Continued*)

Table 3 General Exercise Recommendations for Otherwise Healthy Older Adults with Cancer (*Continued*)

Components of exercise program	Parameter	Recommendation	Comment
Postural stability	Mode	Specific exercises to improve balance or exercise programs such as Tai Chi and dancing to challenge muscles involved in postural stability	Good shoes with adequate heel and foot support are recommended when exercising Exercise should be performed in well-lighted areas, with even floor surface, clear of obstacles May need to move indoors if outdoor surfaces become ice covered If the individual has a history of falls or if posture is unstable, exercise in the seated position is advisable (e.g., recumbent bike)

Abbreviations: RPE, rating of perceived exertion; RM, repetition maximum.

and preferences of the individual and include activities that are enjoyable, build confidence, and incorporate social interaction (48). The exercise session should finish with a gradual cool-down period that includes exercises of diminishing intensities to allow appropriate circulatory adjustments and return of the heart rate and blood pressure to near resting values (53). In older adults, a gradual cool-down is of paramount importance to avoid a sudden drop in blood pressure that may potentially lead to cardiac problems postexercise (52–54).

According to the ACSM Position Stand on Exercise and Physical Activity for Older Adults and the National Institute of Aging, older adults should ideally accumulate at least 30 minutes of moderate-intensity aerobic exercise daily to improve their cardiorespiratory fitness (26,55). Cardiorespiratory fitness is improved by aerobic activities that use large muscle groups, are maintained for a prolonged period of time, and are rhythmic in nature such as walking, swimming, and cycling. Alternate activities include dancing, water exercises, and gardening. Although walking may be the preferred mode of exercise in older adults, cycle ergometry or water exercises may be more suitable alternatives to avoid excessive orthopedic stress on lower extremity joints (in those unable to endure weight-bearing activity) and in individuals with hip or knee joint replacements (56). The goal, in the initial phases of the exercise program, is to first reach target frequency (three to five days per week), then duration (at least 20 minutes; which can be broken into shorter bouts of 5–10 minutes), and finally progress to the desired intensity (40–60% of heart rate reserve or a rating of perceived exertion of 11–13 on the Borg scale) (57). This gradual progression of exercise will allow for adequate cardiovascular and musculoskeletal adaptation and help avoid injury. It is important to recognize that while exercise of lower intensity is effective in improving muscular endurance and attenuating the decline in physiological function of the older individual, moderate intensity exercise is necessary to improve cardiovascular function and cardiovascular disease risk factors (26).

Muscular strength and endurance training (i.e., resistance exercise) is essential for older adults to attenuate the decline in muscle mass, strength, and endurance. Resistance exercise is particularly important for the older cancer survivor where age-related losses in physical strength may be accelerated by factors related to cancer or its treatment. It is recommended that older adults perform one to three sets of 10 to 15 repetitions of 8 to 10 exercises that include all of the major muscle groups. Resistance training should be performed twice per week with a minimum of 48 hours of recovery between training sessions. Older adults may require longer recovery periods between exercises, sets, and sessions when performing resistance exercise in order to avoid excessive delayed muscle soreness (53). The recovery period or rest time between exercises, sets, and sessions is a component of the program that may need to be lengthened, particularly in the first few weeks of an exercise program, to allow for adequate recovery and to avoid fatigue (53). An initial overload of increasing the number of repetitions rather than resistance is recommended to minimize loads on joints and to allow for adaptation of muscle and connective tissue. We recommend initially keeping the resistance low, gradually increasing to 20 to 25 repetitions, and performing only one set. We have also found that it may be necessary in some cancer survivors to limit the number of exercises performed in the first few weeks and to progress more slowly to the desired exercise prescription (two sets of 10–15 repetitions of 8–10 exercises). Importantly, when the intensity (i.e., resistance) is too low, only modest improvements in strength will be realized by older adults. Older adults have the capacity to greatly increase muscular strength if the training stimulus is progressively increased over time (26).

As flexibility declines with age, stretching and range of motion exercises are necessary to increase range of motion of joints and muscles (26,58). A flexibility training program should include a regular set of exercises intended to progressively increase range of motion in a joint or set of joints. Ideally, the choice of exercises should be individualized to meet the functional needs of the older individual (e.g., improve ankle range of motion for stair descent) and to address cancer treatment–specific deficits (e.g., shoulder range of motion following breast surgery). Exercises should always consist of slow, static stretches held for 10 to 30 seconds. At least four repetitions of each stretch should be performed; however, the goal should be to progress to a total stretch time of approximately two minutes per exercise (e.g., four repetitions of 30 seconds duration). Flexibility exercises should be performed at least two days per week and can be incorporated into the cool-down phases of aerobic and/or resistance training sessions.

The National Institute of Aging (55) also recommends balance training for older adults as a means of improving postural stability and reducing the incidence and risk of falls. Balance and coordination, and thus postural stability, may be improved through specific lower body strengthening exercises that focus on the ankle plantar and dorsiflexors, knee flexion, hip extension, and hip abduction. These specific exercises can be incorporated into a resistance training program. Balance and coordination are improved if lateral sway (ability to control balance when center of mass moves away from the base of support) is challenged through exercises such as tandem walking (hand touching wall for support) and one-legged stand (holding onto a counter) (52). Modes of exercise that also involve balance and coordination training are Tai Chi Chuan and dancing (52). At present, the optimal frequency and intensity of exercise to improve postural stability remains unknown; however, positive effects on postural stability have been achieved through a wide range of interventions that include resistance exercise, balance training, and flexibility.

EXERCISE MOTIVATION IN OLDER CANCER SURVIVORS

Motivating individuals to exercise is challenging in any population; however, older cancer survivors may have additional unique barriers as a result of their cancer and its treatments. Several recent studies have suggested that exercise participation rates in cancer survivors decline drastically during treatment and remain lower than pre-diagnosis levels even years after treatments have ended (59,60). For example, recent surveys of non-Hodgkin's lymphoma, endometrial cancer, and multiple myeloma survivors have indicated that 29% to 34% reported exercising pre-diagnosis but only 5% to 7% reported exercising during adjuvant therapy, and only 20% to 31% reported exercising after their treatments (61–63). Motivation and adherence issues may be even further compromised in the older cancer survivor, who may have additional physical, psychological, and social reasons not to exercise.

To date, only one study has specifically examined exercise participation rates in older cancer survivors (64). The study surveyed over 1600 cancer survivors and found that exercise participation rates declined with age. Specifically, 40.7% of cancer survivors in the 18 to 39 years age group reported meeting public health exercise guidelines whereas only 25.2% in the 40 to 64 years age group and 20.6% in the 65 years and above age group reported meeting the guidelines. These data are consistent with the general decline in exercise with age in the broader population. For example, in the United States, 41% of individuals aged 18 to 24 reported getting regular exercise while only 25% and 17% aged 65 to 74 years and 75 years and older, respectively, reported exercising regularly (65). In the Coups and Ostroff (64) study, the exercise participation levels of the older cancer survivors were only marginally lower than adults of the same age in the general population (20.6% vs. 22.1%) but the overall participation rates are poor in both groups.

At least 10 other studies have analyzed the association between age and the adherence/participation in exercise by cancer survivors. These findings have been inconclusive, however, with three of these studies demonstrating a negative association between age and exercise adherence (66–68), five studies finding no significant relationship (59,69–72), and two studies finding a positive association between age and exercise (73,74). One study with an objective measure of exercise adherence involved an RCT of prostate cancer survivors participating in a 12-week supervised resistance training program (74). Results indicated that exercise adherence rates were the lowest for the oldest participants. For participants <65 years of age and those aged 65 to 74, adherence rates were 82% and 83%, respectively. However, for those 75 years and older, adherence was only 65%.

Given the decline in exercise participation with cancer treatments, a number of research studies have examined determinants of exercise behavior in cancer survivors (62,75–78). Overall, these studies have found that social cognitive variables such as attitudes towards exercise, perceived social norms, and perceived control over exercise are more important predictors of exercise than medical and demographic factors. More specifically, many cancer survivors have reported a number of barriers to exercise, including pain or soreness, nausea, fatigue, diarrhea, weakness, poor health, lack of time, work responsibilities, lack of support, and lack of counselling (60,76,77). Cancer survivors also report a number of exercise incentives including that it helps them cope with the stress of cancer and its treatments. Also, exercise helps survivors maintain a normal lifestyle, gain control over their lives, feel better and improve their well-being, get their mind off cancer, recover from surgery and treatment, develop/maintain a positive attitude, improve fitness, increase energy, lose weight, and feel better about themselves (60,70,76,77).

To date, only a few studies have directly examined the effects of age on exercise motivation in cancer survivors (76,77). Courneya et al. (76) found that, in a survey of non-Hodgkin's lymphoma survivors, age interacted with instrumental attitudes toward exercise (i.e., the belief that exercise is beneficial or not) when exercise intention was the dependent measure. The nature of this interaction was such that instrumental attitude was only a significant correlate of intention to exercise in participants less than 60 years of age. In survivors 60 years and older, instrumental attitude did not significantly correlate with exercise intention. Another similar study involving endometrial cancer survivors (77) found that age moderated the association between exercise intentions and exercise behavior. Results indicated that exercise intentions correlated positively with exercise behavior in participants under the age of 70 years, but not in participants 70 years of age and older. These findings suggest that intention to exercise has no association with actual exercise behavior in older endometrial cancer survivors.

Moreover, only one study has examined the utility of an exercise behavior change intervention in cancer survivors (79). This RCT was a primary care–based intervention that involved the oncologist as the potential source of exercise counseling. The Oncologist Recommendation to Exercise trial involved 329 newly diagnosed breast cancer survivors. Participants were randomly assigned to receive (i) an oncologist's recommendation to exercise, (ii) an oncologist's recommendation to exercise plus a referral to an exercise specialist, or (iii) usual care. At five weeks after the initial consultation, results indicated that the group receiving only the oncologist's recommendation reported exercising more than the recommendation/ referral group and significantly more than the usual care group. These findings suggest that exercise interventions through oncologists may be an effective means of increasing exercise participation in cancer survivors. An additional RCT that is currently in progress involves older breast and prostate cancer survivors (80). The results of this study will provide valuable data on exercise intervention strategies for older breast and prostate survivors.

Much more is known about older adults in the general population. A number of individual level factors, such as demographics, physical condition, exercise history, and social cognitive variables may influence exercise participation in older adults. Some of the key barriers to exercise in older adults include time restraints, poor self-discipline, lack of exercise partners, expenses associated with exercise, lack of access to facilities, fatigue, poor health, fear of health complications/injuries, and fear of falling. These barriers, however, may not necessarily be insurmountable, and if approached in this way, may be overcome with the help of health care workers or exercise specialists.

Social-cognitive variables may also influence older adults' choice to exercise. For example, older adults may choose not to exercise because of prevailing social beliefs that exercise may be harmful to or inappropriate for older adults (81). Older adults may also not be aware of the health benefits of regular exercise. For example, one study found that older adults in general do not view regular exercise as a major health determinant (82). Moreover, Booth et al. (83) found that many older women did not exercise regularly because they were influenced by normative beliefs about older women being "too old" to exercise. This kind of misinformation about the role of exercise in maintaining and promoting health may act as a deterrent from exercise for some older adults.

Some research has found that older adults who are high in self-efficacy for exercise are the most likely to adhere to an exercise program (84–86). However, many older adults may lack self-efficacy for exercise for a number of age-related reasons. Perceptions of sickness, frailty, disability, or advanced age may prevent some older adults from exercising (87,88). Arthritis, for example, may cause some older adults to avoid exercise because they feel that it would be painful and/or harmful to their joints despite evidence that exercise may actually be beneficial in alleviating symptoms (89). Fear of injury from falling may also be a reason for not exercising in some older adults. One study found, in a sample of high-functioning, healthy older adults, that fear of falling was independently associated with reduced levels of participation in physical activity (90).

Certain demographic variables have also been found to be associated with exercise participation in older adults. For example, research has shown that higher socioeconomic status and education are related to exercise participation (84,91). Being unmarried and younger in age have also been found to be associated with exercising regularly in older adults (92). Sex also appears to influence exercise behavior in older adults with men being more active than women. For example, in Canada, approximately 64% of men between the ages of 65 and 74 and 48% of men over the age of 75 report regular exercise compared to only 46% of women between 65 and 74 years and 29% of women 75 years and older (93).

A number of studies have examined the effectiveness of different exercise interventions in older adults in the general population (94). Conn et al. (94) recently conducted a systematic review of 17 randomized trials of exercise interventions in older adults. The types of intervention strategies that have been used are self-monitoring, problem solving, general health education, feedback, goal setting, exercise supervision, relapse prevention education, and reinforcement. Ten studies found a significant increase in exercise after the exercise intervention, while seven studies found no significant change in exercise behavior.

Many exercise intervention studies have examined primary care–based strategies. These interventions involve the use of primary care health care practitioners as the source of the intervention. A review of primary care–based exercise intervention studies found that these types of strategies seem to be moderately effective in the short term; however, results are still inconclusive (95). Other kinds of exercise interventions for older adults involve a several week-long exercise program, sometimes in conjunction with an educational program. These programs have been criticized as participants often fall back into previous inactive patterns of behavior following completion of the program (96). A recent review of 57 physical activity intervention studies involving older adults found that interventions are not always effective because older adults often do not adhere to the program and have difficultly remaining physically active in the long term (96). Group-based programs seem to have greater long-term effectiveness than home-based interventions. The effectiveness of behavioral reinforcement techniques (e.g., social support, buddy groups, etc.) was not clear. The authors suggest that, to maintain increased physical activity in the long term, exercise interventions should be tailored to the needs and preferences of the individual and include a variety of exercise choices.

FUTURE RESEARCH DIRECTIONS

Given the paucity of research on exercise in older cancer survivors, there is a significant amount of work that needs to be completed. In general, RCTs of exercise interventions that explicitly target older cancer survivors are needed. It is clear from present research that exercise trials that do not target older cancer survivors will not recruit sufficient numbers of older adults to be able to comment on the utility of exercise in this population. Consequently, researchers must develop specific proactive strategies for recruiting and retaining older cancer survivors in randomized controlled exercise trials.

Given the needs of this population, the most important outcomes for older cancer survivors will likely be physical functioning and QOL. We need research that examines the effects of exercise interventions on all aspects of QOL in older cancer survivors including physical, functional, emotional, cognitive, spiritual, and social well-being. It will also be important to determine if exercise can help control some of the common side effects of cancer treatments in this population including nausea, pain, fatigue, weakness, and/or depression. Research may also be warranted on clinical endpoints such as treatment completion rates, disease recurrence, and mortality, although these outcomes may be considered secondary in importance and are less likely to be realized from an exercise intervention given the age of the population.

For studies that do not target older cancer survivors specifically, it may be possible to conduct subgroup analyses of older adults in the sample. Such analyses may help determine if older cancer survivors respond to an exercise training intervention to the same extent as younger cancer survivors. If possible, it would be ideal to power the study, "a priori," to conduct such a subgroup analysis by stratifying on age prior to randomization and attempting to recruit equal numbers of younger and older cancer survivors.

For all of the above questions, it will be important to determine the optimal type (e.g., aerobic vs. resistance training), volume (i.e., frequency, intensity, and duration), progression, and context (e.g., center-based vs. home-based, individual vs. group format) of exercise for older cancer survivors. This information will allow for evidence-based guidelines for a given endpoint of interest in older cancer survivors. One important question is whether older cancer survivors might benefit from an exercise program that is lower in volume than that required for benefits in younger cancer survivors. Moreover, the optimal guidelines for older cancer survivors are likely to vary based on the cancer site, treatment protocol, co-morbid conditions, baseline fitness levels, past exercise, and even age within the older adult classification.

Lastly, research on exercise motivation and adherence will be necessary. Some research has shown that older cancer survivors may be less able to adhere to a supervised exercise training program (66,97); but this question remains to be definitively answered. We also need information on factors that affect exercise adherence in older cancer survivors both inside and outside of clinical trials. Are these factors the same as those that influence younger cancer survivors or older adults from the general population? These factors may include the type of exercise (e.g., walking, swimming), the context (e.g., group vs. individual, home-based vs. center-based, older adults only vs. mixed age groups), social cognitive variables (e.g., attitudes, perceptions of control), environmental factors (e.g., access to facilities, costs, safe sidewalks), and social influence (e.g., spousal support, perceived norms). Lastly, it will be necessary to develop effective exercise behavior change interventions for older cancer survivors that can be delivered by cancer centers, community cancer care organizations, and fitness centers (80).

SUMMARY AND CONCLUSIONS

Older cancer survivors are at risk of significant morbidities due to the combined effects of aging, disease, and aggressive medical treatments (98). Exercise may play an important role in ameliorating these effects in older cancer survivors but direct evidence is not yet available. Research in middle-aged and younger cancer survivors and other older adult populations suggests that the magnitude of the beneficial effect of regular exercise may be substantial. In the absence of direct evidence, we recommend that older cancer survivors follow the exercise guidelines for older adults available from the ACSM (26). Finally, we emphasize the need for future research that will provide the evidence necessary to refine these guidelines and to better characterize the indications, benefits, and risks of exercise in the growing population of older cancer survivors.

ACKNOWLEDGMENTS

Kerry S. Courneya is supported by the Canada Research Chairs Program and a Research Team Grant from the National Cancer Institute of Canada (NCIC) with funds from the Canadian Cancer Society (CCS) and the CCS/NCIC Sociobehavioral Cancer Research Network. Margaret L. McNeely and Kristina H. Karvinen are supported by Health Research Studentships from the Alberta Heritage Foundation for Medical Research.

REFERENCES

1. Bouchard C, Shephard RJ. Physical activity, fitness, and health: the model and key concepts. In: Quinney HA, Gauvin L, Wall AE, eds. Physical Activity, Fitness, and Health: International Proceedings and Consensus Statement, Champaign. Illinois: Human Kinetics, 1994:77–88.
2. Dutta C. Significance of sarcopenia in the elderly. J Nutr 1997; 127(suppl 5):992S–993S.
3. Kamel HK. Sarcopenia and aging. Nutr Rev 2003; 61(5 Pt 1):157–167.
4. Elia M. Obesity in the elderly. Obes Res 2001; 9(suppl 4):244S–248S.
5. Suh TT, Lyles KW. Osteoporosis considerations in the frail elderly. Curr Opin Rheumatol 2003; 15(4):481–486.
6. Hurley BF, Roth SM. Strength training in the elderly: effects on risk factors for age-related diseases. Sports Med 2000; 30(4):249–268.
7. Hawkins S, Wiswell R. Rate and mechanism of maximal oxygen consumption decline with aging: implications for exercise training. Sports Med 2003; 33(12):877–888.
8. Barnard RJ, Grimditch GK, Wilmore JH. Physiological characteristics of sprint and endurance masters runners. Med Sci Sports 1979; 11(2):167–171.
9. Stevinson C, Lawlor DA, Fox KR. Exercise interventions for cancer patients: systematic review of controlled trials. Cancer Causes Control 2004; 15:1035–1056.
10. Galvao DA, Newton RU. Review of exercise intervention studies in cancer patients. J Clin Oncol 2005; 23(4):899–909.
11. Schmitz K, Holtzman J, Courneya KS, Masse LC, Duval S, Kane R. Controlled physical activity trials in cancer survivors: a systematic review and meta-analysis. Cancer Epidemiol Biomarkers Prev 2005; 14(7): 1588–1595.
12. McNeely M, Campbell KL, Rowe BH, Klassen TP, Mackey JR, Courneya KS. Exercise interventions in breast cancer patients: a meta-analysis of randomized controlled trials. Manuscript submitted for publication.
13. Courneya KS, Vallance JKH, McNeely ML, et al. Exercise issues in older cancer survivors. Crit Rev Oncol Hematol 2004; 51(3):249–261.
14. Fairey AS, Courneya KS, Field CJ, et al. Effects of exercise training on fasting insulin, insulin resistance, insulin-like growth factors, and insulin-like growth factor binding

proteins in postmenopausal breast cancer survivors: a randomized controlled trial. Cancer Epidemiol Biomarkers Prev 2003; 12(8):721–727.

15. Courneya KS, Mackey JR, Bell GJ, Jones LW, Field CJ, Fairey AS. Randomized controlled trail of exercise training in postmenopausal breast cancer survivors: cardiopulmonary and quality of life outcomes. JCO 2003; 21(9):1660–1668.

16. Courneya KS, Friedenreich CM, Sela R, Quinney HA, Rhodes RE, Jones LW. Exercise motivation and adherence in cancer survivors after participation in a randomized controlled trial: an attribution theory perspective. Intern J Behav Med 2004; 11(1): 8–17.

17. Courneya KS, Friedenreich CM, Sela RA, Quinney HA, Rhodes RE, Handman M. The group psychotherapy and home-based physical exercise (group-hope) trail in cancer survivors: physical fitness and quality of life outcomes. Psycho-Oncology 2003; 12(4):357–374.

18. Courneya KS, Friedenreich CM, Sela RA, et al. Correlates of adherence and contamination in a randomized controlled trial of exercise in cancer survivors: an application of the theory of planned behavior and the five factor model of personality. Ann Behav Med 2002; 24(4):257–268.

19. Bean JF, Vora A, Frontera WR. Benefits of exercise for community-dwelling older adults. Arch Phys Med Rehabil 2004; 85:S31–S42.

20. Taylor AH, Cable NT, Faulkner G, et al. Physical activity and older adults: a review of health benefits and the effectiveness of interventions. J Sports Sci 2004; 22:703–725.

21. Skelton DA, Beyer N. Exercise and injury prevention in older people. Scand J Med Sci Sports 2003; 13(1):77–85.

22. Toth MJ, Beckett T, Poehlman ET. Physical activity and the progressive change in body composition with aging: current evidence and research issues. Med Sci Sports Exerc 1999; 31(suppl 11):S590–S596.

23. Berard A, Bravo G, Gauthier P. Meta-analysis of the effectiveness of physical activity for the prevention of bone loss in postmenopausal women. Osteoporos Int 1997; 7(4): 331–337.

24. Gregg EW, Pereira MA, Caspersen CJ. Physical activity, falls, and fractures among older adults: a review of the epidemiologic evidence. J Am Geriatr Soc 2000; 48(8):883–893.

25. Chang JT, Morton SC, Rubenstein LZ, et al. Interventions for the prevention of falls in older adults: systematic review and meta-analysis of randomised clinical trials [see comment]. BMJ 2004; 328:680.

26. Mazzeo RS, Cavanagh P, Evans WJ, et al. American College of Sports Medicine Position Stand. Exercise and physical activity for older adults. Med Sci Sports Exerc 1998; 30(6): 992–1008.

27. Roberts CK, Barnard RJ. Effects of exercise and diet on chronic disease. J Appl Physiol 2005; 98:3–30.

28. Thompson PD, Buchner D, Pina IL, et al. Exercise and physical activity in the prevention and treatment of atherosclerotic cardiovascular disease: a statement from the Council on Clinical Cardiology (Subcommittee on Exercise, Rehabilitation, and Prevention) and the Council on Nutrition, Physical Activity, and Metabolism (Subcommittee on Physical Activity). Circulation 2003; 107(24):3109–3116.

29. Wendel-Vos GC, Schuit AJ, Feskens EJ, et al. Physical activity and stroke. A meta-analysis of observational data. Int J Epidemiol 2004; 33:787–798.

30. Ades PA. Cardiac rehabilitation and secondary prevention of coronary heart disease. N Engl J Med 2001; 345(12):892–902.

31. Vonder Muhll I, Daub B, Black B, et al. Benefits of cardiac rehabilitation in the ninth decade of life in patients with coronary heart disease. Am J Cardiol 2002; 90(6):645–648.

32. Knowler WC, Barrett-Connor E, Fowler SE, et al. Reduction in the incidence of type 2 diabetes with lifestyle intervention or metformin. N Engl J Med 2002; 346(6):393–403.

33. Zinman B, Ruderman N, Campaigne BN, et al. Physical activity/exercise and diabetes. Diabetes Care 2004; 27(suppl 1):S58–S62.

34. Hawley JA. Exercise as a therapeutic intervention for the prevention and treatment of insulin resistance. Diabetes Metab Res Rev 2004; 20:383–393.

35. Boule NG, Haddad E, Kenny GP, et al. Effects of exercise on glycemic control and body mass in type 2 diabetes mellitus: a meta-analysis of controlled clinical trials [see comment]. JAMA 2001; 286(10):1218–1227.

36. Cooper CB. Exercise in chronic pulmonary disease: aerobic exercise prescription. [Erratum appears in Med Sci Sports Exerc 2001; 33(9): following table of contents.] Med Sci Sports Exerc 2001; 33(suppl 7):S671–S679.

37. Sutherland ER, Cherniack RM. Management of chronic obstructive pulmonary disease [see comment]. N Engl J Med 2004; 350(26):2689–2697.

38. Anonymous. Pulmonary rehabilitation-1999. American Thoracic Society. Am J Respir Crit Care Med 1999; 159:1666–1682.

39. American Geriatrics Society Panel on Osteoarthritis. Exercise prescription for older adults with osteoarthritis pain: consensus practice recommendations. A supplement to the AGS Clinical Practice Guidelines on the management of chronic pain in older adults. J Am Geriatr Soc 2001; 49(10):808–823.

40. McAuley E, Kramer AF, Colcombe SJ. Cardiovascular fitness and neurocognitive function in older adults: a brief review. Brain Behav Immun 2004; 18:214–220.

41. Colcombe S, Kramer AF. Fitness effects on the cognitive function of older adults: a meta-analytic study. Psychol Sci 2003; 14(2):125–130.

42. Pope SK, Shue VM, Beck C. Will a healthy lifestyle help prevent Alzheimer's disease? Annu Rev Public Health 2003; 24:111–132.

43. Lindsay J, Laurin D, Verreault R, et al. Risk factors for Alzheimer's disease: a prospective analysis from the Canadian Study of Health and Aging. Am J Epidemiol 2002; 156(5):445–453.

44. Verghese J, Lipton RB, Katz MJ, et al. Leisure activities and the risk of dementia in the elderly [see comment]. N Engl J Med 2003; 348(25):2508–2516.

45. Chen H, Zhang S, Schwarzchild M, et al. Physical activity and the risk of parkinson disease. Neurology 2005; 64:664–669.

46. Bergen JL, Toole T, Elliott RG III, et al. Aerobic exercise intervention improves aerobic capacity and movement initiation in Parkinson's disease patients. Neuro Rehabil 2002; 17(2):161–168.

47. http://www.csep.ca/ (May 10, 2005).

48. Courneya KS, Mackey JR, Rhodes R. Cancer. In: LeMura LM, von Duvillard SP, eds. Clinical Exercise Physiology: Applications and Physiological Principles. Philadelphia, Pennsylvania: Lippincott, Williams & Wilkins, 2004.

49. Humpel N, Iverson DC. Review and critique of the quality of exercise recommendations for cancer patients and survivors. Support Care Cancer 2005; 13(7):493–502.

50. Courneya KS, Mackey JR, McKenzie DC. Exercise for breast cancer survivors. Phys Sports Med 2003; 30(8):33.

51. Courneya KS, Mackey JR, Jones LW. Coping with cancer: can exercise help? Phys Sports Med 2000; 28(5):49.

52. Butler RN, Davis R, Lewis CB, et al. Physical fitness: exercise prescription for older adults. Geriatrics 1998; 53:52–54.

53. Franklin BA. In: Franklin BA, ed. ACSM's Guidelines for Exercise Testing and Prescription. Baltimore: Lippincott Williams & Wilkins, 2000.

54. Shephard RJ. Aging. In: LeMura LM, von Duvillard SP, eds. Clinical Exercise Physiology: Application and Physiological Principles. Philadelphia: Lippincott Williams & Wilkins, 2004:549–564.

55. www.nia.nih.gov (November 1, 2003).

56. Kuster MS. Exercise recommendations after joint replacement: a review of current literature and proposal of scientifically based guidelines. Sports Med 2002; 32(7): 433–445.

57. Borg G. Borg's Perceived Exertion and Pain Scales. Champaign, Illinois: Human Kinetics, 1998.

58. Brody LT. Impaired range of motion and joint mobility. In: Hall CM, Brody LT, eds. Therapeutic Exercise: Moving Toward Function. 2nd ed. Philadelphia: Lippincott Williams & Wilkins, 2005:113.
59. Courneya KS, Friedenreich CM. Determinants of exercise during colorectal cancer treatment: an application of the theory of planned behavior. ONF 1997; 24(10):1715–1723.
60. Courneya KS, Friedenreich CM. Relationship between exercise during treatment and current quality of life among survivors of breast cancer. J Psychosoc Oncol 1997; 15(3/4):35–57.
61. Courneya KS, Karvinen KH, Campbell KL, et al. Associations among exercise, body weight, and quality of life in a population-based sample of endometrial cancer survivors. Gynecol Oncol 2005; 97:422–430.
62. Jones LW, Courneya KS, Vallance JHK, et al. Association between exercise and quality of life in multiple myeloma survivors. Support Care Cancer (Online first 2004).
63. Vallance JKH, Courneya KS, Jones LW, et al. Differences in quality of life between non-Hodgkin's lymphoma survivors meeting and not meeting public health exercise guidelines. Psycho-Oncology 2005; 14(11):979–991.
64. Coups EJ, Ostroff JS. A population-based estimate of the prevalence of behavioral risk factors among adult cancer survivors and noncancer controls. Prev Med 2005; 40:702–711.
65. www.cdc.gov/nchs/about/major/nhis/released200212/figures07_1–7_3.htm (November 1, 2003).
66. Courneya KS, Friedenreich CM. Utility of the theory of planned behavior for understanding exercise during breast cancer treatment. Psycho-Oncology 1999; 8:112–122.
67. Courneya KS, Segal RJ, Reid RD, et al. Three independent factors predicted exercise adherence in a randomized controlled trial of resistance training among prostate cancer survivors. J Clin Epidemiol 2004; 57(6):571–579.
68. Irwin ML, McTiernan A, Bernstein L, et al. Physical activity levels among breast cancer survivors. Med Sci Sports Exerc 2004; 36:1484–1491.
69. Blanchard CM, Courneya KS, Rodgers WM, et al. Determinants of exercise intention and behavior in survivors of breast and prostate cancer: an application of the theory of planned behavior. Cancer Nurs 2002; 25(2):88–95.
70. Courneya KS, Friedenreich CM, Arthur K, Bobick TM. Understanding exercise motivation in colorectal cancer patients: a prospective study using the theory of planned behavior. Rehabil Psychol 1999; 44(1):68–84.
71. Pinto BM, Maruyama NC, Clark MM, Cruess DG, Park E, Roberts M. Motivation to modify lifestyle risk behaviors in women treated for breast cancer. Mayo Clinic Proc 2002; 77:122–129.
72. Young-McCaughan S, Sexton DL. A retrospective investigation of the relationship between aerobic exercise and quality of life in women with breast cancer. Oncol Nurs Forum 1991; 18:751–757.
73. Blanchard CM, Denniston MM, Baker F, et al. Do adults change their lifestyle behaviors after a cancer diagnosis? Am J Health Behav 2003; 27(3):246–256.
74. Courneya KS, Friedenreich CM, Quinney HA, Fields ALA, Jones LW, Fairey AS. Predictors of adherence and contamination in a randomized trial of exercise in colorectal cancer survivors. Psycho-Oncology 2004; 13:857–866.
75. Cooper H. The role of physical activity in the recovery from breast cancer. Melpomene J 1995; 14:18–20.
76. Courneya KS, Vallance JKH, Jones LW, et al. Correlates of exercise intentions in non-Hodgkin's lymphoma survivors: an application of the theory of planned behavior. J Sport Exerc Phsychol 2005; 27:335–349.
77. Karvinen KH, Courneya KS, Campbell KL, et al. Correlates of exercise motivation and behavior in a population-based sample of endometrial cancer survivors: an application of the theory of planned behavior. Manuscript submitted for publication.
78. Leddy SK. Incentives and barriers to exercise in women with a history of breast cancer. Oncol Nurs Forum 1997; 24(5):885–890.

79. Jones LW, Courneya KS, Fairey AS, et al. Effects of an oncologists recommendation to exercise on self-reported exercise behavior in newly diagnosed breast cancer survivors: a single-blind, randomized controlled trial. Ann Behav Med 2004; 28:105–113.

80. Demark-Wahnefried W, Morey MC, Clipp EC, et al. Leading the Way in Exercise and Diet (Project LEAD): intervening to improve function among older breast and prostate cancer survivors. Control Clin Trials 2003; 24(2):206–223.

81. Hardcastle S, Taylor AH. Looking for more than weight loss and fitness gain: psychological dimensions among older women in a primary-care exercise-referral program. J Aging Phys Act 2001; 9:313–328.

82. Alfonso C, Graca P, Kearney JM, et al. Physical activity in European seniors: attitude, beliefs, and levels. J Nutr Health Aging 2001; 5:226–229.

83. Booth ML, Bauman A, Owen N, et al. Physical activity preferences, preferred sources of assistance, and perceived barriers to increased activity among physically inactive Australians. Prev Med 1997; 26:131–137.

84. Clark DO. Age, socioeconomic status, and exercise self-efficacy. Gerontologist 1996; 36(2):157–164.

85. Hellman EA. Use of the stages of change in exercise adherence model among older adults with a cardiac diagnosis. J Cardiopulm Rehabil 1997; 17(3):145–155.

86. Resnick B, Nigg C. Testing a theoretical model of exercise behavior for older adults. Nurs Res 2003; 52(2):80–88.

87. Brassington GS, Atienza AA, Perczek RE, et al. Intervention-related cognitive versus social mediators of exercise adherence in the elderly. Am J Prev Med 2002; 23:80–86.

88. Grembowski D, Patrick D, Diehr P, et al. Self-efficacy and health behavior among older adults. J Health Soc Behav 1993; 34:89–104.

89. Evcik D, Sonel B. Effectiveness of a home-based exercise therapy and walking program on osteoarthritis of the knee. Rheumatol Int 2002; 22:103–106.

90. Bruce DG, Devine A, Prince RL. Recreational physical activity levels in healthy older women: the importance of fear of falling. J Am Geriatr Soc 2002; 50:84–89.

91. Boyette LW, Lloyd A, Boyette JE, et al. Personal characteristics that influence exercise behavior of older adults. J Rehabil Res Dev 2002; 39(1):95–103.

92. Kaplan M, Newsom J, McFarland B, et al. Demographic and psychosocial correlates of physical activity in late life. Am J Prev Med 2001; 21:306–312.

93. www.statcan.ca/english/Pgdb/health46.htm (November 1, 2003).

94. Conn VS, Minor MA, Burks KJ, et al. Integrative review of physical activity intervention research with aging adults. J Am Geriatr Soc 2003; 51:1159–1168.

95. Eakin EG, Glasgow RE, Riley KM. Review of primary care-based physical activity intervention studies: effectiveness and implications for practice and future research. J Fam Pract 2000; 49:158–168.

96. van der Bij AK, Laurant M, Wensing M. Effectiveness of physical activity interventions for older adults. Am J Prev Med 2002; 22:120–133.

97. Courneya KS, Segal RJ, Reid RD, et al. Multiple distinct factors predict exercise adherence in prostate cancer survivors during a randomized controlled trial. J Clin Epidemiol 2004; 57(6):571–579.

98. Hewitt M, Rowland JH, Yancik R. Cancer survivors in the United States: age, health, and disability. J Gerontol A Biol Sci Med Sci 2003; 58(1):82–91.

24

A Review of the Evidence Base of an Evolving Science: Gero-Oncology Nursing

Deborah A. Boyle
Banner Good Samaritan Medical Center, Phoenix, Arizona, U.S.A.

INTRODUCTION

The historic unrecognized problem of cancer and aging was identified in tandem by medicine and nursing over 25 years ago. Although great progress has been made to champion the needs of older adults facing cancer, significant discovery is required to bridge the knowledge gap between the epidemiologic prevalence of cancer with advancing age and the paucity of investigative findings to enhance and optimize elder cancer care. The goal of this chapter is to chronicle the evolution of the field of oncology nursing in its efforts to address the needs of the older adult facing cancer and to provide a review of the important scientific contributions made to gero-oncology by nursing research.

THE EVOLUTIONARY BLUEPRINT FOR GERO-ONCOLOGY NURSING

In analyzing oncology nursing's investment in the specialized care of the older adult over time, three distinct phases can be identified. These phases reflect both increasing recognition and behaviors to address predominantly unmet needs of the older adult facing cancer (Table 1). The phases focus on the recognition of bias, the beginning of advocacy, and the promotion of scientific discovery to provide evidence for nursing care planning and implementation.

Phase 1: Recognition of the Enormity of Bias, 1975–1985

The first phase of nursing's gero-oncology focus can be broadly depicted by small increments of awareness related to the historic magnitude of ageism that characterized elder cancer care. Practice and research exclusionary behaviors were first being identified during this time frame. Pediatric oncology, formally acknowledged since 1975 when the first medical specialty boards were offered to physicians, did not have a geriatric counterpart despite the fact that the elderly were diagnosed with cancer, more than four times the rate diagnosed in children. However, the realization of

Table 1 Phases in Nursing Recognition of the Special Needs of the Older Adult Facing Cancer

Phase I (1975–1981)	Recognition of the enormity of bias
Phase II (1982–1995)	Beginning of advocacy
Phase III (1996–present)	Delineation of action steps to drive nursing science in care

these clinical, educational, and research dilemmas was only discerned by a handful of oncology nurses, who for the most part, distinguished this scenario in their individual clinical practice settings (i.e., during rounds and patient care conferences) or in consideration of eligibility criteria for clinical trial participation.

The greater part of nursing focus during this time converged on symptom management related to the administration of novel systemic therapies, where clinical knowledge was basic at best (1). Hence interventions to minimize treatment-related symptom distress were determined on an empiric basis. Prior to the early 1990s, many older adults were inadequately treated for their malignancy due to significant age bias and the lack of consideration of physiological status (2). This deficit led to undertreating, mistreating, not treating, or substitution of a less optimal treatment. This paradigm resulted from the assumption that due to advanced age, the older adult was not a candidate for the preferred therapy at that time.

Phase 2: The Beginning of Advocacy, 1982–1995

The second phase of nursing attentiveness to the older adult facing cancer is best typified by the concept of an emerging defense of the elderly majority. For most of the 1980s through the early 1990s, small but incremental steps were taken by individual champions to address the needs of older adults with cancer. Begg and Carbone (3) were credited with the initial revelation of considerable ageism within the ranks of medical oncology in their review of 21 Eastern Cooperative Oncology Group clinical trials involving eight primary cancer sites. Awareness of these findings by a small, yet vocal cohort of oncology nurses prompted scrutiny of age-related bias in their own practice settings. In 1982, the first abstract focusing on the elderly with cancer was submitted for presentation at the Annual Oncology Nursing Society (ONS) Congress (4). Not long after, Rose Mary Yancik PhD as Editor-in-chief, published the first text on geriatric oncology (5). The content of this book emanated from a National Institutes of Health/National Institute on Aging-sponsored consensus meeting the year before. The first article citing special needs of the elderly was published in the nursing literature in 1984 (6). During that same year, Adria Laboratories sponsored the publication of a monograph concerning nursing care of the elderly with cancer (7). Weinrich, the first nursing author of an article published in a peer-reviewed journal, published the results of her initial research findings in 1986 (8). A compendium of medical articles was published in "Clinics in Geriatric Medicine" in 1987, whose authors represented a cross-section of oncologists and geriatricians with an early interest in gero-oncology (9). In spite of this early progress however the exclusionary precedent for consideration of older adults eligibility for clinical trials did not change until 1990.

The four years between 1988 and 1992 represented a time of intense enlightenment concerning the older adult with cancer. Of note were the following activities:

- 1988: Both ONS and the International Society for Nurses in Cancer Care sponsored plenary sessions on cancer in the elderly; an entire issue of

    "Seminars in Oncology Nursing" was devoted to the needs of the older adult facing cancer; British oncology nurse leader and editor, Bob Tiffany, added a chapter on the topic of nursing care of the elderly with cancer to the second edition of a nursing text used widely throughout Europe (10,11).

- 1989: Zenser and Coe (12) published the second major interdisciplinary text on cancer and aging; "Seminars in Oncology" devoted an issue to cancer in the elderly (13).
- 1990: A poignant commentary by European medical oncologists was published in "Lancet" calling attention to significant bias in treating older adults (2); The Lancet commentary that cited specific examples of ageism in cancer practice, became a "call to arms" for American oncology professionals, and offered precedent for the reversal of exclusionary practices.
- 1991: The ONS allocated funds to bring together a panel of oncology and gerontology nurse specialists to write a position paper on cancer in the elderly, which was ultimately published in the "Oncology Nursing Forum" in 1992 (14).
- 1992: A third text was published with editorial staffing by three early medical gero-oncologist leaders, Balducci, Lyman, and Ershler (15).

    Hence great effort evolved during this period to reduce the information gap evident within the ranks of oncology professionals. It was the nursing community however, that made the greatest strides in empowering their constituents with knowledge about the prominence of cancer in the elderly. In so doing, the ONS established itself as the leader of professional organizations in formally acknowledging this subset of ignored cancer patients by crafting a position paper on this topic and disseminating publications that called attention to this undeserved population.

Phase 3: Delineation of Action Steps to Drive Nursing Science in Care

The third and current phase of oncology nursing responsiveness to the older adult facing cancer could be best characterized by purposeful progress in advancing the scope of nursing research conducted on behalf of the older adult with or at risk for cancer. By the mid- to late-1990s, cancer nursing efforts were bolstered by a growing national recognition of the need for more comprehensive generic and specialty nursing expertise on older adults with both acute and chronic disease. Collaboration with professional agencies also enhanced more global awareness of the knowledge gap about elders and illness.

    The John A. Hartford Foundation first invested in age-specific nursing education in 1996 (16). They established the John A. Hartford Institute for Geriatric Nursing at New York University as a center of excellence. In 2003, ONS received a grant from this Foundation to evaluate specialty education's inclusion of gerontology content in curricula. This support further enhanced ONS's leadership in gero-oncology. In 2000, the Oncology Nursing Press published a specialty nursing text on care of older cancer patients (17).

    A productive collaboration between oncology nursing and the Geriatric Oncology Consortium (GOC) began with GOC's creation in 2001. Founded with the goal of enhancing opportunities for cancer research on the older adult, this groups interdisciplinary membership fostered collegial investigative endeavors. The GOC subsequently were the coauthors of the second ONS position paper on cancer and aging in 2004 (Table 2) (18).

Table 2 Comparison of ONS Position Statements on Care of the Older Adult Facing Cancer

1992 Ten major imperatives for oncology nurses include the following	2004 It is the position of ONS and GOC that care for older adults with cancer requires
Recognize personal biases toward aging and the elderly, which may interfere with the delivery of quality nursing care	Elimination of ageism in research, education, care, and public policy as it stands against core American values of autonomy and choice
Advocate cancer prevention and early detection activities for older adults	Full and equal access to cancer care across the trajectory (e.g., screening, diagnosis, treatment, rehabilitation, palliative care, survivorship, and wellness care)
Acknowledge the dynamic and complex interrelationship between cancer and aging, which affects cancer nursing care	Education of students and practicing clinicians across health disciplines in both oncology and elder care on the unique physiologic, developmental, psychological, emotional, social, and spiritual needs of older adults with cancer and their families
Intervene to prevent or minimize the unique age-specific sequelae of cancer and its management	Acknowledgment of and assessment for risks related to declining functional reserve as part of normal aging
Integrate comprehensive geriatric assessment into the nursing care of older adults	Incorporation of measurement of age beyond chronology to include biologic, functional, and personal dimensions
Assess the availability and capability of the support networks of elderly patients and their significant others	Interdisciplinary teams and comprehensive geriatric assessment to optimize treatment planning, access, and resulting outcomes
Increase communication with colleagues about older adults with cancer to enhance problem-solving in a variety of different settings and at different points along the cancer continuum	Integration of geriatric oncology care within and across care settings and delivery systems, including primary care, acute and critical care, and long-term institutional, home, and hospice care
Consider age-related factors that affect learning and performance of self-care activities related to the cancer experience	Redefinition of optimal outcomes to extend beyond disease-free survival and to include comorbidity, function, and quality of life
Maximize the advocacy role in ethical decision-making relative to quality of life of elderly people with cancer	Improved education, outreach, and incentives for older adults to participate in clinical research
Recognize the effects of health care policy on the nursing care of older adults who have or who are at risk for cancer	Advocacy, policy, and legislation that recognizes the demographic implications of aging and cancer and mandates necessary research and development of appropriate health and social services
	Increased funding for basic, clinical, and translational research in aging and cancer

Abbreviations: ONS, Oncology Nursing Society; GOC, Geriatric Oncology Consortium.
Source: From Refs. 14, 18.

Although great strides have been evidenced over the past two decades, the delay in recognition of the impact of aging on cancer care has resulted in an ongoing posture of "catch up" as patient needs are addressed. Progress in oncology nursing is further supported by the recent publication of a comprehensive nursing text featuring an evidence-based approach to the care of the elderly with cancer (19). Only in 2003 did the American Society of Clinical Oncology publish its curriculum on aging and develop a pilot program for a joint medical oncology/geriatric fellowship for physicians. A review of elder-specific clinical trials undertaken that same year (by internet data sources and telephone survey) revealed the existence of only 16 active studies. Of these, six addressed acute myeloid leukemia, five were for the treatment of breast cancer in older women, two were for non–small cell lung cancer, and one each were for colorectal and prostate cancers. In addition, there was one supportive care study focusing on the use of growth factors during treatment for breast, lung, and ovarian primaries, and non-Hodgkin's lymphoma. Of particular note was the absence of any elder-specific clinical trials sponsored by the Radiation Therapy Oncology Group, Gynecologic Oncology Group, and National Surgical Adjuvant Breast and Bowel Project. The number of elder-specific trials is increasing in response to federal, cancer center, and industry initiatives. Yet, the Senior Adult Oncology Program at the H. Lee Moffitt Cancer Center remains the rare example of a comprehensive clinical program in gero-oncology in the United States.

TWENTY YEARS OF ONCOLOGY NURSING RESEARCH

Four articles that address the scope of the nursing research agenda relative to elders with or at risk for cancer are particularly noteworthy. In 1990, Given and Keilman (20) posed ideas for nursing investigation clustered within three themes of prominence: prevention and early detection, reactions to treatment (as compared with younger adults), and psychosocial responses of elders and their families. Over a decade later, Boyle (21) readdressed these categories offering specific research questions and considerations for study within thematic subsets. A section on international perspectives for cancer nursing research with the older adult was included. Country- and region-specific epidemiologic trends were identified with recommendations for assimilating these findings into nursing research priorities.

In 2004, Kagan characterized, "The volume and sophistication of research in cancer and aging within nursing and across disciplines are incongruent with the demographics of aging and the epidemiology of cancer" (22, p. 293). Reviewing existing opinion papers and key nurse-generated studies of the older adult with cancer, Kagan analyzed the literature base and divided her chronology into two phases. The first phase focused on awareness of cancer and aging whereby the recognition of the special needs of the older adult were initially outlined. The second phase was identified as focusing on the semantics and appropriate language of gero-oncology. Providing an important analogy with pediatric oncology, Kagan distinguished a conceptual framework for consideration of nursing care specific to the older adult. She postulated that whereas children face cancer within the paradigm of a life yet to live, the older adult faces cancer within the context of a life mostly lived. While the optimum pediatric end point of care is frequently long-term survival, the geriatric equivalent often focuses on quality during age- and disease-adjusted remaining years of life (22). This conceptualization offered much needed direction for targeting meaningful studies that provide the evidence base for developing elder-specific nursing interventions. Based on Kagan's construct, the yet-to-evolve third phase of oncology nursing research with older adults will provide a more sophisticated, age-focused anthology of critical investigative findings.

Recently, Bourbonniere and Kagan (23) delineated existing research findings in an attempt to summarize the evidence base for oncology nursing decision-making and practice planning. While this evidence base was small, heterogeneous, and frequently qualitative in design, it established a beginning framework for future investigation of age-specific nursing interventions. Of note were the results of the most recent survey of the ONS membership on research priorities (24). Doctoral level nurses comprised 23% of the total sample completing the questionnaire and ranked "older adults/elderly" as the top research priority and "cognitive impairment/mental status changes" as the second highest priority for oncology nursing research. This was the first time that care of the elderly was distinguished as a critical target for research within cancer nursing.

ANTHOLOGY OF NURSE-DIRECTED RESEARCH FOCUSING ON THE OLDER ADULT WITH OR AT RISK FOR CANCER: 65 KEY PUBLICATIONS

Medline and Cinahl databases were queried for research articles with a nurse as primary investigator or coinvestigator within an interdisciplinary research team. The primary or majority patient sample had to be elderly ($\geq$60 years of age). Between 1986 and 2005, a total of 65 research papers were identified. These reports were characterized by an evolving frequency and focus over time.

In the period before the ONS assumed a leadership position within cancer care by publishing the first position statement on cancer and aging in 1992, only 5 of the 65 investigations identified as nurse-led were in print. Between 1992 and 2000, along with the recognition of the clinical importance of cancer with advancing age, there was a quadrupling of research publications compared with the early and initial phase of inquiry. Twenty-four published reports targeting the older adult with cancer were identified during this eight-year time frame. Using the anthology of 65 research papers as a reference set, more than half of all nursing research to date on the older adult with or at risk for cancer, has been published in the past five years as evidenced by 36 research papers in print in a variety of journals across disciplines.

The two decades of existing nurse-championed research (the anthology of 65 publications) was reviewed for thematic foci. Using subject headings suggested by the primary focus of the research paper, seven themes were delineated. These included ageism, community-based care, families and caregivers, information and education, symptom distress, physical functioning, and quality of life and patient coping. A synopsis of these studies provides the reader with a brief overview of nursing research in the field of gero-oncology, its intent, selection of sample populations, and key findings.

Ageism

Two international nurse colleagues published study results that addressed age-related bias in cancer care. Despite Sweden having one of the highest populations of elders in the world, older patients in Tishelman's (25) cross-sectional descriptive study perceived less sense of engagement and concern by health care professionals. Using spontaneous narrative responses, this study identified a lack of congruence between the needs of the older patient and the response of the health care providers to these needs. Older cancer patients were characterized as having a greater degree of health care need, yet were less likely to have their needs met by professional staff. Patients themselves also relayed ageist attitudes. When discussing fears about growing older and expectations about symptom prevalence, older patients generally recounted expectations that debilitation and functional decline come with old age. Hence a sense of futility and powerlessness predominated as the future was anticipated by these older patients with cancer.

Kearney et al. (26) implemented a survey at a regional Cancer Center in Scotland to evaluate oncology health care professionals' attitudes toward the elderly. Using the Kogan Old People Scale, persistent negative attitudes about growing old and elderly patients were documented. This cynicism prevailed despite the gender of the respondents, their professional role, clinical experience, and specialist education. Although no specific change strategy was recommended, the researchers called for a radical cultural shift in attitudes within the practice environment, especially in anticipation of evolving age-dominated demographics in the future.

Professional and patient ageism concerning cancer screening in older adults has been addressed in the United States. A retrospective chart review was undertaken for older women ($\geq$60 years of age), receiving care in a Mid-western family practice residency program (27). Charts were reviewed for documentation concerning screening recommendations for breast, gynecologic, and colorectal cancers. While recommendations were generally made to approximately two-thirds of the women in this age group (breast, 70%; gynecologic, 63%; and fecal blood test, 59% for colorectal cancer), less than one-third of the women receiving recommendations actually underwent the screening procedure. Citing numerous obstacles to screening, Blair (27) suggested increasing the knowledge of resident physicians about cancer screening guidelines in the elderly and augmenting existing didactic medical education with geriatric content. This training would increase the opportunity for providing older women with the education about their cancer risk, with particular attention to myths and misinformation, which was needed to empower them to assume greater responsibility for self-care.

Gulitz et al. (28) also addressed reasons why primary care providers miss opportunities to screen older women for breast and cervical cancer. They differentiated between human factors (patient and provider barriers) and system factors (practice, access, and medico-legal issues). Suggested strategies to improve screening were clustered within the categories of patient education and empowerment, professional training, modifications in the practice setting, and increasing accessibility. In the absence of interventions in each of these areas, older women may remain underserved despite their pronounced risk for cancer. Finally, using multiple medical and nursing databases, a research synthesis of the benefits and burdens of breast cancer screening in older women was completed by Yarbrough (29). There was no evidence cited that older women were less able than their younger counterparts to tolerate screening or treatment for breast cancer. Yet, underutilization of screening and suboptimum treatment of breast cancer in older women has consistently been documented (30–32).

Community-Based Care

Six publications about home and community-based care of the older adult with cancer emanated from two research projects. One investigation delineated older women's perceptions of the effectiveness of nurse case managers in the home setting. A second article derived from this study evaluated the effectiveness of nurse case managers on the treatment of older women with breast cancer. The second research project resulted in articles depicting the role of the oncology advanced practice nurse (APN) in the home setting, including a description of effective interventions, patient information needs, and the impact of home care interventions on the family caregiver's psychosocial status.

Along with physician colleagues, Anderson (33) evaluated the effect of nurse case management on the treatment of older women with breast cancer. Three hundred thirty-five women from 60 surgical practices participated in this randomized prospective trial. One hundred sixty-nine older women received an intervention that entailed use of nurse case management services for 12 months following initial diagnosis, while 166 women received usual care. Of note were the following findings: women in the intervention group received more breast-conserving therapy with higher rates of axillary dissection and adjuvant radiation therapy, and also more reconstructive surgery. Two months following surgery, women in the nurse case management group had greater arm mobility and normal arm function than those receiving usual care. Women with advanced disease in the intervention group were more likely to have received chemotherapy. Older women with minimal social support were more likely to benefit from nurse case management interventions at home.

A second report from this study presented findings on the perceptions of older women on the efficacy of nurse case management mediation (34). Positive sequelae included help with the management of comorbid conditions, provision of emotional support and information, assistance with activities of daily living (ADL), and advice on how to navigate the complex health care system. Key characteristics of effective nurse case management in this study included the use of excellent communication skills, possession of an in-depth knowledge about breast cancer, possession of standard gerontology nurse case manager training, and the awareness of and ability to mobilize community resources and support systems as needed.

The results of a significant investigation comparing the length of survival of older postsurgical cancer patients ($n = 375$), who received specialized home care intervention ($n = 190$) provided by APNs with that of patients who received usual follow-up care ($n = 185$) in the ambulatory setting was reported in 2000 (35). The intervention consisted of a standardized protocol that included well-defined patient assessment parameters and postsurgical management guidelines, doses of instructional content, and schedules of contact. The interventions combined physical care and psychosocial support during the acute postoperative period. Two critical phenomena were addressed by these interventions. First, patients and families were assisted during the period of transition from hospital to home by the availability of education, guidance, and reassurance during a time of heightened psychological stress and uncertainty. Second, monitoring of the patient's physical status was undertaken during the initial phase of recovery, which is often characterized by vulnerability to postoperative complications. The interventions prevailed over four weeks and included three home visits and five telephone contacts provided by APNs. Overall, the specialized home care intervention group had significantly increased survival. Of note was a higher percentage (38%) of patients with late-stage cancer in the specialized care group as compared with only 28% with late-stage cancer at initial diagnosis in the usual care group. This was the first study of postsurgical cancer patients to link specialized home care intervention by APNs with improved survival (35). Three companion reports detailed additional study findings.

For the APN intervention study, the four-week course of home care was described in detail by Hughes et al. (36). Types of interventions, frequency, range, and variation over time in intervention emphasis and dose intensity were recounted using the Nursing Intervention Lexicon and Taxonomy categorical classification that captures the content domain of nursing interventions. Teaching represented the highest percentage of documented interventions. This was followed in order of decreasing frequency by the provision of psychosocial support, reassurance, assessment of patient needs and nursing care requirements, appraisal of current status, and indirect care activities (usually in the context of patient advocacy and fact finding). Dose intensity of nursing interventions changed over time, suggesting that the APNs altered their care as patient needs evolved. The greatest diversity in nursing care interventions was noted in the cohort of older women newly diagnosed with breast cancer.

Hughes et al. also elucidated information needs of elderly postsurgical oncology patients by conducting a content analysis of 3280 statements of teaching interventions performed by nurses (37). Major teaching themes included instructing on postoperative self-care, advising on symptom management, clarifying the illness experience, discussing psychological responses, and preparing patients and families to coordinate follow-up care. Focusing on the time frame of transitional care from hospital to home, the scope of elderly postsurgical patient informational needs was extensive. Teaching interventions ranged from the very practical (i.e., offering concrete information about care of surgical wounds) to the predominantly abstract (i.e., analyzing complex information concerning cancer therapy options). The investigators proposed that in the absence of informational support during this time of transitional care, older patients may remain at risk for inadequate postoperative care due to undermanagement, wrongful management, or the absence of any management in spite of indications of need.

Finally, Jepson et al. (38) reported on changes in the psychosocial status of caregivers of the elderly postsurgical patients. The presence of physical problems in caregivers and the patient's receipt of the home care intervention were factored in the analysis of caregiver psychosocial responses. Structured interviews and completion of the Caregiver Reaction Assessment and the Center for Epidemiologic Studies-Depression Scale occurred at the time of discharge and at three and six months. Interesting results were revealed. Of caregivers with physical problems, the psychosocial status of those in the home care intervention group either remained stable or declined between the initial evaluation and at three months, followed by improvement between three and six months. The reverse pattern was observed in the control (no intervention) group. The researchers hypothesized that caregivers with their own physical compromise may experience greater psychosocial burden in the initial three months when early recognition of the numerous expectations of providing home health care are reinforced by a home-care nursing requirement. Hence, interventions to help master transitional care for vulnerable patients and relieve vulnerable caregivers warrant further investigation.

Families and Caregivers

There is a paucity of research on developmental implications of care giving when the patient and spouse are both elderly. Harden (39) reviewed the existing literature and examined the impact of prostate cancer on couples' quality of life within three age subsets: late middle age (50–64 years), the young-old (65–74), and the old-old (75 years and older). Normal developmental changes were reviewed and brief citations of possible cancer-related implications were provided. Three studies have addressed elder caregivers of spouses with cancer along with other disease entities.

General findings emanating from these investigations yield important considerations for future research within gero-oncology.

The goal of research by Given et al. (40) was to predict spouses' reactions to new caregiving roles. Patient variables, details of the caregiving environment, and characteristics of the caregiver were analyzed. Four prominent domains of caregivers' responses were identified: negative emotional reactions, feelings of responsibility for the patient, feelings of abandonment by the family, and impact of caregiving on daily schedules. The prominence of caregiver responses within these four domains was influenced most by the presence of patient cognitive impairment, patient dependencies in instrumental ADLs, older age, and compromised physical health in the spouse caregiver. The researchers noted that their findings validated the complexity and multidimensionality of the caregiving experience for older spouse caregivers. In another study of caregiving, a diverse sample of elders in caregiving roles (for patients with Alzheimer's disease, Parkinson's disease, or cancer) was compared with a control group of elders who were noncaregiving; i.e., with spouses that did not require extra care (41). Fatigue, feelings of having less energy, and more sleep difficulties were increased in caregivers compared with noncaregivers. Even if the patient did not require extensive physical caregiving, the perception of fatigue related to the caregiver role was common.

A secondary analysis by Yang and Kirschling (42) of caregivers of elderly family members receiving hospice care explored factors related to the amount of direct care and outcomes of caregiving (operationally defined as the amount of lifestyle change, role strain, and rewards of caregiving). Eighty-four percent of this patient sample had a malignancy as their primary diagnosis. While all patients were aged 65 years or older, the ages of the caregivers ranged from 39 to 84 years (mean 64.5). Variables that influenced heightened degrees of caregiver distress included the presence of patient behavioral problems and length of time in hospice care. Patient behavioral problems included the caregiver's listening to and answering repetitive questions and dealing with episodes of crying, paranoia or suspiciousness, and aggressive behaviors. As length of stay in hospice increased, caregivers reported an intensification of communication tasks such as relaying news of patient status, particularly news of disease progression. Ongoing monitoring of visitors also caused added strain, as caregivers became intermediaries sensitive to patient needs. The need for formal caregiver support was also highlighted because role strain in caregivers was prominent. Finally, two studies targeted caregivers within the cancer experience.

Lewis et al. (43) explored the scope of decision-making required by elderly cancer patients and their family caregivers. Weekly interviews over a period of four months were completed with five nurse cancer center coordinators. The nurses were queried about the nature and frequency of topics that required decision-making by older patients and their families, requests for assistance, and perceptions of assistance related to telephone contacts. Content analyses revealed 11 categories germane to decision-making and information-support needs within the gero-oncology treatment experience. They included

- symptom management;
- chemotherapy use;
- medical provider choice (other than primary oncologist);
- end-of-life care planning;
- alternative therapies;
- vacation planning;
- respite care;

- discharge planning;
- family survivor issues; and
- involvement of adult children in elder care.

In addition to the provision of information related to these topics, the investigators also identified core requirements of family members during this experience that related to information clarification, reassurance around decisional conflict, having a listener, being offered permission to question the treatment plan, and advocacy assistance with communication difficulties between multiple health professionals and the patient and family. Information was also the focus of another investigation concerning caregiver preparedness and its effect on coping.

Citing multiple negative indices of caregiving within the context of elder care (particularly during protracted times of caregiving requirements), Rusinak and Murphy (44) described their results of an exploratory study to examine the relationship between perceptions of preparedness for caregiving, use of coping strategies, and knowledge about care requirements in caregivers of older patients in the home setting. Moderate scores on instruments measuring preparedness were noted as were relatively high scores on knowledge and skill scales concerning the provision of basic aspects of care required in the home setting. Relatively high scores were also identified on measures evaluating caregiver coping. This study was limited in sample size and in the inclusion of caregivers only at the initiation of home care. The investigators suggested the need for longitudinal assessment of changes in caregivers, which occur in coping, preparedness, knowledge, and skills in relation to the cancer trajectory. Demands on informal caregivers will increase in the future. Consequently, there will be an increased need for data about role strain and the doses of knowledge, skill, and support needed to enhance caregiver effectiveness.

Information and Education

Based on both clinical experience and commentary offered in the sections above, the prominence of information and education quandaries in elder cancer care is unquestionable. Ten studies focusing on this paradigm have addressed knowledge in relation to the nature of cancer, screening, and the management of pain.

Despite older adults' heightened vulnerability to cancer, Weinrich and Weinrich (8) noted inadequate knowledge about cancer related to the belief in common cancer myths, recognition of the American Cancer Society's warning signs, and delineation of frequent symptoms of cancer. A Canadian sample of 158 older adults also demonstrated a lack of recognition that advanced age was an important risk factor for cancer (45). To address awareness of vulnerability to common forms of solid tumors in the elderly, such as colorectal cancer, older adults in another sample stated they were never informed about this malignancy and the need for screening (46). This second study also addressed the influence of an education module on participation in screening by older adults. Weinrich et al. (47) further studied education strategies to enhance screening behaviors by utilizing elderly educators to provide information about colorectal cancer and screening to a group of socioeconomically disadvantaged elders. Four educational methods were studied with the outcome measure being participation in fecal occult blood screening. The two methods that utilized elderly educators had statistically significant improved participation rates over those methods that did not employ peer educators.

Coleman et al. (48) targeted rural primary health care providers (physicians, nurses, and mammography technicians) for the provision of intensive education about breast cancer screening for older primarily African-American women. Following an education intervention, older women in the rural counties where the provider education was offered, received more mammograms than those women cared for in comparison counties. In another study that focused on improved screening for older low-income women, Morrison (49) investigated the frequency and proficiency of breast self-examination (BSE) and BSE predictors to guide clinical discussion and formal teaching agendas. Ten predictors emerged within three categories that included predisposing factors, enabling factors, and reinforcing factors. Again, citing the complexity of understanding motivation to participate in cancer screening, patient involvement can most likely be positively influenced when confidence and knowledge (predisposing factors), awareness, sufficient time and influence of a trusted teacher (enabling factors), and clinician follow-up contact (reinforcing factor) are all operational to promote behavior change.

Another example of customizing education interventions was published by Wood et al. (50). An age- and race-sensitive breast health kit (including a video, mini-lump model, BSE poster, BSE skill checklist, educational pamphlet, and series of calendar reminder stickers) was created to test the kit's influence on knowledge of breast cancer risk, screening, and BSE proficiency. A group of predominantly older (≥ 60 years of age), low-income, African-American volunteers comprised the sample of inner-city women for this quasiexperimental pretest and posttest investigation. Two weeks following kit use, knowledge and BSE proficiency scores had improved significantly for the intervention group. The researchers concluded that using age- and race-sensitive teaching tools positively influenced knowledge and behavioral outcomes. Low income of target populations has been identified as a significant variable influencing participation in screening, particularly with reference to prostate cancer screening. However, Weinrich et al. (51) identified that low income was not an independent significant factor related to participation rates for free prostate cancer screening. Even when the barrier of cost has been removed, other barriers remain for low-income men, which prove influential in determining screening participation. For example, a prominent barrier relates to a fatalistic attitude about what could be found with prostate screening and subsequent hesitancy to impose the potential social and financial burden of cancer on the family. Targeted teaching about benefits of early detection and treatment options related to stage of prostate cancer could help reduce historic and cultural beliefs that foster diagnosis delay and ultimate treatment futility.

Finally, formal instruction on the management of pain in older adults was the focus of two quasiexperimental studies. Ferrell et al. (52) targeted their instruction to family caregivers of older adults experiencing pain due to cancer, while Clotfelter (53) focused on older adult patients receiving ambulatory care in the office setting. Ferrell et al. noted improvements in knowledge and attitudes of family members following education program participation. Clotfelter demonstrated statistically significant improvement in patient pain score intensity ratings following exposure to formal education on pain control including a video presentation and pamphlet, compared with usual instruction only. While the management of pain, particularly chronic pain, is well recognized as problematic within gerontology, pain and its corollaries due to cancer are significantly underrepresented in the scientific literature.

Symptom Distress

The relationship between age and cancer-related symptom distress continues to be characterized by a paucity of scientific findings. In 1989, McMillan (54) first attempted to study this association with specific attention to nausea, vomiting, and pain. While preliminary analysis in a small sample tended to support the theory that older adults may experience decreased symptom distress, McMillan noted that this association was a statistically weak one that required more extensive investigation. Given et al. (55) further studied the impact of age and treatment on symptom distress. Probably of most importance was the finding that the degree of symptom distress in older adults, at initial intake and at six months, had the greatest impact on the patient's functionality and mental health. Building on important early findings about the relationship between quality symptom management and functional status, the additional findings of these researchers have fostered interest in the complex affiliation between age, symptoms, functional status, and outcome from cancer therapies.

In 2000, a profile for elderly lung cancer patients who were most at risk for suffering substantial losses in physical functioning following initial diagnosis was identified (56). Prior physical function, patient age, and symptom severity were variables most predictive of physical compromise for this older subset of lung cancer patients. A later report focusing on symptoms of pain and fatigue in the elderly identified stage of disease, presence of comorbidity, and a diagnosis of a primary lung tumor as being most associated with these debilitating symptoms (57). Duggleby (58) qualitatively researched the concept of suffering and its relationship to pain in elderly hospice patients with cancer. The global impact of pain on function was exemplified by this elderly sample in terms of its enduring nature. Accepting the presence of unrelenting pain, while anticipating death in the near future, represented a daunting example of "pain work" that these elderly patients experienced primarily in isolation. This aspect of mismanaged or undermanaged symptom distress and its affiliation with choice to pursue unconventional therapy within cancer care for the elderly deserves further investigation.

In 1999, Wyatt et al. (59) investigated complementary therapy use by older adult cancer patients, and this study is a rare example of an investigation targeting the consumption or utilization of alternative therapy by the elderly. A survey of nearly 700 elderly patients with solid tumors (i.e., breast, colorectal, prostate, or lung) was undertaken to assess patterns of use and characteristics of patients most likely to utilize complementary therapies. Over one-third of this sample reported using complementary therapies, consisting primarily of exercise, herbal therapy, and spiritual healing. A notable finding was that women with breast cancer having higher education degrees were more likely to utilize these approaches. More recently, two unique components of symptom distress in the elderly with cancer have been reported. They include the report of a secondary analysis of age differences in self-reported symptoms of lymphedema following breast cancer therapy and the evolving recognition of symptom clusters when focusing on the reduction of symptom distress (60–62). Limited investigation of age-related differences in symptom appearance and intensity, and early work identifying common symptom clusters are likely to be augmented by more intense research in the future.

Physical Functioning

Functional status is a central denominator in numerous queries of the older adult's cancer experience. Compromise in physical functioning may prompt increased symptom distress, while the premorbid presence of cancer-related symptoms may promote a worsening variant of functional status. Poor functional status is associated with heightened levels of psychosocial morbidity and negative outcomes from cancer therapy. Duffy et al. (63) also identified the association of functional status with engagement in screening behaviors, including pursuit of early detection testing and proficiency in self-care practices such as BSE. Finally, physical functioning is a critical determinant of patient perceptions of quality of life.

Given and Given with multiple collaborators have reported a series of research findings on functional status in the older cancer patient and its relationships with numerous variables (56,64–68). These investigations have addressed issues related to functional recovery from surgery, the status of physical functioning prior to diagnosis and following initial treatment, the influence of symptoms, age, comorbidity, and cancer type on physical functioning and mental health of older women with cancer, and tumor-specific indices of functional impairment (Table 3, also see Chapter 28). Three other nurse-generated studies have included one that addresses the influence of functional status on hope in the elderly with and without cancer. A second study has investigated physical and psychosocial outcomes of midlife and older women following surgery and adjuvant chemotherapy for breast cancer. A third study describes the use of a specialized instrument to evaluate functional status in older patients with cancer (69–71). This concentration of investigative effort on physical functioning is testimony to nurses' recognition of the importance of this variable in the quality of patient survival, regardless of the projected trajectory.

Quality of Life and Patient Coping

Eighteen nurse-directed studies have covered a diverse range of topics and cohorts of older patients under the broad theme of coping with cancer. They are so diverse in nature and scope that each warrants a brief synopsis so that the reader can further pursue a report of particular interest.

The early work of Edlund and Sneed (72) explored the nature of emotional responses to the diagnosis of cancer as a function of age. Of the 133 newly diagnosed, hospitalized patients in their sample, four adult subsets were identified: 21 to 49 years ($n = 34$), 50 to 59 years ($n = 26$), 60 to 69 years ($n = 39$), and 70 years or older ($n = 34$). Five instruments were used, which measured prediagnosis perceptions and attitudes and postdiagnosis adjustment. Findings included the observation that younger patients (≤ 50 years of age) experienced greater emotional distress in the time immediately following diagnosis in comparison with older subsets. The oldest-old (≥ 70 years of age) patient cohort exhibited the most fatalistic reaction to the news of cancer. Fatalism associated with a diagnosis of cancer was also determined to be a key factor in Powe's (73) descriptive study of elderly Caucasians' and African-Americans' views about cancer.

Qualitative research findings regarding characteristics of living with cancer as an older adult were described by multiple researchers. Thome et al. from Sweden (74) identified some of the existential experiences of older adults who were pondering life and death issues. Via life review, study findings revealed that many older patients dealing with cancer could validate their reality of "living a good life," and recognize the finiteness of life without experiencing overwhelming emotional turmoil. Semi-structured interviews of five older adults with advanced cancer offered insightful narratives on factors influencing the quality of end-of-life care (75). These included genuine caring, compassionate honesty from trusted members of the healthcare team, the use of cautious hopefulness, unquestioned faith, an involvement in desired activities, and positive personal and professional relationships. In lieu of limited

Table 3 Investigations of Functional Status in Older Cancer Patients

References	Research foci/Sample	Major findings	Recommendations
64	Degree symptoms, physical functioning, and mental health are influenced by age and comorbid conditions and how these vary by cancer site; 299 women ($\geq$65 years of age) with breast, colon, or lung primaries	Women with lung cancer experienced greatest losses in physical functioning; there was no difference in mental health scores among tumor sites; correlation analysis revealed a moderately strong relationship between symptom severity and physical functioning and mental health	Role and importance of rigorous control of symptom distress during therapy is underappreciated; by reducing the disabling nature of symptom presence and intensity, overall functional recovery could be enhanced
65	Psychosocial and disease-specific factors influence functional recovery in newly diagnosed elders; 172 community-dwelling elderly ($\geq$65 years of age) surgically treated for lung, prostate, breast, or colorectal primaries	Prostatectomy patients experienced more of a delay in recovery as compared to patients undergoing surgery for breast, lung, or colorectal primaries; pain and fatigue were the most common severe symptoms experienced; psychological well-being influenced functional recovery	Use of APNs could enhance functional recovery postsurgery by aggressively monitoring and managing comorbid conditions and symptom distress
66	Does cancer site and stage predict functional limitations; how well do age, comorbidity, stage, treatment, and cluster of symptoms[a] explain changes in physical function between 3 and 8 mos. postdiagnosis; 826 patients (mean age of 72–75) with a new diagnosis of either breast, colon, lung, or prostate cancer	Site and stage of cancer do not affect functioning; presence of pain, fatigue, and insomnia were significant and independent predictors of change in physical functioning; despite high levels of functioning prior to treatment, 25% of patients in each tumor type grouping deteriorated two quartiles on repeated SF-36 physical subscale scoring during treatment	Interventions to reduce symptom distress (particularly pain, fatigue, and insomnia) early in the course of treatment is paramount; when and how comorbidity affects functioning remains an important area for future research

(Continued)

Table 3 Investigations of Functional Status in Older Cancer Patients (*Continued*)

References	Research foci/Sample	Major findings	Recommendations
67	Relationship between age, gender, comorbidity, site and stage of cancer, and treatment to losses in physical functioning at four evaluation points during the year following diagnosis; 907 older patients ($\geq$65 years of age) newly diagnosed with either breast, colon, lung, or prostate cancer	Men scored higher than women on physical functioning at all observation points; comorbidity ($\geq$3) was predictive of lower functioning; postsurgical patients within 40 days of study intake, had lower function scores than those beyond 40 days; this trend was reversed for patients undergoing chemotherapy (with the exception of older women receiving chemotherapy for breast cancer); patients receiving radiation therapy were least affected in physical functioning at any evaluation time; cumulative increase in number of symptoms was associated with functional decline	Older women with $\geq$3 comorbid conditions may benefit from professional intervention to enhance function and reduce symptom distress within the first month following surgery for breast, lung, or colorectal cancer; instrument use to quantify changes in functional status and measure symptom distress is needed to validate degree of change and efficacy of symptom distress–relieving measures
68	How does symptom severity vary according to treatment type, stage of cancer, and gender; what variable influences longitudinal change in function; 129 older patients with lung cancer	Loss of physical functioning predictors included symptom severity, prior physical functioning, and patient age; a high risk profile for elderly lung cancer patients vulnerable for substantial loss in physical functioning included higher prior level of physical functioning, higher level of symptom distress, and lower patient age	Early recognition strategies for declining functional status should be in place for planning supportive care interventions to enhance patient quality of life

[a]This was one of the first studies to describe the presence of symptom clusters (i.e., pain, fatigue, and insomnia).
Abbreviations: APN, advanced practice nurse; SF, short form.

treatment goals during metastatic disease, explanation of the benefits of interventions promoting tumor stability, the deterrence of progression and optimization of quality of life must be purposeful and reinforced to counter many older adults' perceptions concerning the nature of systemic therapies (76). Also using a phenomenological research design, Thome et al. (77) investigated the meaning of living with cancer in old age. The analysis of findings revealed four themes: transition into a more or less disintegrated existence, sudden awareness of the finiteness of life, meeting disease and illness, and redefinition of one's role in life for good or bad. This issue of redefining oneself was also of interest to Heidrich and Ward (78). They investigated the psychological adjustment of elderly women with cancer and noted a common theme. Their research postulated that the positive adjustment of some elderly women may be the result of their ability to lower their ideal self expectations, thereby reducing self-discrepancies that may result in psychological distress. Fehring et al. (79) correlated hope and positive mood states with intrinsic religiosity and spiritual well-being in older adults coping with cancer. Of note was Houldin and Wasserbauer's (80) survey of 105 older cancer patients where the majority of respondents (69%) cited spiritual help as a major way to enhance personal coping. Gillies and Johnston (81) highlighted role change and loss as indicators of transition to different social groups, limiting responsibilities in older adults with cancer and dementia.

Fitch et al. (82) targeted older women's reactions to living with ovarian cancer while Overcash (83) focused on older women's adaptation to breast cancer. Using both questionnaires and narrative interviews, both studies revealed patient depictions of unrecognized needs for information, enhanced communication, emotional counseling, and tangible support. Fitch et al. proposed that more rigorous assessment of impediments to quality of life over time could assist in the identification of these unmet needs. Additionally, soliciting individual needs within numerous supportive, care domains (i.e., physical, social, practical, informational, psychological and spiritual), fosters the tailoring of interventions within the older adult's life context. Acknowledging older women's pervasive concern regarding sustaining independence, binding and group (84) suggested undertaking comprehensive nursing histories with special attention paid to decision-making preferences. Although quality of life in the elderly is recognized as a potentially nebulous and highly individualized construct, specific concerns about quality of life in the elderly with cancer were the recent genesis for three reports.

Esbensen et al. (85) investigated quality of life of older adults with cancer in relation to patient age, their contact with the health care system, ability to perform ADLs, their degree of hope, and the nature of their social network and support structure. Predictors of low quality of life were considered. Elderly patients diagnosed with cancer within the previous three weeks (75 women and 26 men aged ≥ 65 years of age) were included in the sample recruited from the county of Copenhagen in Denmark. Multiple measures of quality of life, hope, functional status, and social interaction were employed. An at-risk profile for inferior quality of life in older adults recently diagnosed with cancer emanated from this study. Characteristics of these patients included being of low income, having lung cancer, and feeling hopeless about their prognosis. A study of the gender perspective of quality of life in older adults was undertaken by Thome and Hallberg (86) in Sweden. A comparison of older men ($n = 76$) and women ($n = 74$) with cancer (≥ 75 years of age) with a matched control group of peers without cancer (men $= 74$, women $= 64$) was performed using measures of quality of life, functional status, and social support. Older women with cancer were more vulnerable than their male counterparts to problems ensuing from inadequacies in social support (e.g., living alone, fewer adult children to assist with care, etc.), economic security (e.g., reliance on pension as sole source of financial support), and greater symptom burden (e.g., more comorbidity, greater symptom distress related to cancer and cancer therapies, etc.).

A distinct focus on older women's quality of life during the trajectory of breast cancer survivorship was addressed by Sammarco (87). A total of 103 women over the age of 50 participated in this study of the dynamics of social support and feelings of uncertainty and their relationship to quality of life following breast cancer therapy. Consistent with the reality that advancing age brings increased concern about, and need for, social support, older female breast cancer survivors perceived dwindling amounts of support in their lives. A significant relationship between uncertainty and quality of life was evidenced. Sammarco delineated the unique nature of this dyad in the older adult's experience by noting that "the unpredictable nature of breast cancer and treatment coupled with the presence of other diseases or functional disabilities of aging may serve to influence a poorer quality of life in health/functioning, socioeconomic, and psychological/spiritual domains." Of equal importance to study findings were the investigator's suggestions for practice and research specific to older adult cancer survivors. They included

- recognizing requirements for more time for assessment and follow-up care,
- paying special attention to the etiology and differentiation of symptoms,
- advocating assistance for the elderly to identify and expand family and community resources of support,
- offering age-specific support groups, and
- investigating quality of life in older breast cancer survivors beyond the usual patient sampling of middle- to upper-class Caucasian women.

Most recently, Deimling and colleagues investigated the concept of vulnerability in 321 older survivors with a history of breast, prostate and colorectal primary malignancies (88). Citing cancer-related symptom persistence in addition to ongoing health concerns associated with co-morbid illness, women and African-American survivors were most frequently characterized by this concept of vulnerability persistent pain and compromised functional status were more prominent in these two survivor cohorts.

Although of primary importance, many of these practice suggestions will require further investigation to quantify the patient, social, and cost benefits of these interventions. To assist with this important construct, McCorkle et al. (89) proposed a nursing lexicon and taxonomy strategy for classifying elements of nursing interventions that capture multiple domains of nursing expertise in cancer nursing practice. Also related to the survivorship paradigm is further elucidation of the powerful force of fear of cancer recurrence in older adults and the implications of anxiety over time, because watchful waiting in select subpopulations of older patients remains operational (90,91).

A FUTURE TEMPLATE FOR GERO-ONCOLOGY NURSING RESEARCH

The possibilities for continued investigation of issues in gero-oncology are extensive, diverse, enhanced by intradisciplinary collaboration, and highly sensitive to nursing intervention. The ONS recently sanctioned the creation and publication of a white paper on nursing-sensitive patient outcomes (92). Acknowledging that nursing interventions play a vital role in preventing and minimizing symptoms, complications, and other untoward effects across the entire trajectory of cancer care, the collective oncology nursing community must assume responsibility for documenting the

Table 4   Outcome Exemplars from the ONS Outcomes Project Team

Symptom control and management
Pain
Peripheral neuropathy
Fatigue
Insomnia
Nausea
Constipation
Anorexia
Breathlessness
Diarrhea
Altered skin or mucous membranes
Neutropenia
Functional status
ADL
IADL
Role functioning
Activity tolerance
Ability to carry out usual activities
Nutritional status
Safety
Infections
Falls
Skin ulcers
Extravasation incidents
Hypersensitive reactions
Psychological health status
Anxiety
Depression
Spiritual distress
Coping
Economic (incorporated into all categories)
Length of stay
Unexpected readmissions
Emergency room visits
Out-of-pocket costs (family)
Homecare visits
Costs per patient episode

Abbreviations: ADL, activities of daily living; IADL, instrumental activities of daily living; ONS, Oncology Nursing Society.
Source: From Ref. 93.

impact of their contributions on patient outcomes (Table 4). Although many of these outcomes have been the focus of existing research as described in this chapter, there are numerous additional opportunities for nursing query when the target patient population is the older adult facing cancer. The following suggestions represent some considerations for future research within the context of elder cancer care.

The Symptom Experience

It is generally acknowledged that disease and its associated symptoms present differently in older adults as compared to their younger counterparts (94). There is a paucity of evidence addressing the intensity, prevalence, intensity, pattern, duration, contributing factors, management, and prevention of symptom distress in the older adult receiving antineoplastic therapies, particularly as compared to their younger counterparts. Frequently, past experience and assumption, rather than the results of scientific inquiry, guide decision-making in this area. However, recent attention to the deleterious effects of underdosing both supportive and therapeutic drugs in elder cancer care and this phenomenon's impact on symptom distress and ultimate treatment outcomes, has challenged existing age-related bias, particularly related to growth factor support in ever moderately toxic regimens (95). Oncology nurses then must become proficient in teaching older patients the rationale for schedule adherence and reporting of untoward effects and early symptoms related to neutropenia and anemia (96–99). Additionally, the heterogeneity of older adults, by age subset, presence of co-morbidity, and functional status, is rarely synthesised as influencing research outcomes (100). Co-morbidity in particular is an important in the prominance and magnitude of symptom distress (101). Also, attention to the symptom distress associated with the administration of chemotherapy should not preclude investigation of symptom distress during radiation therapy and surgical interventions. Boyle outlined common geriatric syndromes with the identification of critical questioning about the nature of these symptoms within gero-oncology (Table 5) (102). A critique of the general gerontologic literature on symptom management would benefit oncology nurses who are investigating the cancer experience. For example, examination of comorbidity and its effect on fatigue and sleep alterations as well as a review of interventions for chronic insomnia would be worthwhile (103–107). Approaches to the assessment of incontinence (both fecal and urinary) could augment the determination of toxicities associated with pelvic irradiation and obstructive symptoms commonly associated with prostate and bladder tumors in older men (108). Also, evidence-based reports described in the general context of cancer care should be analyzed for their meaning and adaptation to the experience of older adults (109,110). Additionally, older patients perceptions of their cancer care has been only minimally studied (100). The concept of frailty and vulnerability and its application within elder cancer care requires consideration (111–113).

Functional Status

Due to the exclusive nature of biological and chronological age, the determination of functional status assumes great importance will be older adults (114). The appropriate use of instruments to measure this entity in cancer care has not been determined (115). However, the feasibility of using meaningful, practical yet comprehensive assessment guides are currently under investigation (116–118). Unique variables that relate to provider constraints, particularly when specialty teams and/or resources are unavailable, require development and testing of alternatives to, or variations of, traditional comprehensive geriatric assessments. Fitzsimmons (119) advised that methodological adaptations take into account improved ways of understanding and rethinking how the outcomes of the cancer experience are prioritized for the older person with cancer. An important corollary to functional status, which must be considered is the ability to maintain cancer care in the older adults' home setting. Marek et al. (120) elucidated the benefits of aging in place. This ability may not only promote enhanced quality of life but may also impact the reduction of cancer-specific indices of symptom distress such as delirium and falls, as well as the economic burden of cancer care.

Safety

Twenty priorities for improving healthcare quality were recently delineated by the Institute of Medicine committee (121). One area with particular relevance to nursing as well

Table 5 SPPICEES Geriatric Assessment Model and Its Application to Oncology Nursing

	Common problem	Cancer-specific issues
S	Skin integrity	Radiation-related skin compromise
		Postsurgical wound healing
		Skin vulnerability R/T prolonged immobility in conjunction with symptom cluster of pain, fatigue, and anorexia
P	Problems with nutrition	Food intolerances and taste changes
		Suboptimum quantity requirements to boost caloric intake
		Short periods of anorexia associated with weight loss and decreased large muscle mass
P	Problems with pain	Unknown ideal dose requirements of opioids, nonopioids, and adjuvant medications
		Questionable toxicity prevalence and intensity as compared with younger adults
		Potential delirium with pain drugs + metabolic abnormalities
I	Immobility	Heightened infectious corollaries associated with immune compromise + immobility
		Significant implications of falls during bone marrow depression
		Peripheral neurotoxicity prolonged incidence + reversal time frame
C	Confusional states	Absence of physiological multiple risk factor identification + prodromal signs
		Lack of quick screen to recognize early signs
		Unknown protocol for drug + behavioral management
E	Elimination	Prevalence + optimum management of constipation, diarrhea R/T chemo- + radiotherapy
		Tolerance of parenteral nutrition
		Hesitancy to disclose use of OTC medications or complementary approaches to manage symptoms
E	Elder mistreatment	Withholding of pain medications by family for fear of dependency
		Professional age bias in the undertreatment of pain
		Isolation/aversion by family unwilling to assist with care
S	Sleep	Alterations in sleep pattern during hospitalization
		Hesitancy to disclose use of OTC medications to manage symptoms
		Unknown effects of sleep deprivation on symptom intensity

Abbreviation: OTC, over-the-counter.
Source: From Ref. 92.

as medicine and pharmacy relates to improving the global paradigm of safety (122). A major opportunity for oncology nursing that has not been addressed in the research literature to date is the reduction of adverse effects associated with medication consumption in the older patient with cancer. There are numerous opportunities to intervene in this area. Figure 1 portrays the many demands on the older patient to assume responsibility for medications with therapeutic, supportive care, and preventive intentions. The reality of polypharmacy in gero-oncology imposes a plethora of opportunities for adherence problems, medication mismanagement, and iatrogenic effects that require significant attention particularly because age-related altered pharmacokinetics and pharmacodynamics create the milieu upon which these drug related issues evolve

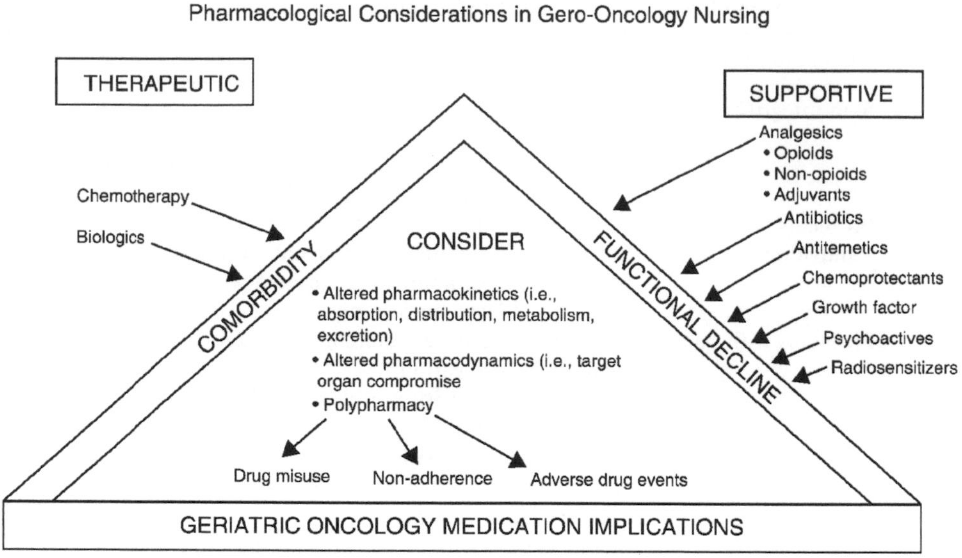

Pharmacological Considerations in Gero-Oncology Nursing

Figure 1 Pharmacological considerations in gero-oncology nursing. *Source*: From Ref. 123.

(123). Because numerous scenarios of falling are related to medications, the promotion of a safe environment of care for older adults compromised by cancer assumes added importance due to the serious consequences of falls such as bleeding, fractures, added requirements for surgery, infection, and acute confusion (124,125). Adapting sensitive risk parameters and utilizing new technology to prevent or minimize adverse falls-related sequelae, are two general gerontological interventions with special significance to gero-oncology (126).

Psychological Distress

There are a myriad of emotional issues that afflict cancer patients and their families when cancer strikes in later years. Some of these issues are shared by both patients and family members while others are more specific to one group (Table 6).

Similar to scenarios previously described, professional reactions to patient coping styles are frequently tempered by ageism. This bias is of particular relevance to the recognition and management of symptoms such as depression and delirium (110,127). Because these symptoms are perceived to be a usual corollary of growing old, both their early recognition and prompt treatment lag far behind what is instituted for other adult cohorts (128).

Depression is *not* an automatic corollary of growing old. However, the reality of multiple losses in the older adults' social circles makes the demands associated with grieving more frequent and intense (129). Variables predictive of vulnerability to cancer-related depression in later life require further investigation. An early study of women with gynecological malignancies noted that the greatest risk factor for depression with advanced age was not chronologic age, but rather a premorbid history of depression (130). Additionally, drug trials of antidepressants in older cancer patients, particularly older patients with comorbid conditions, are necessary (131,132). The differential diagnosis of depression may be difficult due to its association both with the presentation of delirium and dementia. Hence, assessment tools are required to assist nurses with the prompt identification of depression. Assessment tools

Table 6 Coping Dilemmae in Gero-oncology

Patient issues	Common themes of concern	Family issues
Anticipation of death	Presence of cognitive	Caregiving burden
Life review/reminiscence	dysfunction+overall	Demands on elder spouse as the
Worry about spouse	symptom distress	"hidden patient"
Worry about family	Worries R/T long-term care	Role reversal
burden caused by	requirements	Anger over siblings not
illness	Acceptance of home care	involved in parental care
Dependency aversion	Acceptance of hospice care	needs
Survivor guilt	Trust in multiple office-based	Anticipation of widowhood
Neurosensory	health care providers	Long-distance family guilt
compromise affecting	Unresolved family conflict	Anxiety over information
reception of	Cost/financial concerns	deficiencies
information	Reaction to losses/cumulative	Competing demands by own
Transportation	grief	family
Role loss	Fear of recurrence	Multiple family members
		experiencing loss concurrently

distinguishing signs and symptoms can help augment clinical assessment (Table 7). This unmet need is of particular importance for exploring the relationship between depression in later life and functional recovery from cancer and other disease entities (133).

Communication strategies with ill older adults have been the focus of recent attention. This is especially noted in findings related to discussions about advance directives and end-of-life care. A prominent theme has focused on patient and family perceptions of the inadequacy of communication with physicians (134–136). With minimal attempt to ascertain preferred amounts of information desired for disclosure, often too much information (particularly about prognosis) is given or too little is offered, frequently in reference to family needs for information. Gender and ethnicity are critical variables to consider in this context as well (137). In the 65 article anthology, no studies were identified that dealt with oncology nurse communication strategies for older patients and their families. Yet, in reality, communication and the provision of emotional support may consume much of the oncology nurse's time spent with patients and families.

CONCLUDING THOUGHTS

This chapter is in no way intended to be an exhaustive review of research issues of interest to oncology nurses. However, it is meant to reveal the enormity of topics that require further investigative inquiry. Many other questions remain unanswered, such as dilemmas regarding access, use, and benefit of screening the elderly at-risk population nursing considerations in caring for critically ill older cancer patients, optimizing communication with older adults and then families, particularly around treatment and end of life decision making, and interventions to partner with and support primary caregivers in the home setting (138–146). Obtaining the interest of older adults in clinical trial participation will be critical to the testing of interventions specifically tailored for the elderly (147,148). Integrating diversity into all aspects of elder cancer care will be a necessity rather than an afterthought (149). Exactly how best to assimilate this factor into prevention, screening, treatment, survivorship, and end-of-life care is a timely topic for research and novel program development.

Table 7 Clinical Features of Delirium, Dementia, and Depression

Feature	Delirium	Dementia	Depression
Onset	Acute (over hours to days); often at twilight; often a corollary of acute illness	Chronic, generally insidious (over months to years)	Episodic, coinciding with life changes; often abrupt, progressing from weeks to months
Course	Short, diurnal fluctuation in symptoms; worse at night, in the dark, and on awakening; symptoms can fluctuate hourly	Long, no diurnal effects, symptoms progressive yet relatively stable over time	Diurnal effects, typically worse in the morning; situational fluctuations but less than delirium
Progression	Abrupt	Slow but even	Variable, uneven
Duration	Hours to weeks, seldom longer than a month; resolves with treatment	Months to years; progressive and irreversible	At least two weeks, but can be several months to years; resolves with treatment
Awareness	Reduced	Unaffected	Clear but selective
Alertness	Lethargic or hypervigilant; fluctuates	Generally normal	Normal
Attention	Impaired, fluctuates, easily distracted	Generally unaffected	Minimal impairment but may have difficulty concentrating
Orientation	Generally impaired; early disorientation to time and place; fluctuates in severity	Impaired as disease progresses	Selective disorientation
Memory	Recent and immediate impaired	Generally impaired; unable to learn new information; unconcerned about memory deficits	Selective or patchy (i.e., slow recall) impairment; "islands" of intact memory; concerned about memory deficits

Thinking	Disorganized, distorted, fragmented, slowed or accelerated; speech is incoherent	Difficulty with abstraction; thoughts impoverished; judgment impaired; words difficult to find	Intact but laden with negative thoughts of hopelessness, helplessness, or self-deprecation
Perception	Gross distortions; illusions, delusions, and hallucinations; difficulty distinguishing between reality and misperceptions	Misperceptions often absent; may experience hallucinations	Intact but characterized by depressive themes; delusions and hallucinations absent except in severe cases
Psychomotor behavior	Variable, hypokinetic, hyperkinetic, or mixed	Normal, may have apraxia	Variable, psychomotor retardation or agitation
Sleep–wake cycle	Disturbed; cycle may change hourly or be reversed	Disturbed; day/night reversal	Disturbed, often early morning awakening; hypersomnia during the day
Associated features	Variable affective changes; symptoms of autonomic hyperarousal; exaggeration of personality type; associated with physical illness	Affect superficial, inappropriate, and labile; attempts to conceal deficits in intellect; personality changes; aphasia; lack of insight	Affect depressed; exaggerated, and detailed complaints; preoccupation with personal thoughts (usually negative); associated with recent or cumulative loss
Mental status testing	Distracted from task; family describes abrupt change in patient norm; in early phase, patient aware of, yet attempts to hide, abnormality	Failings highlighted by family; frequent "near miss" answers; struggles with test; great effort to find an appropriate reply	Failings highlighted by the patient; frequent "don't know" answers; little effort; frequently gives up; indifferent, does not care or attempt to find answer

Source: From Ref. 110.

In the year 2000, seven million "baby boomers" (born in the two decades following World War II) accounted for nearly 30% of the U.S. population (150,151). By the year 2030, when the last of this generation reaches age 65, the U.S. population aged 65 and older will exceed 70 million, approximately twice the number in 2000 (152). Nearly two-thirds of people in the United States will be older adults and unless major breakthroughs in cancer care occur, by virtue of aging alone, cancer may be of epidemic proportions. Acknowledging this trend, all of health care will be required to have dual expertise in their respective professional and medical specialties as well as in the care of the older adult (153).

There is no greater imperative for nurses than embracing the elder care reality. Knowledge and training to optimize elder care to mandatory mandation particularly for advanced practice nurses (154,155). Additionally, have models of care delivery will be required to nurse older adults with chronic disease, residing in the suburbs, with limited mobility and transportation and dwindling social support (156–158). A dedicated gero-oncology subspeciality will foster age specific scientific discovery generated within a committed team (159). Deliberation about research questions of equal interest to pharmacists, clinicians, social workers, counselors, and physical therapists will only enhance the methodology, analysis, and influence of potential findings emanating from such collaboration (160). In the original position paper from the ONS (14), it was stated that oncology nurses have a clear mandate to establish a formal framework within which nursing care will meet the unique cancer-specific needs of the elderly. Scientific rigor applied to questions in need of answers can only enhance the capability of nurse clinicians to ensure this outcome. Given the progress that has been documented in this chapter, it is apparent that oncology nursing has come of age, and gero-oncology will be a major beneficiary of this transition.

REFERENCES

1. Boyle DA, Engelking C. The evolution and future of breast cancer therapy. Oncol Support Care Quart 2003; 2(2):14–25.
2. Fentiman IS, Tirelli U, Monfardini S, et al. Cancer in the elderly: why so badly treated? Lancet 1990; 335(8696):120–122.
3. Begg CB, Carbone PP. Clinical trials and drug toxicity in the elderly: the experience of the Eastern Cooperative Oncology Group. Cancer 1983; 52(11):1986–1992.
4. Welch DA. Cancer in the elderly: considerations in nursing management. In: Proceedings of the Seventh Annual Oncology Nursing Society. Pittsburgh: Oncology Nursing Society 1982:72.
5. Yancik R, Carbone PP, Patterson WB, Steel K, Terry WD, eds. Perspectives on Prevention and Treatment of Cancer in the Elderly. New York: Raven Press, 1983.
6. Weinrich SP, Nussbaum J. Cancer in the elderly: early detection. Cancer Nurs 1984; 7(6):475–482.
7. Welch-McCaffrey D, ed. Nursing Considerations in Geriatric Oncology. Columbus, Ohio: Adria Laboratories, 1984.
8. Weinrich SP, Weinrich MC. Cancer knowledge among elderly individuals. Cancer Nurs 1986; 9(6):301–307.
9. Cohen HJ, ed. Cancer I: general aspects. Geriatr Med 1987; 3(3); Cancer II: specific neoplasms. Geriatr Med 1987; 3(4).
10. Welch-McCaffrey D, ed. Cancer in the elderly. Semin Oncol Nurs 1988; 4(3).
11. Welch-McCaffrey D. The elderly with cancer. In: Tiffany R, ed. Oncology for Nurses and Health Care Professionals. 2d ed. London: Beaconsfield Press, 1988:261–273.

12. Zenser TV, Coe RM, eds. Cancer and Aging: Progress in Research and Treatment. New York: Springer Publishing, 1989.
13. Ershler WB, ed. Cancer in the elderly. Semin Oncol 1989; 16(1).
14. Welch-McCaffrey D, Engelking C, Blesch K, et al. Oncology nursing society position paper on cancer and aging: the mandate for oncology nursing. Oncol Nurs Forum 1992; 19(6):913–933.
15. Balducci L, Lyman GH, Ershler WB, eds. Geriatrci Oncology. Philadelphia: JB Lippincott; 1992.
16. Regenstreif DI, Brittis S, Fagin CM, et al. Strategies to advance geriatric nursing: The John A. Hartford Foundation initiatives. J Am Geriatr Soc 2003; 51(10):1479–1483.
17. Luggen AS, Meiner SE, eds. Handbook for the Care of the Older Adult with Cancer. Pittsburgh: Oncol Nurs Press, 2000.
18. Oncology Nursing Society and Geriatric Oncology Consortium. Oncology Nursing Society and Geriatric Oncology Consortium joint position on cancer care in the older adult. Oncol Nurs Forum 2004; 31(3):1–2.
19. Cope D, Reb A, eds. An Evidence-Based Approach to the Treatment and Care of the Older Adult with Cancer. Pittsburgh: Oncology Nursing Press, 2006.
20. Given BA, Keilman L. Cancer in the elderly population: research issues. Oncol Nurs Forum 1990; 17(1):121–123.
21. Boyle DM. Establishing a nursing research agenda in gero-oncology. Crit Rev Oncol Hematol 2003; 48(2):103–111.
22. Kagan SH. Gero-oncology nursing research. Oncol Nurs Forum 2004; 31(2):293–299.
23. Bourbonniere M, Kagan SH. Nursing intervention and older adults who have cancer: specific science and evidence-based practice. Nurs Clin North Am 2004; 39(3): 529–543.
24. Berger AM, Berry DL, Christopher KA, et al. Oncology Nursing Society year 2004 research priorities survey. Oncol Nurs Forum 2005; 32(2):281–290.
25. Tishelman C. Who cares? Patients' descriptions of age-related aspects of cancer and care in Stockholm. Cancer Nurs 1993; 16(4):270–282.
26. Kearney N, Miller M, Paul J, et al. Oncology healthcare professionals' attitudes toward elderly people. Ann Oncol 2000; 11(5):599–601.
27. Blair KA. Cancer screening of older women. Cancer Pract 1998; 6(4):217–222.
28. Gulitz E, Bustillo-Hernendez M, Kent EB. Missed cancer screening opportunities among older women. Cancer Pract 1998; 6(5):289–295.
29. Yarbrough SS. Older women and breast cancer screening: research synthesis. Oncol Nurs Forum 2004; accessed at www.ons.org/xp6/ONS/Library.xml/ ONS_Publications.xml/ONF.xml.
30. Boyle DA. The older adult with breast cancer. In: Cope D, Reb A, eds. An Evidence-Based Approach to the Treatment and Care of the Older Adult with Cancer. Pittsburgh: Oncology Nursing Press, 2006; pp. 103–134.
31. Bouchardy C, Rapiti E, Fioretta G, et al. Undertreatment strongly decreases prognosis of breast cancer in elderly women. J Clin Oncol 2003; 21(19):3580–3587.
32. DeMichele A, Putt M, Zhang Y, et al. Older age predicts a decline in adjuvant chemotherapy recommendations for patients with breast carcinoma: evidence from a tertiary care cohort of chemotherapy-eligible patients. Cancer 2003; 97(9):1455–1461.
33. Goodwin JS, Satish S, Anderson ET, et al. Effect of nurse case management on the treatment of older women with breast cancer. J Am Geriatr Soc 2003; 51(9):1252–1259.
34. Jennings-Sanders A, Anderson ET. Older women with breast cancer: perceptions of the effectiveness of nurse case managers. Nurs Outlook 2003; 51(3):108–114.
35. McCorkle R, Strumpf NE, Nuamah IF, et al. A specialized home care intervention improves survival among older post-surgical cancer patients. J Am Geriatr Soc 2000; 48(12):1707–1713.
36. Hughes LC, Robinson LA, Cooley ME, et al. Describing an episode of home nursing care for elderly post-surgical cancer patients. Nurs Res 2002; 51(2):110–118.

37. Hughes LC, Hodgson NA, Muller P, et al. Information needs of elderly post-surgical cancer patients during the transition from hospital to home. Image J Nurs Sch 2000; 32(1):25–30.

38. Jepson C, McCorkle R, Adler D, et al. Effects of home care on caregivers' psychosocial status. Image J Nurs Sch 1999; 31(2):115–120.

39. Harden J. Developmental life stage and couples' experiences with prostate cancer. Cancer Nurs 2005; 28(2):85–98.

40. Given B, Stommel N, Collins C, et al. Responses of elderly spouse caregivers. Res Nurs Health 1990; 12(2):77–85.

41. Teel CS, Press AN. Fatigue among elders in caregiving and noncaregiving roles. West J Nurs Res 1999; 21(4):498–515.

42. Yang C, Kirschling JM. Exploration of factors related to direct care and outcomes of caregiving: caregivers of terminally ill older persons. Cancer Nurs 1992; 15(3):173–181.

43. Lewis M, Pearson V, Corcoran-Perry S, et al. Decision-making by elderly patients with cancer and their caregivers. Cancer Nurs 1997; 20(6):389–397.

44. Rusinak RL, Murphy JF. Elderly spousal caregivers: knowledge of cancer care, perceptions of preparedness, and coping strategies. J Gerontol Nurs 1995; 21(3):33–41.

45. Fitch MI, Greenberg MM, Levstein LB, et al. Health promotin and early detection of cancer in older adults: needs assessment for program development. Cancer Nurs 1997; 20(6):381–388.

46. Weinrich SP, Weinrich MC, Boyd MD, et al. Knowledge of colorectal cancer among older persons. Cancer Nurs 1992; 15(5):322–330.

47. Weinrich SP, Weinrich MC, Stromborg MF, et al. Using elderly educators to increase colorectal screening. Gerontologist 1993; 33(4):491–496.

48. Coleman EA, Lord J, Heard J, et al. The Delta Project: increasing breast cancer screening among rural minority and older women by targeting rural healthcare providers. Oncol Nurs Forum 2003; 30(4):669–677.

49. Morrison C. Determining crucial correlates of breast self-examination in older women with low incomes. Oncol Nurs Forum 1996; 23(1):83–93.

50. Wood RY, Duffy ME, Morris SJ, et al. The effect of an educational intervention on promoting breast self-examination in older African American and Caucasian women. Oncol Nurs Forum 2002; 29(7):1081–1090.

51. Weinrich SP, Ellison GL, Boyd M, et al. Participation in prostate cancer screening among low-income men. Psychol Health Med 2000; 5(4):439–450.

52. Ferrell BR, Grant M, Chan J, et al. The impact of cancer pain education on family caregivers of elderly patients. Oncol Nurs Forum 1995; 22(8):1211–1218.

53. Clotfelter CE. The effect of an educational intervention on decreasing pain intensity in elderly people with cancer. Oncol Nurs Forum 1999; 26(1):27–33.

54. McMillan SC. The relationship between age and intensity of cancer-related symptoms. Oncol Nurs Forum 1989; 16(2):237–241.

55. Given CW, Given BA, Stommel M. The impact of age, treatment, and symptoms on the physical and mental health of cancer patients. Cancer 1994; 74(7):2128–2138.

56. Kurtz ME, Kurtz JC, Stommel M, et al. Symptomatology and loss of physical functioning among geriatric patients with lung cancer. J Pain Symptom Manage 2000; 19(4):249–256.

57. Given CW, Given B, Kozachik S, et al. Predictors of pain and fatigue in the year following diagnosis among elderly cancer patients. J Pain Symptom Manage 2001; 21(6): 456–466.

58. Duggleby W. Enduring suffering: a grounded theory analysis of the pain experience of elderly hospice patients with cancer. Oncol Nurs Forum 2000; 27(5):825–831.

59. Wyatt GK, Friedman LL, Given CW, et al. Complementary therapy use among older cancer patients. Cancer Pract 1999; 7(3):136–144.

60. Armer J, Fu MR. Age differences in post-breast cancer lymphedema signs and symptoms. Cancer Nurs 2005; 28(3):200–207.

61. Gift AG, Jablonski A, Stommel M, et al. Symptom clusters in elderly patients with lung cancer. Oncol Nurs Forum 2004; 31(2):203–210.
62. Kim HJ, McGuire DB, Tulman L, et al. Symptom clusters: concept analysis and clinical implications for cancer nursing. Cancer Nurs 2005; 28(4):270–282.
63. Duffy ME, Wood RY, Morris S. The influence of demographics, functional status and co-morbidity on the breast self-examination proficiency of older African-American women. J Black Nurses Assoc 2001; 12(1):1–9.
64. Kurtz ME, Kurtz JC, Stommel M, et al. The influence of symptoms, age, comorbidity and cancer site on physical functioning and mental health of geriatric women patients. Women Health 1999; 29(3):1–12.
65. Hodgson NA, Given CW. Determinants of functional recovery in older adults surgically treated for cancer. Cancer Nurs 2004; 27(1):10–16.
66. Given B, Given C, Azzouz F, et al. Physical functioning of elderly cancer patients prior to diagnosis and following initial treatment. Nurs Res 2001; 50(4):222–232.
67. Given CW, Given B, Azzouz F, et al. Comparison of changes in physical functioning of elderly patients with new diagnoses of cancer. Med Care 2000; 38(5):482–493.
68. Kurtz ME, Kurtz JC, Stommel M, et al. Symptomatology and loss of physical functioning among geriatric patients with lung cancer. J Pain Symptom Manage 2000; 19(4):249–256.
69. McGill JS, Paul PB. Functional status and hope in elderly people with and without cancer. Oncol Nurs Forum 1993; 20(8):1207–1213.
70. Wyatt GK, Friedman LL. Physical and psychosocial outcomes of midlife and older women following surgery and adjuvant therapy for breast cancer. Oncol Nurs Forum 1998; 25(4):761–768.
71. Overcash J, Extermann M, Parr J, et al. Validity and reliability of the FACT-G scale for use in the older person with cancer. Am J Clin Oncol 2001; 24(6):591–596.
72. Edlund B, Sneed NC. Emotional responses to the diagnosis of cancer: age-related comparisons. Oncol Nurs Forum 1989; 16(5):691–697.
73. Powe BD. Cancer fatalism among elderly Caucasians and African Americans. Oncol Nurs Forum 1995; 22(9):1355–1359.
74. Thome B, Dykes AK, Gunnars B, et al. The experiences of older people living with cancer. Cancer Nurs 2003; 26(2):85–96.
75. Ryan PY. Approaching death: a phenomenologic study of five older adults with advanced cancer. Oncol Nurs Forum 2005; 32(6):1101–1108.
76. Kurtz JE, Dufour P. Strategies for improving quality of life in older patients with metastatic breast cancer. Drugs Aging 2002; 19(8):605–622.
77. Thome B, Esbensen BA, Dykes AK, et al. The meaning of having to live with cancer in old age. Eur J Cancer Care 2004; 13(5):399–408.
78. Heidrich SM, Ward SE. The role of self in adjustment to cancer in elderly women. Oncol Nurs Forum 1992; 19(10):1491–1496.
79. Fehring RJ, Mmiller JF, Shaw C. Spiritual well-being, religiosity, hope, depression and other mood states in elderly people coping with cancer. Oncol Nurs Forum 1997; 24(4):663–671.
80. Houldin AD, Wasserbauer N. Psychosocial needs of older cancer patients: a pilot study abstract. Medsurg Nurs 1996; 5(4):253–256.
81. Gillies B, Johnston G. Identity loss and maintenance: commonality of experience in cancer and dementia. Eur J Cancer Care 2004; 13(5):436–442.
82. Fitch MI, Gray RE, Franssen E. Perspectives on living with ovarian cancer: older women's views. Oncol Nurs Forum 2001; 28(9):1433–1442.
83. Overcash J. Using narrative research to understand the quality of life of older women with breast cancer. Oncol Nurs Forum 2004; 31(6):1153–1160.
84. Sinding C, Wiernikowski J, Aronson J. Cancer care from the perspectives of older women. Oncol Nurs Forum 2005; 32(6):1169–1175.

85. Esbensen BA, Osterlind K, Roer O, et al. Quality of life of elderly persons with newly diagnosed cancer. Eur J Cancer Care 2004; 13(5):443–453.
86. Thome B, Hallberg IR. Quality of life in older people with cancer—a gender perspective. Eur J Cancer Care 2004; 13(5):454–463.
87. Sammarco A. Quality of life among older survivors of breast cancer. Cancer Nurs 2003; 26(6):431–438.
88. Deimling GT, Sterns S, Bowman KF, et al. The health of older adult, long-term cancer survivors. Cancer Nurs 2005; 28(6):415–424.
89. McCorkle R, Hughes L, Robinson L, et al. Nursing interventions for newly diagnosed older cancer patients facing terminal illness. J Palliat Care 1998; 14(3):39–45.
90. Gil KM, Mishel MH, Belyea M, et al. Triggers of uncertainty about recurrence and long-term treatment side effects in older African American and Caucasian breast cancer survivors. Oncol Nurs Forum 2004; 31(3):633–639.
91. Wallace M, Bailey D, O'Rourke M, et al. The watchful waiting management option for older men with prostate cancer: state of the science. Oncol Nurs Forum 2004; 31(6):1057–1064.
92. Given BA, Sherwood PR. Nursing-sensitive patient outcomes—a white paper. Oncol Nurs Forum 2005; 32(4):773–784.
93. ONS Outcomes Project Team, 2004. Accessed via http://onsopcontent.ons.org/tookkits/evidence/Clinical/outcomes.shtml.
94. Amella EJ. Presentation of illness in older adults. AJN 2004; 104(10):40–51.
95. Balducci L, Carreca I. The role of myelopoietic growth factors in managing cancer in the elderly. Drugs 2002; 62(suppl 1):47–63.
96. Hood LH. Chemotherapy in the elderly: supportive measures for chemotherapy-induced myelotoxicity. Clin J Oncol Nurs 2002; 7(2):185–190.
97. Dolan S, Crombez P, Munoz M. Neutropenia Management with granulocyte colony-stimulating factors: from guidelines to nursing practice protocols. Eur J Oncol Nurs 2006.
98. Smyth D, Zumbrink S. Optimising the management of anaemia in patient with cancer with practice guidelines using erythropoiesis-stimulating proteins. Eur J Oncol Nurs 2006.
99. Gillespie TW. Anaemia in cancer. Cancer Nurs 2003; 26(2):119–128.
100. Chouliara Z, Kearney N, Stott D, Molassiotis A, Miller M. Perceptions of older people with cancer of information, decision making and treatment: a systematic review of selected literature. Annals of Oncology 2004; 15(11):1596–1602.
101. Sutton LM, Demark-Wahnefried W, Clipp EC. Management of terminal cancer in elderly patients. Lancet Oncol 2003; 4(3):149–154.
102. Boyle D. Cancer in the elderly: key facts. Oncol Support Care Quart 2003; 2(1):6–21.
103. Ancoli-Israel S, Cooke JR. Prevalence and comorbidity of insomnia and effect on functioning in elderly populations. J Am Geriatr Soc 2005; 53(7):S264–S271.
104. McCall WV. Diagnosis and management of insomnia in older people. J Am Geriatr Soc 2005; 53(7):S272–S277.
105. Krystal AD. The effect of insomnia definitions, terminology and classifications on clinical practice. JAES 2005; 53(7):S258–S263.
106. Berger AM, Parker KP, Young-McCaughan S, et al. Sleep/wake disturbances in people with cancer and their caregivers: state of the science. Oncol Nurs Forum 2005; 32(6):E98–E126.
107. Mock V. Clinical excellence through evidence-based practice: fatigue management as a model. Oncol Nurs Forum 2003; 30(5):790–795.
108. Specht JK. Nine myths of incontinence in older adults. Am J Nurs 2005; 105(6):58–68.
109. Rao A, Cohen HJ. Symptom management in the elderly cancer patient: fatigue, pain and depression. J Natl Cancer Inst Monogr 2004; 32:150–157.
110. Boyle DA. Delirium in older adults with cancer: a review and recommendations for practice and research. Oncol Nurs Forum 2006; 33(1):61–79.

111. Woods NF, LaCroix AZ, Gray SL, et al. Frailty: emergence and consequences in women aged 65 and older in the Women's Health Initiative Observational Study. J Am Geriatr Soc 2005; 53(8):1321–1330.

112. Higashi T, Shekelle PG, Adams JL, et al. Quality of care is associated with survival in vulnerable older patients. J Am Geriatr Soc 2005; 143(4):274–281.

113. Balducci L, Stanta G. Cancer in the trial patient: a coming epidemic Hemat/oncol clinics. N Amer 2000; 14(1):235–250.

114. Amin SH, Kuhle CL, Fitzpatrick LA. Comprehensive evaluation of the older woman. Mayo Clin Proc 2003; 78(9):1157–1185.

115. Gosney MA. Clinical assessment of elderly people with cancer. Lancet Oncol 2005; 6:790–797.

116. Extermann M, Aapro M, Bernabei R, et al. Use of comprehensive geriatric assessment in older cancer patients: recommendations from the task force on CEA of the International Society of Geriatric Oncology (SIOG). Critical Reviews in Oncology/Hematology 2005; 55:241–252.

117. Hurria A, Gupta S, Zauderer M, et al. Developing a cancer specific geriatric assessment: a feasibility study. Cancer 2005; 104(9):1998–2005.

118. Overcash J, Beckstead J, Extermann M, Cobb S. The abbreviated comprehensive geriatric assessment (aCGA): a retrospective analysis. Critical Reviews in Oncology/Hematology 2005; 54(2):129–136.

119. Fitzsimmons D. What are we trying to measure? Rethinking approaches to health outcome assessment for the older person with cancer. Eur J Cancer Care 2004; 13(5):416–423.

120. Marek KD, Popejoy L, Petroski G, et al. Clinical outcomes of aging in place. Nurs Res 2005; 54(3):202–211.

121. Adams K, Corrigan J. Commission on Identifying Priority Areas for Quality Improvement. In: Priority areas for national action: transforming health care quality. Washington, D.C.: National Academy Press, 2003.

122. Naylor MD. Nursing intervention research and quality of care: influencing the future of healthcare. Nurs Res 2003; 52(6):380–385.

123. Boyle D. Cancer in the elderly. In: Gates R, Fink R, eds. Oncology Nursing Secrets. Philadelphia: Hanley & Belfus, 2001:508 514.

124. Lord SR, Tiedemann A, Chapman K, et al. The effect of an individualized fall prevention program on fall risk in older people: a randomized, controlled trial. J Am Geriatr Soc 2005; 53(8):1296–1304.

125. Vassallo M, Stockdale R, Sharma JC, et al. A comparative study of the use of four fall risk assessment tools on acute medical wards. J Am Geriatr Soc 2005; 53(6):1034–1038.

126. Nelson D, Powell-Cope G, Gavin-Dreschnack, et al. Technology to promote safe mobility in the elderly. Nurs Clinics No Amer 2004; 39:649–671.

127. Winell J, Roth DJ. Depression in cancer patients. Oncol 2004; 18(12):1554–1560.

128. Tanner EK. Recognizing late-life depression: why is this important for nurses in the home setting? Geriatr Nurs 2005; 26(3):145–149.

129. Roth AJ, Modi R. Psychiatric issues in older cancer patients. Crit Rev Oncol Hematol 2003:185–197.

130. Breitbart W. Psycho-oncology: depression, anxiety, delirium. Semin Oncol 1994; 21(6):754–769.

131. Buffum MD, Buffum JC. Treating depression in the elderly: an update on antidepressants. Geriatr Nurs 2005; 26(3):138–142.

132. Luggen AS. Pharmacology update: depression. Geriatr Nurs 2005; 26(3):195.

133. Goodwin JS, Zhang DD, Ostir GV. Effect of depression on diagnosis, treatment and survival of older women with breast cancer. J Am Geriatr Soc 2004; 52(1):106–111.

134. Fried TR, Bradley EH, O'Leary J. Prognosis communication in serious illness: perceptions of older patients, caregivers and clinicians. J Am Geriatr Soc 2003; 51(10):1398–1403.

135. Baik WF, Lenzi R, Parker PA, et al. Oncologists' attitude toward and practices in giving bad news: an exploratory study. J Clin Oncol 2002; 20(8):2189–2196.

136. Butow PN, Dowsett S, Hagerty R, et al. Communicating prognosis to patients with meta-static disease: what do they really want to know? Support Care Cancer 2002; 10(2):161–168.

137. Perkins HS, Shepherd KJ, Cortez JD, Hazuda HP. Exploring chronically ill seniors' attitudes about discussing death and postmortem medical procedures. J Am Geriatr Soc 2005; 53(5):895–900.

138. Silverman MA, Zaidi U, Barnett S, et al. Cancer screening in the elderly population. Hematol/Oncol Clin North Am 2000; 14(1):89–112.

139. Mick DJ, Ackerman MH. Critical care nursing for older adults: pathophysiological and functional considerations. Nurs Clin N Am 2004; 39:473–493.

140. Schumacher KL, Marren J. Home care nursing for older adults: state of the science. Nurs Clin N Am 2004; 39:443–471.

141. Overcash J, Balducci L. Social support networks of the older cancer patients. In: Overcash J, Balducci L (eds). The older cancer patients. A guide for nurses and related professionals. New York, Springer 2003:223–242.

142. Northouse LL. Helping families of patients with cancer. Oncol Nurs Forum 2005; 32(4):743–750.

143. Vanderwerker LC, Laff RE, Kadan-Lottick NS, et al. Psychiatric disorders and mental health service use among caregivers of advanced cancer patients. J Clin Oncol 2005; 23(28):6899–6907.

144. Hudson PL, Aranda S, Hayman-White K. A psycho-educational intervention for family caregivers of patients receiving palliative care: a randomized controlled trial. J Pain Symptom Manage 2005; 30(4):329–341.

145. Yin T, Zhou Q, Bashford C. Burden on family members: caring for frail elderly. A meta-analysis of interventions. Nurs Res 2002; 51(3):199–208.

146. Haten WE. Family depression of elderly patients with cancer: understanding and mini-mizing the burden of care. Supportive Oncol 2003; 1(suppl 2):25–29.

147. Ehrenberger HE, Breeden JR, Donovan ME. A demonstration project to increase the awareness of cancer clinical trials among community-dwelling seniors. Oncol Nurs Forum 2003; 30(4):E80–E83.

148. Lewis JH, Kilgore ML, Goldman DP, et al. Participation of patients 65 years of age or older in cancer clinical trials. J Clin Oncol 2003; 21(7):1383–1389.

149. Parke B, Ross D, Moss L. Creating a cultural shift: a gerontological program for acute care. J Nurses Staff Dev 2003; 19(6):305–312.

150. American Geriatrics Society Core Writing Group of the task force on the future of geriatric medicine. Caring for older Americans: the future of geriatric medicine. J Am Geriatr Soc 2005; 53(6):S245–S256.

151. Libow LS. Geriatrics in the United States-Baby boomers' boon? N Engl J Med 2005; 352(8):750–752.

152. Knickman JR, Snell EK. The 2030 problem: caring for aging baby boomers. Health ser-vices Research 2002; 37(4):849–884.

153. Mezey M, Capezuti E, Fulmer T. Care of older adults (preface). Nurs Clinics N Amer 2004; 39:xiii–xx.

154. LaMascus Am, Bernard MA, Barry P, et al. Bridging the workforce gap for an aging society: How to increase and improve knowledge and training. Report of an expert panel. JAGS, 2005; 53(2):343–347.

155. Clark AP, Baldwin K. Best practices for care of older adults: highlights and summary from the preconference. Clin N Specialist 2004; 18(6):288–300.

156. Vladeck BC. Economic and policy implications of improving longerity. JAGS 2005; 53(9):5304–5307.

157. Lee VK, Fletcher KR. Sustaining the Geriatric Resource Nurse Model at the University of Virginia. Geriatr Nurs 2002; 23(2):128–132.

158. Clark JS. An aging population with chronic disease compels new delivery systems focused on new structures and practices. Nurs Adm Q 2004; 28(2):105–115.

159. Monfardini S. Geriatric oncology: a new subspeciality? (letter). J Clin Oncol 2004:4655.

160. McBride AB. Nursing and gerontology. J Gerontol Nurs 2000; 26(7):18–27.

25
Cancer in the Frail Elderly

Arti Hurria and Tara A. Cleary
Memorial Sloan Kettering Cancer Center, New York, New York, U.S.A.

Ronald D. Adelman
Division of Geriatrics and Gerontology, Weill Medical College of Cornell University, New York, New York, U.S.A.

INTRODUCTION

Among the older patient population, there is wide heterogeneity in physical functioning and tolerance to cancer treatment. The term "frail" is often used to describe those patients with the greatest vulnerability for adverse outcomes, including dependency, hospitalization, disability, need for long-term care, and mortality. The American Medical Association estimates that 40% of adults aged 80 and over are frail, and that the majority of the 1.6 million residents in nursing homes are frail (1).

As the older population dramatically expands, so does the subset of frail older patients. Some authors have proposed that older adults with a chronologic age of 85 and over should be considered "frail," based on the progressive deterioration in physical function and the prevalence of dementia in this age group (2–4). Between 1900 and 2000, the population aged 85 and over grew from over 100,000 to 4.2 million and is estimated to grow to nearly 21 million by 2050 (Table 1) (5,6). Much consideration must be given to those who live to the age of 100 and beyond, the "centenarians," who are the fastest growing segment of the older population: by 2050 the number of centenarians will increase 10-fold, so that there will be 834,000 centenarians in the United States (7). This increased proportion of older adults is not just in the United States. In fact, 25 countries in Europe have the world's oldest populations (Fig. 1) (8).

This global expansion of the aged also leads to the recognition of cancer as a health problem that overwhelmingly affects older adults (8–10). People aged 65 and over have an 11-fold increase in the incidence of cancer and a 15-fold increase in cancer mortality compared to people younger than the age of 65. Sixty percent of all cancers and 70% of all cancer deaths occur in people aged 65 and over (10,11). Based on these demographics, oncology health care providers are caring for a growing number of older patients. Within this population, a certain proportion will be frail and at increased risk for adverse health outcomes.

Table 1 The Growing Older Population: U.S. Population ≥Age 65 and ≥Age 85

Year	Age 65 and older (millions)	Age 85 and over (millions)
1900	3.1	0.1
2000	35	4.2
2050	86.7	20.9

Data derived from the Federal Interagency Forum on Aging-Related Statistics.
Source: From Ref. 5.

It is within the context of this chapter to describe the clinical and laboratory correlates of frailty, the physiologic changes associated with aging that can affect tolerance to cancer treatment in the frail older oncology patient, and the use of the comprehensive geriatric assessment to identify the specific needs of this population. To date, there has been little data with regard to the risks and benefits of cancer treatment in this patient population. Implications for future research will be proposed.

DEFINITION OF FRAILTY

Despite the widespread use of the term "frailty," a standardized definition is lacking. The term "frail" holds the connotation of a patient at high risk for adverse health outcomes including mortality, institutionalization, falls, and hospitalization. A broad definition of frailty is as follows: a diminished biologic reserve and resistance to stressors that is caused by cumulative declines across physiologic systems, leading to vulnerability and adverse outcomes (4,12). Frailty is often, but not always, associated with advanced age and can be characterized as being dependent on others and having multiple chronic illnesses with atypical disease presentations, with the potential of benefiting from specialized geriatric programs (13,14). Other authors refer to frailty as a constellation of signs and symptoms that are distinguished by high susceptibility to adverse outcomes, declining physical functioning, and increased risk of death (1,12,15,16). The clinical descriptors and laboratory correlates of frailty are described next.

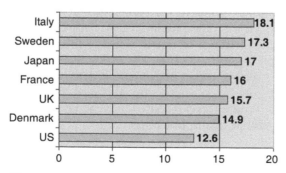

Figure 1 Population of age 65 and over by country in year 2000. *Source*: From Ref. 8.

Clinical Descriptors of Frailty

A Phenotype of Frailty

Fried et al. developed a phenotype of frailty among community-dwelling older adults, using data from a prospective observational study of 5317 men and women aged 65 and over. They performed baseline, four-year, and seven-year assessments of the following outcomes: incident disease, hospitalization, falls, disability, and mortality. The authors describe frailty as a clinical syndrome in which three or more of the following criteria are present: unintentional weight loss ($\geq$10 lbs in the past year), self-reported exhaustion, weakness (the lowest 20th percentile in grip strength adjusted for gender and body mass index), slow walking speed (the lowest 20th percentile on a timed walk of 15 ft), and low physical activity (lowest quintile of kilocalories per week) (Table 2). Patients defined as frail, in comparison to nonfrail, by these criteria had a higher incidence of three- and seven-year mortality, hospitalization, and incident falls, a progressive decline in the ability to complete activities of daily living (ADL), and decreased mobility (Table 3). The proportion of frail individuals increased with age: 7% of community-dwelling individuals aged 65 and over were frail and 30% aged 80 and over were frail. Based on this definition, frailty is a physiologic syndrome, not synonymous with comorbidity or disability (13,17).

A Frailty Scale

In an attempt to measure frailty as a predictor of death and institutionalization, Rockwood et al. prospectively evaluated a group of Canadian community residents stratified by age (aged 65–74 years, 75–84 years, and $\geq$85 years) with initial contact in 1991–1992 and reevaluation in five years. Each participant was initially classified using a frailty scale with ratings from 0 to 3 on the spectrum of fitness to frailty, based upon the degree of dependence in ADL, presence of incontinence, and degree of cognitive impairment (Table 4). At baseline, 67% of the cohort met the criteria for the classification "0," 12% were classified as "1," 16% as "2," and 5% as "3." At follow-up, 24% of the cohort had died and 12% were institutionalized. A relationship between increased frailty and subsequent institutionalization and mortality was demonstrated (Table 4). Patients with a frailty score of "3" had a 9.4-fold increased

Table 2   A Phenotype of Frailty: Fried et al.

Characteristics of frailty	Cardiovascular Health Study Measure
Unintentional weight loss	Baseline: $>$ 10 lbs lost unintentionally in prior year
Sarcopenia (loss of muscle mass)	
Weakness	Grip strength: lowest 20% (by gender, body mass index)
Poor endurance	Exhaustion (self-report)
Exhaustion	
Slowness	Walking time/15 ft: slowest 20% (by gender, height)
Low activity	Kcal/wk of physical activity: lowest 20%
	Males: $<$ 383 Kcal/wk
	Females: $<$ 270 Kcal/wk
Definitions of frailty	
Frailty phenotype	$\geq$3 criteria present
Intermediate or prefrail	1 or 2 criteria present

Source: From Ref. 13.

Table 3 Incidence of Adverse Outcomes Associated with Frailty: Kaplan–Meier Estimates at 3 Years and 7 Years After Study Entry for Both the Cohorts (N = 5317)

Frailty status at baseline	n	Died		First hospitalization		First fall		Worsening ADL disability		Worsening mobility disability	
		3 yr (%)	7 yr (%)	3 yr (%)	7 yr (%)	3 yr (%)	7 yr (%)	3 yr (%)	7 yr (%)	3 yr (%)	7 yr (%)
Not frail	2469	3	12	33	79	15	27	8	23	23	41
Intermediate	2480	7	23	43	83	19	33	20	41	40	58
Frail	368	18	43	59	96	28	41	39	63	51	71
P value		< 0.0001		< 0.0001		< 0.0001		< 0.0001		< 0.0001	

Abbreviation: ADL, activities of daily living.
Source: From Ref. 13.

Table 4 The Frailty Scale

Frailty scale	Definition	Institutionalization RR (95% CI)	Mortality RR (95% CI)
1	Bladder incontinence only	1.7 (1.3–2.1)	1.2 (1.0–1.4)
2	One or more of the following criteria (two or more if incontinent): (a) Needs assistance with mobility or ADL (b) Cognitive impairment with no dementia (c) Bowel or bladder incontinence	3.6 (3.1–4.3)	2 (1.8–2.2)
3	Two or more of the following criteria (need three or more if incontinent) (a) Totally dependent for transfers or one or more ADL (b) Bowel or bladder incontinence (c) Diagnosis of dementia	9.4 (7.7–11.5)	3.1 (2.7–3.6)

Abbreviations: ADL, activities of daily living; RR, relative risk; CI, confidence interval.
Source: From Ref. 18.

relative risk (RR) of institutionalization and a 3.1-fold increased RR of mortality in comparison to those with no frailty. The authors recognize the need for further research to determine if frail patients will benefit from interventions to decrease the risk of adverse outcomes (18,19).

Geriatric Syndromes as a Marker of Frailty

Winograd et al. prospectively evaluated a cohort of hospitalized older adults to develop criteria for frailty, based on the presence of "geriatric syndromes," which are medical problems that put older patients at risk for adverse outcomes. These include polypharmacy, dementia, instability, falls, incontinence, pressure ulcers, sensory impairments, and malnutrition (Table 5). A cohort of patients was screened within 96 hours of hospital admission and then followed for one year to observe for outcomes of mortality, hospital readmission, and nursing home utilization. During the initial screening, patients were categorized as (i) independent, (ii) frail, or (iii) severely impaired. Those classified as frail were significantly older (mean age of the "frail" cohort was 75.2 years while that of the overall population was 71.6 years; $p < 0.0001$). The authors also found that frailty was significantly correlated with increasing length of hospital stay ($P < 0.001$), nursing home utilization ($P < 0.001$), and mortality ($P < 0.001$) (Table 5). All patients were also classified into one of five major diagnostic groups (based on the principal diagnosis responsible for the length of stay): surgery, oncology, cardiovascular, pulmonary, and others. There was an increased risk of mortality with increasing frailty within each diagnostic group. This model suggests that classification of frailty, based on the presence of geriatric syndromes, is predictive of one-year risk of mortality and nursing home utilization (20).

Table 5 Classification of Frailty

Classification	Definition	Admitted to nursing home[a] n (%)	Readmitted to hospital[a] n (%)
Independent	Independent in all ADL with short-term acute illness	6 (3)	120 (49)
Frail	Meets any one of these criteria: Cerebrovascular accident Chronic and disabling illness Confusion Dependence in ADL Depression Falls Impaired mobility Incontinence Malnutrition Polypharmacy Pressure sore Prolonged bedrest Restraints Sensory impairment Socioeconomic/family problems	31 (34)	52 (58)
Severely impaired	Severe dementia and ADL dependence Terminal illness	10 (42)	11 (46)

[a]$P < 0.001$.
Abbreviation: ADL, activities of daily living.
Source: From Ref. 20.

The Geriatrician's View of Frailty

Geriatricians and oncologists often state that they can clinically differentiate between a frail and a nonfrail individual. To identify the clinical indicators used to describe a frail individual, Fried et al. surveyed geriatricians through standardized case scenarios. In evaluating each scenario, each geriatrician was asked to rank the clinical profiles from 0 to 100, representing a spectrum of "nonfrail" to "frail." The clinicians surveyed described frailty as the "presence of a critical mass of consequences of disease and aging related changes," including: (a) generalized weakness, (b) poor endurance, (c) weight loss and/or undernourished, (d) low activity level, and (e) fear of falling and/or unsteady gait. Notably, of those surveyed, individual diseases, any two diseases, or disability alone were not adequate to identify those who are frail. Rather, these geriatricians viewed frailty as a combination of impairments rather than any one condition (1).

Laboratory Markers of Frailty

An area of active research is the identification of laboratory markers of frailty (Table 6) (21). These laboratory markers are discussed below. Further studies are needed to correlate these findings with the clinical classifications of frailty.

Table 6 Potential Laboratory Markers of Frailty

IL-6
C-reactive protein
D Dimer
Factor VIII
Plasma hypertonicity
Hemoglobin

Abbreviation: IL, interleukin.

IL-6 Levels

Cohen et al. described an association of plasma interleukin (IL)-6 levels with functional disability in a sample of 1727 community-dwelling older adults, aged 70 and over. Within this population, increasing age was associated with increased IL-6 levels ($P = 0.001$). There was also a correlation between increased IL-6 levels and functional disability ($P = 0.001$). The authors also reported higher median levels of IL-6 in patients with cancer, heart attacks, and hypertension, but not diabetes or arthritis. These data suggest that dysregulation of IL-6 may be associated with functional disability and that IL-6 may be a useful measure of overall health (22).

Leng et al. also propose that chronic inflammation is associated with frailty and that an increased serum IL-6 level is a marker of chronic inflammation. They conducted a pilot study among 200 community-dwelling older adults aged 74 and over and measured IL-6 levels and hematologic parameters (specifically hemoglobin and hematocrit levels). The subjects were initially screened for frailty using the criteria outlined from the phenotype developed by Fried et al. including weight loss, fatigue, low levels of physical activity, poor grip strength, and slow walking speed (Table 2). Those with three or more criteria were "frail," and those with zero criteria were "nonfrail," based on initial screening. Eight percent of the original cohort met entry criteria: 11 frail and 19 nonfrail patients completed the study. Within this modest sample size, frail patients had higher serum IL-6 levels ($P = 0.03$), lower hemoglobin and hematocrit levels ($P < 0.001$), and an increased number of chronic diseases ($P = 0.05$) than nonfrail patients (23).

C-Reactive Protein, Factor VIII, and D Dimer

Walston et al. established biologic correlates of frailty in 4735 community-dwelling adults aged 65 and over participating in the Cardiovascular Health Study. The authors used the definition of frailty as proposed by Fried et al., described above. Frail participants had an increased level of C-reactive protein, Factor VIII, and D dimer ($P \leq 0.001$) when compared to nonfrail participants. The findings persisted even when individuals with diabetes and cardiovascular disease were excluded from the analysis. The results support the notion that frailty can also be characterized by a physiologic state of increased inflammation with secondary changes in coagulation. It is further hypothesized that chronic inflammation may lead to progressive degradation in vascular integrity (17,24).

Plasma Hypertonicity

Stookey et al. evaluated plasma hypertonicity as a marker of risk for frailty. The authors used data from a cohort of community-dwelling older adults who subjectively reported no disability. Plasma hypertonicity levels were measured at baseline and over a four-year period and were correlated to new functional disability and mortality over an eight-year period. The results indicated that increased plasma hypertonicity correlated with an increased RR of new disability in instrumental ADL (IADL) [RR = 2.3; 95% confidence interval (CI) = 1.2–4.2] and ADL (RR = 2.7; 95% CI = 1.3–5.6). In addition, increased plasma hypertonicity correlated to increased risk of overall mortality at eight years (RR = 1.4, 95% CI = 1.0–1.9). The findings suggest that plasma hypertonicity may be a marker of early frailty; however, the authors acknowledge that further studies are needed to confirm this finding (25).

CHANGES IN PHYSIOLOGY WITH AGING: PRACTICAL RECOMMENDATIONS IN CARING FOR THE FRAIL OLDER PATIENT

Aging is a heterogeneous process that affects each individual at a unique pace. Despite the heterogeneity of the aging process, there are characteristic universal changes with aging that occur in each organ system, leading to a depletion of physiologic reserve over time (Table 7).

Most organ systems undergo a physiological decline beginning at age 30. This decline occurs at variable rates in individuals; however, it is usually evident by the fourth or fifth decade of life. Many clinicians consider those over 85 years as inherently frail because many of these physiological changes will be apparent at this age and need to be considered in treatment planning. The consequence of these changes during normal activity is minimal; yet during times of stress, the decreased reserve becomes more apparent. The following age-related changes in physiology should be considered in caring for a frail older patient (20,26).

Cardiovascular

As the cardiovascular system ages, there is a decrease in cardiac output, a decrease in the maximal heart rate, a decrease in the response to catecholamines during times of stress, and prolonged recovery following exertion. Therefore, in response to stress, an older patient will not be able to mount as brisk a tachycardia as a younger patient. To calculate the maximum estimated heart rate by age, the following formula can be utilized: $208 - (0.7 \times age)$ (26,32).

Anthracycline chemotherapeutic agents have been associated with a dose-dependent risk of cardiomyopathy and congestive heart failure, with increased risk in those who receive a cumulative dose of $500 \, mg/m^2$ or greater. Other common risk factors for doxorubicin-induced cardiomyopathy include older age (age > 70), hypertension, previous cardiac disease, and radiation to the mediastinum (33).

Pulmonary

As the pulmonary system ages, there is a decreased response to hypoxemia or hypercapnia, decreased elasticity in the lung tissue, increased ventilation–perfusion mismatch, and decreased forced expiratory volume. Although total lung capacity remains the same with aging, there is a decrease in vital capacity and an increase in residual volume. The arterial partial pressure of oxygen in arterial blood (PaO_2) concentration also decreases with age and can be calculated using the following formula: $[PaO_2 = 110 - (0.4 \times age)]$ (26–31). Additionally, the cough and

Table 7 Changes in Organ Systems with Aging

Organ system	Sequelae of aging
Cardiovascular	Decreased maximum heart rate
	Decreased pacemaker cell in SA node
	Decreased maximum cardiac output
	Impaired left ventricular filling
	Increased systolic blood pressure, unchanged diastolic
	Increased peripheral vascular resistance
Pulmonary	Decrease FEV_1 and FVC
	Increased residual volume
	Increased ventilation–perfusion mismatch, causing decreased PaO_2
Renal	Decreased creatinine clearance and GFR by 10 mL/decade
	Decreased renal mass
	Decreased concentrating and diluting ability
	Decreased renin and aldosterone
	Accentuated ADH release in response to dehydration
Gastrointestinal	Decreased liver size and blood flow
	Decrease in phase I hepatic reactions
	Decrease in acid production
	Impaired response to gastric mucosal injury
Central nervous system	Small decrease in brain mass
	Decreased brain blood flow and impaired autoregulation of perfusion
	Impaired dark vision
	Inability to focus on near items (presbyopia)
	Decreased contrast sensitivity
	Decreased smell
	Decreased thirst drive
	Loss of high frequency tones
	Difficulty discriminating source of sound

Abbreviations: SA, sinoatrial; FEV_1, forced expiratory volume in one second; FVC, forced vital capacity; ADH, anti-diuretic hormone; GFR, glomerular filtration rate; PaO_2, partial pressure of oxygen in arterial blood.
Source: From Refs. 26–31.

laryngeal reflexes decline with age, possibly predisposing the patient to aspiration or pneumonia. This risk can be minimized by use of an incentive spirometer, early mobilization, and careful attention to pulmonary toilet.

Neurological

Changes in the neurological system that come with aging include a decrease in vision with decreased contrast sensitivity. Therefore, instructions should be written in black ink on white paper in a large font size. Furthermore, with aging there is a loss in high-frequency hearing, and often a preservation of low-frequency hearing (26). Therefore speaking in a low-pitched tone, eliminating background noise, and utilizing a hearing amplifier for those who are hearing impaired can assist in communication. Cisplatin chemotherapy is associated with a risk of ototoxicity (including tinnitus and hearing loss), which is dose related and irreversible (34). In addition, several chemotherapy agents are associated with the risk of neuropathy, including paclitaxel, the vinca alkaloids, and the platinum agents (35). Older patients receiving these therapies should be monitored for the development or progression of neuropathy, which can pose an increased risk of falls or impaired mobility.

As part of the neurological examination, a cognitive assessment is needed. This is particularly important in patients who are self-administering oral chemotherapy, to determine if the patient has decisional capacity to consent and adhere to medication instructions at home. In addition, abrupt changes in cognitive function may be a sign of central nervous system metastases, warranting further evaluation.

Renal

Renal mass decreases by 25% to 30% over a person's life span. Renal blood flow decreases by 1% per year after the age of 50 and glomerular filtration decreases by 1 ml/min/yr after the age of 40. The serum creatinine does not adequately reflect the decline in renal function with aging, secondary to the loss in lean body mass and subsequent decreases in creatinine production (26–28,30,34). Therefore, creatinine clearance is a better measure of renal function and should be considered when dosing medications. Two common formulas for calculating creatinine clearance are the Cockcroft–Gault and Jeliffe formulas:

Cockcroft and Gault method:

$$\frac{[140 - age(yr)] \, [weight \, (kg)]}{72[serum \, creatinine(mg/dL)]} \times 0.85 \text{ if female}$$

Jeliffe method:

$$\frac{98 - 0.8 \, [age(yr) - 20]}{serum \, creatinine \, (mg/dL)} \times 0.9 \text{ if female}$$

For older adults in particular, a 24-hour creatinine clearance is a more accurate measure of renal function than the calculated creatinine clearance. This was demonstrated in a study of octogenarians by Rimon et al., in which calculated creatinine clearance was compared to 24-hour creatinine clearance. In this cohort, only 9% of the calculated creatinine clearance values (by Cockcroft–Gault and Jeliffe formulas) correlated to ±10% of the measured 24-hour creatinine clearance (36,37). Therefore, a 24-hour urine creatinine clearance can provide a more accurate measure of renal function.

Gastrointestinal

Age-related changes in the gastrointestinal tract include decreased acid secretion and fewer villi in mucosal surfaces. Despite these changes, there is no significant change in drug absorption with aging. Previous studies have demonstrated that older patients may be at increased risk for chemotherapy-associated mucositis or diarrhea (38,39). Therefore, careful attention to the fluid status is warranted.

With aging, there is a decrease in liver volume by approximately 25% to 50% and a decrease in hepatic blood flow by 10% to 15% (27). This decline in hepatic function with aging may not be reflected in the serum liver function tests. The phase I hepatic reactions, which include oxidation, deamination, and hydroxylation, decrease with aging. There is no significant change in phase II hepatic reactions (conjugation: acetylation, glucuronidation, and sulfation).

Hematopoietic

With aging, there is a decrease in bone marrow mass and an increase in bone marrow fat. The peripheral blood cell concentrations in healthy older patients are similar to those of younger patients; however, the myelosuppressive effects of chemotherapy are greater in older patients, secondary to the decreased bone marrow reserve. Older patients receiving moderately toxic chemotherapy (of similar dose intensity to CHOP: cyclophosphamide, vincristine, doxorubicin, and prednisone) are at increased risk for neutropenia and neutropenia-associated complications (29–31). Therefore, the National Comprehensive Cancer Network advisory panel for the treatment of older patients with cancer recommends the use of growth factors for primary prophylaxis in older patients receiving treatment with CHOP or a drug combination with similar dose intensity (40).

COMPREHENSIVE GERIATRIC ASSESSMENT: IDENTIFICATION OF THE FRAIL OLDER ONCOLOGY PATIENT

Geriatricians describe the diversity in health status among individuals of the same chronological age through a comprehensive geriatric assessment. The standard domains of a geriatric assessment include an evaluation of functional status, comorbidity, nutritional status, cognition, psychological state, and social support. This comprehensive evaluation identifies the areas of vulnerability among all geriatric patients, not just those with cancer. In fact, to date, there has been no clinical trial that has tested the hypothesis that a geriatric assessment is effective in shaping interventions and clinical decisions among oncology patients (15,41). As future geriatric oncology studies are planned, a baseline geriatric assessment should be incorporated to answer these questions. Below, we will discuss each of the domains of geriatric assessment. Practical ways to address the findings are summarized in Table 8.

Functional Status

Functional status can be measured by subjective self-reported measures or objective physical performance tests. These will be described below.

Subjective Measures of Functional Status

Traditional assessment measures of functional status include questions regarding the need for assistance in ADL and IADL. ADL are basic self-care skills such as ability to bathe, dress, transfer, maintain continence, and feed oneself. The need for assistance with these activities is predictive of risk of mortality, increased length of hospital stay, and progressive loss of function during hospitalization (42,43). Balducci and Stanta describe patients who require assistance in one or more ADL as "frail" (44).

IADL are those self-care skills that are required for independent functioning within the community. These include the ability to telephone, shop, travel, prepare

Table 8 Impact of Geriatric Assessment on Clinical Care Through Intervention

Identification of vulnerability in the following domain	Potential action taken
Functional status	Initiate visiting nurse to assess for home health aide Physical therapy evaluation Assessment of the need and eligibility for transportation services
Comorbidity	Assessment of the impact of the comorbid condition on life expectancy Collaboration with patient's other physicians Review of medication list to look for possible interactions
Cognition	Ruling out of a reversible cause of memory loss (i.e., TSH, B12) Neurological evaluation, including CNS imaging as indicated Providing written instructions
Nutritional status	Nutrition consultation Assessing if patient qualifies for community home-delivered meals
Psychological state	Referral to social worker Referral to support group Treatment with an antidepressant
Social support	Referral to social worker: identification of community resources Referral to a support group

Abbreviations: CNS, central nervous system; TSH, thyroid-stimulating hormone.

meals, do housework, take medications, and manage one's finances. Requiring assistance in IADL is predictive of risk of mortality, cognitive impairment, and loss of ability to maintain independence in the community (45,46).

Performance-Based Measures of Functional Status

Other authors have described objective measures of functional status, to aid in the identification of frailty (47). The physical performance test first described by Reuben and Siu and later by Brown et al., consists of timed performance on the following tasks: writing a sentence, simulated eating, turning 360 degrees, putting on and removing a jacket, lifting a book and putting it on a shelf, picking up a penny from the floor, walking 50 ft, and climbing stairs (Table 9). Performance on the physical performance test correlates with risk of death or nursing home placement ($P < 0.05$) (48,49).

Falls in the older adult have been associated with limited mobility, decreased ability to perform ADL, and increased risk of nursing home placement (50,51). With the deleterious impact of falls on an older person's functional status, many authors have studied the risk factors associated with falling. Tinetti et al. identified risk factors for falls, which include: arthritis; presence of depressive symptoms; orthostasis; cognitive impairment; vision, gait, or balance impairments; impairment of muscle strength; and four or more medications. As the number of risk factors increased, so did the risk of falling ($P < 0.0001$) (50–53).

To further assist in the assessment of physical mobility and muscle strength, the "Timed Up & Go" performance test can be utilized. The test measures the number

Table 9 Modified Physical Performance Test Items

Task	Description
Book lift	A ~7 lbs book is lifted from waist height to a shelf ~12 in. above shoulder level
Put on and take off a coat	Put on and take off a standard lab coat of appropriate size as quickly as able
Pick up a penny	Pick up as quickly as possible a penny that is located ~12 in. in front of the foot
Chair rise	Sit in a chair that has a seat height of 16 in. Then stand fully and sit back down, without using the hands, five times, as quickly as possible
Turn 360	Turn both clockwise and counterclockwise quickly, but safely. Patients are subjectively graded on steadiness and ability to produce continuous turning movement
50 ft walk	Walk 25 ft in a straight line, turn, and return to the initial starting place as quickly as possible, safely
One flight of stairs	The time required to ascend 10 steps
Four flights of stairs	Climb four flights of stairs. One point is given for each flight of stairs completed
Progressive Romberg test	Subjects are scored according to their ability to maintain a reduced base of support: feet together, semi-tandem, and full tandem, for a maximum of 10 sec

of seconds an individual takes to stand up from a standard armchair (approximate seat height of 46 cm), walk a distance of 3 m (10 ft), turn, walk back to the chair, and sit down again. The test was originally reported by Mathias et al., and subsequently modified by Podsiadlo and Richardson to be a timed test (54,55). Guralnik et al. reported gait speed as an important predictor of disability (56).

Grip strength has also been used as a measure of frailty. Sydall et al. studied grip strength in a cross-sectional study of 717 men and women aged 64 to 74 years. Grip strength decreased with increasing age and was associated with other markers of aging, including decreased cognitive function, higher hearing threshold, and increased risk of walking problems. In men, grip strength significantly correlated with all-cause mortality ($P < 0.001$) (57).

Comorbidity

The terms "frailty" and "comorbidity" were previously used interchangeably; however, they are more recently being recognized as distinct, but interrelated clinical entities (1). Comorbidity is defined as concurrent medical problems that are competing causes of morbidity or mortality (58,59). The number of comorbid conditions increases as one ages and adversely impacts on the projected life expectancy (Fig. 2) (60,61). For the oncologist, a thorough understanding of comorbid medical conditions is important in order to: (i) determine whether another competing cause of mortality will limit an individual's life expectancy more than the cancer, and

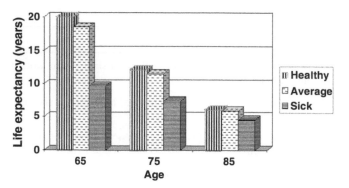

Figure 2 Life Expectancy Based on Age and Comorbidity. *Source*: From Ref. 60.

(ii) consider the impact of these coexisting medical problems on the patient's ability to tolerate treatment (44). Certain comorbid diseases have been associated with increased risk of frailty, in particular cardiovascular disease and depression (62,63). There is no clear link between the diagnosis of cancer and the increased risk of frailty (44).

Nutrition

Poor nutritional status, defined as a body mass index less than $22\,kg/m^2$, is associated with increased dependence in ADL (odds ratio = 1.21; 95% CI = 1.01–1.45) and decreased one-year survival [RR = 0.85 (95% CI = 0.74–0.97)] (64). In addition, unintentional weight loss is associated with lower chemotherapy response rates and decreased performance status. Weight loss of 5% or greater is associated with an increased risk of mortality (hazard ratio = 1.67, 95% CI = 1.29–2.15) (65,66).

Sarcopenia is the loss of muscle mass and strength associated with aging. Reduced muscle mass and strength are evident in all older adults, but if sarcopenia progresses beyond what is needed for functional requirements, it can lead to disability and frailty. The mechanisms leading to sarcopenia are multifactorial, the most notable causes being central nervous system decline, intrinsic loss of muscle contractile function, and humoral factors (decline in growth hormone, testosterone, and estrogen). The most widely utilized treatment of sarcopenia is progressive resistance training, which has been shown to increase muscle mass at any age, even in the presence of chronic disease. Progressive resistance training will not only reverse, but may also partially prevent sarcopenia (67).

Cognition

Dementia is an independent prognostic indicator for mortality (68,69). For older patients with cancer, the degree of cognitive impairment needs to be considered when devising the treatment plan. Oral chemotherapy should be used with caution in older patients with cognitive dysfunction (35). A patient with cognitive impairment will need assistance to remember instructions regarding use of supportive medications such as antiemetics. The patient's family or caregiver can be critical in maintaining safety and assessing for signs of toxicity. Furthermore, the caregiver will need to be aware of the potential side effects of treatment that would necessitate medical attention.

Psychological State, Social Support, and Frailty

The psychological state of the older patient correlates with the presence of social support (70,71). Social isolation is a predictor of mortality independent of physical functioning, health status, and cognitive functioning (72). To address the issue of the frail older adult lacking social support, McCorkle et al. utilized oncology advance practice nurses (APN) and developed a standardized protocol to provide specialized home care interventions to older postsurgical cancer patients. The specific components of this APN model included patient education, assessment of patient problems, providing psychological support and coordinating community support services. The findings indicated that the specialized home care intervention group was found to have increased survival even when adjustments were made for age, race, depressive symptoms, symptom distress, and enforced social dependency ($P = 0.002$) (73,74).

THE FRAIL GERIATRIC ONCOLOGY PATIENT

Few authors have applied the definitions of frailty to the older oncology patient or delineated how characterizing an oncology patient as frail would affect treatment. To guide the clinician in this evaluation, Balducci and Stanta describe a frail oncology patient as having the following criteria: aged 85 years or over, dependent in one or more ADL, presence of comorbidity (defined as serious cardiovascular, respiratory, or cerebrovascular conditions; three or more comorbid conditions), and presence of one or more geriatric syndromes (moderate to severe dementia with a Folstein Mini-mental Status exam score of 25 or less; three or more falls during one month; delirium secondary to an upper respiratory tract infection, coronary ischemia, or medication induced; urinary incontinence unrelated to stress and fecal incontinence; history of osteoporotic fractures or compression vertebral fracture; and failure to thrive, neglect, or abuse).

To determine whether to proceed with cancer treatment, Balducci and Stanta recommend that the clinician first evaluate whether the patient will die of the malignancy or experience disease-related morbidity during the anticipated life expectancy. If life expectancy is shorter than cancer survival, then palliation is appropriate. If life expectancy is greater than cancer survival, then the clinician must estimate whether the patient can tolerate treatment of the disease without sustaining life-threatening complications (44).

The data regarding the optimal treatment of the frail geriatric oncology patient is sparse because few clinical trials have included the frail elderly. Efforts are needed to operationalize the definition of frailty within the oncology patient population. The Interventions on Frailty Working Group developed recommendations to screen and recruit frail older patients in clinical trials. The authors recommend that patients aged 70 and over be included in these trials, due to the higher prevalence of physical disability in this age group. The trials should also include a screening measure for frailty. This would include focusing on the domains of mobility, muscle strength, nutritional intake, weight change, balance, endurance, fatigue, and physical activity. Exclusion criteria should be minimized to include patients with competing medical problems. Additionally, collecting the performance-based measures of physical function, along with the self-reported measures of disability is recommended to be included in clinical trials. An intention-to-treat study design should be utilized to reduce the potential effect of drop out bias. Just as important is the need for clinical trials to develop a uniform assessment of an older individual's baseline physiological status, which can serve as a predictive model for tolerance to cancer treatment (15,40). Also, it is critical to emphasize that an independent, robust elderly patient who undergoes cancer treatment may be quickly rendered frail due to the lack of physiologic reserve often manifested in older patients under stress. Therefore, future research also needs to address the role of comprehensive geriatric assessment as a form of anticipatory guidance for the nonfrail older cancer patient about to undergo treatment.

In summary, the population of older patients is rapidly growing, leading to an increasing number of older frail oncology patients. The geriatric literature provides clinical and laboratory indicators of frailty, which can be utilized in the care of the geriatric oncology population. Data with regard to the risks and benefits of cancer treatment in the frail oncology population are sparse. Clinical trials including and focusing on this population are needed in order to determine the optimal care for the frail older patient. In clinical care and trials, a comprehensive geriatric assessment can be used to identify areas of vulnerability, initiate interventions based on the findings, and potentially improve outcomes.

REFERENCES

1. Fried LP, Ferrucci L, Darer J, et al. Untangling the concepts of disability, frailty, and comorbidity: implications for improved targeting and care. J Gerontol 2004; 59(3):255–263.
2. Balducci L. Geriatric oncology challenges for the new century. Eur J Cancer 2000; 36(14):1741–1754.
3. Balducci L, Extermann M. Management of the frail person with advanced cancer. Crit Rev Oncol/Hematol 1999; 33:143–148.
4. Fried LP, Walston J. Frailty and failure to thrive. In: Hazzard WR, Blass JP, Ettinger WH, Halter JB, Ouslander JG, eds. Principles of Geriatric Medicine and Gerontology. New York: McGraw-Hill, 1999:1387–1402.
5. Federal Interagency Forum on Aging-Related Statistics. Older Americans 2004: Key Indicators of Well-Being. Federal Interagency Forum on Aging-Related Statistics, P2–140. Washington D.C.: U.S. Government Printing Office, November 2004.
6. Population Projections Program. Population Division, US Census Bureau, Washington D.C., 2002. Available at: http://www.census.gov/population/projections/nation/summary/np-t3-b.pdf (accessed: January 10, 2004).
7. Day JC. Population projections of the United States by age, sex, race, and hispanic origin: 1995 to 2050, U.S. Bureau of the Census, Current Population Reports, P25–1130. Washington D.C.: U.S. Government Printing Office, 1996.
8. Yancik R, Ries LA. Cancer in older persons: an international issue in an aging world. Semin Oncol 2004; 31(2):128–136.
9. Misra D, Seo PH, Cohen HJ. Aging and cancer. Clin Adv Hematol Oncol 2004; 2(7):457–464.
10. Yancik R. Cancer burden in the aged. Cancer 1997; 80:1273–1283.
11. Yancik R, Ries LA. Aging and cancer in America: demographic and epidemiologic perspectives. Hematol/Oncol Clin North Am 2000; 14(1):17–23.
12. Buchner DM, Wagner EH. Preventing frail health. Clin Geriatric Med 1992; 8:1–7.
13. Fried LP, Tangen CM, Walston J, et al. Frailty in older adults: evidence for a phenotype. J Gerontol 2001; 56A(3):M146–M156.
14. Repetto L, Venturino A, Fratino L, et al. Geriatric oncology: a clinical approach to the older patient with cancer. Eur J Cancer 2003; 39:870–880.
15. Ferruci L, Guralnik JM, Cavazzini C, et al. The frailty syndrome: a critical issue in geriatric oncology. Crit Rev Oncol Hematol 2003; 46:127–137.

16. Wymenga ANM, Slaets JPJ, Sleijfer Dth. Treatment of cancer in old age, shortcomings and challenges. Neth J Med 2001; 59:259–266.
17. Fried LP, Kronmal RA, Newman AB, et al. Risk factors for 5-year mortality in older adults: the Cardiovascular Health Study. J Am Med Assoc 1998; 279(8):585–592.
18. Rockwood K, Stadnyk K, MacKnight C, et al. A brief clinical instrument to classify frailty in elderly people. Lancet 1999; 353:205–206.
19. Rockwood K, Hogan DB, MacKnight C. Conceptualisation and measurement of frailty in elderly people. Drugs Aging 2000; 17(4):295–302.
20. Winograd CH, Gerety MB, Chung M, et al. Screening for frailty: criteria and predictors of outcomes. J Am Geriatr Soc 1991; 39:778–784.
21. Cohen HJ. In search of the underlying mechanisms of frailty. J Gerontol Med Sci 2000; 55A(12):M706–M708.
22. Cohen HJ, Pieper CF, Harris T, et al. The association of plasma IL-6 levels with functional disability in community-dwelling elderly. J Gerontol A Biol Sci Med Sci 1997; 52 (4):M201–M208.
23. Leng S, Chaves P, Koenig K, et al. Serum interleukin-6 and hemoglobin as physiological correlates in the geriatric syndrome of frailty: a pilot study. J Am Geriatr Soc 2002; 50: 1268–1271.
24. Walston J, McBurnie MA, Newman A, et al. Frailty and activation of the inflammation and coagulation systems with and without clinical comorbidities; results from the Cardio-vascular Health Study. Arch Int Med 2002; 162:2333–2341.
25. Stookey JD, Purser JL, Pieper CF, Cohen HJ. Plasma hypertonicity: another marker of frailty?. J Am Geriatr Soc 2004; 52:1313–1320.
26. Cobbs EL, Duthie EH, Murphy JB, eds. Geriatric Review Syllabus. 5th ed. Blackwell Publishing, 2002:171, 253, 316, 375.
27. Avorn J, Gurwitz JH. Principles of pharmacology. In: Cassel C, Cohen HJ, Larson EB, Meier DE, Resnick NM, Rubenstein L, eds. Geriatric Medicine. 3rd ed. Springer-Verlag, 1997:55–70.
28. Balducci L, Extermann M. Management of cancer in the older person: a practical approach. Oncologist 2000; 5(3):224–237.
29. Repetto L, Carreca I, Maraninchi D, Aapro M, Calabresi P, Balducci L. Use of growth fac-tors in the elderly patient with cancer: a report from the Second International Society for Geriatric Oncology (SIOG) 2001 meeting. Crit Rev Oncol Hematol 2003; 45(2):123–128.
30. Dees EC, O'Reilly S, Goodman SN, et al. A prospective pharmacologic evaluation of age-related toxicity of adjuvant chemotherapy in women with breast cancer. Cancer Invest 2000; 18(6):521–529.
31. Balducci L, Lyman GH. Patients aged ≥70 are at high risk for neutropenic infection and should receive hemopoietic growth factors when treated with moderately toxic che-motherapy. J Clin Oncol 2001; 19(5):1583–1585.
32. Tanaka H, Monahan KD, Seals DR. Age-predicted maximal heart rate revisited. J Am Coll Cardiol 2001; 37(1):153–156.
33. Singal PK, Iliskovic N. Doxorubicin-induced cardiomyopathy. N Engl J Med 1998; 339(13):900–905.
34. Naeim A, Reuben D. Geriatric syndromes and assessment in older cancer patients. Oncology 2001; 15(12):1–19.
35. Lichtman SM. Chemotherapy in the elderly. Semin Oncol 2004; 31(2):160–174.
36. Rimon E, Kagansky N, Cojocaru L, Gindin J, Schattner A, Levy S. Can creatinine clear-ance be accurately predicted by formulae in octogenarian in-patients? Quart J Med 2004; 97:281–287.
37. Fehrman-Ekholm I, Skeppholm L. Renal function in the elderly (> 70 years old) measured by means of iohexol clearance, serum creatinine, serum urea and estimated clearance. Scand J Urol Nephrol 2003; 38:73–77.
38. Popescu RA, Normans PJ, Parikh RB, et al. Adjuvant or palliative chemotherapy for colorectal cancer in patients 70 years or older. J Clin Oncol 1999; 17(8):2412–2418.

39. Gelman RS, Taylor SG. Cyclophosphamide, methotrexate, and 5-fluorouracil chemotherapy in women more than 65 years old with advanced breast cancer: the elimination of age trends in toxicity by using doses based on creatinine clearance. J Clin Oncol 1984; 2(12):1401–1413.

40. National Comprehensive Cancer Network Guidelines in oncology. Guidelines in supportive care; senior adult oncology. Available at: http://www.nccn.org/professionals/physician. Accessed March 10, 2005.

41. Ferrucci L, Guralnik JM, Studenski S, et al. Designing randomized, controlled trials aimed at preventing or delaying functional decline and disability in frail, older persons: a consensus report. J Am Geriatr Soc 2004; 52:625–634.

42. Naglie G. Fraility. In: Evans JG, Williams TF, Beattie BL, Michel JP, Wilcok GK, eds. Oxford Textbook of Geriatric Medicine. New York: Oxford University Press, Inc., 2000:1181–1192.

43. Narain P, Rubenstein LZ, Wieland GD, et al. Predictors of immediate and 6 month outcomes in hospitalized elderly patients. The importance of functional status. J Am Geriatr Soc 1988; 36:775–783.

44. Balducci L, Stanta G. Cancer in the frail patient: a coming epidemic. Hematol/Oncol Clin North Am 2000; 14(1):235–249.

45. Reuben DB, Rubenstein LV, Hirsch SH, Hays RD. Value of functional status as a predictor of mortality: results of a prospective study. Am J Med 1992; 93(6):663–669.

46. Barberger-Gateau P, Fabrigoule C, Helmer C, Rouch I, Dartigues JF. Functional impairment in instrumental activities of daily living: an early clinical sign of dementia? J Am Geriatr Soc 1999; 47(4):456–462.

47. Brown M, Sinacore DR, Binder EF, Kohrt WM. Physical and performance measures for the identification of mild to moderate frailty. J Gerontol Med Sci 2000; 55A(6):M350–M355.

48. Reuben DB, Siu AL. An objective measure of physical function of elderly outpatients. The Physical Performance Test. J Am Geriatr Soc 1990; 38(10):1105–1112.

49. Reuben DB, Siu AL, Kimpau S. The predictive validity of self-report and performance based measures of function and health. J Gerontol Med Sci 1992; 47(4):M106–M110.

50. Tinetti ME, Williams CS. The effect of falls and fall injuries on functioning in community-dwelling older persons. J Gerontol A Biol Sci Med Sci 1998; 53:M112–M119.

51. Tinetti ME, Williams TF, Mayewski R. Fall risk index for elderly patients based on number of chronic disabilities. Am J Med 1986; 80(3):429–434.

52. Tinetti ME, Speechley M, Ginter SF. Risk factors for falls among elderly persons living in the community. N Engl J Med 1998; 319:1701–1707.

53. Tinetti ME. Preventing falls in elderly persons. N Engl J Med 2003; 348(1):42–49.

54. Mathias S, Nayak US, Issacs B. Balance in elderly patients: the "get up and go" test. Arch Phys Med Rehabil 1986; 67:387–389.

55. Podsiadlo D, Richardson S. The timed "Up & Go": a test of basic functional mobility for frail elderly persons. J Am Geriatrics Soc 1991; 39(2):142–148.

56. Guralnik JM, Ferrucci L, Pieper CF, et al. Lower extremity function and subsequent disability: consistency across studies, predictive models, and value of gait speed alone compared with the short physical performance battery. J Gerontol A Biol Sci Med Sci 2000; 55(4):M221–M231.

57. Syddall H, Cooper C, Martin F, Briggs R, Aihie Sayer A. Is grip strength a useful single marker of frailty? Age Ageing 2003; 32(6):650–656.

58. Lattanzio F, Zuccala G, Bernabei R. Comorbidity and cancer in the aged: the geriatrician's point of view. Rays(suppl) 1997; 22(1):12–16.

59. Extermann M. Measuring comorbidity in older cancer patients. Eur J Cancer 2000; 36:453–471.

60. Extermann M, Balducci L, Lyman GH. What threshold for adjuvant therapy in older breast cancer patients? J Clin Oncol 2000; 18:1709–1717.

61. Yates JW. Comorbidity considerations in geriatric oncology research. Cancer J Clin 2001; 51(6):329–336.

62. Newman AB, Gottdiener JS, McBurnie MA, et al. Associations of subclinical cardiovascular disease with frailty. J Gerontol 2001; 56A(3):M158–M166.

63. Kop WJ, Gottdiener JS, Tangen CM, et al. Inflammation and coagulation factors in persons > 65 years of age with symptoms of depression but without evidence of myocardial ischemia. Am J Cardiol 2002; 89:419–424.

64. Landi F, Giuseppe G, Gambassi G, et al. Body mass index and mortality among older people living in the community. J Am Geriatr Soc 1999; 47(9):1072–1076.

65. Newman AB, Yanez D, Harris T, et al. Weight change in old age and its association with mortality. J Am Geriatr Soc 2001; 49:1309–1318.

66. Dewys WD, Begg C, Lavin PT, et al. Prognostic effect of weight loss prior to chemotherapy in cancer patients. Am J Med 1980; 68:491–497.

67. Roubenoff R. Sarcopenia and its implications for the elderly. Eur J Clin Nutr 2000; 54(suppl 3):S40–S47.

68. Eagles JM, Beattie JAG, Restall DB, et al. Relationship between cognitive impairment and early death in the elderly. Br Med J 1990; 300:239–240.

69. Wolfson C, Wolfson DB, Asgharian M, et al. A reevaluation of the duration of survival after the onset of dementia. N Engl J Med 2001; 344:1111–1116.

70. Rao A, Cohen HJ. Symptom management in the elderly cancer patient: fatigue, pain, and depression. J Natl Cancer Inst Monogr 2004; 32:150–157.

71. Kornblith AB, Herndon JE II, Zuckerman E, et al. Cancer and Leukemia Group B. Social support as a buffer to the psychological impact of stressful life events in women with breast cancer. Cancer 2001; 91(2):443–454.

72. Seeman TE, Berkman LF, Kohout F, Lacroix A, Glynn R, Blazer D. Intercommunity variations in the association between social ties and mortality in the elderly. A comparative analysis of three communities. Ann Epidemiol 1993; 3:325–335.

73. McCorkle R, Strumpf NE, Nuamah IF, et al. A specialized home care intervention improves survival among older post-surgical cancer patients. J Am Geriatr Soc 2000; 48(12): 1707–1713.

74. Bourbonnicre M, Evans LK. Advanced practice nursing in the care of frail older adults. J Am Geriatr Soc 2002; 50:2062–2076.

26

End-of-Life Care

Joyce Liu and Ursula Matulonis
Department of Medical Oncology, Dana Farber Cancer Institute, Boston,
Massachusetts, U.S.A.

INTRODUCTION

Many unique issues arise in the end-of-life care of elderly patients with cancer. Although there are similarities with end-of-life care of younger individuals, end-of-life care for the elderly cancer patient is complicated by difficulties with assessing and managing pain, toxicities of medications, and depression. Furthermore, care of the elderly is sometimes delivered in unique settings such as the nursing home, and special attention must be given toward advance directives that specify levels of care to be provided at the end of life. Properly assessing and managing these issues in the elderly can be difficult in the face of impaired cognitive status, financial pressures, or the desire not to be perceived as a burden on the family. In this chapter, we will discuss the issues that surround the end-of-life care of the elderly patient with cancer, as well as the approach toward management.

PAIN

Successful pain control is a critical part in the care of the dying patient. Management of pain is required, to allow patients to die comfortably, as well as to allow patients' families to recover from their grief without potentially upsetting memories of their loved ones suffering. Pain is a very common symptom in the dying elderly patient; up to 66% of dying patients have pain in the last month of life, and 33% experience pain in the last 24 hours (1). With appropriate assessment and management, pain in most patients can be successfully treated with a combination of nonpharmacologic and pharmacologic interventions. Pain in the elderly is often underestimated by health care providers and families, as well as by patients themselves (1). However, studies suggest that the qualitative experience of pain does not differ greatly between elderly populations and younger ones (2). Nonetheless, pain in the elderly continues to be undertreated, and studies have shown that elderly patients are less likely to be prescribed analgesic medications for their pain than younger patients (3).

   Many barriers exist that lead to the underestimation and undertreatment of pain in the elderly. Studies have demonstrated that oncologists often feel undertrained in pain assessment (4), and may not address the issue unless the patient first initiates discussion. Patients themselves may be reluctant to introduce the issue, because they fear that discussion of pain may distract clinicians from addressing their primary oncologic diagnosis (5). Elderly patients also tend to have greater concerns regarding analgesics, including fear of addiction and other side effects. Of note, fear of addiction is a primary concern for older patients, and may influence their willingness to initiate discussions regarding pain control with their oncologist (4).

For those cancer patients living in a long-term care (LTC) facility, pain is prevalent, and assessment and management can be challenging (6,7). However, these patients are able to provide reliable information about their pain and can be reliably assessed (7,8). Despite this, many investigators have shown that LTC residents experience untreated and undiagnosed pain (3,9). This may be partly because the residents of nursing homes often believe that pain should be expected with aging and that complaining could negatively affect their care (6,7). In addition, pain assessment in LTC facilities may be compromised by patients' cognitive states, and studies have suggested that common tools used to assess pain in LTC residents underestimate pain in those patients with severe cognitive impairment (10). However, cognitive impairment does not "mask" pain complaints, and although these patients may underreport pain, self-reports of pain are as valid as in those without cognitive impairment (11). Nonetheless, pain remains undertreated, and studies suggest that pain rates are higher in those who have dementia or are noncommunicative (9).

Pain control in LTC facility residents has been found to be suboptimal. Various studies have shown that between 33% and 83% of nursing home residents have ongoing pain that affects mobility, promotes depression, and diminishes quality of life (11–14). In a study specific to cancer patients of all ages admitted to LTC facilities in the United States, Barnabei et al. demonstrated that one in three cancer patients had daily pain, and that no analgesic medications were prescribed for one in four of these individuals (3). Elderly patients were especially less likely to be treated with stronger analgesics such as morphine. Accurate assessment of pain in LTC facilities has been demonstrated to be reliable with use of the minimum data set (MDS) used in LTC (15). Of note, when compared with hospice staffs, nursing home staffs tend to underestimate the rating and severity of pain on the MDS (16).

Nonpharmacologic Management of Pain

Nonpharmacologic therapies can be incorporated into the pain management regimens of older patients, to improve pain control (17). Therapies that have been used in the treatment of pain in the elderly include acupuncture and transcutaneous electrical nerve stimulation, as well as physical modalities such as heat, cold massage, positioning, and exercise (18). Cognitive therapies are also encouraged and include education and reassurance, counseling, relaxation, music and art therapy, and hypnosis. Proper positioning alone can reduce discomfort in dying patients (19).

Pharmacologic Management of Pain

Use of analgesic medications in the elderly patient should follow the World Health Organization (WHO) analgesic ladder (20), which remains an effective tool in providing pain relief for patients experiencing mild, moderate, and severe pain. Specifically, the WHO ladder divides analgesics into three classes, and suggests using nonopioid medications such as aspirin, acetaminophen, or nonsteroidal anti-inflammatory drugs (NSAIDs) for mild pain (class 1), low-dose oxycodone or the weaker opioids, alone or combined with class 1 agents, for moderate pain (class 2), and potent opioids such as morphine, oxycodone, hydromorphone, fentanyl, or methadone for patients with severe pain (class 3).

Concerns exist regarding the metabolism and efficacy of pain medications in the elderly patient. Table 1 outlines some of the unique clinical concerns when treating the elderly cancer patient for pain. Acetaminophen is likely the safest medication for control of mild to moderate pain (21), although there are few clinical trials that have included patients older than 65 years. NSAIDs, which are highly protein bound, prove problematic, particularly in the elderly, due to their lower serum albumin levels. This can lead to higher free NSAID serum levels as compared to younger patients receiving the same dose, placing the elderly patient at greater risk of toxic side effects such as hyperkalemia and renal toxicity. Furthermore, most NSAIDs are metabolized through both phase I (oxidation or reduction) and phase II (glucuronidation or acetylation) reactions in the liver, which may be significantly reduced in the elderly patient (22), resulting in higher circulating drug levels. Thus, the elderly using NSAIDs may be at higher risk of gastrointestinal bleeding, confusion, and salt and water retention. Other drugs may be problematic as well; because older patients have less muscle and more fat (21), the half-lives of lipid-soluble drugs such as diazepam and opioids can be prolonged, and these medications should be used with caution.

Treatment with nonopioid medications alone is often inadequate for successful pain management, which requires the use of opioids. Opioid use in the elderly patient should be carefully monitored. Typically, older patients require smaller doses of opioids than their younger counterparts because of increased fat:muscle ratio, decreased renal and hepatic clearance of medications, higher plasma concentrations of opioids, and increased sensitivity to peak plasma concentrations of the drug (23). Similarly, studies have shown that the elderly can achieve similar pain relief with markedly lower opioid doses in comparison to those required for younger patients (2). Because of these alterations in opioid metabolism and sensitivity, opiate therapy in the elderly should be initiated at low doses and slowly titrated to clinical effect (1). Initial doses should be 25% to 50% lower than those used for younger patients. Rescue doses, which are usually dosed at approximately 10% of the total daily opioid dose for younger patients, should be no more than 5% in the elderly. Furthermore, rescue medications should be initially administered at intervals of four hours instead of the two-hour interval recommended for younger patients.

Several opioid medications are particularly difficult to use in the elderly and should be used with caution. For example, recommendations for the usage of transdermal fentanyl in the elderly include avoiding its use in opioid-naïve patients and watching for excess toxicities in patients with low serum albumin (23). Because transdermal fentanyl may travel more quickly through the skin in the elderly (24), the

Table 1 Unique Clinical Concerns Regarding Use of Pain Medications in the Elderly

Lowered serum albumin levels
Altered hepatic and renal clearance of drugs
Preexisting comorbid illnesses
Lowered muscle/fat ratio
Increased sensitivity to toxicities of medications, including opioids
Increased transdermal transit of medications

transfentanyl patch may need to be changed every 48 hours rather than every 72 hours. However, if the patch is removed in order to transition to oral opioids, lower doses should initially be used and then titrated upwards over the course of three days due to the continued infusion of fentanyl through a subcutaneous reservoir that accumulates under the patch (18).

Opioids such as methadone and meperidine are not recommended in the elderly population because of active metabolites with long and variable half-lives. Specifically, meperidine has been associated with numerous adverse events in seniors and should be avoided in the elderly population (25). Meperidine toxicity is due to a metabolite of meperidine, normeperidine, which accumulates beyond the analgesic duration of meperidine and can lower the seizure threshold when meperidine is used chronically. The accumulation of long-acting metabolites can also lead to myoclonus. Furthermore, meperidine has been associated with a higher incidence of falls and sedation when compared with other opioids (26,27).

Adverse Drug Reactions

In general, the elderly have increased vulnerability to adverse drug reactions. A study of adverse drug events among patients over 65 years of age found that both non-opioid analgesics and opioids were frequent causes of adverse drug events (28). NSAIDs in the elderly may cause an increased incidence of hypertension, hyperkalemia, renal failure, and gastrointestinal bleeding. Patients on NSAID medication should be monitored carefully, and consideration should be made toward empiric gastrointestinal prophylaxis. Because of the increased risk of hyperkalemia or renal failure in the elderly, they should also have laboratory studies evaluated two weeks after beginning an NSAID. Like NSAIDs, cyclooxygenase-2 (COX-2) inhibitors are extensively metabolized in the liver, and circulating drug levels can be up to 50% higher in elderly patients (22). The risks of gastrointestinal bleeding with COX-2 inhibitors are thought to be lesser when compared to those associated with standard NSAIDs, but risks of hyperkalemia and renal failure are very similar (22). No specific studies in the elderly have been performed with regard to recent findings linking COX-2 use and cardiac events. Overall, COX-2 inhibitors do appear to reduce the risk of significant gastrointestinal bleeding, but carry similar risks with regard to renal function and possibly increased cardiac risks. In the elderly patient with significant gastrointestinal risk factors, COX-2 inhibitors may provide benefit, but they should be started at a low dose, given their reduced metabolism in the elderly.

Opioids also cause increased toxicity in the elderly, and these effects can include urinary retention, pruritus, and gastrointestinal effects such as nausea, vomiting, and constipation (17,23,29). When an opioid regimen is initiated in an elderly patient, senna should be started prophylactically, in addition to other laxatives if appropriate (23,29). Nausea and vomiting, if prolonged, may require the addition of an antinausea medication, but typically, this toxicity is self-limited. If nausea and vomiting persist, switching to another opioid may be helpful in managing toxicities (30). Urinary retention is also observed more in the elderly and may be compounded by concomitantly administered medications (23). Myoclonus may occur and can often be troubling to patients and family members; myoclonus often ceases or improves with a change to another narcotic (30), or alternatively, it may be treated with clonazepam (23).

In summary, pain management in the elderly is complicated by multiple issues and must be individualized. Pain assessment can be difficult, and barriers include physicians' lack of comfort in assessing and initiating discussion of pain, as well as the patient's concerns and preconceptions regarding pain and pain medications. In LTC facilities, these issues can be further complicated by cognitive disabilities, and many patients are undertreated for pain. Important considerations when treating the elderly with pharmacologic therapy include altered drug metabolism, increased toxicities associated with medications in the elderly, and the prevalence of comorbid conditions. "Start low and go slow" (2,23) is a safe philosophy when treating pain in the elderly patient with cancer.

HYDRATION

Controversy exists regarding the decision to provide nutrition and hydration to terminally ill cancer patients. In healthy subjects, dehydration can lead to symptoms of headache, nausea, vomiting, cramps, thirst, and dry mouth (31), a finding that may prompt concern that dehydration in the dying patient causes similar distress. However, in the dying patient, dehydration has not been clearly associated with these symptoms. With the evolution of palliative care, there has been growing support for managing the terminally ill patient without artificial fluid therapy. Some have suggested that dehydration is not distressing to the dying patient and may reduce other symptoms such as increased respiratory secretions (32).

Due to logistic, ethical, and statistical issues, it is unlikely that prospective or randomized trials will be developed to examine the effects of artificial hydration in the dying patient. Nonetheless, in a systematic review of the effect of fluid status in the dying cancer patient, only 6 of 21 publications described the clinical effect of hydration, whether negative or beneficial (33). Thirst and dry mouth are very common complaints in the dying cancer patient (34,35). However, no clear correlation can be drawn between these symptoms and fluid status, as determined by serum osmolality and the levels of sodium, creatinine, and urea (34–36). Instead, symptoms of a dry mouth may be related to or exacerbated by medications used in palliation, such as opioids and antidepressants, or through mouth breathing. Symptoms of thirst and dry mouth respond well to sips of water, administration of ice chips, and mouth care (34,37). All of these findings have formulated a general consensus in palliative medicine that, regardless of age, artificial hydration is unnecessary and potentially distressing to the dying cancer patient.

DEPRESSION

Major depressive disorders are common in the older community, with a prevalence estimated at 4.4% in women and 2.7% in men (38). However, although common, depression is often underdiagnosed in older patients, or is attributed to the effects of normal aging. In one study, physicians only recognized depression in 51% of depressed elderly patients (39). Depression is also common in cancer patients, with an estimated prevalence of 17% to 25% (40). Nonetheless, depression in the elderly dying population is commonly diagnosed, but underappreciated and undertreated (41–43). One study determined that only 3% of terminal cancer patients were being given antidepressant medication, while the prevalence of depression was between 20% and 50% (42).

In the terminally ill, depressive symptoms may seem appropriate, given the clinical outlook. However, identification and treatment of depression in these individuals remain important and can significantly affect the quality of life and outcomes. A study in elderly patients suffering from severe depression and requiring psychiatric hospitalization found that therapy could alter their outlook as well as their attitude toward clinical outcome and desire for death (44), suggesting that depression itself can alter the patient's desires. As with depression in the general populace, depression in individuals at the end of life is associated with hopelessness and persistent suicidal thoughts (45), which if untreated, can result in earlier admission to hospice or inpatient care (46). One study demonstrated that among oncology outpatients, hoarding of drugs to prepare for a possible suicide attempt was related more to depression than to pain (47). Thus, it remains important to assess and treat the symptoms of depression in the dying cancer patient.

Various barriers have been identified in the diagnosis and treatment of depression in patients with cancer (Table 2). Cancer can often cause symptoms that mimic those traditionally seen with the diagnosis of depression, such as fatigue, anorexia, and weight loss. Often, clinicians have difficulty in differentiating symptoms associated with depression from those that occur from cancer or are a normal reaction to the diagnosis of cancer (48,49). This uncertainty in diagnosis may lead physicians to undertreat and/or underdiagnose depression in their patients. Furthermore, the issue of depression is often avoided in the clinical setting. Patients may avoid initiating discussion due to the concern that depression will be seen as a weakness and may lead their oncologist to pursue less aggressive management (50,51). Physicians themselves often do not initiate discussion of depression symptoms and treatment. One study of British general physicians found that clinicians generally assumed that cancer patients would seek their aid if they developed psychological problems that required help (50). However, unless patients initiated the conversation, physicians tended not to ask patients about their psychological state.

The diagnosis of depression in the elderly cancer patient may also be hindered by underlying variability in many of the typical symptoms used to diagnose depression, including fatigue, decreased appetite, weight loss, and sleep disturbances (52). Because of this, somatic symptoms have typically been removed from criteria for making a diagnosis of depression in the elderly cancer patient, and other more psychological features such as pervasive anhedonia, loss of contact with family and friends, and pessimism have been used instead (53,54). The elderly may also have other comorbid illness, such as dementia, delirium, or cognitive impairment, which makes the assessment of depression more difficult (55).

Assessment of depression has traditionally been obtained by the clinical interview. There are several, commonly used structural clinical interviews, including the Schedule for Affective Disorders and Schizophrenia (56), Structured Clinical Interview for diagnostic and statistical manual of mental disorders (DSM) (57),

Table 2   Barriers in Diagnosis and Treatment of Depression in the Elderly Cancer Patient

Symptom overlaps between depression and cancer
Clinical uncertainty by providers in identifying
Patient reluctance to initiate discussion due to fear of appearing weak
Lack of physician-initiated discussion regarding depression symptoms and treatment
Underlying variability in depressive symptoms in the elderly
Increased prevalence of comorbidities such as dementia, delirium, or cognitive impairment

Table 3 Risk Factors for Depression in the Elderly Cancer Patient

Low social support
Increased physical disability
Increased inability for self-care
Pain
Cancer type (less clear)

Research Diagnostic Criteria (58), and the diagnostic interview schedule (59). The use of structured interviews requires specific training to attain sufficient proficiency in administration and scoring. In addition, some clinicians utilize unstructured interviews that target DSM (60,61), or Endicott (62) criteria, to establish a diagnosis of depression. However, although these interviews may establish a diagnosis of depression, it has been suggested that they are not the most effective means of identifying those patients who may be at greater risk of depression (52). The latter goal appears to be better served by the usage of written self-report measures. Many self-report measures exist to help identify symptoms of depression in patients. These include the Hospital Anxiety and Depression Scale (63), the Rotterdam Symptom Checklist (64), the Beck Depression Inventory (65,66), the Brief Symptoms Inventory-Depression scale (67–69), Center for Epidemiologic Studies Depression Scale (70), and the Zung Self-Rating Depression Scale (71,72). Because of the reduced usefulness of somatic symptoms in the elderly, several additional questionnaires have been designed to help with the identification of depression in these patients, most notably the Geriatric Depression Scale, a 30-item questionnaire with binary yes or no response choices (73).

Many of the risk factors for depression in the elderly patient with cancer overlap with risk factors for the nonelderly cancer population (Table 3). It is not clear if gender is a risk factor for depression. Population studies do show a higher incidence of depression in women compared with men, in the general population (74). In the cancer population, however, studies are mixed, and some have found women to have higher incidence of depression while others have shown that men are more at risk (75). More definitive risk factors for depression in the elderly population include low social support (41), increased physical disability and inability to care for oneself (76), pain (77), and certain cancers such as pancreatic cancer, although this may be solely related to the pain induced by the cancer (23).

Management of Depression

The management of depression in the elderly involves both pharmacologic and non-pharmacologic therapies. Because of the multiple comorbidities that are more common in the elderly population, clinicians are sometimes more hesitant to initiate pharmacologic treatment of depression in the elderly. Studies have shown that a patient's education regarding symptoms and expectations can be an important factor in the treatment of depression, and a meta-analysis of various studies showed that educational interventions directed toward these purposes reduced depressive symptoms in patients with cancer (78). These studies focused on the general population of cancer patients; currently, there are no specific educational interventions that have been detailed for the elderly patient with cancer. Similarly, there have been suggestions that various forms of psychotherapy such as interpersonal therapy, behavior therapy, cognitive behavior therapy, and dynamic psychotherapy may be beneficial. But these interventions have also not been examined with regard to the elderly cancer patients (79). However, while mild to moderate depression can typically be treated with psychotherapy or counseling, management with medication is indicated for those not responding and for patients with major depression.

Antidepressant use in older patients can be complicated by several factors (Table 4). Older individuals are much more likely to use other prescription medications, which increase the potential for drug interactions (80). Furthermore, the elderly may be more sensitive to adverse drug events related to the antidepressants themselves, due to changes in metabolism and excretion, which can alter plasma drug concentrations (81,82). Aging is also associated with several changes in the neuroendocrine system (83), which may alter the individual's response to the drug and increase the risk of side effects.

Older patients appear to benefit from antidepressant therapy as much as younger individuals do, but response to therapy may occur more slowly (84). In efficacy trials conducted in older patients, most studies have demonstrated equivalence between various selective serotonin uptake inhibitors (SSRIs) and tricyclic antidepressants (TCAs) (85). With these treatments, at least six weeks of therapy are needed to achieve an optimal therapeutic effect. Within the SSRIs themselves, most clinical trials show no differences in remission rates, which range from 45% to 60% (86,87). Venlafaxine (88), mirtazipine (89), and buproprion (90) have also been studied in the elderly patient, and have demonstrated both efficacy and safety comparable with that of SSRIs.

In a meta-analysis of adverse effect data obtained from clinical trials in older patients, venlafaxine and SSRIs appeared to have fewer adverse effects and superior tolerability as compared with TCAs (91). Generally, most categories of antidepressants, including SSRIs and TCAs, tend to be well tolerated, and in efficacy trials, there was no difference in discontinuation of medication due to adverse events (85). However, TCAs were associated with more cholinergic side effects such as dry mouth, constipation, and impaired accommodation (92–94). The most common side effects of the SSRIs include nausea, gastrointestinal upset, and headaches; the toxicities of SSRIs can be dose related (41). Although most studies suggest that the SSRIs have very similar side effect rates, one study did demonstrate greater incidences of severe adverse events and of central nervous system–related side effects for fluoxetine, when compared with the effects of paroxetine (86). The most common side effects associated with mirtazapine included dry mouth and weight gain (95), and both the SSRIs and venlafaxine may be associated with hyponatremia.

Due to their more favorable side effect profile and equal efficacy, SSRIs are the first-line choice of antidepressant medication for the elderly (96,97). The recommended initial dose for the elderly patient is lower compared to that for younger patients, and SSRIs should be started at the minimal effective dose, which is often half the dose typically used in the nonelderly patient (41). Increases in the dosage should be slow and individualized. If the patient has an inadequate response or a

Table 4 Clinical Concerns Regarding Antidepressant Use in the Elderly

Altered metabolism and excretion
Increased probability of drug interactions due to increased likelihood of concomitant use of
   multiple prescription medications
Age-associated changes in the neuroendocrine system

contraindication to SSRIs, venlafaxine, mirtazapine, and buproprion are considered second-line drugs, and nortriptyline or desipramine can be used as third-line drugs (49). Medical conditions can also affect drug elimination, and special consideration should be given to the patient's renal (paroxetine) and hepatic (citalopram, fluoxetine, fluvoxamine, and sertraline) function (98,99). Specific antidepressant drugs cited in a consensus panel in 1997, which are to be avoided in the elderly included amitriptyline, amoxapine, clomipramine, doxepin, imipramine, maprotiline, protriptyline, and trimipramine (100).

SUICIDE

Epidemiological studies have suggested that the risk of suicide among patients with cancer is higher than that of the general population (193). Furthermore, this risk is increased in patients with more advanced disease (101). Studies directed toward the elderly population confirm this trend, showing that the incidence of suicide in the elderly cancer patient is higher than in elderly patients without cancer (102,103). However, it is important to note that many factors outside of the diagnosis of advanced cancer alone can contribute to the patient's "desire for death," and that identifying them and treating them may help improve the patient's quality of and outlook on life (104). Several studies have shown that the prevalence of "desire for death" in patients who are terminally ill with cancer can be fairly significant, ranging from 8.5% to 22.2% (47,105–109). These studies have found possible associations between the desire for death and a number of factors, including pain, weakness, loss of control, and psychological distress. Patients have also been observed to have specific concerns regarding clinical symptoms, such as adequate control of pain or anxiety. From a psychological standpoint, feelings of depression, hopelessness, or a fear of becoming a burden to others appear to be associated with a stronger desire for death. Some have suggested that cognitive dysfunction and delirium may also increase the likelihood of suicide (110,111).

Although studies have clearly shown an increased prevalence in the desire for death and in suicide rates in both elderly and nonelderly, terminally ill cancer patients, there is a paucity of data addressing the appropriate clinical evaluation and treatment of these concerns. Several self-written report questionnaires such as the Desire for Death Rating Scale (107) and the Schedule of Attitudes Toward Hastened Death (112,113) have been developed by researchers in palliative medicine and validated in oncology patients to help better assess risks for suicide. However, these questionnaires have been designed primarily for use in research studies and are not easily applied in the nonresearch setting. Furthermore, no guidelines exist regarding treatment of the terminally ill cancer patient expressing suicidal thoughts or desires. Some studies have suggested that increased spirituality is associated with a decreased desire for death, and have advocated that clinicians focus on providing patients with spiritual interventions (114). Because of a relatively strong association between depression and suicidal thoughts, others have suggested that treatment of underlying depression may decrease patients' desire for death. One Japanese study examined the use of TCA medications in six terminally ill cancer patients, and found that five of these patients showed marked improvement of their mood with no further suicidal thoughts after treatment (115). However, guidelines regarding this issue remain unclear, and the overall consensus suggests that patients should be monitored carefully for risk factors, with a focus on treating the risk factors that are identified (116).

ADVANCE DIRECTIVES

Physicians and other caregivers have often struggled with decisions about the appropriate care for patients at the end of life. Patients and their families have become increasingly more involved in this decision-making process, and often conflicts arise regarding what care should be provided for patients who are near death. Advance directives have evolved as a method of helping to address the difficulties of this decision-making. Advance directives have traditionally comprised two main components: the health care proxy and medical directives (117). The health care proxy is a legal mechanism by which the patient can transfer decision-making capabilities to the person(s) the patient chooses when the patient is incapable of making decisions. These individuals are sometimes referred to as surrogate decision makers. The medical directive or living will provides instructions about how decisions regarding patients' medical care should be made should they be unable to actively participate. Some medical directives also ask patients to include information about their values, to aid the interpretation of their wishes and instructions (118). Specifically, advance directives should ensure that treatments provided to patients are consistent with their values and goals, and that providers do not pursue treatments the patient would not have desired. Thus, when discussing advance directives, it is important to have patients describe any specific situations they wish to avoid. This documentation may also ease the burden for health care providers and family members trying to make difficult decisions for incompetent patients (117).

Many states have enacted specific or preferred instruments that state the wishes of the patient during complex medical situations (117). End-of-life care decisions ranging from do-not-resuscitate orders, and the use of potentially life-prolonging treatments such as antibiotics, intravenous fluids, and total parenteral nutrition may be addressed. However, the complexities of care in various medical situations may or may not be reflected in these state-mandated or crafted documents. This has led patients and their families to create their own documents, in addition to participating in open and frank conversations about end-of-life care. Many patients will include explicit stipulations about the type of care they desire at the end of life to relieve family members of the burden of making decisions, which can result in less complex, intrusive, and costly medical care (119). Thus, it is extremely important that physicians caring for the terminally ill elderly initiate and be included in discussions regarding their end-of-life desires or be made aware of the results of these discussions.

Although advance directives are potentially very beneficial to the patient at the end of life, their effectiveness in the clinical setting has several limitations (117,119,120). Because of the complexity of medicine, directives may not capture the full complexity of the patient's medical issues and the interventions or treatments that the patient would have desired or not desired in a particular situation (121,122). These documents can cause caregivers to struggle with questions such as what constitutes "life-sustaining treatments," and at what point an individual should be considered "terminally ill" (117). However, directives that are very specific and those that delve into specific interventions and scenarios have also been criticized. Critics of these types of directives argue that patients have limited knowledge and experience with these scenarios and are therefore unlikely to be able to provide informed or meaningful answers regarding their wishes (123). A study that examined patients' knowledge and understanding after discussion of advance directives with physicians demonstrated that patients leave these discussions with serious misconceptions about life-sustaining treatments (121). In this study, after a standard discussion regarding advanced directives, 66% of patients did not know that most patients needed mechanical ventilation after undergoing resuscitation; 67% did not know that patients generally cannot talk while on ventilators. Furthermore, the study showed that, despite these discussions, physicians continued to have a poor understanding of patient preferences and were unable to accurately predict the patient's desires in 18 of 20 scenarios.

Traditionally, physicians receive little formal training in how to conduct advance directive discussions. One study demonstrated that discussions between physicians and patients regarding these issues often lack depth or address easy issues, without probing for situations in which the decision-making may be less straightforward. Furthermore, the authors found that physicians often discussed medical scenarios in ways that could lead to patient misunderstanding and rarely attempted to truly understand patients' values (124). Examination of discussions of do-not-resuscitate orders conducted by resident physicians demonstrated similar weaknesses in their ability to successfully convey the medical issues to patients (125). In discussions, physicians tended to focus on treatment descriptions rather than listening to patient concerns (125–128), which can lead to a misunderstanding of patient wishes.

To successfully establish an advance directive that will be beneficial to the patient, several points need to be addressed. As discussed above, it is essential that the advance directive accurately reflects the patient's goals and desires. Studies have shown that patients are often more influenced by what the expected health outcome is than by the details of the interventions themselves (129,130). Because the potential for many clinical scenarios exists, it is often more useful to focus less on specific scenarios and more on the patient's own values and goals. Physicians can then check their understanding of a patient's goals by focusing on a few potential scenarios or interventions (117). Questions that merit specific discussion include the question of reversibility of the patient's illness, and whether that would change the patient's views about the type of treatment the patient would desire. A second related issue is that of medical uncertainty, where physicians cannot accurately predict the effectiveness of a chosen therapy. This issue occurs because physicians often do not know whether or not a specific treatment will be of benefit to the patient. However, patients are often less aware of this uncertainty and express their treatment desires based upon the assumption that the outcomes are easily predictable. Thus, they will express a desire for treatment if the intervention will help them, but do not wish to be treated if there will not be a benefit. It can be helpful to explore this issue and the concept of uncertainty with patients (117), because treatment uncertainty can often cause physicians to pursue more aggressive treatment (131), which may not be congruent with the patient's desires.

Other limitations to advance directives also exist (Table 5). Discussion of advance directives is sometimes impaired by hesitation on the part of the patient, family members, and/or the physician to discuss issues. Furthermore, some patients

Table 5 Limitations of and Complications Associated with Advance Directives

Lack of formal physician training in conducting advance directive discussions
Frequent miscommunication between patients and care providers regarding patient goals and values
Reluctance of physicians to initiate advance directive discussions
Lack of patient knowledge regarding advance directives
Completion of advance directives without communication to physicians
State-to-state variability in advance directive requirements and validity

are not aware that advance directives exist. Other patients may complete advance directives without discussing them with their physicians, and physicians may be unaware that this issue has been addressed (122,126). This problem can be further exacerbated by the fact that existing directives may not travel with the patient during institution transfer. The type of health care directives allowable from state to state varies, as does the legality of the health care proxy. Because directives vary from state to state, some may be vague and therefore not useful in actual clinical settings (117,121). Some individuals have even questioned whether the directive makes a difference given its limitations, and currently only 15% to 20% of patients have a completed directive (117,121).

Despite their potential benefits, there is a low rate of use of advance directives, even in elderly patients at the end of life. For example, in a survey of long-term care (LTC) facility residents, 63% of those interviewed had no documented discussion of advanced-care directives (132). Several studies have examined whether clinical interventions can increase the percentage of patients using advanced directives. Intervention methods have included increased patient education about life-sustaining treatments and their right to express preferences about use of these treatments, increasing physician-initiated conversations regarding advanced-care planning through physician education, or a combination of interventions directed at both patients and physicians. A review of 16 studies suggests that these interventions as a whole were able to increase patients' awareness and use of advanced-care planning, including creation of advance directives and appointment of health care proxies. However, despite this, the effect of these interventions on medical treatment decisions was somewhat more limited, and review of clinical outcomes such as use of treatments, pain control, satisfaction with care, and cost demonstrated no changes after intervention.

There are several studies conducted in the elderly that suggest that clinical interventions and education can successfully increase the use and understanding of advanced-care planning. One study randomized 61 patients who were either over the age of 65 with a life-threatening illness or over 75 years of age, healthy and ambulatory, to standard care versus an intensive, personalized intervention. The standard care arm consisted of the Massachusetts Health Care Proxy form, which was completed by patients at home. The intervention arm included written brochures on end-of-life care and scheduled meetings with a facilitator, the patient, and the patient's family. Patients in the intervention arm showed increased knowledge about advanced planning and were less willing to undergo life-sustaining treatments for new serious medical problems compared with those who had only completed the Health Care Proxy form (133). In addition, health care proxies designated by the patients were more likely to be accurate in their understanding of patients' end-of-life preferences.

Although interventions may increase the use of advanced-care planning, other studies have shown that these interventions do not appear to increase physician understanding of patient preferences or to affect other clinical outcomes. The Study to Understand Prognoses and Preferences for Outcomes and Risks of Treatment (SUPPORT) tested the impact of a nurse-administered advanced-care planning initiative in 4301 patients, with a median age of 65 years, admitted to teaching hospitals in the United States, who had a life-threatening diagnosis (134). The objectives of the first phase of this study were to discover shortcomings with communication practices, determine the frequency of aggressive treatment, and describe the characteristics of the hospital death. The second phase, with 4804 patients enrolled, was a randomized trial to test the effectiveness of a nurse-driven intervention that facilitated advanced-care planning. Findings from phase I showed that (i) physicians accurately knew their patients' preference to avoid cardiopulmonary resuscitation (CPR) only 47% of the time, (ii) 46% of the do-not-resuscitate orders were written within 48 hours before death, and (iii) close to 40% of patients with terminal illnesses spent at least 10 days in the intensive care unit. The nursing intervention in phase II did not improve targeted goals and areas compared with the control. These targeted areas included incidence and timing of the do-not-resuscitate order, physicians' knowledge of patients' resuscitation preferences, days spent in the intensive care unit, and reported pain levels.

The failure of clinical interventions to affect targeted clinical outcomes despite their efficacy in increasing the awareness and use of advance directives has led to discussion of the possible barriers in fully understanding patient preferences. Possible reasons for the failure of the nurse-directed intervention to improve end-of-life parameters in the SUPPORT study included that the end-of-life discussions had not been initiated at an earlier point of time, and that the leaders of the discussion were nurses unknown to the patient and not the patient's physician. Furthermore, while nurses in the study stated that they had communicated with the treating physicians in nearly all of the cases, physicians recalled receiving the information on patient preferences only 34% of the time (134). Other reasons for the interventions failing to affect the use of treatment or cost of medical care may include the possibility that these interventions do not promote meaningful communication between patients and physicians, or that other determinants of physicians' behavior such as beliefs about treatment efficacy, perceived standards of care, or prognostic uncertainty are more influential than patient preferences (120).

Despite uncertainty about the effectiveness of advance directives in directing end-of-life treatment, evidence suggests that patients in fact do want to talk about advanced-care planning with their doctors (135). Furthermore, these discussions should occur before the patient becomes acutely ill, and despite some discomfort with the topic, patients want their physicians to initiate discussions about advanced-care planning and end-of-life care (136). Advance directive discussions early during the elderly patient's illness can be empowering to patients and allow them to learn more about their disease and prognosis.

TREATMENT PREFERENCES

As discussed above, it is extremely important for both family and medical providers to understand patients' treatment preferences so that their wishes are maintained and respected at the end of life. For the elderly with advanced cancer, treatment preferences involve options for active treatment in addition to management of the dying process. Studies have shown a lower rate of referral to oncologists from general practitioners (137) in the elderly. In addition, analyses of treatment patterns of cancer patients have demonstrated that increasing age is associated with less aggressive treatment (138–143). Many factors are thought to contribute to this, including the presence of more comorbid conditions in the elderly, toxicities of treatment, and patient preferences (144).

For the elderly patient at the end of life, treatment preferences and decisions are strongly influenced by possible outcomes (118,145–147). Avoidance of pain, loss of cognition, loss of function (148), and maintaining dignity (149) are all important to the elderly patient. A series of interviews with elderly informants revealed that a range of personal and interpersonal outcomes, including cognitive and physical function, self-care, productivity, and emotional or caretaking burden on loved ones, influenced their attitudes toward resuscitation and ventilation (147). In this series, an open-ended, in-depth interview was conducted with 14 independently living elderly with at least one chronic health condition and seven informants with a greater level of functional impairment. Analysis of the interviews suggested that informants judged medical interventions as being more desirable if the patient would still be able to pursue valued life activities afterwards and maintain his or her functional status. Furthermore, informants felt that advanced age and the perception of having lived a "full life" made them less willing to tolerate pain and functional loss as trade-offs for possible increased longevity.

However, although older patients may be less willing to tolerate pain and functional loss, studies have shown that even for elderly patients with a limited life expectancy, treatments are sought unless the treatment will result in severe cognitive or physical dysfunction. This tendency was demonstrated in a questionnaire administered to 226 patients above the age of 60 years with a life expectancy of six months or less (148). Participants in the study were interviewed in their home and were asked about the burden their illness imposed, possible treatment outcomes, and the likelihood that the treatments would be successful. For a low-burden treatment that would restore current health, 98.7% of participants would choose that treatment. If the treatment was highly burdensome, but would guarantee survival, 89% of patients would accept the therapy. Interestingly, when the adverse outcome of the treatment was death, the number of subjects in the study who wanted treatment declined significantly only when the possibility of death reached 90% or higher. However, if the outcome of the treatment was survival but with it came severe functional impairment or cognitive impairment, 74.4% and 88.8%, respectively, would not choose the treatment. Preferences did not differ according to whether the primary diagnosis was cancer, chronic obstructive pulmonary disease, or congestive heart failure.

This desire to pursue treatments that offer hope for improved survival is also corroborated in other studies (150,151). A study of 106 newly diagnosed cancer patients with a median age of 60 years demonstrated that patients and oncologists had differing perspectives on whether they would accept medical treatment for small survival benefits (151). For a treatment which would extend life by three months and which was described as "intensive," 40% of the interviewed patients expressed that they would accept this treatment while only 6% of oncologists would agree to accept to provide the therapy. Similarly, another study of patient preferences in older and middle-aged patients with late-stage cancer found that a preference to extend life was related to the patient's estimate for survival, which in most cases, was significantly more optimistic than physician estimates (152). These studies point out the importance of explaining all the risks and realistic benefits of treatments to patients, especially to elderly patients with limited life spans, because there is evidence that many patients will choose minimally effective treatment. A patient's desire for restorative treatments may relate to a number of issues, including relieving their perceived burden on their family, a desire not to die, misunderstanding of their prognosis, and misunderstanding of the degree of the toxicities associated with therapy.

Some patients, family members, and hospital staff may have a more realistic expectation of the results of treatment. In an analysis of SUPPORT data of 9105 patients, all of whom had a serious medical problem or were ≥80 years of age, most patients and their family members, as opposed to findings from other studies (148,149), preferred a comfort care approach (153). This was especially true in the population above 80. Patient preferences for intensive treatment such as CPR can be influenced by providing the patient with outcome data; one study of nursing home residents found that although 60% of patients desired CPR at the end of life, this desire for intervention dropped by 14% after an education program that defined the risks of CPR (154). In a separate study of 287 outpatients over the age of 60, similar effects were observed; initially 41% of those responding opted for CPR in the setting of an acute illness, but this percentage dropped to 22% after learning the probability of survival. In the setting of an acute illness, only 6% of those patients over the age of 85 would prefer CPR (155).

In summary, an understanding of patients' treatment preferences remains critical to the provision of appropriate medical care. The evidence suggests that patient desires regarding medical intervention are heavily influenced by outcome and results as opposed to the actual mechanics of the intervention. In elderly patients, interviews and questionnaires suggest that a high value is placed on being able to perform valued life activities, and that severe cognitive or functional impairment would discourage patients from pursuing aggressive treatment. However, in comparison to practitioners, patients appear to be more willing to pursue aggressive treatments for small survival benefits. This may be due to misunderstanding of toxicities and benefits of treatment, and studies have shown that in the case of CPR, patient preference can be greatly reduced by provision of survival and outcome data. Thus, when discussing treatment and end-of-life preferences with the elderly cancer patient, it remains essential to achieve a good understanding of their individual goals and outcome preferences, as well as to provide full information regarding treatment toxicities and benefits.

DIGNITY

One concept that can influence patients' treatment and end-of-life preferences is the concept of dignity, and considerations of dignity are often raised in the discussion of end-of-life care (156,157). The notions of dignity, defined in the literature as an "inherent respect to be granted patients in preparation for death" (158) and death with dignity can have a pronounced influence on the treatment provided by health care providers at the end of life. Studies have shown that support for assisted suicide or euthanasia often centers around concerns about dignity (47,159–162). When asked why they agreed to the patient's requests for euthanasia or some form of self-assisted suicide, physicians often cited the loss of dignity as one of the leading reasons (160,161,163). Concerns about dignity are important to cancer patients; in one study of 213 patients with terminal disease, 46% of patients reported at least some or occasional loss of dignity, and 7.5% of patients indicated that this loss of dignity was a significant problem (164).

To better define the concept of dignity, studies have surveyed patients with terminal disease. Chochinov et al. conducted 60-minute interviews in 50 patients with advanced terminal cancer, focusing on what defined and maintained the patient's sense of dignity (158). Major themes that emerged as contributing heavily to the sense of dignity included illness-related concerns, as well as concerns regarding individuality, pride, and autonomy. When discussing illness-related concerns, patients expressed that things that would have a significant effect on their sense of dignity included the loss of independence or cognitive function due to effects of their disease. In addition, patients expressed that symptoms related to their disease, such as severe pain, would have a significantly negative effect on maintaining a sense of dignity. Similarly, patients felt strongly that the maintenance of a sense of self and of being able to perform simple tasks of living were important contributions to preserving dignity. When questioned about whether dignity was an intrinsic quality or whether it could be affected by others, most individuals in the outpatient setting supported the notion of dignity as an intrinsic quality, whereas a majority of patients in the hospital setting felt that dignity could be "taken away" by other individuals and expressed frustration at experiencing some of that loss (158).

The concept of dignity has been linked with the notion of the "the good death." Patient views on what constitutes a good death have not been extensively explored in the medical literature. In one study, which utilized descriptive interviews with 16 patients over the age of 65 with heart disease or cancer and a life expectancy of greater than six months, patient preferences and values regarding the end-of-life were found to be heterogeneous, although there were a few prevalent themes (165). In general, patients were more likely to associate good death as being without pain, in one's sleep, occurring quickly, free of suffering, and occurring without the knowledge of impending death. However, responses varied, and no theme was mentioned by more than half the participants. Similarly, characteristics that were associated with a "good death" in some patients were cited by other patients as features of a "bad death," and although many patients identified the support of their family as an important part of a good death, several individuals also expressed that they would not want their family present at the time of death itself.

In summary, the concepts of dignity and good death have influenced the treatment preferences of patients and the care provided by physicians. The notion of "death with dignity" has been a significant influence in movements regarding euthanasia and self-assisted suicide, and can inform patient decisions regarding end-of-life preferences. However, patient perceptions of the themes and principles that constitute dignity and define "good death" remain heterogeneous. An understanding of the patient's concept of dignity, including concerns such as symptoms and pain from disease, as well as loss of autonomy or self-awareness, must be carefully tailored through discussion with the individual patient. Similarly, discussions regarding treatment preferences at the end-of-life should also address the patient's perception of "the good death," as preferences and values surrounding this topic may vary greatly.

HOSPICE

Hospice care was developed in order to provide relief from pain and suffering and to help patients regain control of events at the end of life. Originally pioneered in Great Britain, hospice care was first introduced as a pilot project in the United States in 1979 and was firmly established in 1982 with the creation of the Medicare Hospice Benefit (166). The Medicare Hospice Benefit defines core services to be provided by any hospice program accepting Medicare patients. These services include nursing, social work, physicians, and counseling services, as well as the use of volunteers to aid in care. To be eligible for hospice care, the patient must be entitled to Medicare Part A and be certified as being terminally ill, with a prognosis of six months or less if the disease runs its normal course. Once they enter hospice care, patients receive no further active treatment for their cancer or noncancer life-threatening illness, with the emphasis of care shifting to palliative care, bereavement counseling for family members, and creating a peaceful and "good death" for the patient.

Table 6 Levels of Hospice Care

Routine care	Care provided in the patient's home; can be private residence or an intermediate or skilled-care facility
Respite care	Care in a 24-hr skilled nursing facility; provided for 5 days per benefit period, or when caretaker is absent or requires a few days rest
General inpatient care	Hospital level care
Continuous (crisis) care	High level care in the patient's home when hospital level care is not available or desired

Hospice care is initiated by the patient and the physician together. The patient's physician must certify the presence of a terminal illness with a prognosis of six months or less, and this must be cocertified by the hospice physician. The patient then signs an election statement agreeing to palliative care of the terminal illness and no resuscitation. The certification of terminal illness is valid for 90 days, after which a second 90-day period may be certified. If the patient continues to require hospice care beyond the initial six months, serial 60-day periods of certification can be provided. If the patient's prognosis appears to improve at any point during their hospice care, the hospice may discharge the patient. Similarly the patient is free to choose to be removed from hospice care at any time.

The Medicare Hospice Benefit provides for four levels of care (166–168), as outlined in Table 6. *Routine care* encompasses care provided in the patient's home. This may be a private residence or an intermediate or skilled-care facility. *Respite care* is available for five days per benefit period and allows the patient to be cared for in a facility with 24-hour, skilled nursing care. This level of care is designed for times when the caregiver will be absent or to provide a few days of rest for the caregiver. *General inpatient care* refers to hospital-level care and is required when the patient has symptoms that cannot be controlled at home as well as for deaths that cannot occur in the home. The final level of care is termed *continuous care* or *crisis care* and allows for high-level care to be provided in the patient's home, when general inpatient care is not available or desired.

Since the establishment of the Medicare Hospice Benefit, the number of hospices in the United States has risen to over 3000, and the number of patients receiving hospice care has increased from 25,000 to 775,000 in 2001. However, despite these increasing numbers, overall, very few patients are ever enrolled into hospice. It is estimated that only one out of four people who died in the United States in the year 2000 was enrolled into hospice (169). Moreover, 34% of those patients served by hospice in 2000 died within seven days of enrollment, and the median length of stay was 20.5 days. This suggests that many patients and health care providers are underutilizing this service.

Barriers to Hospice Care

Table 7 outlines some of the barriers to enrollment in hospice care in the terminally ill elderly patient. However, a full understanding of these issues remains unclear. McCarthy et al. (170) conducted a study of 120,000 patients over the age of 65 dying with lung and colorectal cancer. In this study group, 27% of patients with lung cancer and 20% of patients with colorectal cancer received hospice care before death.

Table 7 Barriers to Hospice for the Terminally Ill Elderly

Certain states in the United States
Male gender
Residence in a rural community
Having fee-for-service health insurance
Racial group besides white or African-American
Poor physician education about hospice
Physicians unwilling to deem a patient "terminally ill"
Poor patient education about hospice
Unrealistic expectations of treatment

Different referral patterns among states were apparent; Utah had the lowest hospice use, while New Mexico had the highest. Women with lung cancer used hospice services more than men did (30% vs. 20%), but in colorectal cancer patients, both genders were equally unlikely to use hospice services (20%). One fifth of patients enrolled in hospice one week before death and 50% enrolled within one month before death. Factors associated with delayed enrollment included male gender, residing in a rural community, having fee-for-service insurance, and being from a racial group other than white or black.

Several other studies have also found that fee-for-service insurance has been a barrier to enrollment in hospice care (171,172). These studies have demonstrated that patients with fee-for-service insurance have lower rates of hospice usage and shorter length of stays when compared with patients enrolled in managed care organizations. One potential explanation for this discrepancy may be the different financial incentive structures that exist in managed care and fee-for-service systems. Because the Medicare program assumes the costs of hospice care, managed care organizations are relieved of the end-of-life costs once the patient enrolls in hospice. For this reason, it is possible that managed-care programs have better systems to facilitate the transfer of the dying patient to hospice care with better end-of-life care.

Other investigators have researched influences on the decision to enroll in hospice care. Chen et al. conducted a series of interviews of 234 patients with advanced lung, breast, prostate, or colon cancer with a life expectancy of less than one year, 173 of whom had elected to enroll in hospice and 61 of whom were pursuing traditional hospital care. In this study, patients who elected hospice care were significantly older (average age 69 years vs. 65 years), less educated (on an average, one less year of schooling), and had a greater number of individuals living with them in their household. Patients choosing hospice also had more comorbidities and poorer functional status than their nonhospice counterparts. Analysis of the data found that patients who entered hospice care were more likely to agree to sacrifice length of life for quality of life (173). Another interesting finding of this study was the difference between hospice and nonhospice patients regarding their perceived disease course. Those patients choosing to pursue additional medical treatment were less realistic about their likely survival than those electing hospice, with more than one-third believing that there was a chance of cure or improvement.

Overall, hospice care remains an underutilized option in the care of the dying patient. Although hospice use has increased over the past decade, it is still estimated that only one-quarter of dying patients in the United States in 2000 were enrolled in hospice programs. Other potential barriers to enrollment into hospice programs include the physician's unwillingness to deem a patient "terminally ill" (which is a hospice requirement), causing them to appear to be "giving up" on the patient. Discussions have suggested that factors such as perception of hospice as "medical failure" (174), denial by patients' families and health care providers (175,176), and poor communication and education about hospice and what it entails (166,177,178) may all play a role. Continued education of patients, families, and providers regarding the benefits of hospice is necessary to increase both overall enrollment and earlier referral to maximize the benefit of this service.

LTC FACILITIES

With the aging of American society, LTC facilities have increasingly become a place for care and the site of death for older patients. Currently, it is estimated that approximately 20% of older people in the United States will die in LTC facilities, and approximately 40% of people who reach the age of 65 will spend at least some time in a LTC facility (179,180). One future projection is that by 2020, 40% of all Americans will die in a nursing home (181). The quality of care in LTC facilities has improved since the passage of the Nursing Home Reform Act in 1987. This act mandates that patients be assessed using a Resident Assessment Instrument, which includes a MDS and Resident Assessment Protocol; these are assessments required at the time of LTC admission, quarterly, and if a clinical change occurs. However, although there have been significant improvements in the quality of care at LTC facilities, many challenges still exist in caring for the patient at the end of life in this setting. For example, despite the extensive amount of palliative care provided at LTC facilities, advance directives, comfort, palliative care, bereavement issues, and imminent death are not covered in the MDS (182).

Inadequate response to family concerns during a loved one's terminal illness has sometimes been cited as a concern regarding care in the LTC setting. In a study that surveyed individuals whose family members had died in the LTC setting, Teno et al. found that one in four of the respondents felt that their loved one's dyspnea had not been adequately treated. One-quarter of the respondents also expressed concerns with lack of physician communication. In contrast to families of patients who had died at home with hospice care, family members of patients who had died in a LTC facility reported higher rates of unmet needs, insufficient emotional support, and dissatisfaction with care (183). Interviews conducted by Miller et al. with the next-of-kin of patients treated in LTC facilities near or at the end of life revealed additional concerns. Families expressed that they felt that the symptoms and needs of dying individuals were insufficiently recognized. In addition, low expectations from nursing homes and poor experiences led many family members to feel as if they needed to become vigilant advocates for their loved ones. Furthermore, physicians were perceived to be largely absent, and family members expressed a need for more and better-trained staff (184).

Similar to the non-LTC community, barriers exist in the LTC setting for enrollment in hospice services. It is estimated that approximately one-third of the 1.6 million current nursing home residents will die each year; however, only 1% of them are enrolled in hospice programs (185). Even so, in the years 1996 through 1999, approximately 45% of Medicare Hospice Benefit claims were for hospice care in the nursing home (186). One barrier to hospice referral was a paucity of collaborations between nursing homes and hospice providers; a study analyzed data from 1995 to 1997 and concluded that only 30% of U.S. nursing homes contracted with

Medicare hospices (187). However, collaboration has increased since that time, and in 2000, estimates show that approximately 76% of nursing homes have contracts with hospice providers (188).

Other barriers to hospice referral in LTC settings include administrative overview. LTC facilities are overseen by Title 19, which mandates improvements in functions of LTC facilities. Hospice programs are required to abide by Title 18 regulations. This difference in administrative overview has served to accentuate the care and philosophy differences between hospice and LTC facilities. Financial barriers also exist for hospice enrollment within LTC facilities. Because of the provisions of the Medicare Hospice Benefit, once the patient chooses to enter into a hospice program, only the costs associated with treatment of the terminal illness are reimbursed. Thus, not infrequently, when a patient in a LTC facility changes to a hospice benefit, the patient and/or the family becomes responsible for the room and board of the facility (182), a situation that can be a significant financial burden and a barrier to care.

Although barriers to hospice referral exist, once patients are referred to hospice care in the LTC setting, they do experience significant benefits. Studies have shown that hospice LTC residents experience fewer hospitalizations near the end of life, have fewer invasive treatments, and receive pain management that adheres more closely to the guidelines for management of chronic pain in LTC settings (189,190). Family members of patients who died in nursing homes while enrolled in hospice in LTR acknowledged improvements in care after hospice admission (191,192). Furthermore, some studies have suggested a "spillover" effect from the presence of hospice patients in LTC facilities, with nonhospice patients in facilities with a greater hospice presence also having a reduced number of hospitalizations, more frequent pain assessments, and increased frequency of analgesic administrations as compared to residents in facilities with a limited hospice presence (189).

Overall, terminally ill older patients in LTC facilities represent a large proportion of all dying elderly patients, and the percentage of individuals who will die in the nursing home setting is likely to increase as the U.S. population continues to age. Special attention must be paid to the diagnosis and management of pain in the LTC setting, as well as to management of other issues such as dyspnea. Families often are concerned that physicians are not easily accessible, and also express concerns regarding emotional support for both the dying patient and themselves. Management of these issues has been shown to be improved in patients who are entered in a hospice program; however, the percentage of LTC facility patients who are enrolled in hospice is very small. Barriers to hospice referral exist, and efforts must be made to better educate and train LTC facility staff, as well as patients and their families, in order to increase hospice referrals.

CONCLUSION

Elderly, terminally ill patients require a unique and specialized approach to end-of-life care. A multidisciplinary team should be assembled to care for these patients, given the multifaceted and complex care they require. Special attention to early recognition and intervention for pain and depression needs to occur. In addition, elderly patients are more vulnerable to toxicities of medications, and certain medications should be avoided. Patients and their physicians need to discuss realistic treatment options, if any, and discuss these treatments and end-of-life care in language that is realistic, compassionate, and easy to understand. Discussion of advance directives and end-of-life care should also focus more on what the patient goals and preferred outcomes are, instead of merely the mechanics of treatment. Many of the terminally ill elderly will be cared for in LTC facilities at the end of their lives, so patients and their families need to ascertain the availability of hospice and make decisions with their physician based on advance directives and health care proxy information early in the course of illness. Although the efficacy of advanced-care directives remains somewhat unclear, patients and families desire to discuss these issues with their doctors, and physicians should initiate and facilitate these discussions.

REFERENCES

1. Abrahm J. Advances in pain management for older adult patients. Clin Geriatr Med 2000; 16:269–289.
2. Vigano A, Bruera E, Suarez-Almazor M. Age, pain intensity, and opioid use in patients with advanced cancer. Cancer 1998; 83:1244–1250.
3. Barnabei R, Gambassi F, Lapane K, et al. Management of pain in elderly patients with cancer. JAMA 1998; 279(23):1877–1882.
4. Cleary J, Carbone P. Palliative medicine in the elderly. Cancer 1997; 80(7):1335–1347.
5. Ward S, Goldberg N, Miller-McCauley V, et al. Patient-related barriers to management of cancer pain. Pain 1993; 52:319–324.
6. Ferrell B. Pain evaluation and management in the nursing home. Ann Intern Med 1995; 123:681–687.
7. Ferrell B, Ferrell B, Osterweil D. Pain in the nursing home. J Am Geriatr Soc 1990; 38:409–414.
8. Parmelee P. Pain in the cognitively impaired older person. Clin Geriatr Med 1996; 12:473–487.
9. Sengstaken E, King S. The problems of pain and its detection among geriatric nursing home residents. J Am Geriatr Soc 1993; 41:541–544.
10. Cohen-Mansfield J. The adequacy of the minimum data set assessment of pain in cognitively impaired nursing home residents. J Pain Symptom Manage 2004; 27(4):343–351.
11. Parmelee P, Smith B, Katz I. Pain complaints and cognitive status among elderly institution residents. J Am Geriatr Soc 1993; 41:517–522.
12. Ferrell B, Ferrell B, Rivera L. Pain in cognitively impaired nursing home patients. J Pain Symptom Manage 1995; 10:591–598.
13. Wagner A, Goodwin M, Campbell B, et al. Pain prevalence and pain treatments for residents in Oregon nursing homes. Geriatr Nurs 1997; 18:268–272.
14. Won A, Lapane K, Gambassi G, et al. Correlates and management of nonmalignant pain in nursing home. SAGE Study Group. Systematic assessment of geriatric drug use via epidemiology. J Am Geriatr Soc 1999; 47:936–942.
15. Hawes C, Morris J, Phillips C, et al. Reliability estimates for the minimum data set for nursing home resident assessment and care screening (MDS). Gerontologist 1995; 35:172–178.
16. Wu N, Miller S, Lapane K, et al. The problem of assessment bias when measuring the hospice effect on nursing home residents' pain, care in nursing homes. J Pain Symptom Manage 2003; 26:998–1009.
17. A.C.P. Committee. Management of cancer pain in older patients. J Am Geriatr Soc 1997; 45:1273–1276.
18. Gloth F. Pain management in older adults: prevention and treatment. J Am Geriatr Soc 2001; 49:188–199.

19. McCaffery M, Wolff M. Pain relief using cutaneous modalities, positioning, and movement. Hospice J 1992; 8:121–153.

20. World Health Organization. Cancer Pain Relief: With a Guide to Opioid Availability. 2nd ed. Geneva: World Health Organization, 1996.

21. Gloth F. Concerns with chronic analgesic therapy in elderly patients. Am J Med 1996; 101(suppl 1A):19S–24S.

22. Bell G, Schnitzer T. Cox-2 inhibitors and other nonsteroidal anti-inflammatory drugs in the treatment of pain in the elderly. Clin Geriatr Med 2001; 17(3):489–502.

23. Ingham J, Foley K. Pain and the barriers to its relief at the end of life. A lesson for improving end of life health care. Hospice J 1998; 13:89–105.

24. Holdsworth M, Forman W, Nystrom K. Transdermal fentanyl disposition in elderly subjects. Gerontology 1994; 40:32–37.

25. Stein W. Cancer pain in the elderly. In: Ferrell B, ed. Pain in the Elderly. Seattle, WA: IASP Press, 1996:69–90.

26. Mercantonio E, Juarez G, Goldman L, et al. The relationship of post-operative delirium with psychoactive medications. JAMA 1994; 272:1518–1522.

27. Shorr R, Griffin M, Duaughterty J, et al. Opioid analgesics and risk of hip fracture in the elderly. J Gerontol Med Sci 1992; 47:M111–M115.

28. Gurwitz J, Field T, Harrold L, et al. Incidence and preventability of adverse drug events among older persons in the ambulatory setting. JAMA 2003; 289(9):1107–1116.

29. Portenoy R. Constipation in the cancer patient: causes and management. Med Clin North Am 1987; 71:303–311.

30. Ashby M, Martin P, Jackson K. Opioid substitution to reduce adverse effects in cancer pain management. Med J Aust 1999; 170:68–71.

31. Nadal J, Pederson J, Maddock W. A comparison between dehydration from salt loss and from water deprivation. J Clin Invest 1941; 20:691–713.

32. Regnard C, Mannix K. Reduced hydration or feeding in advanced disease. Palliat Med 1991; 5:161–164.

33. Viola R, Wells G, Peterson J. The effects of fluid status and fluid therapy on the dying: a systematic review. J Palliat Care 1997; 13:41–52.

34. McCann R, Hall W, Groth-Juncker A. Comfort care for terminally-ill patients: the appropriate use of nutrition and hydration. JAMA 1994; 272:1263–1266.

35. Musgrave C, Bartal N, Opstad J. The sensation of thirst in dying patients receiving IV hydration. J Palliat Care 1995; 11:17–21.

36. Ellershaw J, Sutcliffe J, Saunders C. Dehydration and the dying patient. J Pain Symptom Manage 1995; 10:192–197.

37. Billings J. Comfort measures for the terminally ill. Is dehydration painful? J Am Geriatr Soc 1985; 33:808–810.

38. Steffens D, Skoog I, Norton M, et al. Prevalence of depression and its treatment in an elderly population: the Cache County study. Arch Gen Psychiat 2000; 57:601–607.

39. Crawford M, Prince M, Menezes P, et al. The recognition and treatment of depression in older people in primary care. Int J Geriatr Pscyhiat 1998; 13:172–176.

40. Bukberg J, Penman D, Holland J. Depression in hospitalized cancer patients. Psychosom Med 1984; 46:199–212.

41. Lander M, Wilson K, Chochinov H. Depression and the dying older patient. Clin Geriatr Med 2000; 16:335–356.

42. Goldberg R, Mor V. A survey of psychotropic use in terminal cancer patients. Psychosomatics 1985; 26:745–751.

43. Blazer D, Kessler R, McGonagle K, et al. The prevalence and distribution of major depression in a national community sample: The National Comorbidity Survey. Am J Psychiat 1994; 151:979–986.

44. Ganzini L, Lee M, Heintz R, et al. The effect of depression treatment on elderly patients' preferences for life-sustaining medical therapy [comment]. Am J Psychiat 1994; 151:1631–1636.

45. Chochinov H, Wilson K, Enns M, et al. Depression, hopelessness, and suicidal ideation in the terminally ill. Psychosomatics 1998; 39:366–370.

46. Christakis N. Timing of referral of terminally ill patients to an outpatient hospice. J Gen Intern Med 1994; 9:314–320.

47. Emmanuel E, Fairclough D, Danels E, et al. Euthanasia and physician-assisted suicide: attitudes and experience of oncology patients, oncologists, and the public. Lancet 1996; 347:1805–1810.

48. Greenberg D. Barriers to the treatment of depression in cancer patients. J Natl Cancer Inst Monographs 2004(32):127–135.

49. Rao A, Cohen H. Symptom management in the elderly cancer patient: fatigue, pain, and depression. J Natl Cancer Inst Monographs 2004(32):150–157.

50. Maguire P. Improving the detection of psychiatric problems in cancer patients. Soc Sci Med 1985; 20:819–823.

51. Valente S, Saunders J, Cohen M. Evaluating depression among patients with cancer. Cancer Pract 1994; 2:65–71.

52. Trask P. Assessment of depression in cancer patients. J Natl Cancer Inst Monographs 2004(32):80–92.

53. Endicott J. Measurement of depression in patients with cancer. Cancer 1984; 53:2243–2249.

54. Lynch M. The assessment and prevalence of affective disorders in advanced cancer. J Palliat Care 1995; 11:10–18.

55. Ferrell B, Ferrell B. The older patient. In: Holland J, ed. Psychooncology. New York, NY: Oxford University Press, 1998:839–844.

56. Endicott J, Spitzer R. A diagnostic interview: the schedule for affective disorders and schizophrenia. Arch Gen Psychiat 1978; 35:837–844.

57. Spitzer R, Williams J, Gibbons M, et al. Structured Clinical Interview for DSM-III-R (SCID). User's Guide for the Structured Clinical Interview for DSM-III-R. Washington, DC: American Psychiatric Press, 1990.

58. Massie M, Popkin M. Depressive disorders. In: Holland J, ed. Psychooncology. New York, NY: Oxford University Press, 1998:518–540.

59. Robins L, Helzer J, Croughan J, et al. National Institute of Mental Health Diagnostic Interview Schedule: its history, characteristics, and validity. Arch Gen Psychiat 1981; 38:381–389.

60. Alexander P, Dinesh N, Vidyasagar M. Psychiatric morbidity among cancer patients and its relationship with awareness of illness and expectations about treatment outcome. Acta Oncol 1993; 32:623–626.

61. Berard R, Boermeester F, Viljoen G. Depressive disorders in an out-patient oncology setting: prevalence, assessment, and management. Psychooncology 1998; 7:112–120.

62. Ciaramella A, Poli P. Assessment of depression among cancer patients: the role of pain, cancer type and treatment. Psychooncology 2001; 10:156–165.

63. Zigmond A, Snaith R. The hospital anxiety and depression scale. Acta Psychiat Scand 1983; 67:361–370.

64. DeHaes J, Van Knippenberg F, Nejit J. Measuring psychological and physical distress in cancer patients: structure and application of the Rotterdam Symptom Checklist. Br J Cancer 1990; 62:1034.

65. Beck A, Beck R. Screening depressed patients in family practice: a rapid technique. Postgrad Med 1972; 52:595–605.

66. Beck A, Ward C, Mendelson M, et al. An inventory for measuring depression. Arch Gen Psychiat 1961; 4:561–571.

67. Boulet J, Boss M. Reliability and validity of the Brief Symptoms Inventory. Psychol Assess 1991; 3:433–437.

68. Derogatis L. The Brief Symptoms Inventory (BSI) Administration, Scoring and Procedures Manual-II. Baltimore, MD: Clinical Psychometric Research, 1992.

69. Derogatis L, Melisaratos N. The Brief Symptom Inventory: an introductory report. Psychol Med 1983; 13:595–605.

70. Radloff L. The CES-D scale: a self-report depression scale for research in the general population. Appl Psychol Measure 1977; 1:385–401.

71. Zung W. Depression in the normal aged. Psychosomatics 1967; 8:287–292.

72. Zung W. Factors influencing the self-rating depression scale. Arch Gen Psychiat 1967; 16:543–547.

73. Yesavage J, Brink T, Rose T, et al. Development and validation of a geriatric depression screening scale: a preliminary report. J Psychiat Res 1982–1983; 17:37–49.

74. Weissman M, Bland R, Canino G, et al. Cross-national epidemiology of major depression and bipolar disorder. JAMA 1996; 276:293–299.

75. Plumb M, Holland J. Comparative studies of psychological function in patients with advanced cancer. II. Interviewer-rated. Psychosomatics 1981; 43:243–254.

76. Williamson G, Schultz R. Activity restriction mediates the association between pain and depressed affect. A study of younger and older cancer patients. Psychol Aging 1995; 10:369–378.

77. Glover J, Dibble S, Dodd M, et al. Mood states of oncology outpatients: does pain make a difference? J Pain Symptom Manage 1995; 10:120–128.

78. Barsevick A, Sweeney C, Haeny E, et al. A systematic qualitative analysis of psychoeducational interventions for depression in patients with cancer. Oncol Nurs Forum 2002; 29:73–84.

79. Fawzy F, Fawzy N, Arndt L, et al. Critical review of psychosocial interventions in cancer care. Arch Gen Psychiat 1995; 52:100–113.

80. Rosholm J, Bjerrum L, Hallas J, et al. Polypharmacy and the risk for drug-drug interactions among Danish elderly. Dan Med Bull 1998; 45:210–213.

81. De Vane C, Pollock B. Pharmacokinetic considerations of antidepressant use in the elderly. J Clin Psychiat 1999; 60(suppl 20):38–44.

82. McDonald W, Salzman C, Schatzberg A. Depression in the elderly. Psychopharmacol Bull 2002; 36(suppl 2):112–122.

83. Rehman H, Masson E. Neuroendocrinology of ageing. Age Ageing 2001; 30:279–287.

84. Reynolds C, Farank E, Kupfer D, et al. Treatment outcome in recurrent major depression: a post hoc comparison of elderly ("young old") and midlife patients. Am J Psychiat 1996; 153:1288–1292.

85. Rabheru K. Special issues in the management of depression in older patients. Can J Psychiat 2004; 49(3 suppl 1):41S–50S.

86. Cassano G, Puca F, Scapicchio P, et al. Paroxetine and fluoxetine effects on mood and cognitive functions in depressed nondemented elderly patients. J Clin Psychiat 2002; 63:396–402.

87. Newhouse P, Krishnan K, Doraiswamy P, et al. A double-blind comparison of sertraline and fluoxetine in depressed elderly outpatients. J Clin Psychiat 2000; 61:559–568.

88. Mahapatra S, Hackett D. A randomised, double-blind, parallel-group comparison of venlafaxine and dothiepin in geriatric patients with major depression. Int J Clin Pract 1997; 51:209–213.

89. Hoyberg O, Maragakis B, Mullin J, et al. A double-blind multicentre comparison of mirtazapine and amitriptyline in elderly depressed patients. Acta Psychiat Scand 1996; 93:184–190.

90. Gloth F. Geriatric pain. Factors that limit pain relief and increase complications. Geriatrics 2000; 55:46–48, 51–54.

91. Katona C, Livingston G. Safety and efficacy of antidepressants in older people. Abstract number S.09.05. J Eur Coll Neuropsychopharmacol 2002; 12(suppl 3):S108.

92. Bondareff W, Alpert M, Friedhoff A, et al. Comparison of sertraline and nortriptyline in the treatment of major depressive disorder in late life. Am J Psychiat 2000; 157:729–736.

93. Gasto C, Navarro V, Marcos T, et al. Single-blind comparison of venlafaxine and nortriptyline in elderly major depression. J Clin Psychopharmacol 2003; 23:21–26.

94. Navarro V, Gasto C, Torres X, et al. Citalopram versus nortriptyline in late-life depression: a 12-week randomized single-blind study. Acta Psychiat Scand 2001; 157:729–736.

95. Schatzberg A, Kremer C, Rodrigues H, et al. Double-blind, randomized comparison of mirtazapine and paroxetine in elderly depressed patients. Am J Geriatr Psychiatry 2002; 10:541–550.

96. Flint A. Choosing appropriate antidepressant therapy in the elderly. A risk-benefit assessment of available agents. Drugs Aging 1998; 13:269–280.

97. Reynolds C. Depression: making the diagnosis and using SSRIs in the older patient. Geriatrics 1996; 51:28–34.

98. Baumann P. Care of depression in the elderly: comparative pharmacokinetics of SSRIs. Int Clin Psychopharmacol 1998; 13(suppl 5):S35–S43.

99. Muijsers R, Polosker G, Noble S. Sertraline: a review of its use in the management of major depressive disorder in elderly patients. Drugs Aging 2002; 19:377–392.

100. Beers M. Explicit criteria for determining potentially inappropriate medication use by the elderly. Arch Intern Med 1997; 157:1531–1536.

101. Harris E, Barraclough B. Suicide as an outcome for medical disorders. Medicine (Baltimore) 1994; 73:281–296.

102. Bolund C. Suicide and cancer: medical and care factors in suicides by cancer patients in Sweden 1973–1976. J Psychosocial Oncol 1985; 3:31–52.

103. Linda G, Demi A, Camann M, et al. The health status of elderly persons in the last year of life: a comparison of deaths by suicide, injury, and natural causes. Am J Public Health 1997; 87(3):434–437.

104. Akechi T, Okuyama T, Sugawara Y, et al. Suicidality in terminally ill Japanese patients with cancer. Cancer 2004; 100(1):183–191.

105. Akechi T, Okamura H, Nishiwaki Y, et al. Predictive factors for suicidal ideation in patients with unresectable lung carcinoma: a 6-month follow-up study. Cancer 2002; 85:1085–1093.

106. Breitbart W, Rosenfeld B, Pessin H, et al. Depression, hopelessness, and desire for hastened death in terminally ill patients with cancer. JAMA 2000; 284(22):2907–2911.

107. Chochinov H, Wilson K, Enns M, et al. Desire for death in the terminally ill. Am J Psychiat 1995; 152:1185–1191.

108. Kelly B, Burnett P, Pelusi D, et al. Terminally ill cancer patients' wish to hasten death. Palliat Med 2002; 16:339–345.

109. Wilson K, Scott J, Graham I, et al. Attitudes of terminally ill patients toward euthanasia and physician-assisted suicide. Arch Intern Med 2000; 160:2454–2460.

110. Pessin H, Rosenfeld B, Burton L, et al. The role of cognitive impairment in desire for hastened death: a study of patients with advanced AIDS. Gen Hosp Psychiat 2003; 25:194–199.

111. Rosenfeld B, Krivo S, Breitbard W, et al. Suicide, assisted suicide, and euthanasia in the terminally ill. In: Breitbart W, ed. Handbook of Psychiatry in Palliative Medicine. New York, NY: Oxford University Press, 2000:51–62.

112. Rosenfeld B, Breitbart W, Galietta M, et al. The Schedule of Attitudes Toward Hastened Death: measuring desire for death in terminally ill cancer patients. Cancer 2000; 88:2868–2875.

113. Rosenfeld B, Breitbart W, Stein K, et al. Measuring desire for death among patients with HIV/AIDS: the Schedule of Attitudes Toward Hastened Death. Am J Psychiat 1999; 156:94–100.

114. McClain C, Rosenfeld B, Breitbart W. Effect of spiritual well-being on end-of-life despair in terminally-ill cancer patients. Lancet 2003; 361:1603–1607.

115. Kugaya A, Akechi T, Nakano T, et al. Successful antidepressant treatment for five terminally ill cancer patients with major depression, suicidal ideation and a desire for death. Support Care Cancer 1999; 7(6):432–436.

116. Matulonis U. End of life issues in older patients. Semin Oncol 2004; 31(2):274–281.

117. Fischer G, Arnold R, Tulsky J. Talking to the older adult about advance directives. Clin Geriatr 2000; 16:239–254.
118. Doukas D, McCullough L. The values history: the evaluation of the patient's values and advance directives. J Fam Pract 1991; 32:145–153.
119. Weeks W, Kofoed L, Wallace A, et al. Advance directives and the cost of terminal hospitalization. Arch Intern Med 1994; 154:2077–2083.
120. Hanson L, Tulsky J, Danis M. Can clinical interventions change care at the end of life? Ann Intern Med 1997; 126:381–388.
121. Fischer G, Tulsky J, Rose M, et al. Patient knowledge and physician predictions of treatment preferences after discussion of advance directives. J Gen Intern Med 1998; 13:447–454.
122. Teno J, Lynn J, Wenger N, et al. Advance directives for seriously ill hospitalized patients: effectiveness with the patient self-determination act and the SUPPORT intervention. J Am Geriatr Soc 1997; 45:500–507.
123. Brett A. Limitations of listing specific medical interventions in advance directives. JAMA 1991; 266:825–828.
124. Tulsky J, Fischer G, Rose M, et al. Opening the black box: how do physicians communicate about advance directives. Ann Intern Med 1998; 129:441–449.
125. Tulsky J, Chesney M, Lo B. How do medical residents discuss resuscitation with patients? J Gen Intern Med 1995; 10:436–442.
126. Layson R, Adelman H, Wallach P, et al. Discussions about the use of life-sustaining treatments: a literature review of physicians' and patients' attitudes and practices. End of Life Study Group. J Clin Ethics 1994; 5:195–203.
127. Miller D, Coe R, Hyers TM. Achieving consensus on withdrawing or withholding care for critically ill patients. J Gen Intern Med 1992; 7:475–480.
128. Sullivan K, Hebert P, Logan J, et al. What do physicians tell patients with end-stage COPD about intubation and mechanical ventilation? Chest 1996; 109:258–264.
129. Frankl D, Oye R, Bellamy P. Attitudes of hospitalized patients toward life support: a study of 200 medical inpatients. Am J Med 1989; 86:645–648.
130. Pfeifer M, Sidorov J, Smith A, et al. The discussion of end-of-life medical care by primary care patients and physicians: a multicenter study using structured qualitative interviews. J Gen Intern Med 1994; 9:82–88.
131. Detsky A, Stricker S, Mulley A, et al. Prognosis, survival, and the expenditure of hospital resources for patients in an intensive-care unit. N Engl J Med 1981; 305:667–672.
132. Bradley E, Peiris V, Wetle T. Discussions about end of life care in nursing homes. J Am Geriatr Soc 1998; 46:1235–1241.
133. Schwartz C, Wheeler B, Hammes B, et al. Early intervention in planning end-of-life care with ambulatory geriatric patients. Arch Intern Med 2002; 162:1611–1618.
134. T.S.P. Investigators. A controlled trial to improve care for seriously ill hospitalized patients. The study to understand prognoses and preferences for outcomes and risks of treatments (SUPPORT). JAMA 1995; 274(20):1591–1598.
135. Edinger W, Smucker D. Outpatients' attitudes regarding advance directives. J Fam Pract 1992; 35:650–653.
136. Smerling R, Bedell S, Lilienfeld A. Discussing cardiopulmonary resuscitation: a study of elderly outpatients. J Gen Intern Med 1998; 3:317–321.
137. Townsley C, Naidoo K, Pond G, et al. Are older cancer patients being referred to oncologists? A mail questionnaire of Ontario primary care practitioners to evaluate their referral patterns. J Clin Oncol 2003; 21(24):4627–4635.
138. Goodwin J. Factors affecting the diagnosis and treatment of older persons with cancer. In: Ershler W, ed. Comprehensive Geriatric Oncology. London: Harwood, 1998:115–121.
139. Potosky A, Saxman S, Wallace R, et al. Population variations in the initial treatment of non-small-cell lung cancer. J Clin Oncol 2004; 22(16):3261–3268.
140. Ramsey S, Howlader N, Etzioni R, et al. Chemotherapy use, outcomes, and costs for older persons with advanced non-small-cell lung cancer: evidence from surveillance, epidemiology and end results—Medicare. J Clin Oncol 2004; 22(24):4971–4978.

141. Samet J, Junt W, Key C, et al. Choices of cancer therapy varies with age of patient. JAMA 1986; 255:3385–3390.

142. Turner N, Haward R, Mulley G, et al. Cancer in old age—is it inadequately investigated and treated? BMJ 1999; 319:309–312.

143. Wright J, Gibb R, Geevarghese S, et al. Cervical carcinoma in the elderly: an analysis of patterns of care and outcome. Cancer 2005; 103(1):85–91.

144. Chen H, Cantor A, Meyer J, et al. Can older cancer patients tolerate chemotherapy? A prospective pilot study. Cancer 2003; 97(4):1107–1114.

145. Patrick D, Pearlman R, Starks H, et al. Validation of preferences for life-sustaining treatment: implications for advance care planning. Ann Intern Med 1997; 127:509–517.

146. Pearlman R, Cain K, Patrick D, et al. Insights pertaining to patient assessments of states worse than death. J Clin Ethics 1993; 4:33–41.

147. Rosenfeld K, Wenger N, Kagawa-Singer M. End-of-life decision making: a qualitative study of elderly individuals. J Gen Intern Med 2000; 15:620–625.

148. Fried T, Bradley E, Towle V, et al. Understanding the treatment preferences of seriously ill patients. N Engl J Med 2002; 346:1061–1066.

149. Chochinov H, Hack T, Hassard T, et al. Dignity in the terminally ill: a cross-sectional, cohort study. Lancet 2002; 360:2026–2030.

150. Danis M, Patrick D, Southerland L, et al. Patients' and families' preferences for medical intensive care. JAMA 1988; 260:797–802.

151. Slevin M, Stubbs L, Plant H, et al. Attitudes to chemotherapy: comparing views of patient with cancer with those of doctors, nurses, and general public. BMJ 1990; 300:1458–1460.

152. Rose J, O'Toole E, Dawson N, et al. Perspectives, preferences, care practices, and outcomes among older and middle-aged patients with late-stage cancer. J Clin Oncol 2004; 22(24):4907–4917.

153. Lynn J, Teno J, Phillips R, et al. Perceptions by family members of the dying experience of older and seriously ill patients. Ann Intern Med 1997; 126:97–106.

154. O'Brien L, Grisso J, Maislin G, et al. Nursing home residents' preferences for life-sustaining treatments. JAMA 1995; 274:1775–1779.

155. Murphy D, Burrows D, Santilli S, et al. The influence of the probability of survival on patients' preferences regarding cardiopulmonary resuscitation. N Engl J Med 1994; 330:545–549.

156. C.o.S. Affairs. Good care of the dying patient. JAMA 1996; 275:474–478.

157. Pannuti F, Tanneberger S. Dying with dignity: illusion, hope or human right? World Health Forum 1993; 14:172–173.

158. Chochinov H, Hack T, McClement S, et al. Dignity in the terminally ill: a developing empirical model. Soc Sci Med 2002; 54.

159. Back A, Wallace J, Starks H, et al. Physician-assisted suicide and euthanasia in Washington state: patient requests and physician responses. JAMA 1996; 275:919–925.

160. Ganzini L, Johnston W, Hoffman W. Correlates of suffering in amyotrophic lateral sclerosis. Neurology 1999; 52:1434–1440.

161. Meier D, Emmons C, Wallenstein S, et al. A national survey of physician-assisted suicide and euthanasia in the United States. N Engl J Med 1998; 338:1193–1201.

162. Sullivan A, Hedberg K, Fleming D. Legalized physician-assisted suicide in Oregon—the second year. N Engl J Med 2000; 342:598–604.

163. Van der Maas P, Van Delden J, Pijnenborg L, et al. Euthanasia and other medical decisions concerning the end of life. Lancet 1991; 338:669–674.

164. Hack T, Chochinov H, Hassard T, et al. Defining dignity in terminally ill cancer patients: a factor-analytic approach. Psychooncology 2004; 13(10):700–708.

165. Vig E, Davenport N, Pearlman R. Good deaths, bad deaths, and preferences for the end of life: a qualitative study of geriatric outpatients. J Am Geriatr Soc 2002; 50:1541–1548.

166. Medicare program. Hospice care—HCFA, final rule, 1983:56008–56036.

167. Smits H, Ryndes T, Demel B, et al. The Medicare Hospice Benefit. New York: Institute for Medicare Practice, 2002.
168. Herbst L. Hospice care at the end of life. Clin Geriatr Med 2004; 20:753–765.
169. T.N.H.a.P.C. Organization. Facts and figures on hospice care in American [On-line].
170. McCarthy E, Burns R, Davids R, et al. Barriers to hospice care among older patients dying with lung and colorectal cancer. J Clin Oncol 2003; 21:728–735.
171. McCarthy E, Burns R, Ngo-Metgher Q, et al. Hospice use among Medicare managed care and fee-for-service patients dying with cancer. JAMA 2003; 289:2238–2245.
172. Vernig B, Persily N, Morgan R, et al. Do Medicare HMO's and Medicare FFS differ in their use of the Medicare hospice benefit? Hospice J 1999; 14:1–12.
173. Chen H, Haley W, Robinson B, et al. Decisions for hospice care in patients with advanced cancer. J Am Geriatr Soc 2003; 51(6):789–797.
174. Rhymes J. Hospice care in America. JAMA 1990; 264:369–372.
175. Berry D, Boughton L, McNamee F. Patient and physician characteristics affecting the choice of home based hospice, acute care inpatient hospice facility, or hospitals as last site of care for patients with cancer of the lung. Hospice J 1994; 9:21–38.
176. Weggel J. Barriers to the physician decision to offer hospice as an option for terminal care. WMJ 1999; 98:49–53.
177. Siegler E, Levin B. Physician-older patient communication at the end of life. Clin Geriatr Med 2000; 16:175–204.
178. Slomka J. The negotiation of death: clinical decision making at the end of life. Soc Sci Med 1992; 35:251–259.
179. Hanson L, Henderson M. Care of the dying in long-term care settings. Clin Geriatr Med 2000; 16:225–237.
180. Kemper P, Murtaugh C. Lifetime use of nursing home care. N Engl J Med 1995; 324:595–600.
181. Brock D, Foley D. Demography and epidemiology of dying in the US with emphasis on deaths of older persons. Hospice J 1998; 13:49–60.
182. Keay T, Schonwetter R. The case for hospice care in long-term care environments. Clin Geriatr Med 2000; 16:211–223.
183. Teno J, Clarridge B, Casey V, et al. Family perspectives on end-of-life care at the last place of care. JAMA 2004; 291(1):88–93.
184. Miller S, Teno J, Mor V. Hospice and palliative care in nursing homes. Clin Geriatr Med 2004; 20:717–734.
185. Patrisek A, Mor V. Hospice in nursing homes: a facility level analysis of the distribution of hospice beneficiaries. Gerontologist 1999; 39:279–290.
186. Campbell D, Lynn J, Louis T, et al. Medicare program expenditures associated with hospice use. Ann Intern Med 2004; 140(4):269–277.
187. Petrisek A, Mor V. Hospice in nursing homes: a facility level analysis of the distribution of hospice beneficiaries. Gerontologist 1999; 39:279–290.
188. Gage B, Dao T. Medicare's hospice benefit: use and expenditures 1996 cohort. In: Synthesis and Analysis of Medicare's Hospice Benefit. Washington, DC: US Department of Health and Human Services, Assistant Secretary for Planning and Evaluation, Office of Disability, Aging and Long-Term Care Policy, 2000.
189. Miller S, Gozalo P, Mor V. Hospice enrollment and hospitalization of dying nursing home patients. Am J Med 2001; 111:38–44.
190. Miller S, Mor V, Teno J. Hospice enrollment and pain assessment and management in nursing homes. J Pain Symptom Manage 2003; 26:791–799.
191. Baer W, Hanson L. Families' perception of the added value of hospice in the nursing home. J Am Geriatr Soc 2000; 48:879–882.
192. Wetle T, Teno J, Shield R, et al. End of Life in Nursing Homes: Experiences and Policy Recommendations. Washington, DC: AARP Public Policy Institute, 2004.
193. Hem E, Loge JH, Edeburg O. Suicide risk in cancer patients from 1960–1999. J Clin Onc 2004; 22:4209–4216.

27

Family Support for the Older Cancer Patient

Barbara A. Given
College of Nursing, Michigan State University, East Lansing, Michigan, U.S.A.

Paula R. Sherwood
School of Nursing, University of Pittsburgh, Pittsburgh, Pennsylvania, U.S.A.

Charles W. Given
Department of Family Practice, College of Human Medicine,
Michigan State University, East Lansing, Michigan, U.S.A.

INTRODUCTION

As the population ages, the number of older adults with cancer continues to grow. In the United States, 60% of all malignancies occur in persons aged 65 to 95 (1,2) and the median age of diagnosis is 68 years (3). Higher mortality rates from cancer have been reported in older adults; death rates from cancer for people older than 75 may be two times higher than for those aged 65 to 74. In addition, changes in the older patient's physical, emotional, socio-economic, and cognitive function (4–7) may complicate cancer treatment, making disease and symptom management for older adults more challenging.

Due to cost concerns within the health care system, there has been a shift in oncology services from the hospital to the outpatient ambulatory and home setting (8,9). More responsibility now lies with family members to provide care in the home. Family care, as described in this chapter, goes beyond usual family activities such as cooking or household chores that are a required part of normal daily life, and involves therapeutic health care activities aimed at alleviating distress caused by cancer or cancer treatment. Family caregivers of older patients, typically spouses who are older themselves, are often responsible for maintaining comfort in spite of symptoms, managing equipment, coordinating medical treatments, and reporting changes in the patient's condition to health care providers, all while facing uncertainty about the patient's future and their own.

Family members must often deal with the physical, social, and financial dimensions of providing care while simultaneously trying to cope with their own emotional responses to the patient's diagnosis. When older spouses are the caregivers, the dyad of care recipient and caregiver is typically based on 40 years or more of shared living experience. The impact of cancer and cancer treatment can alter family functioning, social roles, and communication patterns, the impact of which may continue across the treatment trajectory (10). In turn, the distress that a family caregiver undergoes may affect the health of the patient. For example, during advanced stages of illness when aggressive chemotherapy is part of the treatment regimen, changes in family roles may create multiple time demands for the caregiver (11,12). Unless family members have the time and skills to become actively involved in the patient's therapeutic plan, patient care and comfort may be in jeopardy.

In addition to the effect of caregiver distress on the quality of care delivered to the patient, providing care to an older patient with cancer can also affect the caregiver's physical and emotional health. Providing care for a family member with cancer can result in positive consequences such as a better relationship with the patient and feeling honored to provide care (13–15). However, negative consequences are also cited as a result of providing care, particularly when caregivers feel unprepared to deliver care and receive little guidance from health care providers (16–18). Family caregivers may be unfamiliar with the type or amount of care needed, may not have adequate information to make decisions or solve problems, and may not know how to access and utilize needed community resources. Caregivers may also lack the time to provide care (particularly when care demands are heavy), the ability to prioritize care demands, and the skills to navigate the health care system. Finally, lack of communication between members of the health care team, the dyad's financial status, and the ever increasing distance of secondary caregivers to help provide support, are all obstacles to caring for an older person with cancer. All of these challenges to providing care, such as being unprepared and underinformed to provide care, increases both the time required to perform care tasks and the distress that may accompany care provision. Caregivers who are distressed, then, may be more apt to neglect their own needs, which can result in emotional burnout and declining physical health (19–21).

Although the cancer care system has recently recognized the importance of a family approach to cancer care, there are few documented guidelines for providing support to family members caring for older patients with cancer. Because family members are now expected to actively participate in helping older cancer patients achieve treatment goals and manage side effects, health care providers must become adept at developing family plans of care (rather than a single patient plan-of-care) and providing assistance to family members to deliver care in the home (22). The quality of care provided by family members will have a significant effect on outcomes for the older patient. Health care professionals must continually integrate family members into the patient's treatment plan-of-care, assisting them in managing patients' symptoms, prioritizing patients' problems, and collaborating with the health care system.

It is against this backdrop that we describe the challenges that face family caregivers of older persons with cancer and identify potential avenues of caregiver support. We begin by describing family caregivers' needs for support and care needs of the older patient with cancer that can increase the complexity of care or caregivers' distress. Then, strategies to provide support aimed at alleviating distress and enabling caregivers to provide high quality care are presented.

FAMILY CAREGIVER SUPPORT

Providing support to the family caregiver encompasses assisting them to gain the necessary knowledge and skills to perform care tasks, information to monitor symptoms and make care decisions, and the resources to meet care demands. Caregivers must provide support in a multitude of areas, as their role in patient care has shifted from one of custodial care and general support to a far more direct and complex care role. Family care includes overall coordination of treatment regimens, symptom monitoring and management, recognizing complications early, accessing community services, managing comorbid conditions, and participating in the decision-making processes. In addition, care related to the use of technical equipment such as infusion pumps, taking time to provide transportation to the patient's treatment, assuring nutritional support, and dealing with the disability that may occur with older age or numerous comorbidities are all components of the family care.

The focus of cancer care is not on the disease, age, and treatment alone, but concerns the interplay between how the disease and treatment affect the older patient and how these care demands affect caregivers' health and well-being. Planning and direction from health care providers can assist family members to more appropriately assume the caregiver role and respond to patient care demands. Provider support should attend to how a family caregiver can respond to psychosocial needs and promote the physical and emotional well-being of the patient without detriment to their own health. The ultimate goals and plan-of-care for the older patient with cancer should help family members to collaborate with health care providers during cancer diagnosis and survivorship.

To provide the necessary support to the dyad, a partnership must be developed (optimally, an interdisciplinary oncology health care team) between the family members and the patient in order to generate a plan-of-care. Supportive care should focus on strategies to assist with patient care while meeting the caregiver's own psychological, social, and spiritual needs (23,24). By engaging and eliciting the support of family members, health care providers can improve the quality of patient assessment, diagnosis of patient problems, implementation of treatment strategies, and evaluation of patient care, ultimately leading to improved overall care. We start the discussion on family support of older persons with cancer by focusing on patient-related needs and care demands.

CARE NEEDS OF THE OLDER PATIENT WITH CANCER

Patients' needs during cancer care are influenced by factors such as age, number and severity of comorbid conditions, preexisting functional status, previous cancer diagnoses and treatment, psychological disposition, and cultural traditions. A multidimensional comprehensive geriatric assessment (CGA) that includes family resources is strongly recommended for the care of the older person with cancer (Table 1) (25,26). Tailoring plans of care to the older cancer patient with attention to each of these areas (several of which are detailed in the following sections), and then monitoring how family members implement plans of care is essential. In addition, the capacity of the family member to care for the patient should be evaluated as a part of the CGA (27).

Physiological age-related changes, comorbid conditions, and the incidence of polypharmacy contribute to the challenges for older patients with cancer and their families. Due to the growing body of literature that suggest that chemotherapy can be safe and effective in older patients (28), it is anticipated that in the future, more family members will be providing care for older patients undergoing complex and potentially aggressive treatment. However, age-related physiologic changes such

Table 1 Areas of Assessments and Related Instruments for the Older Patient with Cancer

Domain	Instrument
Health	Number of comorbid conditions, comorbidity indices such as: Charlson, Cumulative Illness Rating Scale—Geriatrics
Pharmacy	Drug list and interaction
Cognition	Folstein, Mini-Mental Status, DRS
Function	Performance status, IADL, ADL
Emotions	Geriatric Depression Scale
Social	Living conditions, marital adjustment, caregiver adequacy, caregiver stress, income, transportation
Nutrition	Mini-Nutritional assessment

Abbreviations: ADL, activities of daily living; DRS, dementia rating scale; IADL, instrumental activities of daily living.

as alterations in the gastrointestinal and renal systems, body composition, and fluid and electrolyte balance can impact the patient's ability to tolerate chemotherapy (29). Hence, older adults may have varied responses and side effects from treatment, making "typical" symptom management techniques less effective. Health care providers may need to work more closely with caregivers to manage complications of treatment because caregivers of older adults may be particularly challenged in trying to lessen the severity of side effects as well as the impact of side effects on the patient's usual roles.

Age-related changes in the patient's health may also lead to the presence of multiple comorbid conditions (such as diabetes or cardiovascular disease), which deplete the body's reserves to control side effects, making the older patient more susceptible to treatment-related complications. In turn, treatment of multiple comorbid conditions often requires multiple medications, placing older patients with cancer at increased risk for developing drug interactions. Reduced or enhanced drug absorption metabolism may lead to increased toxicities, dose reductions, or altered distribution of the chemotherapeutic agent (30,31). Due to altered pharmacokinetics and pharmocodynamics of antineoplastic drugs, radiation, or biological therapeutics, the older cancer patient may have reduced tolerance to drugs, resulting in treatment complications (25). Side effects more common in older cancer patients are described in Table 2.

Table 2 Side Effects from Cancer Treatment Seen in Older Individuals

Myelodepression
  Neutropenia
  Thrombocytopenia
  Anemia
Mucositis
Cardiopulmonary problems
Depression
Peripheral neuropathy
Central neurotoxicity
  Cognitive decline
  Delirium
  Cerebellar dysfunction

Each of these poses care demands for the patient and their family members. Family members need information and assistance regarding patients' physical care: information as to which symptoms need to be monitored, what interventions should be used, how to address emotional responses, and what community resources might be of assistance. The needs for information will vary across the cancer-care trajectory (32). It may not be the amount or the complexity of care delivered, but the "change" in care demands and the associated adjustments in the demands of care that contribute to caregiver distress and signal the need for patient and family support from the health care provider (33,34). The amount and type of required care change as the number and nature of symptoms change, and as patients' functional status improves, deteriorates, or changes in status. Stage of cancer, response to therapy, and phase of treatment are important transition points and add to the complexity of care. The demands of care are also influenced by the frequency with which tasks have to be completed, i.e., hourly versus one-time per day; the predictability of the task, for example, cooking versus dealing with diarrhea or vomiting, which is more unpredictable; and the nature of the skill and judgment required for the task (35,36). Some of the care demands that family members face when caring for older patients with cancer will be described.

Care demands can be classified as either direct or indirect. Direct care includes tasks that are carried out directly with patients, such as symptom management, medication administration, wound care, and assistance with physical functioning. Indirect care include tasks that are carried out "on behalf" of the patient, such as providing supervision, obtaining medications, transporting the patient, communicating with providers, scheduling and coordinating appointments and services, and assisting with the medical bills and finances. Counseling and supporting the patient are also considered types of indirect care. Health care providers tend to recognize the need for support in the direct care activities, but are less apt to recognize that the caregiver needs support with indirect activities such as helping to identify and obtain secondary support for care. As the plan-of-care is completed for the patient, the indirect care demands should be considered.

Symptom Management

Cancer patients can experience multiple and severe symptoms as the result of cancer or cancer treatment, which includes pain, nausea, fatigue, shortness of breath, anorexia, and increased functional dependence (Table 3). Family members attempt to

Table 3 Common Symptoms Experienced by the Older Cancer Patient from Treatment

Pain	Alopecia
Nausea	Peripheral neuropathy
Vomiting	Cognitive changes
Diarrhea	Mucositis
Insomnia	Anxiety
Constipation	Depression
Fatigue	Dizziness
Anorexia	Infection
Shortness of breath	Weakness
Dry mouth	

provide symptom management but report being bothered by the presence of some symptoms more than others. Fatigue, anorexia, depression (37), and pain (38,39) are particularly problematic for caregivers (40,41). Patients' psychological symptoms such as anxiety and depression may also complicate care tasks for the caregiver, who is experiencing his/her own emotions and reactions (33,42,43).

A major role for family members involves monitoring and assisting with symptom management, which is often due to complex cancer treatments and can be exacerbated by changes from aging and comorbid conditions (44,45). Fatigue, for example, increases the risk of functional dependence in older patients with cancer (46), and the mucosa of older individuals is more vulnerable to cytoxic chemotherapy than that of younger persons, leading to an increased risk of mucositis, which in turn affects appetite and comfort. Cytotoxic chemotherapy with drugs such as anthracyclines have demonstrated an increased risk of nephrotoxicity in older patients, which then poses a problem for the patient and caregiver (25,47,48). Increased symptom severity may occur in the cancer patients with comorbid conditions, because approximately 80% of persons over 65 have been diagnosed with at least one chronic condition (49). An increase in the number and/or severity of symptoms often accompanies cycles of treatment or progressive disease, and can affect both the patient's emotional and physical functioning, creating more care demands for the caregiver (42,50–52). Caregivers need support and information to meet these care demands and to provide symptom management. Pain, results of myelosuppression, such as neutropenia, fever and fatigue, and neurologic changes that can result in coordination and cognitive changes can be challenging to the caregiver of an older person with cancer.

Pain

Pain management is a pervasive and distressing problem for family members and requires pharmacologic and nonpharmacologic interventions (38,42,53). Pharmacology-specific interventions include choosing the appropriate medication and dosing frequency, monitoring for side effects, supervision of medication, administering and keeping a pain diary, and monitoring pain relief. Knowing when and how to report side effects or ineffective dosing is a critical measure among older cancer patients (53). Nonpharmacologic activities related to pain management may include distraction, emotional support, positioning, or heat or cold therapy. The challenges of administering narcotics, managing infusion pumps, and making decisions about the dosage and effectiveness of medicines can produce anxiety and distress among family members. Families report that they would like more assistance from the formal system to understand how best to provide care to their family members. The use of complementary therapy may add another complexity. Health care providers play an integral role in supporting the caregiver to ensure acceptable pain relief.

Myelosuppression

Myelosuppression may occur more frequently, with greater severity, and with varied clinical presentations in older patients with cancer (54). Older adults may not present with the usual signs of infection such as an elevated temperature, but may initially present with delirium. Severe anemia (hemoglobin levels lower than 8 g/dL associated with myelosuppression) has been associated with dyspnea, headache, fatigue, dizziness, decreased cognition, sleep disturbances, and weakness with debilitation and increased dependence (46,55). These secondary symptoms can further exacerbate the older patient's physical functioning. Family members need to understand the role of myelosuppression because it may influence other side effects from cancer treatment, and clearly affect and alter the care demands (22). Recent supportive care drugs are used to manage myelosuppression, which adds to the scheduling and coordination for the dyad.

Neurologic Dysfunction

Older patients with cancer have an increased risk for changes in neurologic status during treatment due to factors such as preexisting neurologic disorders (e.g., dementia and stroke), drug interactions, comorbidities or other side effects, dehydration, and infection. Neurotoxicity from drugs such as vincristine can result in cerebellar dysfunction and peripheral neuropathy (56), and sequelae such as cognitive deterioration. Dizziness and delirium may result from polypharmacy or anemia (57,58). Neurologic symptoms can place older patients at risk for physical injury such as those caused by falling.

The presence of neuropsychiatric and cognitive symptoms such as agitation, dysphoria, confusion, irritability, delusions, depression, inappropriate behavior, violence, and apathy (59,60) are particularly difficult to deal with for family members. Managing neurologic sequelae produces higher family distress and burden than assisting with impaired physical functioning alone (61). Caregivers report that "other" family members are less likely to assist with care demands when the patient has cognitive or neuropsychiatric dysfunction (62–64), which can isolate the patient and caregiver, decreasing social support. Neurologic changes often involve changes in the patient's personality, and caregivers may report that they feel as if they are providing care for a stranger, rather than a family member (63). Neurologic dysfunction may affect care demands by influencing the patient's ability to perform activities of daily living (ADL), thereby increasing the time demands and distress of the caregiver and limiting the caregiver's social network if inappropriate behavior or change in the care recipient's personality occurs (63).

Caregivers of persons with neurologic dysfunction need support with managing neurologic symptoms and coping with their own emotional reactions. Caregivers should to be taught how to recognize and monitor changes in neurologic status, be aware of potential causes for changes in behavior, and integrate strategies for decreasing the severity and impact of neuropsychiatric symptoms. Organizing secondary caregivers to provide respite by watching the patient may be helpful. Pharmacologic strategies such as the use of antipsychotics may also be beneficial in reducing the severity of the care recipient's neuropsychiatric symptoms and in enabling problem management. A dual approach—pharmacologic therapy to affect the care recipient's symptom severity and education/counseling to help the caregiver cope—may offer effective management. Caregivers need to be educated regarding possible triggers for abnormal patient behaviors, environmental modification, and ways to prioritize and divide tasks for patient care. Stress management relaxation techniques for coping with negative emotions may be needed (65,66).

As the previous sections have highlighted, symptom management can be a major struggle for older patients with cancer and their caregivers, one that becomes an even greater concern as the disease progresses and treatments become less effective (20,45,64). In order to support family members in symptom management, health care providers must first assess family members' ability to recognize the symptoms that are problematic and then provide information so that caregivers are able to manage these symptoms effectively or seek assistance from the health care system.

When symptoms are severe or when current symptom-control measures are ineffective, it is critical that family members intervene promptly so that dosages do not have to be reduced or delayed, and treatment goals can be achieved.

Physical Function

Diagnostic procedures and treatment (including surgery, chemotherapy, and/or radiation) may serve to further compromise patients' functional status, which can exacerbate preexisting comorbid conditions. In fact, all of the symptoms and side effects described in the previous sections (e.g., comorbid conditions, symptom severity, and myelosuppression) can accelerate functional decline. Alterations in physical function, then, will dictate the ability to perform ADL, which in turn predicts care demands (42,67). Severity of functional impairment (e.g., ADL and personal care) increases care demands and the need for the family's involvement in care (13,62,68). At the initial phase of treatment, few cancer patients report dependencies in ADL and instrumental ADL; but over time, with long-term treatment regimens or progressive disease, dependencies may occur. Family members often compensate for patients' loss of energy and endurance from pain, fatigue, and other symptoms that compromise and restrict functional and social activities (69). Caregivers should be encouraged to facilitate patient's return to normal physical function and encourage the patients to maintain physical function.

Guidelines of the National Comprehensive Cancer Network recommend using the Vulnerable Elders Survey-13 (VES-13) to see if patients are at risk for negative outcomes from limitations in physical functioning. The VES-13 assesses limitations in physical function and functional disabilities by evaluating patients' level of difficulty with walking, lifting, doing housework, and shopping. Patients who demonstrate high levels of physical disability and immobility will need assistance from family caregivers. Family caregivers, then, need assistance in implementing interventions to assist patients to either return to usual function or prevent deterioration. However, most caregivers of older persons are older spouses, who may not be physically able to provide assistance with heavy tasks (36,64).

Caregiver demands change as patients' treatment plans shift. For example, patients' physical function changes as their disease abates, as well as when the disease progresses (70). Even after patient symptoms and functional abilities improve, family members report that they continue to provide assistance and are "on call" (10,13). When care demands lessen, transition back to previous roles may be difficult. Furthermore, older spouse caregivers center their life activities around care—adjusting their schedules and relinquishing valued personal activities to provide care (42,71). Health care providers must continue to provide support at key transition points during treatment and as patients and their family members recover and return to their customary roles.

In addition to the patient's care demands, characteristics of the family caregivers, such as their age, gender, living arrangements, income, and relationship to the patient may influence the amount and support caregivers carry for older adults with cancer (42).

CAREGIVER-RELATED ISSUES

Gender

Overall, caregiving is reported to be more stressful for women (wives and daughters) than for men (husbands and sons) (10,13,72,73). Men may take on the caregiving role with little or no normative pressure and perform fewer personal care and household chores—overall a more narrow range of care tasks (27). Women, however, may feel a stronger obligation to assume the caregiver role, and experience distress as a result of not only the caregiving requirements, but also the pressures to assume the caregiver role as well.

Age

Age has also been related to caregiver distress (8,13,74). Younger caregivers who may be adult children of older cancer patients have more negative reactions than older spouse caregivers. This is due to the greater commitment of spouses and to the competing roles that affect caregivers' ability to meet care demands. Older family caregivers, though, may have other problems such as decreased physical capacity from their own comorbid health conditions and physical decline (75,76). These conditions are likely to add to the complexity of family/caregiver needs for information, support, and assistance as deterioration in either the emotional or physical health can limit the resources that family members call upon to meet patient-care demands. In addition, older caregivers, particularly spouse caregivers, tend to be more isolated in the caregiver role, becoming enmeshed in the care situation through a strong sense of role obligation (13,27).

Prior Relationships

Family care of the older patient must be placed within the context of prior family relationships; relationships during cancer care often reflect the way families usually function. For example, patterns of decision-making are often established previous to the illness, which can make it easier for older spouses (77) to become involved in care and decision-making. Adult children and their parents may have conflicts over care decisions, especially if siblings become involved. The quality of marital relationships moderates the association between functional impairment, interference in spousal relationships, spousal negativity, and negative behaviors (78). Caregivers with more satisfaction in marital relationships may report less distress from providing care, while discordance among family members may cause aggravation of the distress and affect decision-making related to the care process (20,43).

Socioeconomic Status

Low personal and household incomes, loss of income from taking time away from work to provide care, and other limits in financial resources can make providing care more challenging, particularly if substantial out-of-pocket costs are incurred (13,79–82). Cancer treatment for older adults has been associated with high out-of-pocket expenses for prescription medication and home care services (83), and patients may be forced to choose between the high costs for treatments such as symptom management medications and going without. Langa et al. (83) found that low-income older adults with cancer spent nearly 27% of their yearly income on out-of-pocket expenses for health care compared to 5% of the yearly income expended by older adults with high incomes and no cancer. Caregivers with low socioeconomic status may deplete their resources more quickly, causing them to feel threatened in their capacity to provide care (74,84,85). Caregivers with lower incomes may also display higher role captivity, increasing the difficulty in providing care. Together, the competing stress of care demands and other life stressors may be overwhelming (27). Higher incomes allow patients and caregivers to purchase care resources. Health care providers should consider the socioeconomic status to identify those older families that are most in need of financial assistance.

In the previous sections, we have described factors that influence care needs of the older person with cancer as well as examined caregiver characteristics that influence the ease with which care is delivered. When patients have multiple care demands, or when caregivers lack the necessary resources to meet those demands, negative reactions to providing care may ensue. In the next section, we examine potential reactions of family members to the tasks of caregiving and identify the support that they may need from health care professionals.

CAREGIVER REACTIONS TO PROVIDING CARE

Family caregivers often experience emotional distress such as depression, anxiety, helplessness, fear, psychosomatic symptoms, restriction of activities, role strain, and strain in marital relationships (10,43,73,86). The multiple dimensions of distress that may occur as a result of providing care are referred to as caregiver burden. Caregiver burden is an emotional reaction that occurs when the demands of care outweigh the caregivers' social, psychological, or physical resources to meet those demands (87,88). Family members who are unable to use resources or effective coping strategies to meet care demands may feel burdened, which, in turn, may lead to depression (63). Disruption of daily activities and competing demands such as work and physical care demands have been shown to contribute to caregiver burden (36,79,89–91). Regardless of the amount of care provided, when caregivers are unable to participate in their valued activities and interest, they became more distressed (42,90).

Depression may also develop in family caregivers and is considered to be a secondary or long-term mood disturbance that may develop as a consequence of sustained burden (92–94). The rate of use of mental health services by caregivers was reported by to be twice that of noncaregivers. Spousal caregivers appear to be at a higher risk for distress because they live with the patient and typically provide more extensive and comprehensive care, maintain their role longer, and tolerate greater levels of patient disability (42,74,77). Screening for caregiver burden and depression should be assessed at regular intervals, particularly in conjunction with changes in the patient's condition, so that appropriate counseling or respite care can be implemented.

Caregivers may also have changes in their physical health as a result of providing care. Declines in physical health and premature death in caregivers who perceive themselves as burdened have been reported (21,42,70,87,95), and caregivers have also been found to be at risk for fatigue, sleep disturbances, and altered immune functioning (90,96,97). Providing care can interfere with having time for exercise and may increase the need to take prescription medication for depression and sleep. Caregivers who are distressed tend to report a decrease in overall health, increased health risk behaviors (such as smoking), and higher use of prescription drugs (98,99).

In summary, we have highlighted patient needs and caregiver characteristics that can increase the risk of negative emotional and physical consequences from providing care. The ability of family caregivers to use family, personal, and social resources such as communication skills, and their mastery in meeting care demands will influence the caregiver's risk for distress. As part of the initial CGA, family, personal, and social resources need to be determined, so that supports can be provided to the older patient and their family members.

FAMILY, PERSONAL, AND SOCIAL RESOURCES

Family Communication

Health care providers are better able to integrate family members into the plan-of-care when families have a history of open communication and working with and supporting each other in crisis situations. Families with poor patterns of communication are less able to identify and obtain assistance from a group of friends and family members who can provide emotional and physical support to the older patient and themselves.

"Conspiracies of silence" about cancer and fear of outcomes among family members (especially spouses) may impede coping (100). Family members may be hesitant to communicate with each other because they want to avoid causing distress, remain "positive" about the diagnosis and treatment, and because of the difficult nature of cancer issues, particularly in late-stage disease (101,102). Open communication can help families to identify, prioritize, obtain assistance, and assign care tasks, which can decrease the stress of providing care by maximizing available resources (103).

In transferring care responsibilities to families, health care providers need to consider the family's pre- and post-diagnosis communication patterns and family functioning. It is important to note that methods of communication and avoidance, as well as established roles within the family, develop over decades and may not be easily changed. Interventions, then, may be directed toward assisting families with poor communication patterns to find needed resources. Interventions for families with poor communication patterns may involve teaching basic communication skills or teaching patients and caregivers to identify alternative resources for support.

Family Dynamics

Family communication patterns, roles, and coping methods are components of family dynamics. Similar to communication patterns, family dynamics are typically established well in advance of the patient's diagnosis and will determine a crucial source of patient and caregiver support. Families who have a history of dysfunctional relationships may not only be a lack of support to the patient with cancer, but also may actually hinder the patient's trajectory through the cancer treatment. A dysfunctional family can require more time from the health care team to deal with issues and as a result decrease the time that could be spent formulating and implementing the patient's plan-of-care (104). Health care provider interventions will not be able to alter preexisting family dynamics during the cancer treatment phase, but they have to deal with the conflict to minimize the interference with cancer care. For the older cancer patient, this might involve conflicts between and among the spouse and adult children. Interventions may need to focus on understanding the source of conflict and identify ways to decrease the way in which family conflict will affect the patient's ability to participate in cancer therapeutic plans.

Optimism and Mastery

The way in which caregivers perceive life in general has been associated with their response to the cancer-care situation. Caregivers with higher levels of optimism tend to have better overall emotional health when faced with care demands than those with lower levels of optimism (20,87,105). Caregivers with greater feelings of reward and optimism have also reported less overload, role captivity, and loss of intimate exchange than those with lower levels of optimism (27). In fact, optimism has been shown to be one of the variables that predicts whether caregiver depression will improve after the care situation ends (106). Optimism, used as a screening tool, may help to specify which family members will be less susceptible to the negative emotional effects of providing care. Optimism is an important trait to assess when targeting caregivers at risk for distress (107).

The caregiver's sense of mastery plays a role in caregivers' susceptibility to distress that may result from providing care. Caregivers with higher levels of mastery feel more in control of the care situation and feel that they are meeting the challenges of providing care, which can result in lower levels of emotional distress (27) and more positive responses to providing care (108–110), because they have available coping strategies to meet care demands (14,111,112).

Characteristics such as mastery and optimism are typically viewed as enduring dispositional characteristics, which function as personal resources for the caregiver. Support interventions may not be able to improve levels of mastery and optimism over time, but screening caregivers at the inception of the care situation can help target those caregivers who are more likely to experience distress as a result of providing care (14,27). Caregivers bring different sets of resources and coping strategies to the care situation, and interventions to improve the health of caregivers must be individualized to their characteristics.

Social and Family Support

Social support plays a role in alleviating caregiver distress and results in more positive adjustments to care demands (14,72,73,113,114). As care demands increase, the need for support from others in the caregiver's social networks may increase. Caregivers who perceive that social support is available and accessible may use it to maintain needed levels of care and feel less oppressed (14). A lack of perceived support may increase caregiver's sense of distress. For example, caregivers who report low social support may be at greater risk for caregiver burden, which can lead to depression (27,115).

The previous sections highlight the care needs of older patients with cancer and discuss how caregiver distress may result from trying to meet those needs. The final section addresses interventions to support and assist family caregivers in an effort to facilitate their capacity and ability to provide care to older patients with cancer, while minimizing their own distress.

INTERVENTIONS TO SUPPORT FAMILY CAREGIVERS

To support family members and facilitate patients' quality of care, health care providers need to implement interventions that address both the patient's and the caregiver's needs. A CGA such as the one detailed in Table 1 should be completed—one that goes beyond identifying patient disability and care needs to include family components and evaluates the availability and adaptability of secondary caregivers in supporting the primary family caregiver. The social section of the CGA should assess housing conditions, marital adjustment, caregiver adequacy, caregiver distress, income, and transportation. The family member designated as caregiver is key to the successful cancer management plan for the older patient with cancer.

Health care providers should use the information from the CGA to design a plan-of-care and then implement interventions focused on symptom management, assistance with physical functioning, mobilizing formal and informal resources, and strategies to maintain the caregivers' own physical and emotional health, while acquiring the necessary information and skills to provide patient care. Health care providers must recognize that families possess different levels of knowledge and skill, different levels of burden, and different levels of care demands during the cancer-care trajectory. Further, caregivers differ in the amount of support and assistance they receive from other family members. As a result, the amount of support they need from the health care system must be tailored to the interventions along each of these elements (105).

Families require a variety of knowledge, skills, and judgment to carry out tasks of care. Providers need to assist families to enhance role acquisition and feelings of preparedness as they assume complex care responsibilities (17). Each form of direct or indirect involvement demands different skills, knowledge, organizational capacities, role demands, and social and psychological strengths (18,71). Supportive interventions to be discussed include strategies for improving communication with the health care system, educational and informational interventions, psychotherapeutic interventions to manage caregiver distress and enhance coping skills, and strategies to assist caregivers to mobilize personal and community resources on behalf of the patient for whom they are caring.

Communication

Patients and family members bring established patterns of communication to the diagnosis and treatment of cancer. Understanding communication patterns between the patient and his/her family members is an important step toward supporting the family who is providing care. Patients with cancer have emphasized the importance of including family members in physician–patient conferences and physicians, in turn, have reported that family members often significantly affect how treatment decisions will be selected (104).

Caregivers and other family members may not be included in or encouraged to attend physician–patient conferences and, when they are present, their perspectives and questions may not be acknowledged or addressed. When older caregivers are included in conferences, they may be overwhelmed by the care situation and unable to communicate their needs. Older caregivers may not have prepared their questions or may be unaware of what questions should be asked and are afraid to speak up. Family members may not request that health providers address their own educational information or psychological needs. Caregivers need to be guided in how to communicate with the health care system and how to obtain the information they need to care. In turn, health care providers must assist caregivers to formulate questions about the patient's plan-of-care, while ensuring that they understand care and treatment expectations.

Open communication should be encouraged and some caregivers may need to be given permission to ask questions freely. Health care providers can help caregivers communicate effectively by suggesting the use of daily records of symptoms and changes in the patient's condition (e.g., diaries and logs) so that caregivers can accurately describe problems and are aware of who and when to call when problems arise. Tailored written material should be provided when problems arise, but selected carefully to prevent caregivers from feeling overwhelmed. Simple logs may be welcome. Finally, caregivers need clear details regarding the varying roles of members of their oncology care team, including the role of the primary care physician, so that they are aware of who will be responsible for answering questions about treatment.

Educational and Informational Interventions

Specific information is essential if family caregivers are to "participate" effectively in the care of older patients with cancer. Families report doing much of their care by trial and error with a sense of uncertainty that exacerbates their distress. Information that is tailored to the problems of the older patient and to the learning needs of the caregiver not only helps the caregiver implement appropriate interventions, but also concurrently reduces the distress that arises from feelings of inadequacy and helplessness. Family members need information on how to prepare for medical visits, how to seek and reconcile different medical opinions, and how to best support the patient. Specific actions and guides that caregivers can follow can reduce the uncertainty about care.

Primary care providers and oncologists should collaborate to design a coherent plan-of-care, particularly as the older patient with cancer often has multiple care providers due to comorbidities. Structured and ongoing education and information about treatment goals should be an integral part of the plan-of-care. Acquiring information regarding disease- and treatment-related expectations from health care providers can help caregivers plan care, anticipate possible problems, and detect changes in the trajectory of the illness. In addition, early signs of complications may be identified through the use of "help" sheets or "guides" (e.g., web references, toolkits, guidebooks, CD-ROM, DVD, etc.). Providing specific guidelines with detailed suggestions for care gives caregivers a sense of control. Simple guides or tool kits that have proven helpful to patients contain standardized sections on various symptoms. Each section should contain definitions, information on how patients identify and describe the symptom or problem, possible causes, tips and strategies to help manage the symptom or problem, suggestions for communicating about the symptom or problem with health care professionals and how to enlist their help with symptom management or problems resolution, and what specifically should be reported to the physician or nurse. Giving caregivers and patients specific ranges for symptoms, such as "report a temperature higher than 101.5°F to the health care provider," provides clear direction. Without this direction, family members may not know if they should report a fever of 99.8°F or only 102°F and what other signs to look for.

While books, videos, and mass-produced materials are useful, family members want "patient-specific and tailored" information based on the patient's care situation from their health care team. Although patients and caregivers can show a long-term improvement in retaining and integrating knowledge about treatment and symptom management (116,117), caregivers do not want to be overwhelmed with massive amounts of nonspecific information that is not pertinent to their situation. Health care providers must tailor information to address individual expectations regarding patients' symptoms, treatment, and disease trajectory; and what patients and caregivers can expect.

Providing information and education supports caregivers to feel more in control of the care situation. Family members describe how a sense of competency, mastery, and preparedness as well as a sense of control and confidence in care roles imparts feelings of satisfaction, reduces uncertainty, enhances coping, and provides for a sense of meaning associated with delivering care (71,118,119). Finally, clinicians need to provide information regarding the changes and transitions that are likely to occur in the care situation, and anticipate the problems and needs of family caregivers during these transitions.

Problem-Solving Programs

Problem-solving programs are another type of intervention that have proven useful for caregivers and are a way of both meeting care demands and alleviating distress. Steps in the problem-solving process begin with problem definition and formulation, followed by generating alternative solutions, decision-making, and implementing strategies that provide caregivers with specific guidance. Houts et al. (120) designed a program of caregiver support—the Prepared Family Caregiver model (summarized by the acronym COPE: Creativity, Optimism, Planning, and Expert Information)—which helps uninformed family caregivers. Increasing caregiver competence requires training family caregivers in the skills they need to provide care including information about care tasks and problem solving. The goals of the COPE model are to maximize caregivers' effectiveness and self-efficacy. Information empowers family members, and a problem-solving approach can help reduce feelings of distress and burden, promoting positive patient and caregiver outcomes (71).

Support/Counseling and Cognitive Behavioral Interventions

Families may need interventions designed to help them manage their own emotional reactions such as depression, anxiety, and anger (121), and support/counseling and cognitive behavioral interventions (CBIs) can be particularly effective. Support interventions for family caregivers should be designed to enhance morale, self-esteem, coping, and sense of control while caring for an older adult with cancer. The use of telephone counseling has been reported to assist family caregivers in coping with demands of care and reducing burden by increasing their confidence in care management, identifying resources and support, and assisting them in problem solving (24,74,122,123). The family member involved with care should be assessed for psychological-emotional distress (such as screening for depression and burden), and specific sources of distress should be identified. In addition, assessment of the quality of the family relationship and communication patterns is necessary if interventions are to be effective. If warranted, a referral should be made to outside resources, such as a counselor or psychologist, who has experience in counseling caregivers and/or older adults.

CBIs have also shown promise in improving symptom management and reducing caregiver distress. CBIs operate based on the beliefs that a person's behavior and ability to manage a situation is influenced by their perceptions; so distress and symptom management in patients with cancer and their caregivers can be improved by changing their perceptions (124). Given et al. [(Given B, Given C, Sherwood P, et al. The impact of providing symptom management assistance on caregiver negative reaction: results of a randomized trial. Psychol Aging 2004 (127)] designed a CBI to assist patients and their caregivers in symptom management, physical function, and emotional reactions to the cancer diagnosis and treatment. A nurse with specialized experience in oncology assessed the severity and impact of common symptoms in patients who were undergoing chemotherapy. Once severe or troubling symptoms are identified, the team (nurse, patient, and caregiver) worked together to generate, implement, and evaluate strategies aimed at decreasing symptom severity or impact. Interventions targeted toward the patient and caregiver in this way have shown promise in decreasing symptom severity and caregiver distress (127). The impact of providing symptom management assistance on caregiver negative reaction: results of a randomized trial.

Mobilizing Community Resources and Support Services

Another way to assist caregivers is by identifying support groups and resources to help provide care and respite. Much of the day-to-day care of the older person with cancer rests in the hands of family caregivers, when they are less able to care for themselves. Therapeutic interventions that enhance caregivers' capacity to manage their own reactions to caring can have benefits for both caregivers and patients. Family conferences, particularly for spouse caregivers with adult children, may be a useful strategy to help older family caregivers examine and address the current and expected future demands of care.

The feasibility of maintaining the individual with cancer in the home is largely dependent upon the availability, capacity, and willingness of the family member to provide patient care. The questions in Table 4 can be helpful in determining whether providing care in the home will be feasible. If care demands exceed the caregiver's capacity to provide care, health care providers must help families acquire coping skills and needed formal care resources. In extreme cases, long-term care may be needed when family resources cannot be made available.

It may be more feasible for older caregivers to provide care in the home if outside resources are in place to assist with care demands. Although community services may be able to provide assistance with patient care, arranging these resources adds to the complexity of coordinating the patient's care. In addition, family caregivers, especially an elderly spouse, may be reluctant to seek or accept assistance even when they are unable to adequately meet care demands by themselves. Family members must also interact and negotiate with the formal care system to schedule appointments, report changes in the patient's condition, request alterations in medications, or ask for assistance. Unfortunately, few caregivers receive assistance on how, when, and why to communicate with the health care team, which may prevent health care providers from knowing how to provide support to them. Gatekeepers

Table 4 Determining Feasibility or Ability of Family to Provide Home Care

What resources are needed?
What resources are available?
Is care by the family adequate?
What patient risk factors predispose the care situation to have negative consequences?
When is the family member at risk for financial, emotional, social, or physical problems?
When are resources, information, and formal support needed? Are they available?
Is the family able to provide the care?

and electronic answering systems in the health care system also make access to information and coordination of care challenging for family members. Using new technology such as interactive voice responses or symptom-monitoring technology might facilitate family dyad communication with the system. Teaching communication skills to caregivers at the onset of the care situation can help caregivers feel better equipped to provide care.

Older caregivers may feel they need "permission" from family members and health care providers to use resources. Caregivers may require guidance on how different types of supportive community care services can assist them and which services are most appropriate and useful to their particular situation. Changes in treatment protocols as well as changes in the patient's condition such as disease progression, recurrence, advanced disease, or end of life, necessitate adjustments in care demands. Likewise, caregivers are often confronted with deterioration and dependency over time with their own aging and disease. As patients become more dependent on the caregiver for assistance and supervision as their disease progresses, caregivers may be more likely to need, and perhaps accept, formal assistance. Family members must be able to adapt to changes in the amount, level, and intensity of care demands and changes in the nature of tasks. Even if at earlier points in the care trajectory family members did not accept or need assistance, this option needs to be evaluated and recommendations made to caregivers as the illness/care progresses (36). Brazil et al. (125) found that caregivers of persons over 50 years of age valued resources such as in-home nursing care, housekeeping, respite, and social workers. Data from the study also suggested that younger caregivers of older persons with cancer perceived greater needs for resources than did the older caregivers.

Interventions that help families mobilize resources are important, such as chore services, transportation, or asking for help from other family members. In addition, older caregivers may need to overcome perceived and real barriers to using and accepting assistance, such as lack of referral, lack of acceptability, lack of knowledge, or lack of awareness of their potential benefit to care (126). Health care providers should help caregivers mobilize the support they need as changes and care demands increase.

Ideally, for older cancer patients and their families, a case manager within the oncology care system would be responsible for helping the older family caregiver to utilize community resources for managing their patient's care. A geriatric nurse practitioner or case manager could facilitate communication and care by a multi-disciplinary oncology care team. In this case, the caregiver and patient would have one person on whom to rely for information and evaluation. A complete caregiver/care recipient evaluation could be done at the onset of the care situation. Potential resources could be identified, as well as areas in which the caregiver felt less comfortable performing care tasks. As the care situation continued, the case manager would be responsible for reevaluating the care situation, reinforcing and providing new information, and evaluating the care provided by the family member. Caregivers could communicate in person and via the telephone as care needs changed. Oncology practices that provide care to a large number of older patients might benefit from adding these services to their practice.

Health care providers should watch for signs of caregiver distress and burden and help families to set limits on their care responsibilities. Caregivers need assistance to reevaluate their commitment and capacity to care, especially as the patient's disability increases and the care demands rise. Support groups may be beneficial, but often family members find it difficult to attend them when care demands are high.

Table 5 Caregiver Assessment

Patient needs	Complete a CGA. Identify tasks of care, skills, and knowledge that the caregiver will require. For example: • Is the patient undergoing active cancer treatment? Which side effects are likely and which does the dyad identify as most troublesome or difficult? • Does the patient have comorbid conditions that limit physical function? • Does the patient have underlying neurological dysfunction such as short-term memory loss?
Caregiver gender	Does the caregiver feel external pressure to assume a caregiving role because she is female? Will there be assistance to the caregiver?
Caregiver age	Is the caregiver older and at risk for social isolation? What comorbidities does the caregiver have?
Caregiver physical function	How might the caregiver's physical function limit him/her in the type or amount of care that will be required?
Prior caregiver–care recipient relationship	What was the quality of the dyad's relationship prior to the diagnosis of cancer? Was the dyad able to communicate effectively? What were the decision-making processes prior to treatment and how have those been affected by the care recipient's illness?
Socioeconomic status	What is the socioeconomic and insurance status of the dyad? Will cancer treatment affect available income, retirement benefits, or insurance coverage? Will care demands affect the caregiver's ability to fulfill occupational obligations? Will the dyad have the resources they need to manage the cancer treatment experience?
Caregiver emotional health	Does the caregiver have a history of mental or emotional problems? Has the caregiver had a history of previous depression and have they been treated for it?
Family roles and communication	Who are the other key family members that can be involved in providing care? What are the communication patterns among family members?
Caregiver mastery and optimism	How much control does the caregiver feel over the care situation? Is the caregiver fairly optimistic about life events?
Social support	What is the availability and quality of social support available to the caregiver and care recipient? If this is an adult child, caregiver sibling support needs to be assessed
Health care communication	Does the caregiver know which health care provider to contact for various treatment-related issues? Does the caregiver feel comfortable asking questions and seem to retain information that is provided?
Education and information	What knowledge does the caregiver require in order to provide care and monitor disease progress? What methods of learning are most effective for the caregiver?
Problem solving skills	Does the caregiver feel that he/she is able to impact the symptoms and side effects that occur as a result of cancer treatment? Is the caregiver able to identify problem areas, generate potential solutions, and evaluate interventions?
Community resources	What resources are available in the community? What resources are acceptable to the caregiver? Does the caregiver have the economic stability (income or insurance coverage) to purchase or regularly access these resources?
Competing demands	For the adult child caregiver, competing demands such as their own family, employment, and social activities have to be determined to see how it will impose on caregiving demands

Abbreviation: CGA, comprehensive geriatric assessment.

The utilization of respite services may be necessary. Respite may include relief from care and assistance with laundry, cooking, shopping, or transportation, or it may involve periods when the caregiver is relieved from all responsibilities and can go outside, leaving the home for short periods to shop, go to the library, or enjoy nature. A few hours of respite scheduled each week allows the family members some personal time. The lack of personal time is frequently reported as contributing to caregiver burden (24).

CONCLUSION

In summary, health care providers should examine the demands of care, family roles, social and work roles, and available social and personal resources when anticipating support needs for caregivers (Table 5). Sources of support may include the formal health care system, where support is provided either by health care providers, skilled home care nurses, and chore workers, or by informal support through family and friends. Health care providers must plan patient care based on the assumption that the family is a system and that the behavior and response of one member affects the family as a unit and particularly the patient with cancer. The well-being of family members must be of concern because they have a legitimate and critical role in the cancer-care team. They are partners in care who support the older individual with cancer, and health care professionals must unite with them as team members for cancer care.

REFERENCES

1. Ries LAG, Eisner MP, Kosary CL, et al. SEER cancer situations review, 1975–2000. http://seer.cancer.gov/csr/1975_2000 (accessed June 2005).
2. Balducci L, Extermann M. Management of cancer in the older person: a practical approach. Oncologist 2000; 5:224 237.
3. Edwards BK, Howe HL, Ries LA, et al. Annual report to the nation on status of cancer, 1973–1999, featuring implications of age and aging on U.S. cancer burden. Cancer 2002; 94:2766–2792.
4. Markson EW. Functional, social and psychological disability as causes of loss of weight and independence in older community-living people. Clin Geriatr Med 1997; 13:639–652.
5. Extermann M. Assessment of comorbidity. CRC Crit Rev Hematol Oncol 2000; 14:63–78.
6. Satariano WA, Ragland DR. The effect of comorbidity on 3-year survival of women with primary breast cancer. Ann Intern Med 1994; 120:104–110.
7. Coebergy JW, Janssen-Heijnen ML, Razenberg PP. Prevalence of co-morbidity in newly diagnosed patients with cancer: a population-based study. Crit Rev Oncol Hematol 1998; 27:97–100.
8. Kristjanson L, Leis A, Koop P, et al. Family members' care perceptions, and satisfaction, with advance cancer care: results of a multi-site pilot study. J Palliat Care 1997; 13(4):5–13.
9. Haley WE, LaMonde LA, Han B, et al. Predictors of depression and life satisfaction among spousal caregivers in hospice: application of a stress process model. J Palliat Med 2003; 6:215–224.
10. Northouse L, Mood D, Templin T, et al. Couples' patterns of adjustment to colon cancer. Social Sci Med 2000; 50(2):271–284.
11. Pasacreta JA, Picket M. Psychosocial aspects of palliative care. Semin Oncol Nurs 1998; 14(2):110–120.
12. McCorkle R, Robinson L, Nuamah I, et al. The effects of home nursing care for patients during terminal illness on the bereaved's psychological distress. Nurs Res 1998; 47:2–10.

13. Nijboer C, Triemstra M, Tempelaar R, et al. Patterns of caregiver experiences among partners of cancer patients. Gerontologist 2000; 40(6):738–746.
14. Nijboer C, Tempelaar R, Triemstra M, et al. The role of social and psychological resources in caregivers of cancer patients. Cancer 2001; 89(5):1029–1039.
15. Picot S, Youngblut J, Zeller R. Development and testing of a measure of perceived caregiver or adults. J Nurs Measure 1997; 5(1):33–52.
16. Bucher J, Loscalzo M, Zabora J, et al. Problem-solving cancer care education for patients and caregivers. Cancer Pract 2001; 9(2):66–70.
17. Scherbring M. Effect of caregiver perception of preparedness on burden in an oncology population. Oncol Nurs Forum 2002; 29(6):70–76.
18. Schumacher K, Stewart B, Archbold P, et al. Family caregiving skill: development of the concept. Res Nurs Health 2000; 23(3):191–203.
19. McCorkle R, Yost L, Jepson C, et al. A cancer experience: relationship of patient psychosocial responses to caregiver burden over time. Psycho-Oncology 1993; 2(1):21–32.
20. Northouse L, Kershaw T, Mood D, et al. Effects of a family intervention on the quality of life of women with recurrent breast cancer and their family caregivers. Psycho-Oncology 2005; 14(6):478–491.
21. Schulz R, Beach SR. Caregiving as a risk factor for mortality: the caregiver health effects study. J Am Med Assoc 1999; 282(23):2215–2219.
22. Lueckenotte AG. Gerontologic assessment. In: Lueckenotte AG, ed. Gerontologic Nursing. St. Louis, Missouri: Mosby, 2000:63–95.
23. Grunfeld E, Coyle D, Whelan T, et al. Family caregiver burden: results of a longitudinal study of breast cancer patients and their principal caregivers. Can Med Assoc J 2004; 170(12):1795–1801.
24. Given B, Wyatt G, Given C, et al. Burden and depression among caregivers of patients with cancer at the end of life. Oncol Nurs Forum 2004; 31(6):1105–1115.
25. Balducci L. The geriatric cancer patient: equal benefit from equal treatment. Cancer Control 2001; 8(2 suppl):1–25.
26. Balducci L. Guidelines for the management of the older cancer patient. Cancer Treat Res 2005; 124:233–256.
27. Gaugler J, Hanna N, Linder J, et al. Cancer caregiving and subjective stress: a multisite, multi-dimensional analysis. Psycho-Oncology 2005; 14(9):771–785.
28. Crivellari D, Bonetti M, Castiglione-Gertsch M, et al. Burdens and benefits of adjuvant cyclophosphamide, methotrexate, and fluorouracil and tamoxifen for elderly patients with breast cancer: The International Breast Cancer Study Group Trial VII. J Clin Oncol 2000; 18:1412–1422.
29. Aalami O, Fang T, Song H, et al. Physiological features of aging persons. Arch Surg 2003; 138(10):1068–1076.
30. Luckey AE, Parsa CJ. Fluid and electrolytes in the aged. Arch Surg 2003; 138:1055–1060.
31. Vestal RE. Aging and pharmacology. Cancer 1997; 80:1302–1310.
32. Hileman JW, Lackey NR. Self-identified needs of patients with cancer at home and their home caregivers: a descriptive study. Oncol Nurs Forum 1990; 7:907–913.
33. Given B, Given CW. Health promotion for family caregivers of chronically ill elders. Annu Rev Nurs Res 1998; 16:197–217.
34. Kurtz M, Kurtz J, Given C, et al. Concordance of cancer patient and caregiver symptom reports. Cancer Prac 1996; 4(4):185–190.
35. Aranda S, Hayman-White K. Home caregivers of the person with advanced cancer: an Australian perspective. Cancer Nurs 2001; 24(4):300–307.
36. Stommel M, Given BA, Given C, et al. The impact of frequency of care activities on the division of labor between primary caregivers and other care providers. Res Aging 1995; 17(4):412–433.
37. Newton M, Bell D, Lambert S, et al. Concerns of hospice patient caregivers. Official J Assoc Black Nurs Faculty Higher Educ 2002; 13(6):140–144.

38. Yurk R, Morgan D, Franey S, et al. Understanding the continuum of palliative care for patients and their caregivers. J Pain Symptom Manage 2002; 24(5):459–470.
39. Miaskowski C, Kragness L, Dibble S, et al. Differences in mood states, health status, and caregiver strain between family caregivers of oncology outpatients with and without cancer-related pain. J Pain Symptom Manage 1997; 13(3):138–147.
40. Given CW, Given B, Stommel M, et al. The impact of new demands for assistance on caregiver depression: tests using an inception cohort. Gerontologist 1999; 39(1): 76–85.
41. Dodd MJ, Onishi K, Dibble SL, et al. Differences in nausea, vomiting, and retching between younger and older outpatients receiving cancer chemotherapy. Cancer Nurs 1996; 19(3):155–161.
42. Kurtz M, Kurtz J, Given C, et al. Depression and physical health among family caregivers of geriatric patients with cancer—a longitudinal view. Med Sci Monitor 2004; 10(8):CR447–CR456.
43. Nijboer C, Triemstra M, Tempelaar R, et al. Determinants of caregiving experiences and mental health of partners of cancer patients. Cancer 1999; 86(4):577–588.
44. Given B, Given C. Family caregiver burden from cancer care. In: McCorkle R, Baird S, Grant M, eds. Cancer Nursing: A Comprehensive Textbook. 2nd ed. Philadelphia, Pennsylvania: Saunders, 1996:93–104.
45. Kozachik S, Given C, Given B, et al. Improving depressive symptoms among caregivers of patients with cancer: results of a randomized clinical trial. Oncol Nurs Forum 2001; 28(7):1149–1157.
46. Gabrilove JL, Cleeland CS, Livingston RB, et al. Clinical evaluation of once-weekly dosing of epoetin alfa in chemotherapy patients: improvements in hemoglobin and quality of life are sin three-times-weekly dosing. J Clin Oncol 2001; 19:2875–2882.
47. John V, Mashru S, Lichtman S. Pharmacological factors influencing anticancer drug selection in the elderly. Drugs Aging 2003; 20:737–759.
48. National Cancer Center Network (NCCN). http://www.nccn.org (accessed June 2005).
49. Skirvin JA, Lichtman SM. Pharmacokinetic considerations of oral chemotherapy in elderly patients with cancer. Drugs Aging 2002; 19:25–42.
50. Weitzner M, McMillan S, Jacobsen P. Family caregiver quality of life: differences between curative and palliative cancer treatment settings. J Pain Symptom Manage 1999; 17(6):418–428.
51. Andrews S. Caregiver burden and symptom distress in people with cancer receiving hospice care. Oncol Nurs Forum 2001; 28(9):1469–1474.
52. Morita T, Chihara S, Kashiwagi T. Family satisfaction with inpatient palliative care in Japan. Palliat Med 2002; 16(3):185–193.
53. Ferrell BR, Rhiner M, Grant M. Pain as a metaphor for illness. Part I: Impact of cancer pain on family caregivers. Oncol Nurs Forum 1991; 18:1303–1309.
54. Morrison VA, Picozzi V, Scott S, et al. The impact of age on delivered dose intensity and hospitalizations for neutropenia in patients with intermediate-grade non-Hodgkin's lymphoma recent initial CHOP chemotherapy: a risk factor analysis. Clin Lymphoma 2001; 2(1):47–56.
55. Gillespie TW. Anemia in cancer: therapeutic implications and interventions. Cancer Nurs 2003; 26:119–128.
56. Klasa RJ, Meyer RM, Shustik C, et al. Randomized phase III study of fludarabine phosphate versus cyclophosphamide, vincristine, and prednisone in patients with recurrent low-grade non-Hodgkin's lymphoma previously treated with an alkylating agent or alkylator-containing regimen. J Clin Oncol 2002; 20:4649–4654.
57. Corcoran MB. Polypharmacy in the older patient. In: Balducci L, Lyman GH, Ershler WB, eds. Comprehensive Geriatric Oncology. London: Harwood Academic Publishers, 1997:525–532.
58. Tinetti ME, Speechley M, Ginter SF. Risk factors for falls among elderly persons living in the community. N Engl J Med 1988; 31:1701–1707.

59. Calhoun P, Beckham J, Bosworth H. Caregiver burden and psychological distress in partners of veterans with chronic posttraumatic stress disorder. J Traumatic Stress 2002; 15(3):205–212.

60. Fillit H, Gutterman E, Brooks R. Impact of donepezil on caregiving burden for patients with Alzheimer's disease. Int Psychogeriatr 2000; 12(3):389–401.

61. Pinquart M, Sörensen S. Associations of caregiver stressors and uplifts with subjective well-being and depressive mood: a meta-analytic comparison. Aging Mental Health 2004; 8(5):438–449.

62. Breitbart W, Gibson C, Tremblay A. The delirium experience: delirium recall and delirium-related distress in hospitalized patients with cancer, their spouses/caregivers, and their nurses. Psychosomatics 2002; 43(3):183–194.

63. Sherwood P, Given B, Doorenbos A, et al. Forgotten voices: lessons from bereaved caregivers of persons with a brain tumor. Int J Palliat Nurs 2004; 10(2):67–75.

64. Given CW, Given BA, Stommel M. The impact of age, treatment, and symptoms on the physical and mental health of cancer patients and their family. A longitudinal perspective. Cancer 1994; 74(7):2128–2138.

65. Burns R, Nichols LO, Martindale-Adams J, et al. Primary care interventions for dementia caregivers: 2-year outcomes from the REACH study. Gerontologist 2003; 43(4):547–555.

66. Mahoney DF, Tralow BJ, Jones RN. Effects of an automated telephone support system on caregiver burden and anxiety; findings from the REACH for TLC intervention study. Gerontologist 2003; 43(4):556–567.

67. Yates M, Tennstedt S, Chang B. Contributors to and mediators of psychological well-being for informal caregivers. J Gerontol: Psychol Sci 1999; 54(1):12–22.

68. Pinquart M, Sörensen S. Associations of stressors and uplifts of caregiving with caregiver burden and depressed mood: a meta-analysis. J Gerontol: Psychol Sci 2003; 58B(2):112–128.

69. Given C, Given B, Azzouz F, et al. Comparison of changes in physical functioning of elderly patients with new diagnoses of cancer. Med Care 2000; 38(5):482–493.

70. Kurtz M, Given B, Kurtz J, et al. The interaction of age, symptoms, and survival status on physical and mental health of patients with cancer and their families. Cancer 1994; 74(7 suppl):2071–2078.

71. Barg F, Pasacreta J, Nuamah R, et al. A description of a psychoeducational intervention for family caregivers of cancer patients. J Fam Nurs 1998; 4(4):394–413.

72. Baider L, Kaufman B, Peretz T, et al. Mutuality of fate: adaptation and psychological distress in cancer patients and their partners. In: Baider L, Cooper C, Kaplan De-Nour A, eds. Cancer and the Family. New York, New York: John Wiley & Sons, 1996:187–224.

73. Raveis V, Karus D, Siegel K. Correlates of depressive symptomatology among adult daughter caregivers of a parent with cancer. Cancer 1998; 83(8):1652–1663.

74. Given CW, Given B, Rahbar M, et al. Effect of a cognitive behavioral intervention on reducing symptom severity during chemotherapy. J Clin Oncol 2004; 22(3):507–516.

75. Given BA, Given CW. Family home care for individuals with cancer. Oncology 1994; 8(5):77–83.

76. Administration on Aging. Older population by age: 1900 to 2050. http://www.aoa.gov/prof/statistics/online_stat_data/popage2050.xls (accessed June 2005).

77. Coristine M, Crooks D, Grunfeld E, et al. Caregiving for women with advanced breast cancer. Psycho-Oncology 2003; 12:709–719.

78. Manne SL, Alfieri T, Taylor KL, et al. Spousal negative responses to cancer patients: the role of social restriction, spouse mood, and relationship satisfaction. Consult Clin Psychol 1999; 67(3):352–361.

79. Stephens M, Townsend A, Martire L, et al. Balancing parent care with other roles: interrole conflict of adult daughter caregivers. J Gerontol Ser B Psychol Sci Social Sci 2001; 56(1):24–34.

80. Given B, Given C, Stommel M, et al. Predictors of use of secondary carers used by the elderly following hospital discharge. J Aging Health 1994; 6(3):353–376.

81. Hayman J, Langa K, Kabeto M, et al. Estimating the cost of informal caregiving for elderly patients with cancer. J Clin Oncol 2001; 19(13):3219–3225.

82. Stommel M, Given C, Given B. The cost of cancer home care to families. Cancer 1993; 71(5):1867–1874.

83. Langa KM, Fendrick AM, Chernew ME, et al. Out-of-pocket health-care expenditures among older Americans with cancer. Value Health 2004; 7:186–194.

84. Mor V, Guadagnoli E, Wool M. An examination of the concrete service needs of advanced cancer patients. J Psychosoc Oncol 1987; 5:1–7.

85. Oberst M, Thomas S, Gass K, et al. Caregiving demands and appraisal of stress among family caregivers. Cancer Nurs 1989; 12(4):209–215.

86. Weitzner M, Meyers C, Stuebing K, et al. Relationship between quality of life and mood in long-term survivors of breast cancer treated with mastectomy. Support Care Cancer 1997; 5(3):241–248.

87. Given C, Stommel M, Given B, et al. The influence of the cancer patient's symptoms, functional states on patient's depression and family caregiver's reaction and depression. Health Psychol 1993; 12(4):277–285.

88. Schulz R, Williamson G. A 2-year longitudinal study of depression among Alzheimer's caregivers. Psychol Aging 1991; 6(4):569–578.

89. Cooley M, Moriarty H. An analysis of empirical studies examining the impact of the cancer diagnosis and treatment of an adult on family functioning. J Fam Nurs 1997; 3(4):318–347.

90. Cameron J, Franche R, Cheung A, et al. Lifestyle interference and emotional distress in family caregivers of advanced cancer patients. Cancer 2002; 94(2):521–527.

91. Pavalko E, Woodbury W. Social roles as process: caregiving careers and women's health. J Health Social Behav 2000; 41(1):91–105.

92. Fortinsky R, Kercher K, Burant C. Measurement and correlates of family caregiver self-efficacy for managing dementia. Aging Mental Health 2002; 6(2):153–160.

93. Harris J, Godfrey H, Partridge F, et al. Caregiver depression following traumatic brain injury: a consequence of adverse effects on family members? Brain Injury 2001; 15(3):223–238.

94. Clyburn L, Stones M, Hadjistavropoulos T, et al. Predicting caregiver burden and depression in Alzheimer's disease. J Gerontol Ser B Psychol Sci Social Sci 2000; 55(1):S2–S13.

95. Schulz R, Beach S, Lind B, et al. Involvement in caregiving and adjustment to death of a spouse: findings from the Caregiver Health Effects Study. J Am Med Assoc 2001; 285(24):3123–3129.

96. Kiecolt-Glaser J, Glaser R, Gravenstein S, et al. Chronic stress alters the immune response to influenza vaccine in older adults. Proc Natl Acad Sci USA 1996; 93(2):3043–3047.

97. Jensen S, Given B. Fatigue affecting family caregivers of cancer patients. Support Care Cancer 1993; 1(6):321–325.

98. Beach S, Schulz R, Yee J, et al. Negative and positive health effects of caring for a disabled spouse: longitudinal findings from the Caregiver Health Effects Study. Psychol Aging 2000; 15(2):259–271.

99. Burton L, Newsom J, Schulz R, et al. Preventive health behaviors among spousal caregivers. Preventative Med 1997; 26(2):162–169.

100. Northhouse PG, Northhouse L. Communication and cancer: issues confronting patients, health professionals and family members. J Psychosoc Oncol 1987; 5:17–46.

101. Zhang A, Siminoff L. The role of the family in treatment decision making by patients with cancer. Oncol Nurs Forum 2003; 30(6):1022–1028.

102. Fried T, Bradley E, O'Leary, et al. Unmet desire for caregiver-patient communication and increased caregiver burden. J Am Geriatr Soc 2005; 53(1):59–65.

103. Kotkamp-Mothes N, Slawinsky D, Hindermann S, et al. Coping and psychological well being in families of elderly cancer patients. Crit Rev Oncol Hematol. In press.
104. Speice J, Harkness J, Laneri H, et al. Involving family members in cancer care: focus group considerations of patients and oncological providers. Psycho-Oncology 2000; 9(2):101–112.
105. Kurtz M, Kurtz J, Given C, et al. Relationship of caregiver reactions and depression to cancer patients' symptoms, functional states and depression—a longitudinal view. Social Sci Med 1995; 40(6):837–846.
106. Kurtz M, Kurtz J, Stommel M, et al. Loss of physical functioning among geriatric cancer patients: relationships to cancer site, treatment, comorbidity and age. Eur J Cancer 1997; 33(14):2352–2358.
107. Northouse L, Templin T, Mood D. Couples' adjustment to breast disease during the first year following diagnosis. J Behav Med 2001; 24(2):115–136.
108. Bookwala J, Schulz R. The role of neuroticism and mastery in spouse caregivers' assessment of and response to a contextual stressor. J Gerontol 1998; 53B:155–164.
109. Moody L, McMillan S. Dyspnea and quality of life indicators in hospice patients and their caregivers. Health Qual Life Outcomes 2003; 1(1):9.
110. Pearlin L, Schooler C. The structure of coping. J Health Social Behav 1978; 19(1):2–21.
111. Gitlin L, Corcoran M, Winter L, et al. A randomized, controlled trial of a home environmental intervention: effect on efficacy and upset in caregivers and on daily function of persons with dementia. Gerontologist 2001; 41(1):4–14.
112. Szabo A, Strang V. Experiencing control in caregiving. Image 1999; 31:71–75.
113. Ferrario SR, Zotti AM, Ippoliti M, et al. Caregiving-related needs analysis: a proposed model reflecting current research and socio-political developments. Health Social Care Community 2003; 11(2):103–110.
114. Morse SR, Fife B. Coping with a partner's cancer: adjustment at four stages of the illness trajectory. Oncol Nurs Forum 1998; 25(4):751–760.
115. Kim Y, Duberstein PR, Sorensen S, et al. Levels of depressive symptoms in spouses of people with lung cancer: effects of personality, social support, and caregiving burden. Psychosomatics 2005; 46(2):123–130.
116. Wells N, Hepworth J, Murphy B, et al. Improving cancer pain management through patient and family education. J Pain Symptom Manage 2003; 25(4):344–356.
117. Ferrell BR, Grant M, Chan J, et al. The impact of cancer pain education on family caregivers of elderly patients. Oncol Nurs Forum 1995; 22(8):1211–1218.
118. Archbold P, Stewart B, Greenlick M, et al. Mutuality and preparedness as predictors of caregiver role strain. RINAH 1990; 13:375–384.
119. Cartwright J, Archbold P, Stewart B, et al. Enrichment processes in family caregiving to frail elders. Adv Nurs Sci 1994; 17(1):31–43.
120. Houts P, Nezu A, Nezu C, et al. The prepared family caregiver: a problem-solving approach to family caregiver education. Patient Educ Counsel 1996; 27(1):63–73.
121. Northouse L, Peters-Golden H. Cancer and the family: strategies to assist spouses. Semin Oncol Nurs 1993; 9(2):74–82.
122. Toseland R, Blanchard C, McCallion P. A problem solving intervention for caregivers of cancer patients. Social Sci Med 1995; 40(4):517–528.
123. Herr H. Quality of life in prostate cancer patients. CA Cancer J Clin 1997; 47(4):207–217.
124. Dobson K. Dobson K, ed. Handbook of Cognitive Behavioral Therapies. Manhattan, New York: Guilford Press, 2001.
125. Brazil K, Bedard M, Krueger P, et al. Service preferences among family caregivers of the terminally ill. J Palliat Med 2005; 8(1):69–78.
126. Given B, Given CW. Family caregiving for the elderly. Annu Rev Nurs Res 1991; 9:77–101.
127. Sherwood P, Given B, Given C, et al. A cognitive behavioral intervention for symptom management in patients: advanced cancer oncology nursing forum 2005; 32(6):1–9.

Index

Milton Keynes UK
Ingram Content Group UK Ltd.
UKHW052030071024
449327UK00027B/2500